Color Atlas of Vascular Diseases

Springer

Berlin
Heidelberg
New York
Barcelona
Hong Kong
London
Milan
Paris
Singapore
Tokyo

C. Diehm
J.-R. Allenberg
K. Nimura-Eckert
F. J. Veith

Color Atlas of Vascular Diseases

With 1035 Figures

Springer

Prof. Dr. Curt Diehm, MD
Klinikum Karlsbad-Langensteinbach GmbH
University of Heidelberg
Guttmannstraße 1, D-76307 Karlsbad
Germany

Prof. Dr. Jens-Rainer Allenberg, MD
Department of Vascular Surgery, University of Heidelberg
Im Neuenheimer Feld 110, D-69120 Heidelberg
Germany

Dr. Keiko Nimura-Eckert, MD
Leibnitzstraße 3, D-74889 Sinsheim
Germany

Prof. Dr. Frank J. Veith, MD
Montefiore Medical Center, Vascular Services
111 East 210th Street, NY 10467 Bronx
New York, USA

Translator:
Prof. Dr. Walter H.C. Burgdorf, MD
Traubinger Straße 45 A, D-82327 Tutzing
Germany

ISBN 3-540-62619-0 Springer-Verlag Berlin Heidelberg New York

Library of Congress Cataloging-in-Publication Data

Color atlas of vascular diseases / C. Diehm ... [et al.] ; [translator, Walter Burgdorf].
p. cm. Includes bibliographical references and index.
ISBN 3-540-62619-0 (alk. paper)
1. Blood-vessels–Diseases–Atlases. I. Diehm, C. [DNLM: 1. Vascular Diseases–Atlases.
WG 17 C7186 1999] RC691.4 .C64 1999 616.1'3'00222 21–dc21]

Springer-Verlag is a company in the BertelsmannSpringer publishing group.

Printed in Italy

Production editor: W. Bischoff, Heidelberg
Cover design: e Studio Calamar, Pau/Girona
Typesetting: Fotosatz-Service Köhler GmbH, Würzburg
Reproduction of the figures: Schneider Repro, Heidelberg
Illustrators: R. u. A. R. Gattung, Edingen-Neckarhausen; G. Hippmann, Nürnberg
Printing and binding: Printer, Trento srl

SPIN: 10491821 24/3134 – 5 4 3 2 1 0 – Printed on acid-free paper

Preface

The industrialized world has witnessed a steady increase in diseases of the arteries, veins, and lymph vessels in recent years. The prevalence and incidence of arteriosclerotic vascular disease has taken on the character of an epidemic. Diseases of the superficial and deep veins are widespread.

Every practicing physician is confronted daily by arterial circulatory disorders of the supra-aortic vessels, the thoracic and abdominal aorta, and the pelvic and leg arteries as well as by venous and lymphatic diseases. Today vascular disease is best managed in an interdisciplinary way; interventional radiologists and neurologists should be part of the team at any established vascular center.

Many older colleagues were forced to acquire their knowledge of vascular diseases on their own. There are still many medical schools and hospitals that lack vascular specialists who are capable of passing on their expertise to students. For many years there was no expertise in medical angiology in countries such as Great Britain or the United States. All of vascular medicine resided in the hands of vascular surgeons. It is only in the last few years that vascular internists have appeared in these countries as well.

In vascular disease as in few other areas of specialization, diagnosis as well as evaluation of the success of therapy requires a well-trained clinical eye. This book focuses on the presentation of visual material relevant to the most important vascular diseases. The accompanying text is limited to a short presentation of the essentials and introduces each set of illustrations, which are then discussed in detail. The illustrative material provided by this atlas in conjunction with the succinct legends encourages the reader to browse through its pages; it is impossible to study vascular disease in a more vivid or entertaining manner.

We have intentionally included a presentation of the scientific history of the most important vascular diseases and original quotes from the scientists involved. This is not only the individual style of the book; it may also be helpful in preparing a seminar or stimulating lecture.

We hope that the visual material offered by this atlas serves to train the clinical eye of all those interested in vascular disease. This book should be of value to general practitioners, internists, diabetic specialists, vascular internists and phlebologists, as well as all cardiologists, surgeons and radiologists who deal with vascular disease. However, it should also be of interest to practitioners of related areas of specialization, such as neurologists, dermatologists, and orthopedic surgens. We also hope that this book helps in the training of medical students worldwide.

We owe thanks to our colleagues specializing in angiology, phlebology, vascular surgery, and radiology who have made visual material available to us. This includes G. Kaufmann and G. Richter from the Department of Radiology at the University Hospital in Heidelberg.

It also encompasses K.H. Simon, head of the Department of Radiology at the Bretten District Hospital; F.J. Roth, head of the Department of Radiology of the Aggertal Hospital; W. Heger, head of the Department of Vascular Surgery at the Arcus Hospital in Pforzheim; and, last but not least, all of our fellow staff members and especially E. Hsu. We would also like to extend our gratitude to all those involved in the publication of the book in the copyediting and production departments at Springer-Verlag and especially to Monika Schrimpf. A special note of thanks goes to Heike Ruck, the member of our staff involved in book publication. All of the above attached a unique blend of perseverance and forbearance to the creation of this book.

Karlsbad, Heidelberg and New York City
Spring 2000

Curt Diehm
Jens-Rainer Allenberg
Keiko Nimura-Eckert
Frank J. Veith

Contents

Part B: Venous System

Part C: Lymphatic System

Part D: Vascular Malformations

Appendix

Part A: Arterial System

Chapter 1: Disease Processes Involving Arteries

Contents

A: Introduction

1. Morphology of the Arterial Wall and Types of Vessels

Morphology of the Arterial Wall

Intima

The intima is formed by endothelial cells and the sub-endothelial internal elastic lamina, as well as a connective tissue matrix and small numbers of smooth muscle cells (myo-intimal cells).

Endothelium

The endothelium is a single continuous sheet of cells that covers the inside of the arteries and other vessels. Adults have a total endothelial surface of about 1000 m^2, while the total weight of the endothelium is estimated at about 2 kg. The endothelial cells form a barrier preventing foreign substances from migrating out of the blood into the vessel wall. In addition, by manufacturing both clotting and fibrinolytic factors, the endothelial cells contribute to hemostasis. In addition, they can inhibit platelet adhesion and in the spleen and bone marrow they have phagocytic properties. It is also known that the endothelium-derived vascular relaxing factor mediates the relaxation of vascular smooth muscle. According to the „response-to-injury" theory, endothelial cell damage is the first step in the process of arteriosclerosis. The endothelial cell layer is separated from the media by the internal elastic lamina.

Media

The media consist primarily of smooth muscle cells which run in a spiral pattern surrounding the vessel. Depending on the type of artery, there is a varying number of layers of smooth muscle cells. The smooth muscle cells, when damaged, can produce components of the extracellular matrix, such as proteoglycans, elastic fibers and collagen bundles. Normally this is a task of fibroblasts or myofibroblasts. In arteries such as the aorta or pulmonary arteries, the elastic fibers predominate in order to modulate marked variations in luminal pressure in systole. Muscular arteries have fewer elastic fibers and more smooth muscle cells, whose role is to regulate the flow of blood through vasoconstriction and vasodilatation. Thus, from centrally to peripherally, elastic fibers decrease and smooth muscle cells increase. The external elastic lamina provides the border between the media and the adventitia.

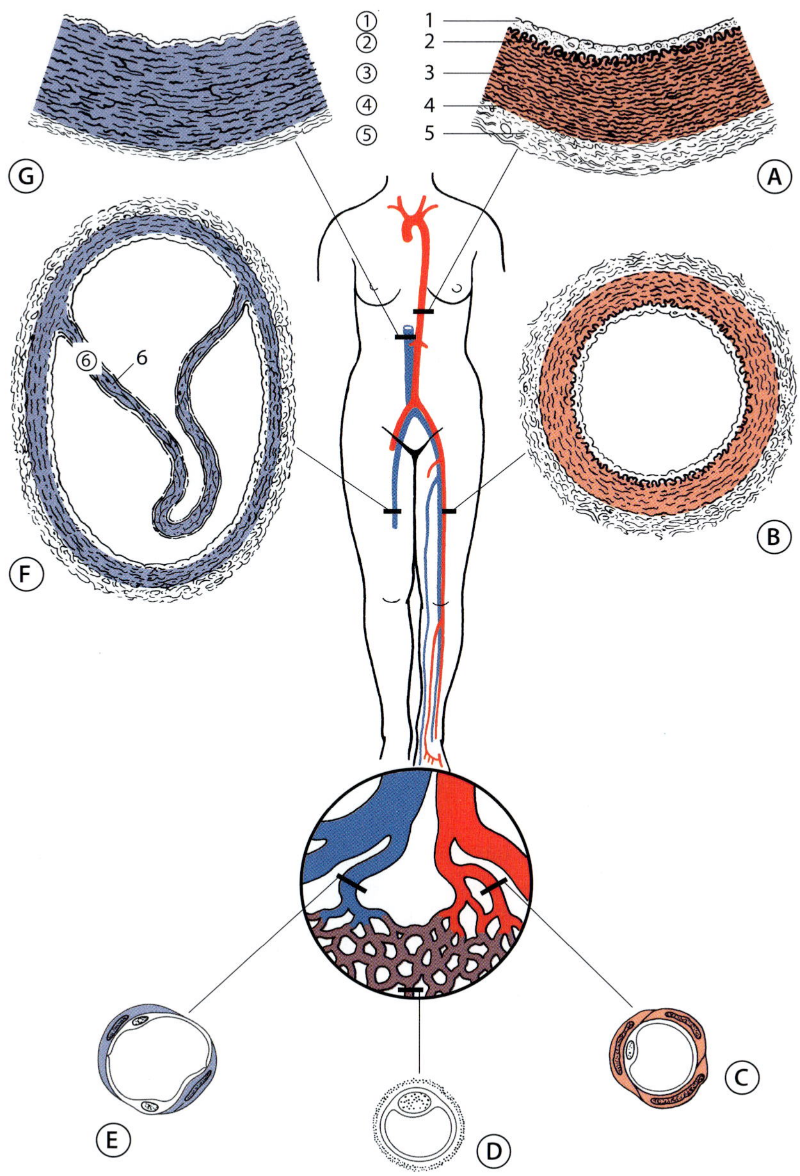

Fig. 1-1. Structure of the vessel wall in cross-section.

Ⓐ Aorta
Ⓑ Muscular artery
Ⓒ Arteriole
Ⓓ Capillary
Ⓔ Venule
Ⓕ Large vein
Ⓖ Vena cava
① Endothelium
② Internal elastic lamina
③ Media
④ External elastic lamina
⑤ Adventitia
⑥ Venous valve

(Modified from Pocket Atlas of Anatomy, Thieme, Stuttgart)

Adventitia

The adventitia forms the outer coat of the artery. It consist of a loose network of collagen fibers, elastic fibers and smooth muscle. The nerves, lymphatics and vasa vasorum are also found here. The adventitia merges imperceptibly with the connective tissue of the adjacent structures. Veins have a thick outer layer with connective tissue bundles running in the direction of the vessel's long axis. The adventitia is separated from the media by the external elastic lamina.

Pericytes (Rouget cells) are found in the adventitia. They are multi-potential mesenchymal cells which, under the appropriate stimulus, can differentiate into smooth muscle cells (vessel wall budding), fibroblasts (wound healing) and phagocytes or macrophages (inflammation).

Types of Vessels

Microscopically one can distinguish several different types of vessels, based primarily on the nature of the media as well as the width of the lumen.

Elastic Arteries

The large vessels near the heart, such as the aorta, common carotid, subclavian, common iliac and pulmonary arteries with a diameter of >1 mm are distinguished by a high elastic fiber content in the media and adventitia.

Muscular Arteries

The more distal large arteries, such as the femoral arteries, show the transition from an elastic to a muscular artery. The latter type is predominant in the various organs and the more peripheral parts of the arterial system. Muscular arteries help control blood pressure by regulating lumen size and thus resistance.

Arterioles

Arterioles help to regulate the peripheral resistance. Their media consist of one to two cell layers of smooth muscle cells which are relatively thick and quite effective because of the small (<50 µm) lumen.

Capillaries

These tiny (~4 m) vessels have no media. They are the narrowest and thinnest vessels, consisting only of endothelial cells, basement membrane and a variable number of pericytes. Variations in these structures characterize the quite different capillaries seen in various organs.

Sinusoids

This variant of capillary has spaces or windows between the endothelial cells and also an irregular or even missing basement membrane.

Venous System

The capillaries flow via their venous arms (8 µm) into the post-capillary venules which are 8–30 µm in diameter. They have no media but increased numbers of pericytes and are the usual site of inflammatory exudates. Smooth muscles first re-appear in the media of the collecting venules (30–50 µm) and in the smallest veins (muscular venules with 50–100 µm lumina). In the still larger veins, the thickness and muscle content of the media is markedly influenced by the local physiological factors. The high hydrostatic and mechanical pressures on the veins of the calves produces an almost artery-like media, while the relatively unstressed veins of the dura mater have almost no media.

Special Forms

Pre-capillary sphincters have circular or ring-like, thickened, often epithelioid, smooth muscle cells which have direct contact with endothelial cells, an increased nerve supply and an increased alkaline phosphatase activity. There are also post-capillary sphincters which are analogous to the pre-capillary form. In addition arterio-venous anastomoses connect the arterial and venous limbs without an intervening capillary bed, providing a mechanism for shunting. There structures also have a thickened media, epithelioid smooth muscle cells and increased adventitial nerve supply but lack elastic fibers.

2. Pathology of Arteriosclerosis

Definition

Arteriosclerosis is a common but imprecise term which refers to thickening and hardening of the arterial wall. The loss of elasticity leads to an increased length and diameter of the aorta and major arteries. As a result there may be kinking or even coiling of these large vessels.

Arteriosclerosis (LOBSTEIN 1833) and atherosclerosis (MARCHAND 1904) are sometimes used as synonyms. This is incorrect. The main term is arteriosclerosis which includes

1. Atherosclerosis
2. Medial calcific sclerosis (Mönckeberg's syndrome)

Atherosclerosis is the most important form and also the more informative term. The Greek origin of the word more accurately describes the pathological process: (athere = gruel or even grit; oma = mass, skleros = hard). Atherosclerosis involves primarily the intima.

Epidemiology

Atherosclerotic cardiac and circulatory diseases are the main cause of death in Western countries. However, atherosclerosis is not a new disease reflecting the advances in civilization. Egyptian mummies from 3000 B.C. have also been shown to have severe atherosclerotic vascular changes. The main problems associated with atherosclerosis are coronary artery disease (CAD), cerebrovascular insufficiency with strokes, peripheral arterial occlusive disease and aneurysms of the aorta and other large vessels. A specific therapy for arteriosclerosis is not available.

Pathogenesis

Despite extensive research, the exact cause of atherosclerosis remains unclear. Arguments center around whether elevations in lipid levels alone are sufficient or if an endothelial injury is first required.

Past and Current Hypotheses

Thrombogenic Incrustation (VON ROKITANSKY 1844)

Membranes are formed on the lumen surface, primarily through fibrin. Cholesterol granules produce soft plaques which tend to rupture and induce further fibrin deposition.

Injury Reaction (VIRCHOW 1856)

Inflammatory injury induces cellular proliferation and plaque formation; the latter imbibe plasma lipids.

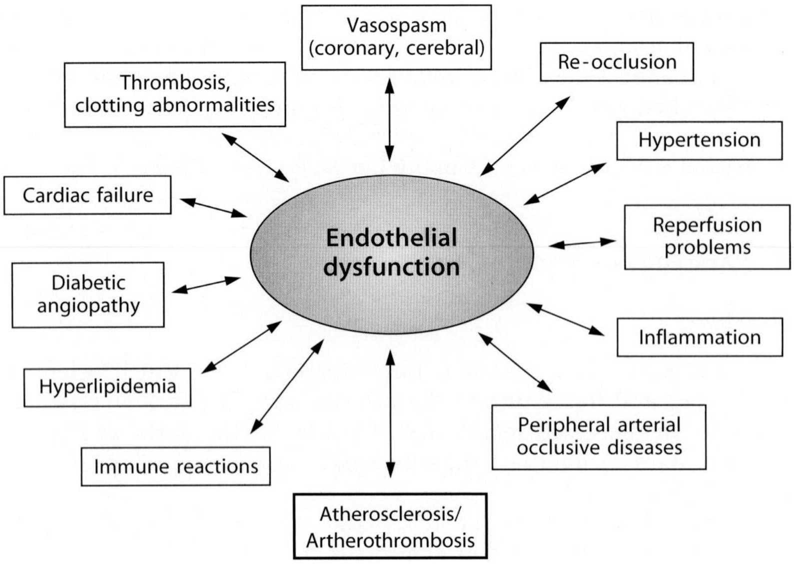

Fig. 1-2. Endothelial dysfunction is a central factor in atherogenesis. Many risk factors and associated diseases influence endothelial function

Duguid's Platelet Theory (Duguid 1949)

A repeated cycle of endothelial injury, platelet deposition, thrombus formation and then organization is coupled with deposition of fibrin layers blocking the lumen.

Monoclonal Hypothesis (Benditt and Benditt 1972)

Mutagens or viruses induce the proliferation of smooth muscle cells, producing monoclonal intra-arterial accumulations. This hypothesis was proposed because of the homogeneity of the smooth muscle cells. More recent research has confirmed the monoclonal nature, but suggests that it is a secondary phenomenon in the sense of natural selection, rather than a primary factor.

Lipid Hypothesis (Goldstein 1979; Mahley 1979)

Modified LDL and β-VLDL are taken up by monocytes/macrophages and myo-intimal cells and convert these cells into lipid-filled foam cells. The elevated blood lipids are primarily responsible for the changes; a precursor endothelial injury is not required.

Response to Injury Hypothesis (Ross and Glomset 1971, 1974, 1984)

Endothelial injury is the key factor. Platelets attach at the site of an injury and release platelet-derived growth factor (PDGF) which stimulates the growth of the myo-intimal smooth muscle cells. These produce less elastin and increased amounts of collagen and proteoglycans, forming the matrix of the atheroma. LDL and LDL-filled macrophages are then deposited. The initial injury can be caused by mechanical, immunological, infectious or toxic factors. Recent interest has centered on bacteria (*Helicobacter pylori*), Chlamydiae and viruses (herpes simplex, cytomegalovirus) as possible triggers.

Chlamydia pneumoniae Hypothesis

There bacteria are currently thought to play a significant role in the development of atherosclerosis. Evidence is accumulating that infec-

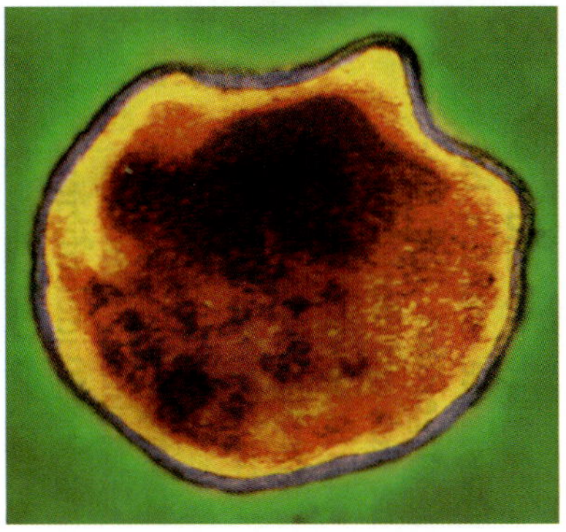

Fig. 1-3. *Chlamydia pneumoniae*

tions are a meaningful factor in the pathogenesis of this disease. *Chlamydia pneumoniae* was first identified in 1989. The working theory is that monocytes transfer this agent from the airways to the peripheral vessels. There the bacteria stimulate the monocytes to attach to the endothelial cells, which they then infects. This represents the start of a chronic inflammatory process influenced by many other risk factors. Many authors have suggested that the quick re-stenosis of a bypass, the rapid closing of a stent or the accelerated atherosclerosis in a transplanted heart are all caused by chronic chlamydial infections. While the concept that atherosclerosis is triggered by Chlamydiae or other organisms is fascinating, it has raised a number of unanswered questions.

Table 1-1. Factors causing initial endothelial damage

High shear forces from hypertension
Changing flow directions or impaired flow
Diabetes mellitus
Elevated lipids (especially LDL)
Toxic substances (for example, contents of cigarette smoke)
Viruses (herpes, cytomegalovirus?)
Bacteria (*Helicobacter pylori, Chlamydia pneumoniae*)
Activation of platelets and clotting factors
Adhesion of monocytes and lymphocytes
Autoimmune mechanisms
Angiotensin II, catecholamines, homocysteine

Unified Hypothesis (Jackson and Gotto 1976; Cathcart 1985)

In this approach the endothelial and lipid pathways are joined together. The high LDL levels can damage endothelial cells triggering the following cascade:

- Platelet aggregation
- PDGF release
- Proliferation of smooth muscle cells

In addition macrophages and myo-intimal cells are activated and LDL is changed via oxidative mechanisms. Chemotactic factors attract monocytes which take up oxidized LDL and β-VLDL becoming foam cells and losing their mobility. Thus lipids accumulate in the vessel wall. The first visible sign of atherosclerosis is the accumulation of these foam cells, known as a fatty streak, in the past often called a milk spot by pathologists. Fatty streaks can even be identified in some children.

Formation of an Atheroma

Atheroma refers to a region of the vessel wall changed or damaged by atherosclerosis. It includes supra-endothelial, endothelial and sub-endothelial changes, such as fibrin deposits, accumulations of macrophages and debris, fat deposits, collagen proliferation and non-physiological proliferation of altered smooth muscle cells.

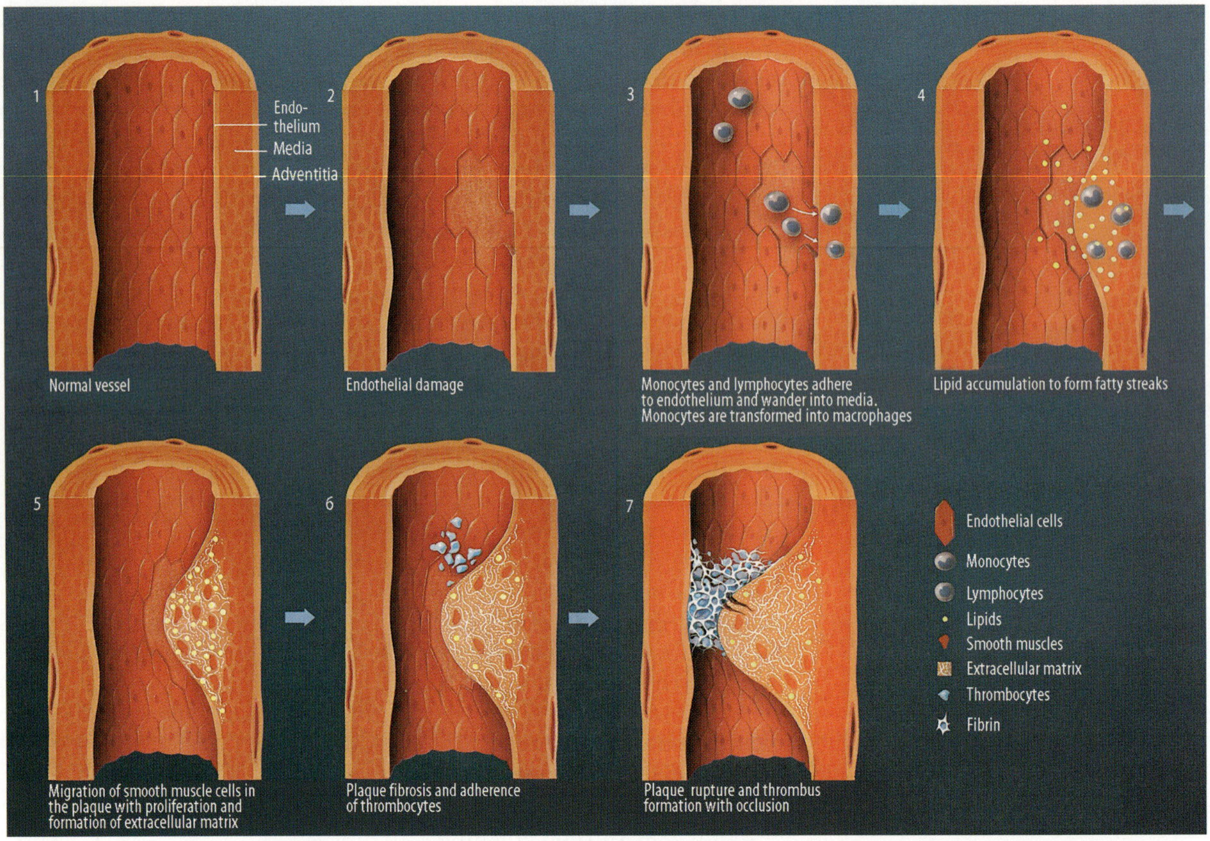

Fig. 1-4. Pathological changes during atherogenesis

Table 1-2. Important steps in atherogenesis

Endothelial damage
Formation of adhesion molecules
Adhesion of monocytes on endothelial cells
Leakage of serum lipids and cellular blood components into vessel wall
Formation of fatty streaks
Lipid accumulation in the intima
Migration of monocytes into the intima and conversion into macrophages
Phagocytosis and oxidation of lipids by macrophages
Formation of a neointima
Migration of smooth muscle cells
Plaque growth through proliferation of smooth muscle cells and macrophages
Formation of an extra-cellular connective tissue matrix
Vessel closure
Organization and calcification of plaques
Retraction and plaque rupture
Deposition of platelets and further thrombosis

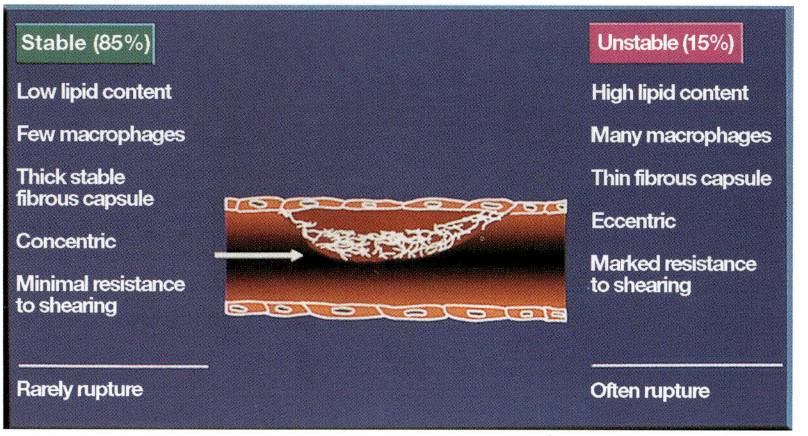

Fig. 1-5. Atherosclerotic plaques. One of the most important questions about coronary artery disease is whether the characteristics are reversible when therapeutic agents such as lipid-lowering agents are employed. (Modified from BROWN et al.)

Risk Factors for Arteriosclerosis

The term „risk factor" comes from epidemiological studies. The authors of the long-term Framingham study, following coronary artery disease in a Boston suburb, first used the expression in the early 1960s. Risk factor refers to the ability to predict the development of a given disease based on the presence of potentially damaging factors. The association must be statistically coupled in a significant fashion.

The following risk factors are today well-accepted for the different types of vascular diseases:

Myocardial infarction
1. Hypercholesterolemia (elevated LDL)
2. Smoking
3. Hypertension
4. Hyperglycemia and hyperinsulinemia (diabetes mellitus)
5. Hyperfibrinogenemia
6. Obesity (indirectly)

Stroke
1. Hypertension
2. Diabetes mellitus
3. Obesity
4. Elevated hematocrit
5. Heart diseases
6. Smoking
7. Alcohol

Peripheral arterial (PAD) disease
1. Smoking
2. Diabetes mellitus
3. Hypertension
4. Hypertriglyceridemia and hypercholesterolemia

3. Mönckeberg's Syndrome

Synonyms. Medial calcific sclerosis, MÖNCKEBERG's arteriopathy, MÖNCKEBERG's medial sclerosis, MÖNCKEBERG's medial calcinosis, MÖNCKEBERG's calcification, Mönckeberg's degeneration (JOHANN GEORG MÖNCKEBERG, German pathologist, 1877–1925)

Mönckeberg's syndrome is a type of arteriosclerosis in which the media of middle-caliber arteries of the muscular type calcify. In contrast to ordinary arteriosclerosis, in which the intima is primarily involved, here the smooth muscle cells of the media are the site of damage, producing extensive ring or pipe-like calcium deposits. The arteries become stiff and can even be palpated as firm cylindrical objects when they are superficial, as is the case with the radial artery, which may resemble a lead pencil. In German the even more descriptive term „Gänsegurgel," or goose's throat, is used to describe the changes.

In most cases the changes are asymptomatic because the lumen is not constricted. Sometimes the leg arteries will have both medial calcification and luminal narrowing or occlusion. Often the extensive calcification is discovered during a routine radiological examination for some other problem. The forearms, legs below the knees and the feet are the most common sites. The coronary, renal and CNS arteries are almost never affected. Factors which accelerated medial calcification include:

- Diabetes mellitus
- Chronic renal insufficiency
- Chronic excessive vitamin D ingestion
- Pseudoxanthoma elasticum

Fig. 1-6 – 1-8. MÖNCKEBERG'S medial calcification in the thigh, the foot and the forearm, respectively

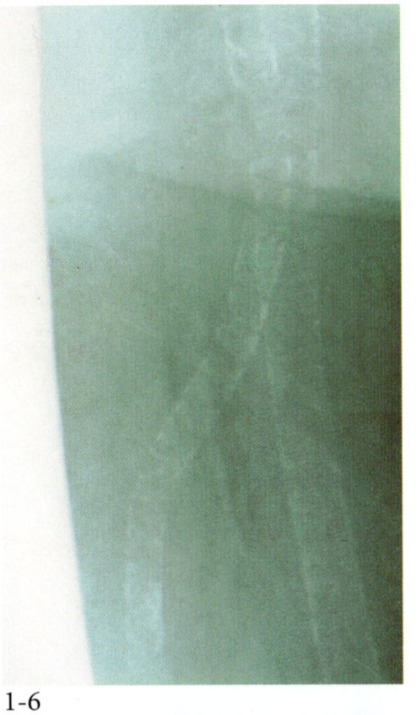

1-6

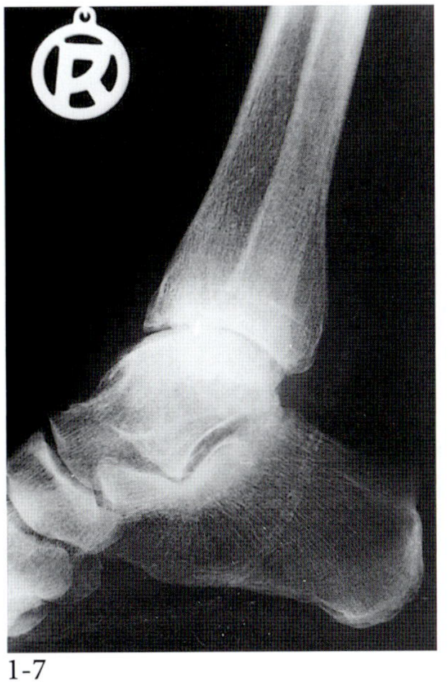

1-7

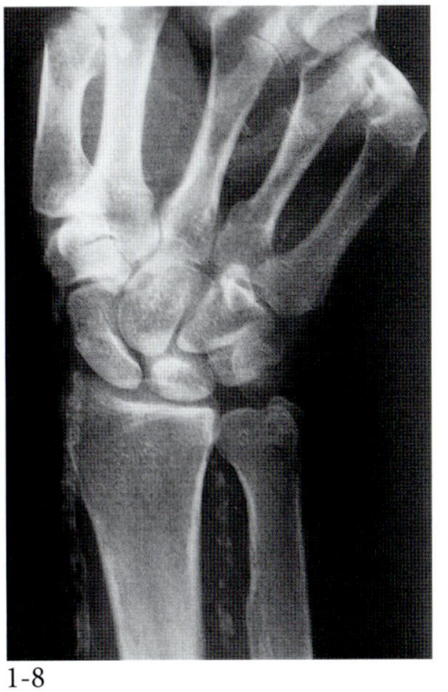

1-8

B: Supplementary Figures and Legends

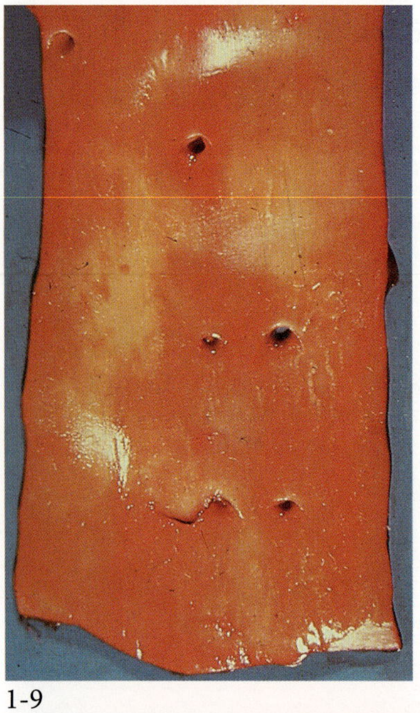

1-9

Fig. 1-9. Abdominal aorta in a 12 year old boy who was autopsied following a traffic accident. The first fatty streaks can be seen

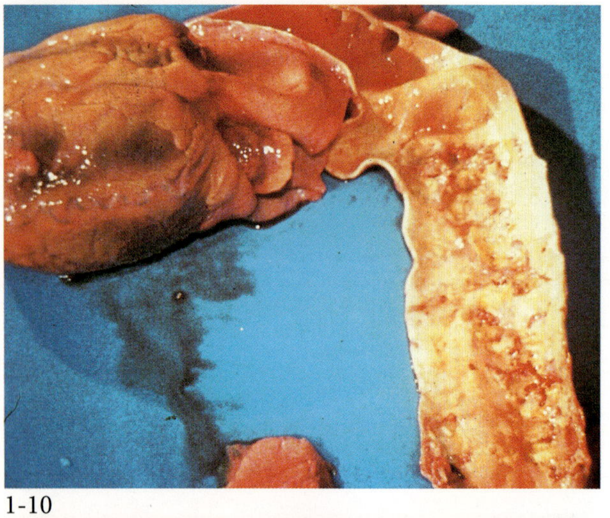

1-10

Fig. 1-10. Severe atheroma formation in the ascending aorta (autopsy specimen)

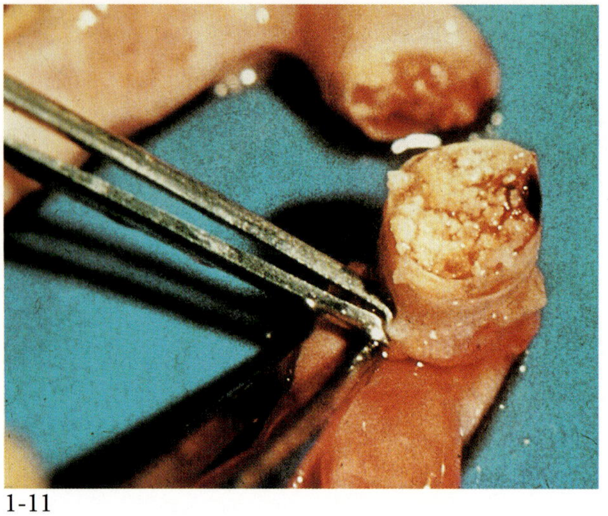

1-11

Fig. 1-11. Massive arteriosclerosis with complete obliteration of the lumen of the artery

Fig. 1-12. Erosive arteriosclerosis in the abdominal aorta

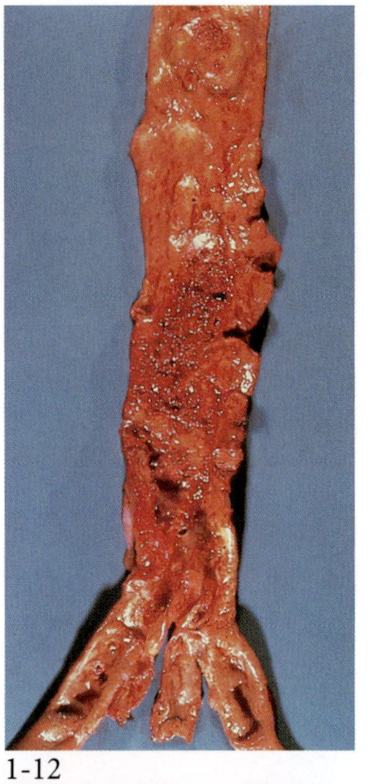

1-12

Fig. 1-13. Complex aortic lesion with crater-like, torn, arterio-sclerotic patches with partial remodeling into connective tissue

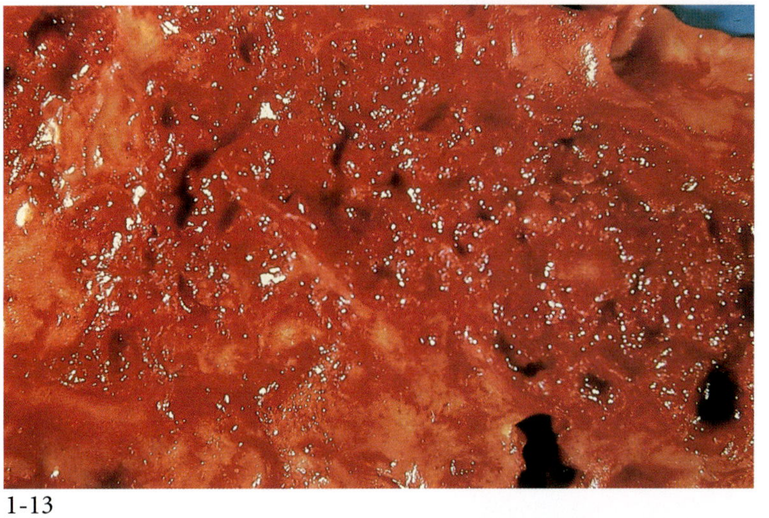

1-13

Fig. 1-14. Plastic-like abdominal aorta with aneurysm and massive atherosclerotic changes

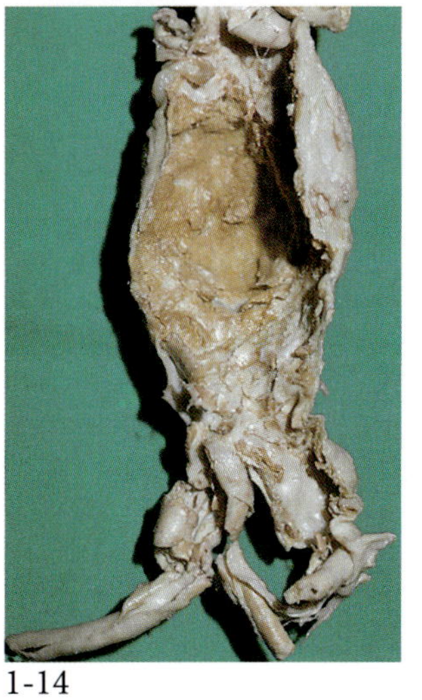

1-14

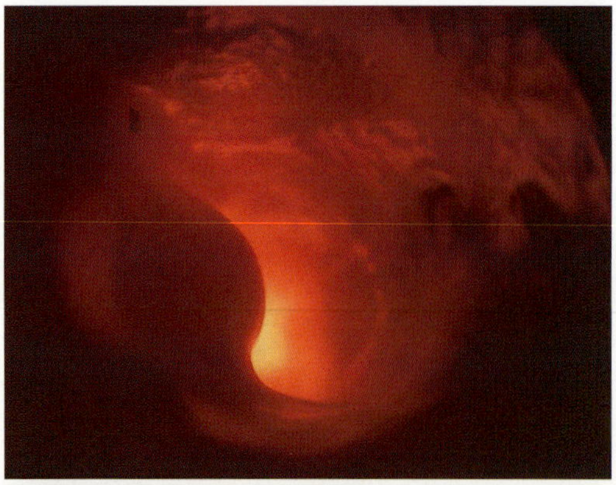

1-15

Fig. 1-15. Atherosclerotic changes in a coronary artery producing luminal stenosis. (From Lennart Nilsson, Boehringer Ingelheim, Germany)

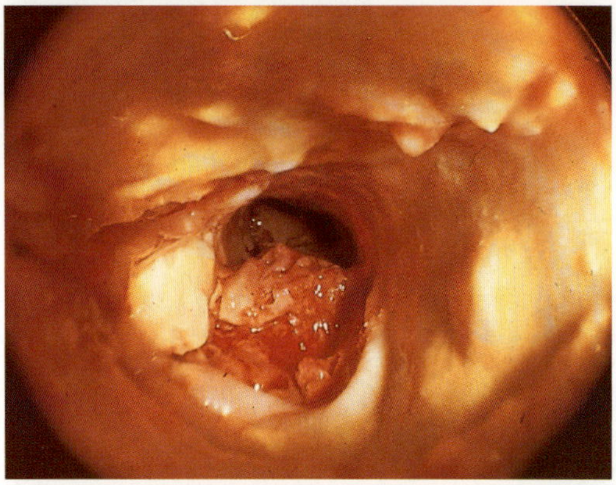

1-16

Fig. 1-16. Endothelial damage and thrombotic repair are part of the entire process of arteriosclerosis and lead to thromboses, as shown here in a coronary artery. (From Lennart Nilsson, Boehringer Ingelheim, Germany)

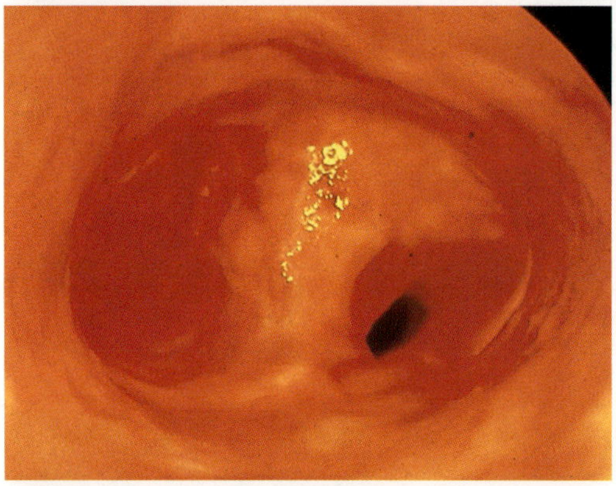

1-17

Fig. 1-17. Arteriosclerosis first occurs at sites of high mechanical pressure, such as here at the aortic bifurcation. (From from Lennart Nilsson, Boehringer Ingelheim, Germany)

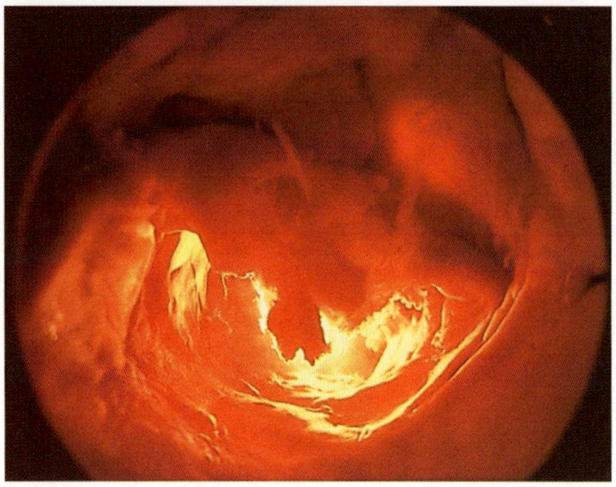

1-18

Fig. 1-18. Thrombus in an aorta with marked arteriosclerotic damage. (From Lennart Nilsson, Boehringer Ingelheim, Germany)

Fig. 1-19. Scanning electron microscopy shows a tiny ulceration in an otherwise healthy aorta. (From Lennart Nilsson, Boehringer Ingelheim, Germany)

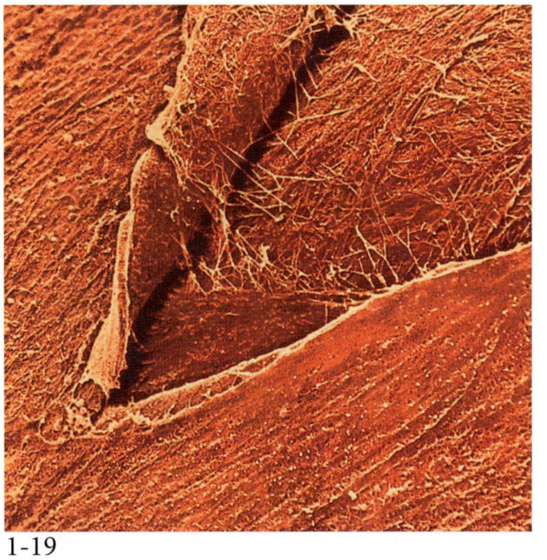

1-19

Fig. 1-20. A deeper crater-like ulceration is shown filled with cellular blood elements. At the edge fibrin threads can be seen. Thrombosis always leads to fibrin formation. (From Lennart Nilsson, Boehringer Ingelheim, Germany)

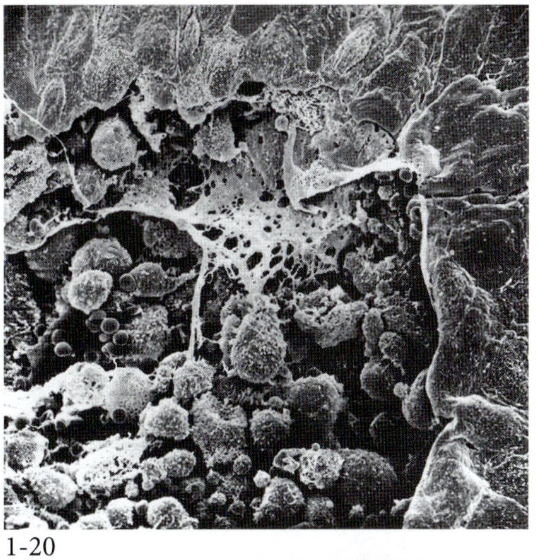

1-20

Fig. 1-21. A 56 year old patient with severe generalized arteriosclerosis. Routine radiological examination of the thorax identifies the coronary arteries because they are so heavily calcified. The patient presented with unstable angina.

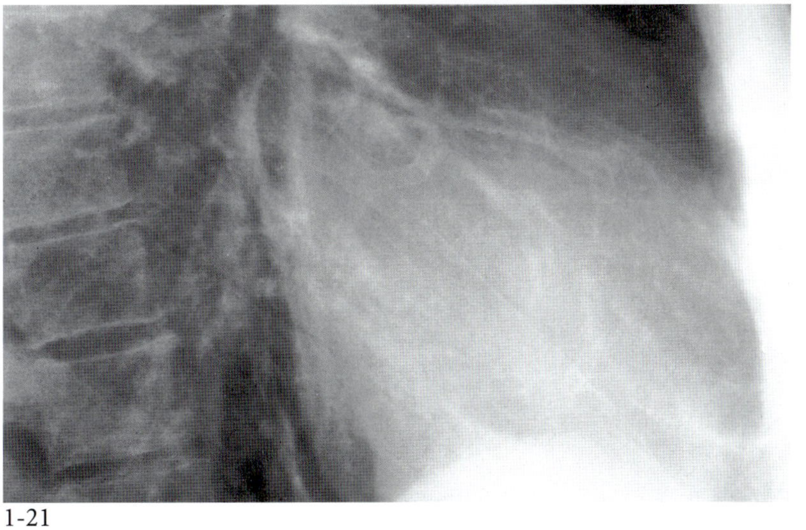

1-21

Chapter 2
Diseases of the Cerebral Arteries

Contents

A: Introduction

Stroke

Synonyms. Apoplexy brain attack, cerebral vascular accident (CVA)

Definition

Following the definitions of the World Health Organization, a stroke can be the result of localized cerebral ischemia, an intracerebral hemorrhage, a subarachnoid hemorrhage or a cerebral venous obstruction (sinus thrombosis). When ischemia is present, the disturbed function is described as an ischemic insult. If the ischemia persists, morphologic changes of an ischemic infarct develop.

Epidemiology

- Strokes are the third leading cause of death, following cardiac and circulatory disturbances. They are a major cause of invalidism.
- Over 80% of the patients are older than 65 years.
- About one-third of strokes are associated with arterial stenoses and occlusions, usually secondary to arteriosclerosis.
- Unlike the situation in Europa, the age-adjusted death rate for stroke in the United States has been steadily declining, dropping from 89 per 100,000 population in 1950 to 28 in 1990.
- In Germany about 350,000 people experience a cerebral insult yearly. About 100,000 die and another 120,000 are disabled or require nursing care. The numbers are approximately twice as large in the United States.

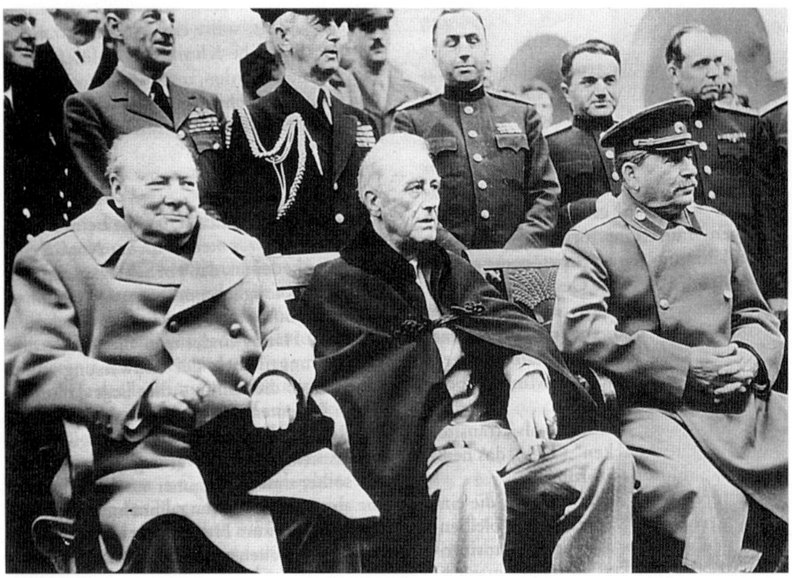

Fig. 2-1. Churchill, Roosevelt and Stalin at the Yalta Conference. All three politicians died from strokes. Roosevelt had a cerebral hemorrhage; Stalin, a cerebral embolus with bleeding and Churchill, a cerebral microangiopathy

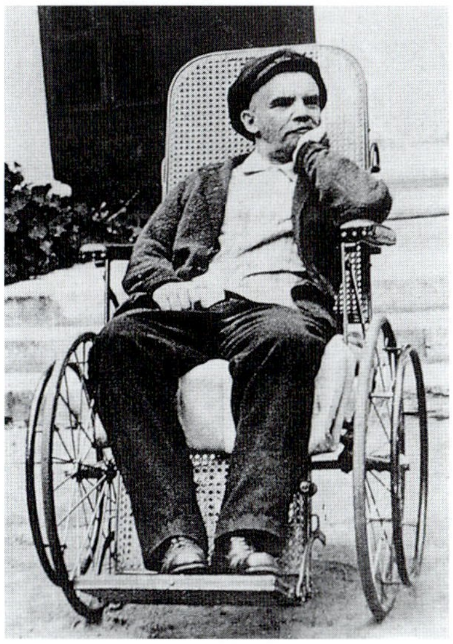

Fig. 2-2. Lenin in a wheelchair. Hemiparesis and loss of speech were the sequelae of Lenin's third stroke. This is one of the last photographs taken of him. He had his first stroke in 1922 and died in January, 1924. The study of Lenin's brain was considered so important that the Moscow State Institute for Brain Research was established. A "genius locus" in his brain had been suggested by many scientists but was not found

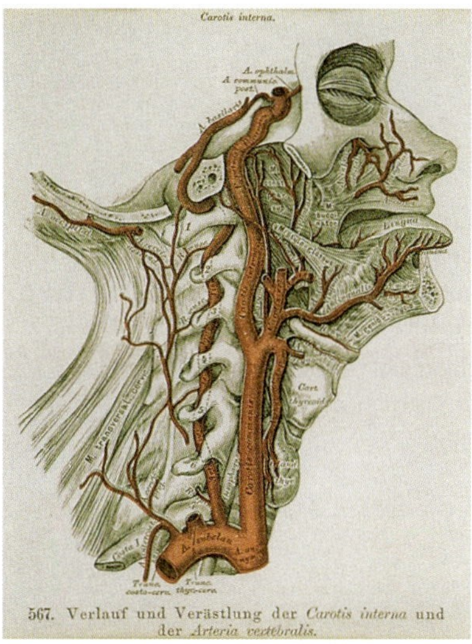

Fig. 2-3. Anatomy of the cerebral arteries. (From Descriptive und topographische Anatomie des Menschen, C. Heitzmann 1893)

Major Risk Factors for Strokes

- increasing age
- being male
- a prior stroke
- Heredity
- Hypertension
- Cardiac disease
- Smoking
- Diabetes mellitus
- Alcohol abuse
- Hyperfibrinogenemia
- Hyperhomocysteinemia
- Race. Afro-Americans have a greater stroke risk than Anglo-Americans

Clinical Features

Cerebral circulatory disturbances are subdivided according to the location and course of the neurological damage they cause.

Classification of Cerebral Circulatory Disturbances

A: Based on Location

1. Carotid artery distribution
2. Vertebral artery distribution

Symptoms

Both reversible and irreversible neurological deficits arise.

1. Carotid artery involvement
   - Ipsilateral visual problems, including hemianopsia
   - Hemiparesis, monoplegia and paresthesias
   - Aphasia
   - Seizures (petit mal)
2. Vertebral artery involvement
   - Drop attacks (dizziness and fainting)
   - Double vision
   - Tinnitus
   - Dysarthria

B: Based on Clinical Course

Functional classification of ischemic cerebrovascular disease (after VOLLMAR)

Stage I Asymptomatic carotid narrowing

Stage II Transient ischemic attacks (TIA). The symptoms resolve within 24 h. Amaurosis fugax is common.

Stage III Progressive stroke (stroke in evolution) lasting 6 – 48 h
(a) Without recovery
(b) With recovery (RIND = reversible ischemic neurologic deficit)
(c) With prolonged (or delayed) recovery (PRIND = prolonged reversible ischemic neurologic deficit)

Stage IV Completed stroke with partial or no recovery
(a) Minor stroke, small injury with minimal disability
(b) Major stroke, large injury, leaving a disabled patient who is unable to work and requires nursing help or care

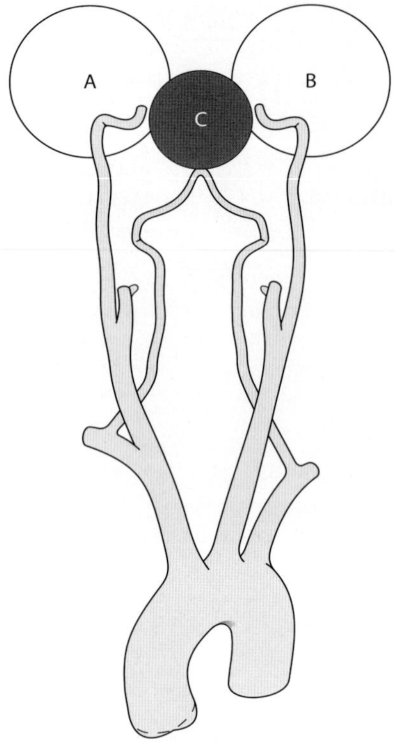

Fig. 2-4. The three sections of the brain that are dependent on a single arterial source: the left and right carotid regions (*A*, *B*) and the central area served by the vertebral system (*C*)

Diagnosis

- General investigation of vessels
  - Palpation of the temporal, subclavian and radial arteries (Fig. 2-6)
  - Auscultation of the carotid and subclavian arteries and above the orbit (Fig. 2-7)
- Cardiologic evaluation, looking for sources of emboli
- Neurological evaluation
- Doppler ultrasonography
  - Extracranial/transcranial Doppler ultrasonography, spectral analysis, B-mode ultrasonography, color duplex ultrasonography, Doppler CO_2 reactivity measurement (Figs. 2-8 – 2-13)
- Cerebral angiography: catheter angiography using both conventional and digital image techniques, but only when therapeutic consequences can be expected from the angiographic results
- Computerized tomography (CT) with contrast material
  - Every stroke patient should have this study. It is the best way to distinguish between ischemia and hemorrhage. CT identification of ischemia is first possible 5 – 8 h after the clinical signs of cerebral insult.

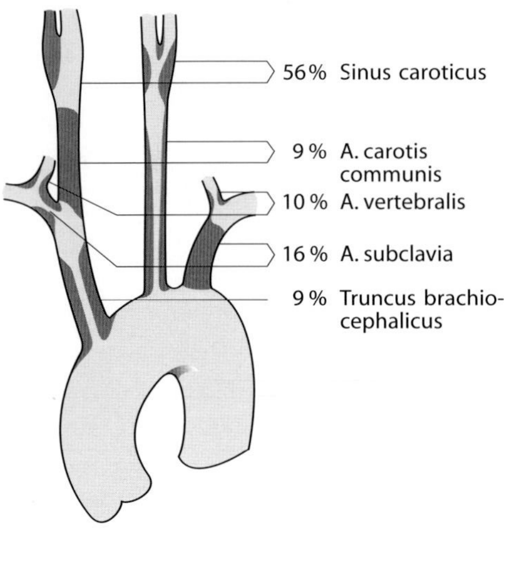

Fig. 2-5. Distribution of supra-aortic arterial occlusion (after VOLLMAR). The predilection sites are the internal carotid artery just after the bifurcation, the carotid artery at the bifurcation and the trunks as they leave the aorta

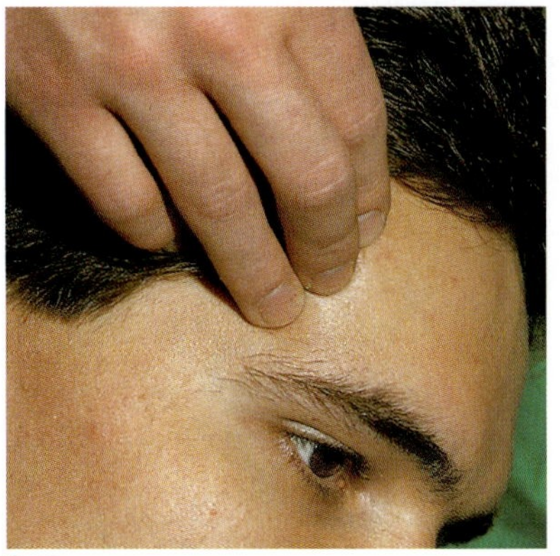

2-6

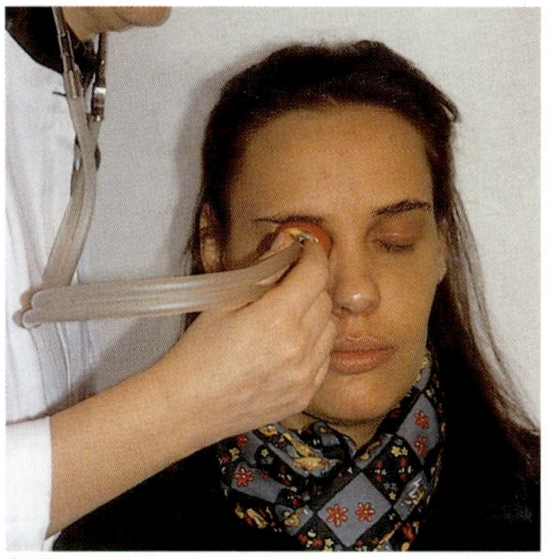

2-7

Fig. 2-6. A palpable temporal pulse indicates that the common and external carotid arteries are patent

Fig. 2-7. A systolic bruit over the orbit suggest a siphon stenosis

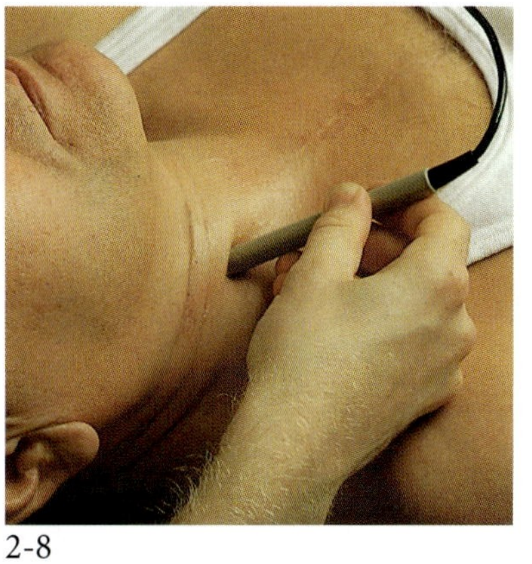

2-8

Fig. 2-8. Evaluating the cervical vessels with continuous wave Doppler ultrasound

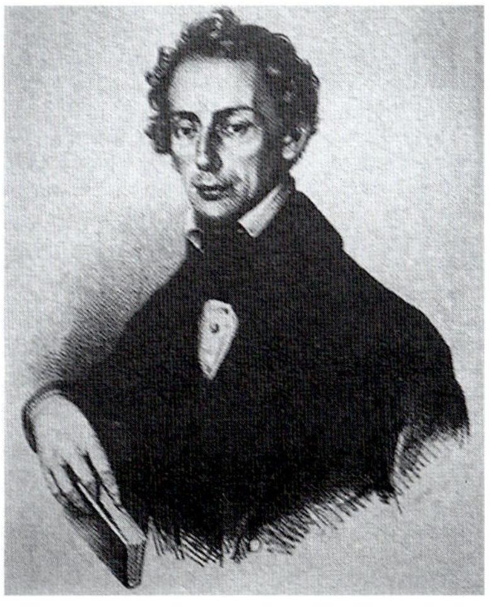

Fig. 2-9.
Christian Andreas Doppler (1803–1853, born in Salzburg, Austria)

- Magnetic resonance imaging (MRI): also helpful as it can show cerebral changes sooner and with more accuracy than CT

Principle of Continuous Wave Doppler Ultrasonography
Doppler, in 1842, observed that when sound waves strike a moving body and are reflected, there is a shift in the echo which correlates with the speed and direction. The Japanese and American bioengineers SATAMURA (1959) and FRANKLIN (1961) developed Doppler instruments for analyzing blood flow.

Transcranial Doppler Ultrasonography
This technique is primarily used to identify high-grade stenotic lesions of the middle cerebral artery and also the internal carotid artery at the level of the carotid siphon. Usually one employs a trans-temporal approach because the skull is relatively thin in this area. The Doppler probe is placed perpendicular to the skull. The axis of the ultrasound beam goes through the main branch of the middle cerebral artery, the distal part of the internal carotid artery and the proximal branches of the anterior and posterior cerebral arteries.

A trans-nuchal approach is also possible, allowing one to assess the vertebral and often the basilar arteries. A trans-orbital approach can also be employed effectively.

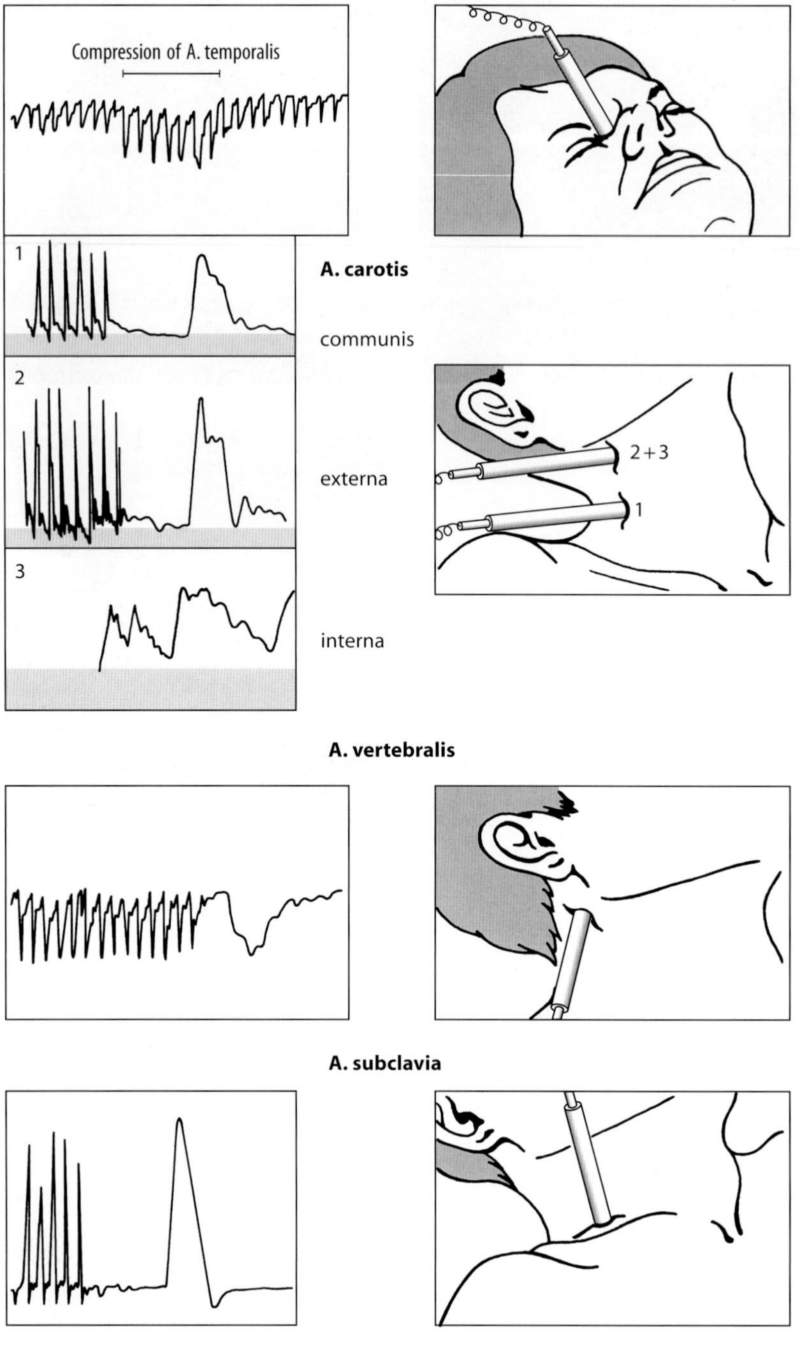

Fig. 2-10. Doppler ultrasound techniques for the relevant arteries. *Left*: the normal pulse curves with slow (5 mm/s) and fast (50 mm/s) paper speed. *Right*: the proper sites for the placement of the probe

Therapy

A: Therapeutic Possibilities in Different Stages

Stage I (asymptomatic carotid narrowing)

- Medical: inhibitors of platelet function (aspirin, ticlopidine clopidogrel)
- Surgical: appropriate for stenoses exceeding 80%, rapidly progressive carotid stenoses, ulcerated high-grade stenotic lesions and soft plaques. Best used in patients with multiple lesions who are at a good anesthetic risks and have a reasonable life expectancy
- Percutaneous transluminal angioplasty (PTA)

Fig. 2-11. Duplex ultrasonography: work station for Doppler and duplex ultrasonography in vascular diagnosis

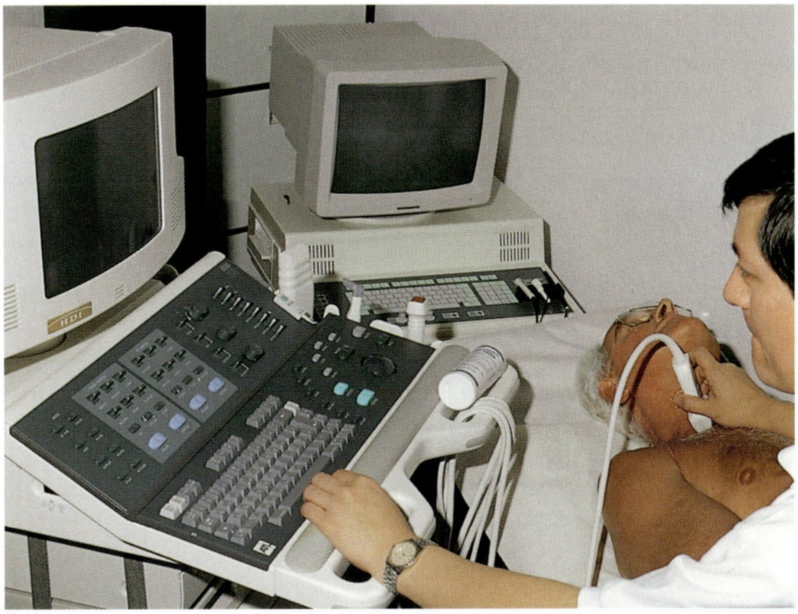

2-11

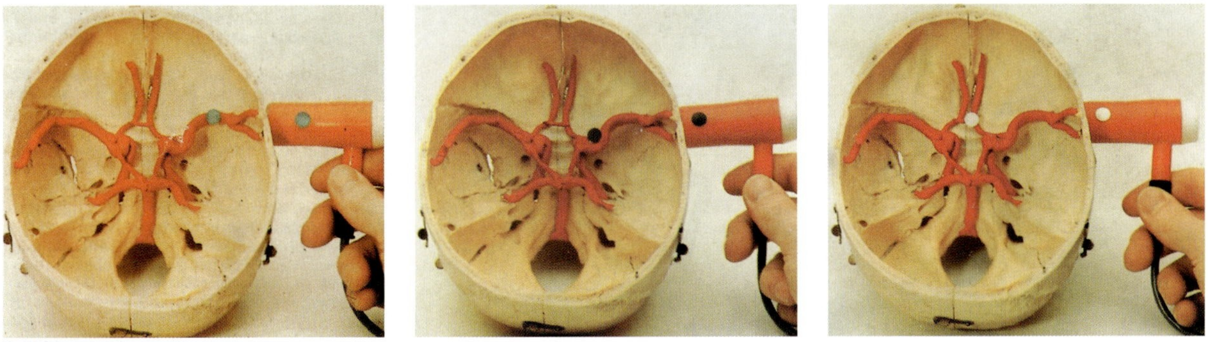

2-12

Fig. 2-12. Transcranial Doppler ultrasonography. Schematic representation showing how the middle cerebral artery, anterior cerebral artery and anterior communicating ramus are studied with a trans-temporal approach. (After Rautenberg et al. 1987)

Fig. 2-13. Trans-nuchal approach for Doppler ultrasonography allowing evaluation of the vertebral and in most cases the basilar arteries

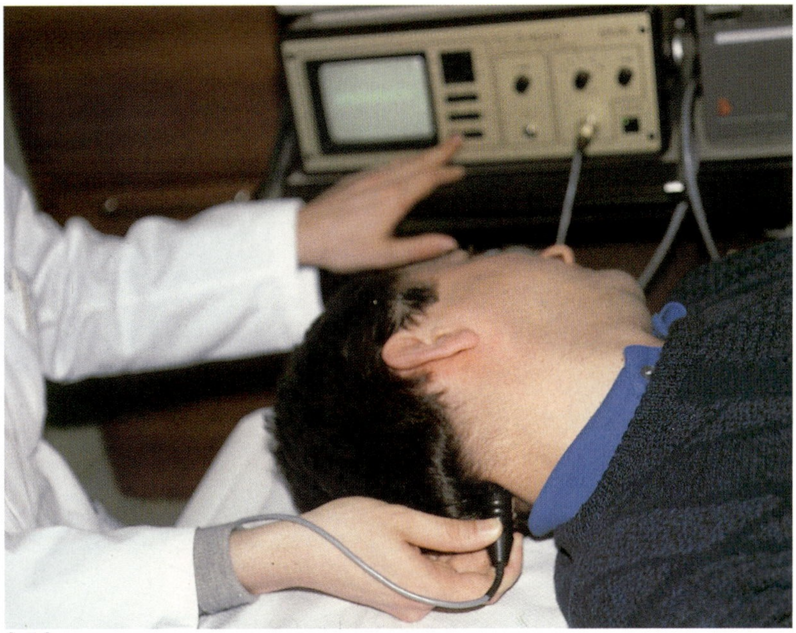

2-13

Stage II (transient ischemic attacks)

- Primary role for reconstructive vascular surgery (carotid endarterectomy) once cardiac disease has been excluded

Stage III (progressive insult)

- Operation in patients in whom full heparinization has not stopped the progression and who still are alert and oriented

Stage IV (completed stroke)

- Surgery following satisfactory rehabilitation to avoid or reduce the risk of a second stroke

History of the Carotid Endarterectomy
The first carotid endarterectomies were performed by CARREA (1951) and De Bakey (1953). However, DE BAKEY did not publish his work until 1959 while in November 1954 EASTCOTT, PICKERING and ROB published

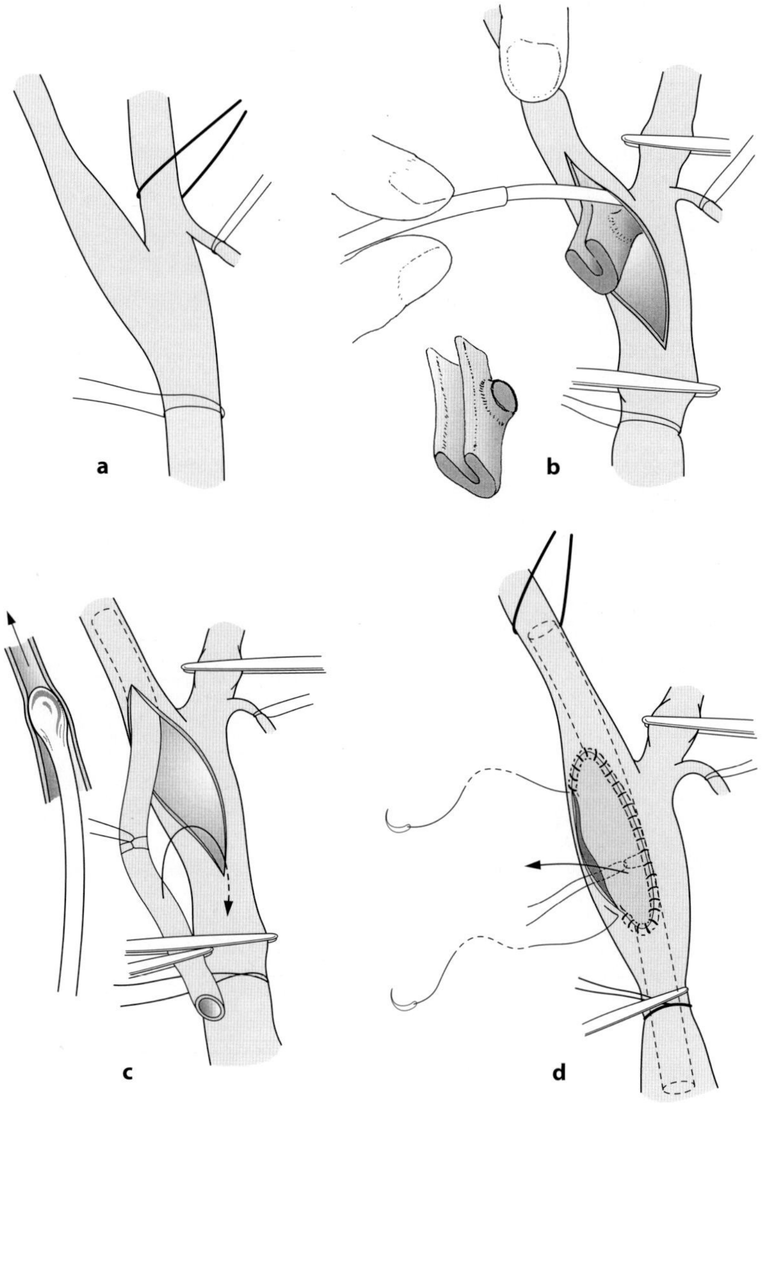

Fig. 2-14 a–d. Technique of carotid endarterectomy (after VOLLMAR).
a Exposure and longitudinal incision;
b Removal of the stenotic intimal cylinder;
c Insertion of a plastic tube as an intraluminal shunt;
d Sewing a vein or synthetic patch in the arteriotomy, removal of the shunt prior to closure

their work in Lancet, describing a carotid endarterectomy in a patient with transient ischemic attacks. They used a direct end-to-end anastomosis between the common carotid and internal carotid arteries. The operation was done with hypothermia, as the patient's body temperature was held at 28°C. In 1957 WARREN and TRIEDMAN published a second case and then there was an explosion of interest in the procedure of carotid endarterectomy. The main pioneers in developing this new procedure were De Bakey, Rob and Wheeler.

B: General Therapeutic Measures

- Treatment of cardiac failure and arrhythmias
- Platelet inhibitors have replaced oral anticoagulants for secondary prevention
- Heparinization and systemic fibrinolysis
- Local fibrinolysis in the case of basilar artery thrombosis (window of opportunity up to 6 h)

C: Rehabilitation

The goal of rehabilitation is to reduce the patient's functional disability and minimize its effects on his or her life. Rehabilitation starts ideally as soon the patient is stable. The three phases of the process are acute rehabilitation on the medical-surgical ward, in-patient rehabilitation in a special unit and then ambulatory services.

B: Supplementary Figures and Legends

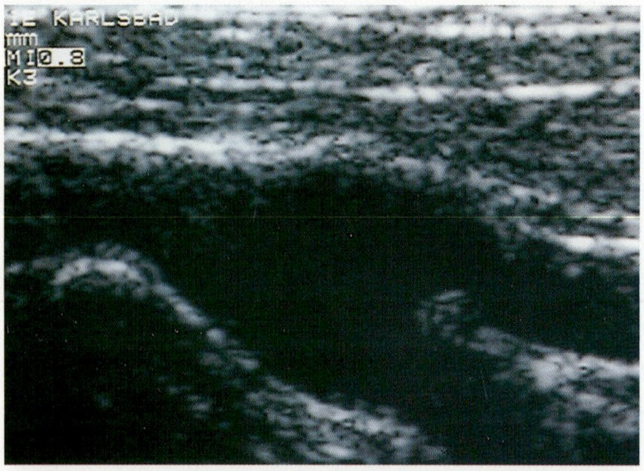

2-15

Fig. 2-15. B-mode ultrasonography of a normal carotid bifurcation without plaque

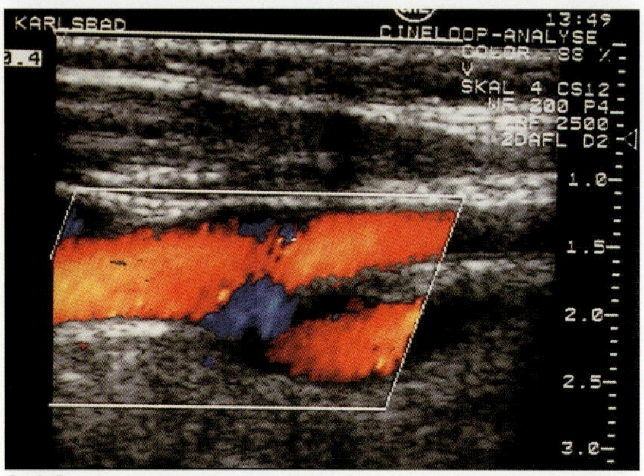

2-16

Fig. 2-16. Color duplex ultrasonography of an unremarkable carotid bifurcation

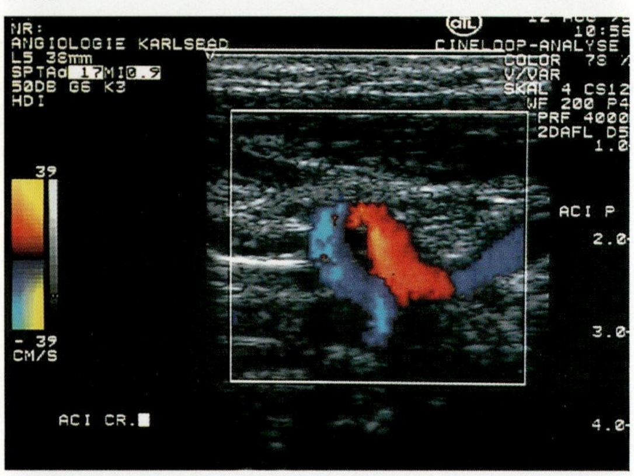

2-17

Fig. 2-17. Color duplex ultrasonography of a striking kink in the internal carotid artery

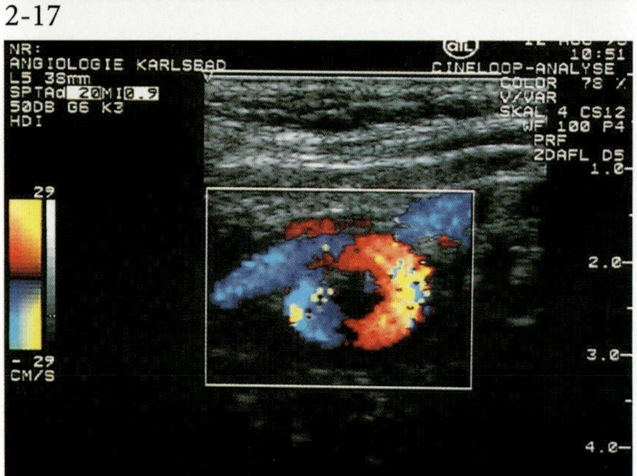

2-18

Fig. 2-18. Color duplex ultrasonography shows marked coiling of the internal carotid artery

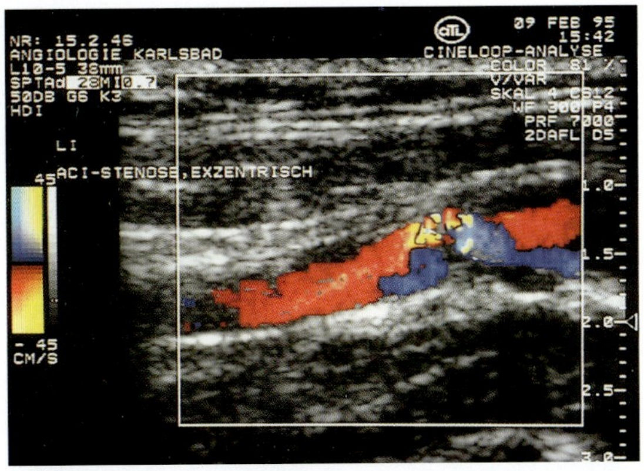

2-19

Fig. 2-19. Color duplex ultrasonography of a mid-grade eccentric stenosis of the internal carotid artery

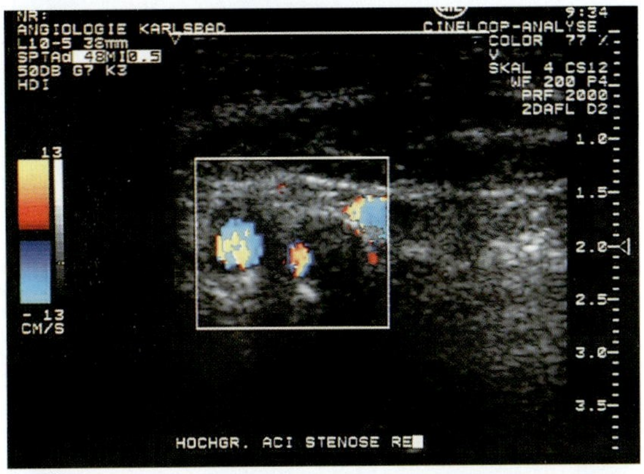

2-20

Fig. 2-20. Color duplex ultrasonography showing subtotal (~90%) obstruction of the internal carotid artery. In the *middle* a tiny residual lumen can be seen

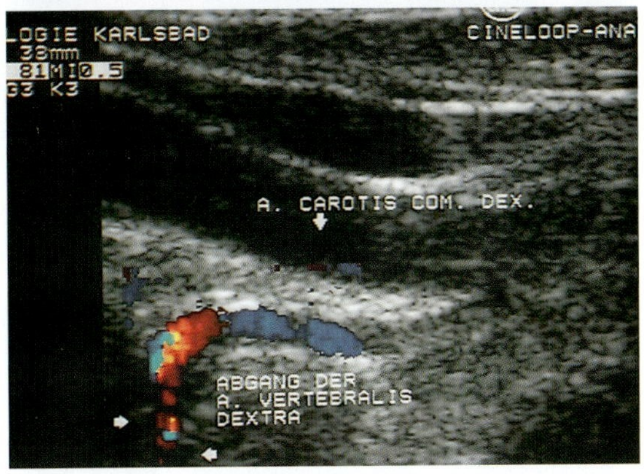

2-21

Fig. 2-21. Color duplex ultrasonography showing complete occlusion of the common carotid artery. Starting at the *arrow* and moving towards the *right*, the echo density increases. Inferiorly, the origin of the vertebral artery is shown

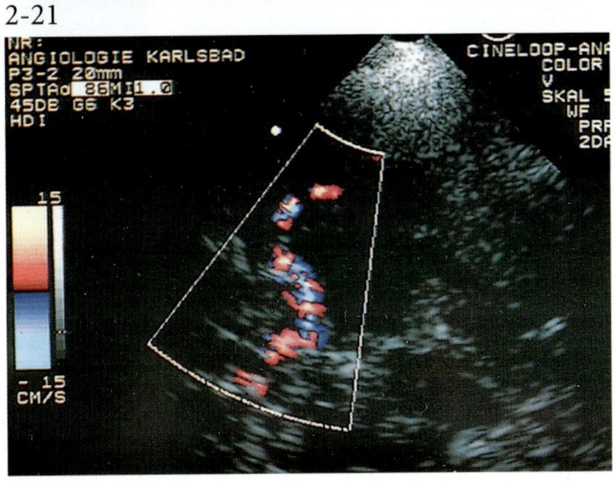

2-22

Fig. 2-22. Color duplex ultrasonography of a normal middle cerebral artery

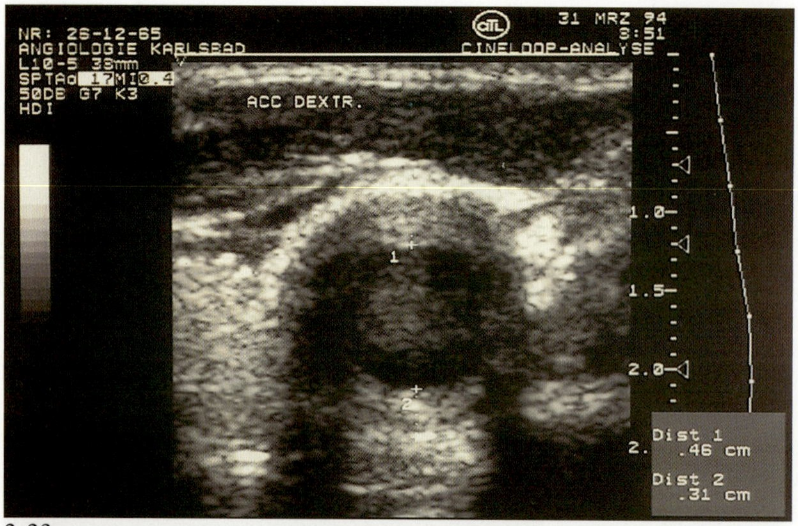

2-23

Fig. 2-23. B-mode ultrasonography (cross-section) of a common carotid artery in a 28 year old patient with Takayasu's disease. The arterial wall shows a massive inflammatory thickening

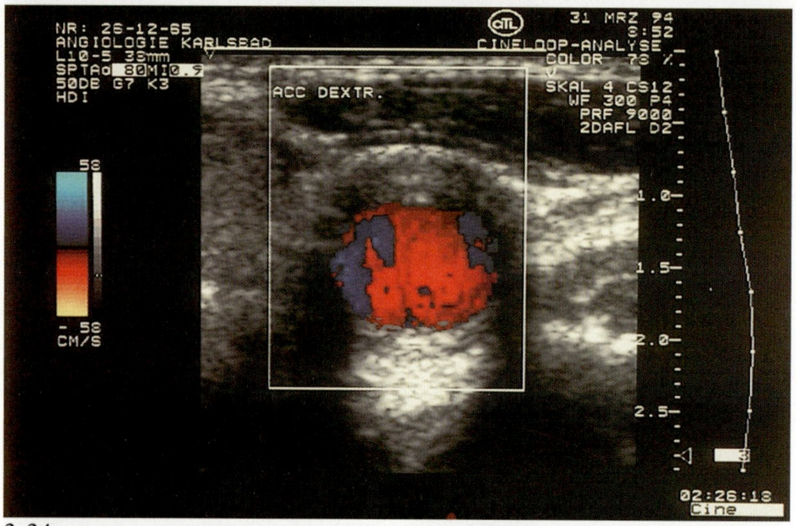

2-24

Fig. 2-24. Color duplex ultrasonography (cross-section) of a common carotid artery in the same patient

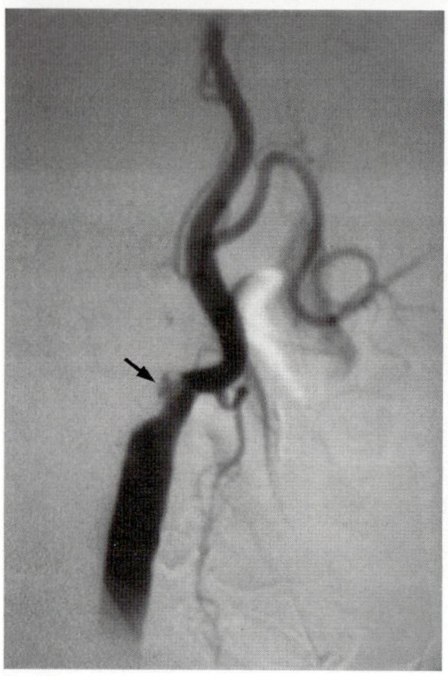

2-25

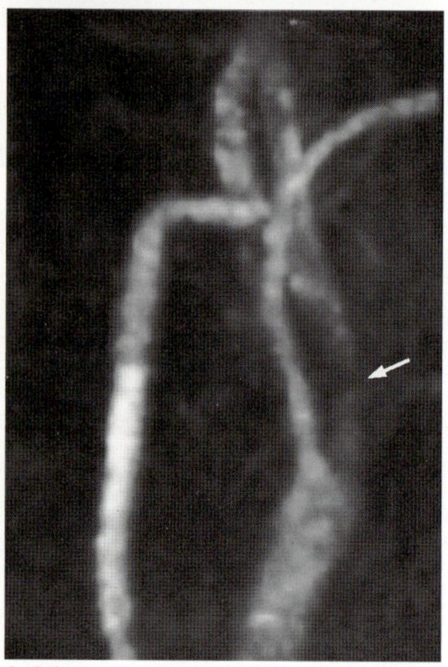

2-26

Fig. 2-25. Digital subtraction angiography demonstrating an occlusion of the internal carotid artery

Fig. 2-26. Magnetic resonance angiography used to show a high-grade recurrent stenosis at the carotid bifurcation

Fig. 2-27. The three dimensional presentation of this spiral computerized tomogram clearly shows the 70% stenosis of the distal internal carotid artery in a non-invasive fashion

Fig. 2-28. Single photon emission computerized tomogram demonstrates the perfusion defect in the right parietal region as a sequel to a stenosis of the right internal carotid artery

Fig. 2-29. Computerized tomography showing temporal lobe ischemia

Fig. 2-30. Computerized tomography showing a cerebral hemorrhage

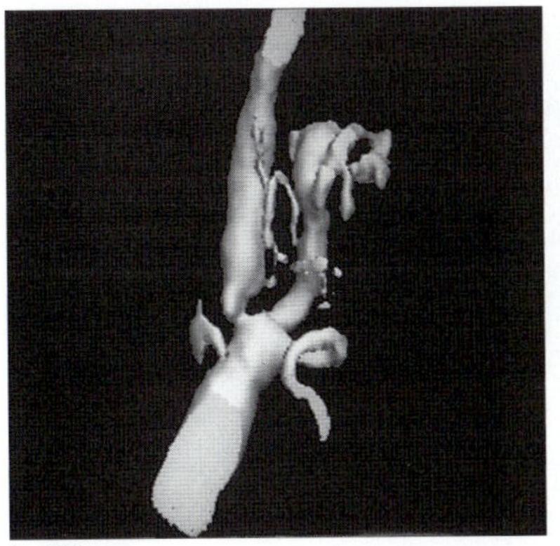

2-27

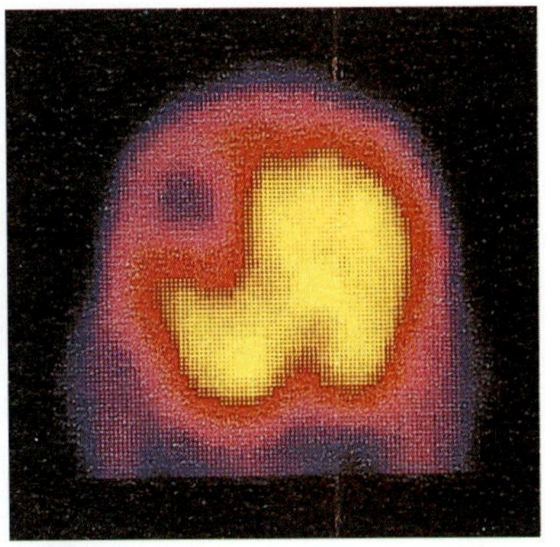

2-28

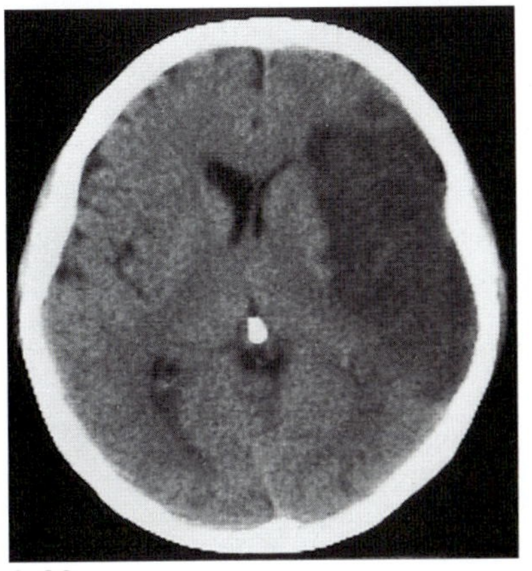

2-29

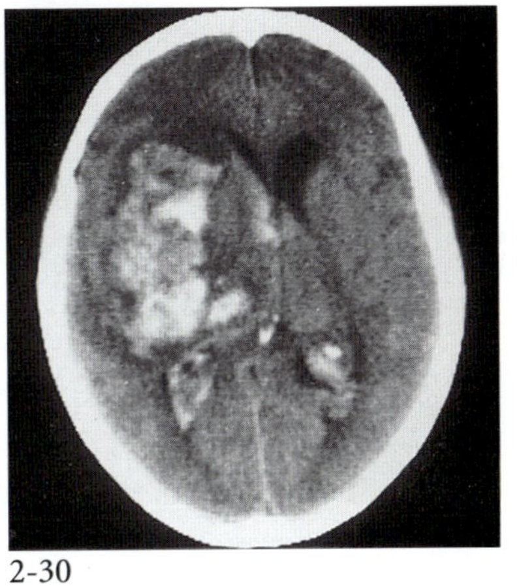

2-30

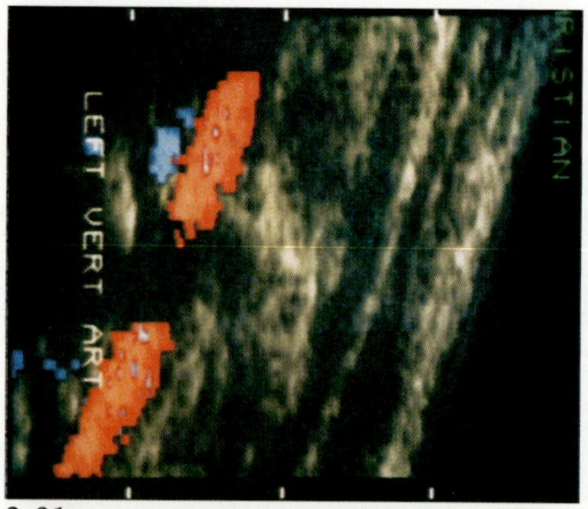

2-31

Fig. 2-31. Color duplex ultrasonography of a normal vertebral artery at its origin from the subclavian artery

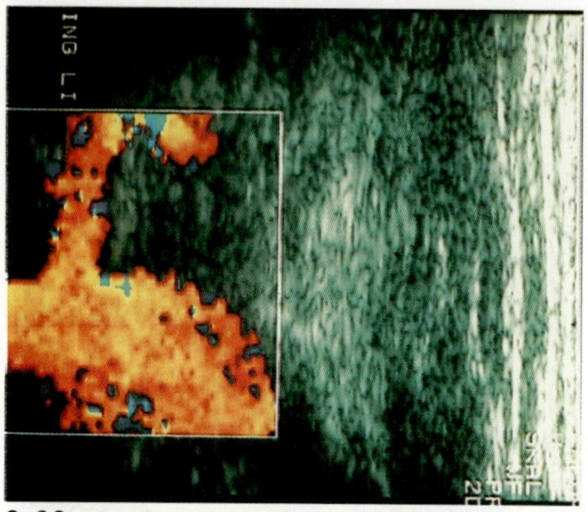

2-32

Fig. 2-32. Color duplex ultrasonography showing kinking of the vertebral artery in a 30 year old patient with drop attacks

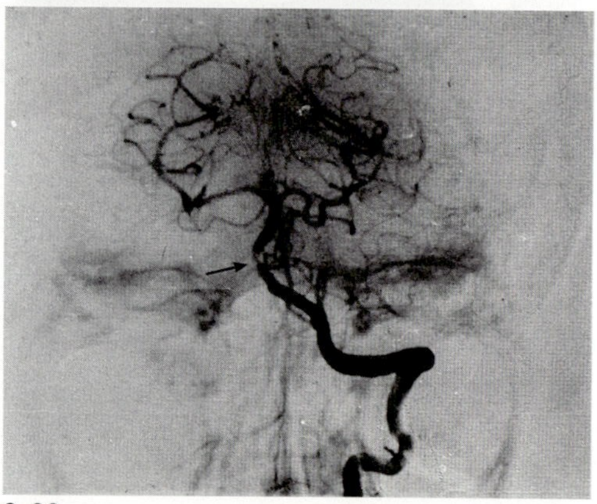

2-33

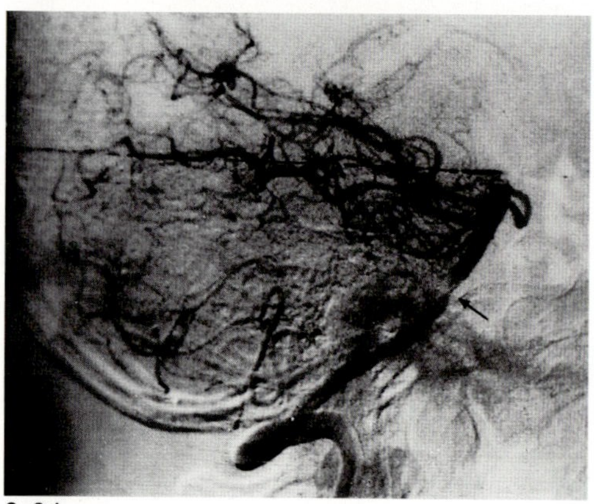

2-34

Figs. 2-33, 2-34. Angiographic demonstration of the basilar artery with filiform stenosis in the antero-posterior and lateral views. When such stenoses are symptomatic, dilatation may be indicated

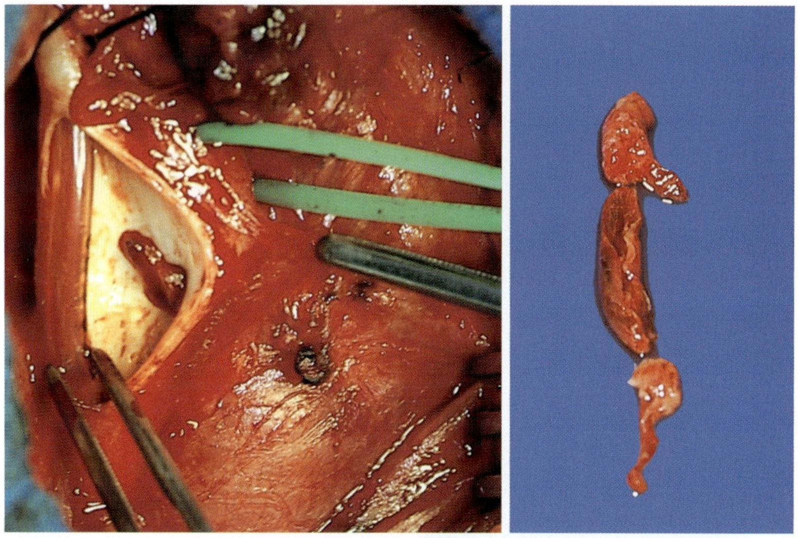

2-35

Fig. 2-35. Intraoperative view of the opened carotid bifurcation with an embolus protruding from the external carotid artery. At the *right*, the embolus is shown

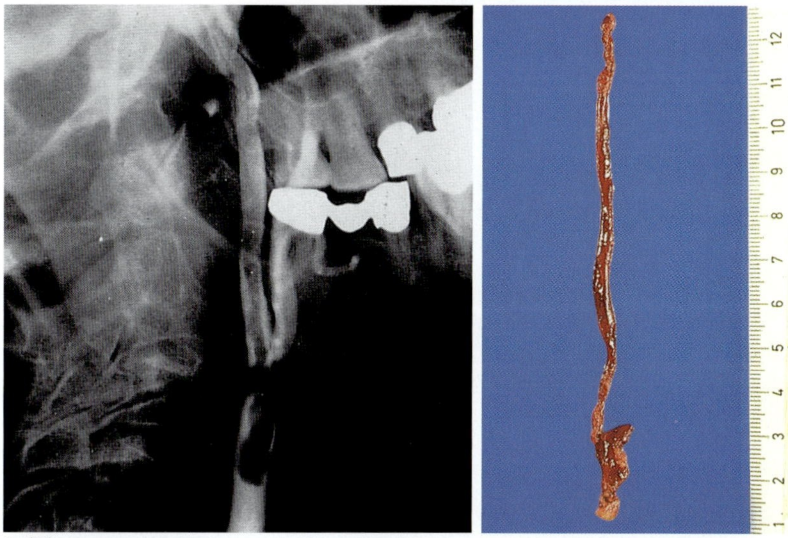

2-36

Fig. 2-36. Embolus from the heart in the carotid bifurcation. At the *right*, the operative specimen

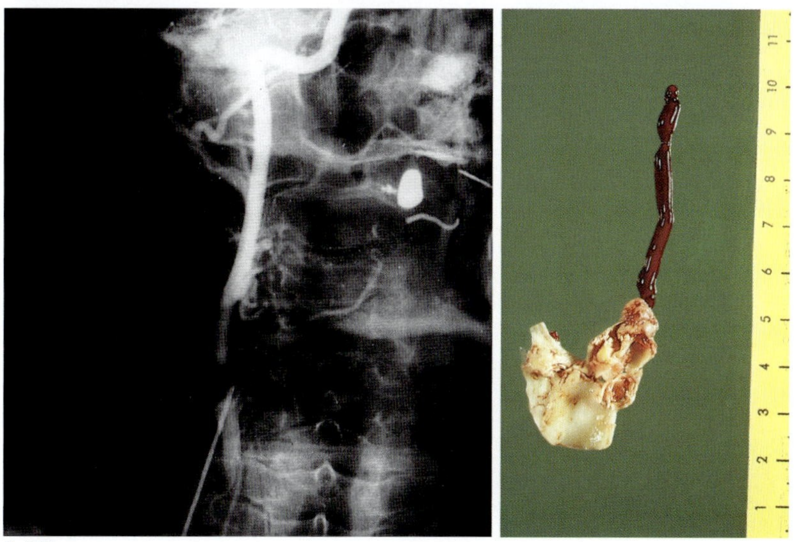

2-37

Fig. 2-37. Acute closure of a high-grade stenosis of the carotid bifurcation. *Right*, the operative specimen showing part of the external carotid artery with a thrombus, often called an apposition thrombus

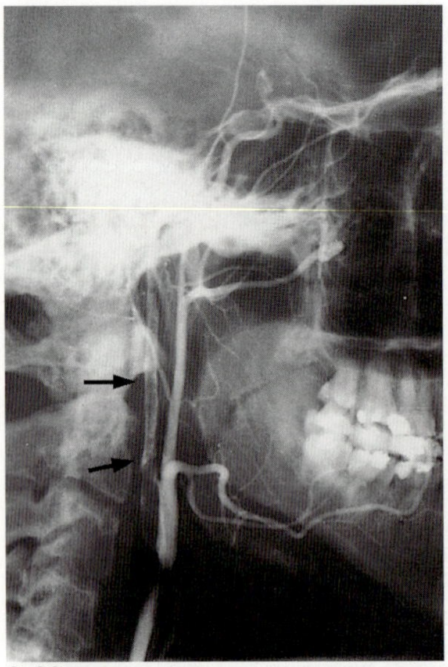

2-38

Fig. 2-38. Thrombosis of the internal carotid artery in a 26 year old man associated with a soft plaque (*arrow*) in the external and internal carotid arteries

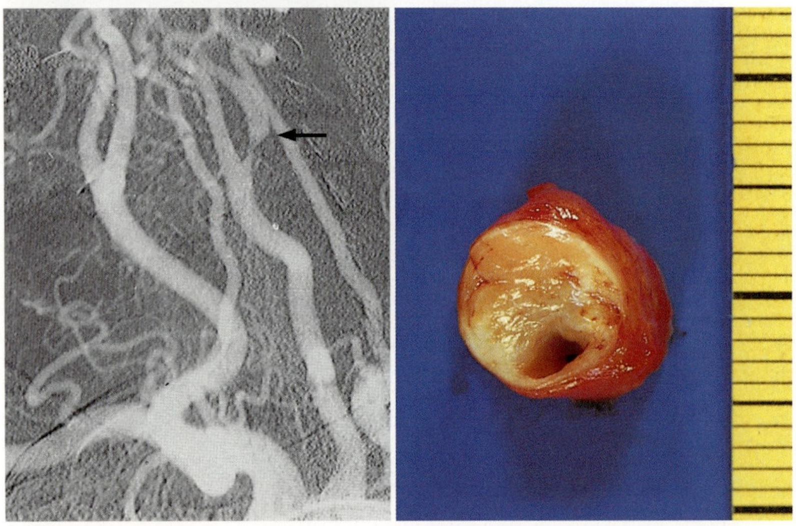

2-39

Fig. 2-39. High-grade stenosis (*arrow*) of the internal carotid artery. The operative specimen shows a mixed plaque with soft and calcified areas

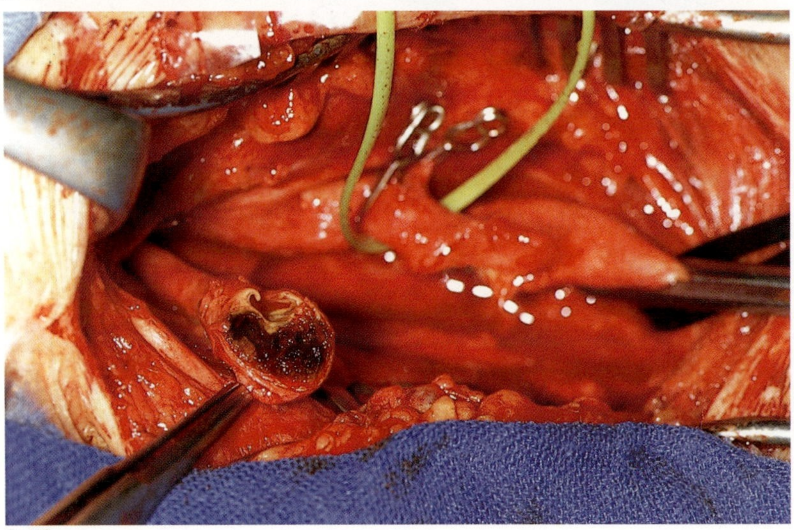

2-40

Fig. 2-40. Operative view of a carotid procedure for a blocked internal carotid artery. One can see the stenosed cylinder with subintimal bleeding and a fresh thrombus. Doppler ultrasonography revealed a sudden increase in the degree of stenosis

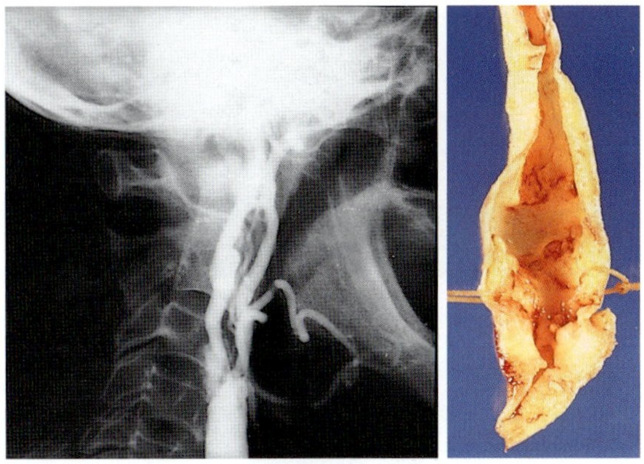

2-41

Fig. 2-41. Carotid angiography showing high-grade progressive stenosis at the bifurcation. The operative specimen following an endarterectomy with thrombus removal is shown

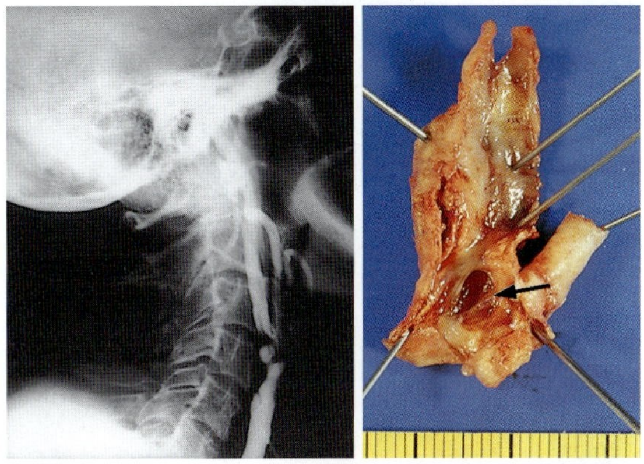

2-42

Fig. 2-42. Ulceration at the carotid bifurcation, shown in both the angiogram and the operative specimen (*arrow*)

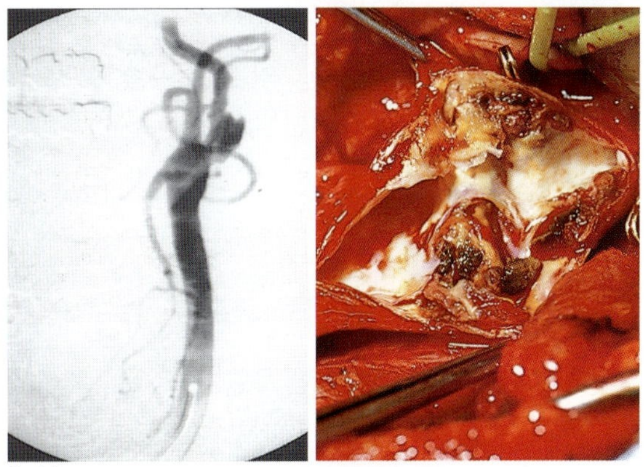

2-43

Fig. 2-43. Ulcerated arteriosclerotic plaque at the take-off of the internal carotid artery. The intraoperative view shows the ulcerations and the thrombotic deposits

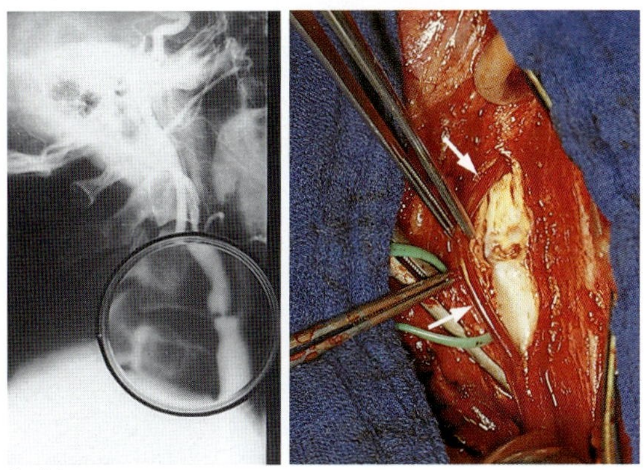

2-44

Fig. 2-44. Septum-like stenosis of the internal carotid artery, shown on angiography and during the operation. An intraluminal shunt is being inserted with the forceps (*arrows*)

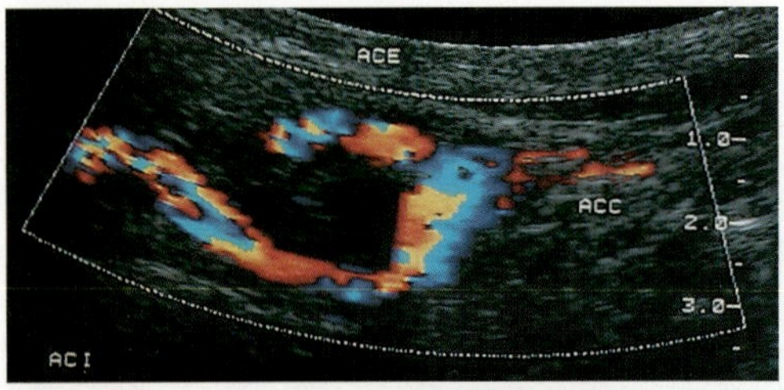

2-45

Fig. 2-45. Color duplex ultrasonography of a marked kinking of the internal carotid artery. Different terms are applied to several closely related conditions: *Tortuosity*, S- or C- shaped elongation; *Coiling*, formation of loops twisting about an axis; *Kinking*, sharp folding of the vessel with a visible narrowing of the lumen

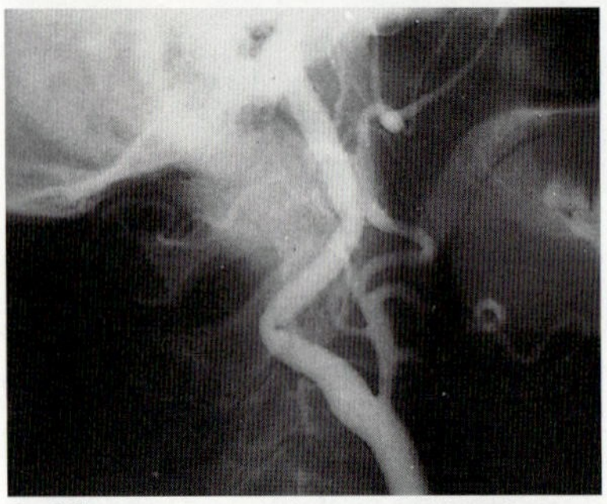

2-46

Fig. 2-46. Angiographic demonstration of kinking of the internal carotid artery with stenosis

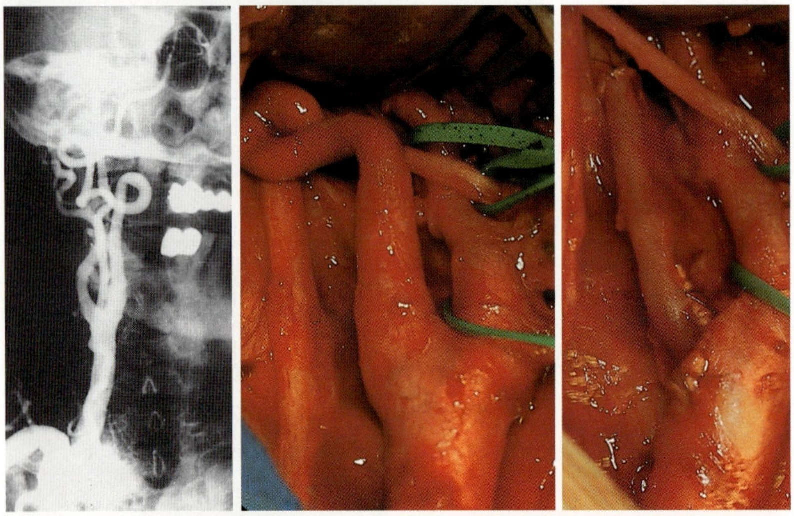

2-47

Fig. 2-47. Marked coiling of the internal carotid artery. From *left*, preoperative angiogram, intraoperative view after exposure and post-operative condition after excision and vein implant

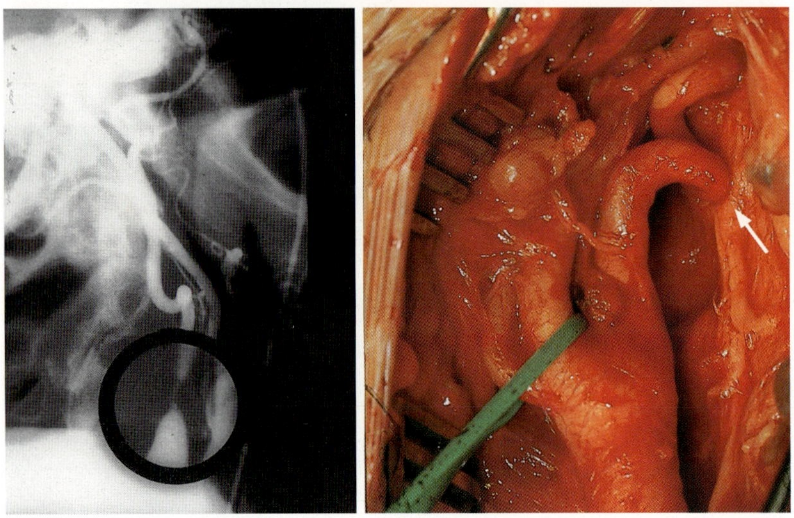

2-48

Fig. 2-48. High-grade kinking and coiling (*arrow*) of the internal carotid artery in combination with filiform stenosis shown in the enlarged view of the angiogram on the *left*

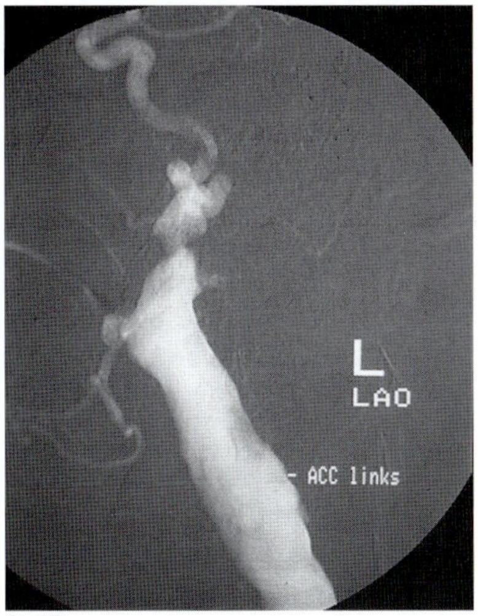

2-49

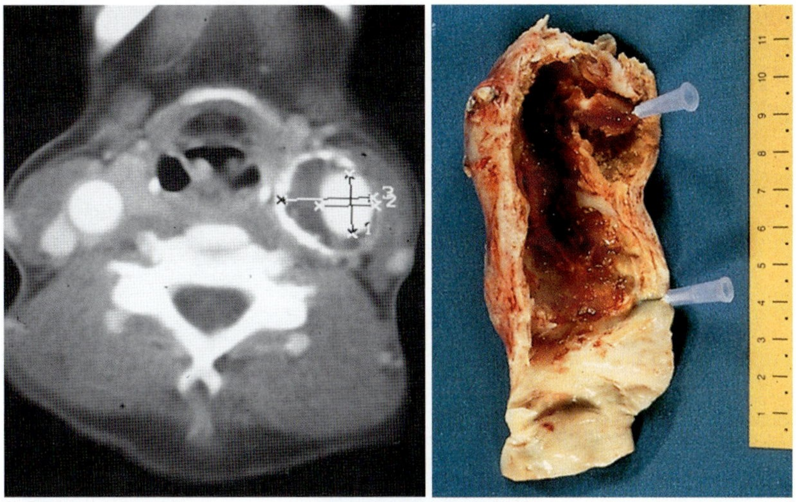

2-50

Fig. 2-49. A 32 year old patient with multiple aneurysms. Angiographic view of aneurysm of the left common carotid and internal carotid arteries

Fig. 2-50. Two-dimensional representation of the aneurysms in the neck with spiral computerized tomography. The changes in both common carotid arteries are easily seen

Fig. 2-51. Two- and three-dimensional longitudinal view of the bilateral carotid artery aneurysms

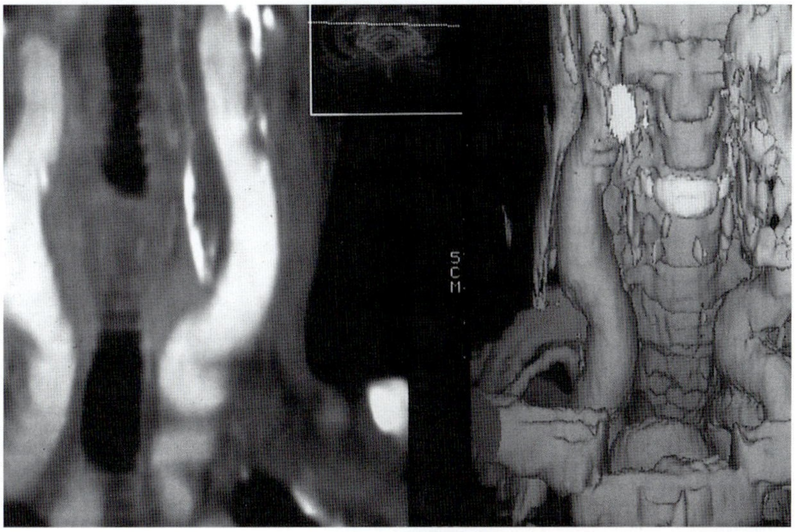

2-51

Fig. 2-52. Intraoperative angiography following vein graft from the proximal common carotid artery to the internal carotid artery with occlusion of the external carotid artery

Fig. 2-53. Post-operative view of scar extending from the jugular notch to behind the ear. The same procedure was carried out on the other side. The patient was not left with any neurological deficits

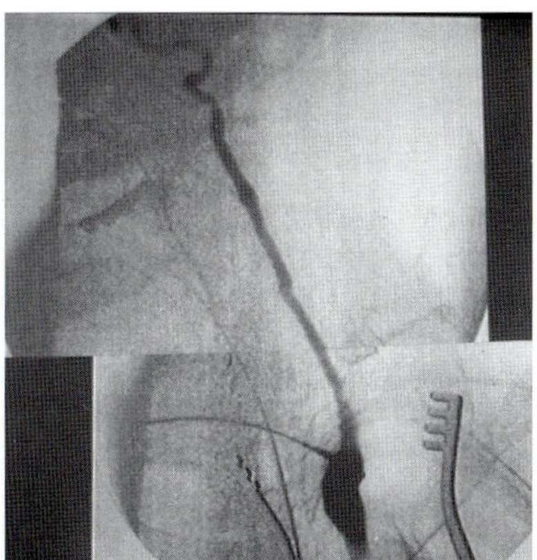

2-52

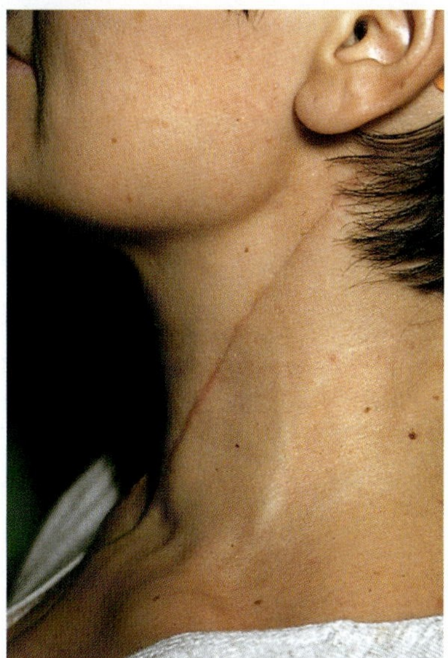

2-53

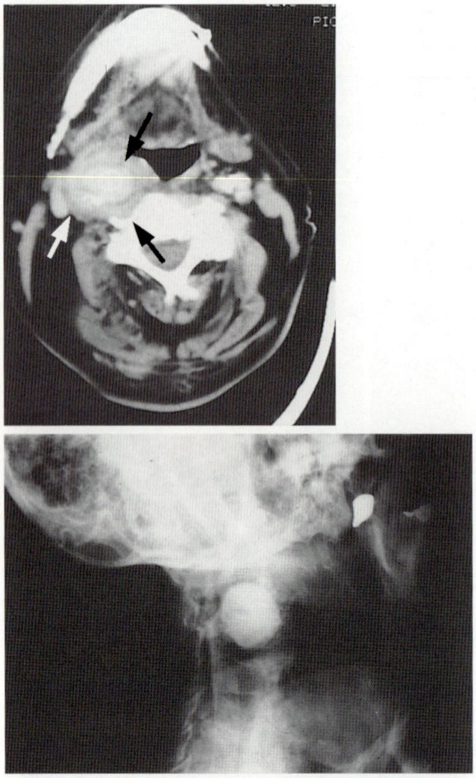

2-54

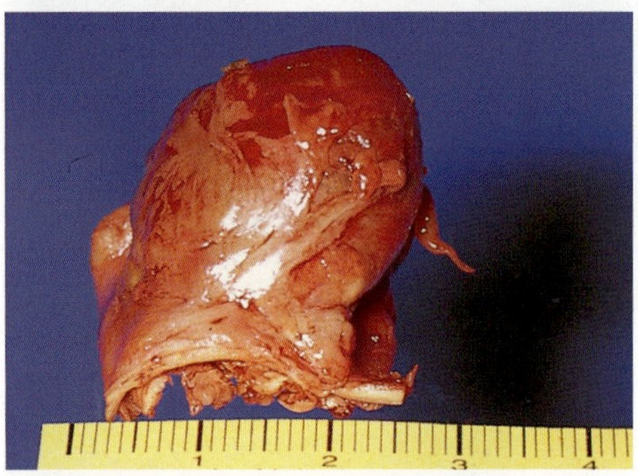

2-55

Figs. 2-54, 2-55. Aneurysm of the carotid artery shown with computerized tomography (*arrows*) and angiography. A delayed view reveals residual contrast material in the sack of the aneurysm. The operative specimen is shown *below*. Most extracranial aneurysms are the result of arteriosclerosis. False aneurysms can develop after an endarterectomy

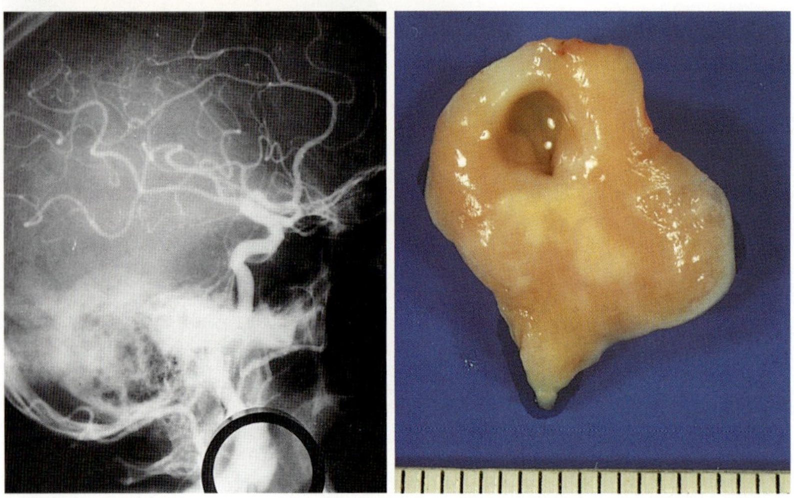

2-56

Fig. 2-56. Angiographic visualization of a small saccular aneurysm of the internal carotid artery in a patient with crescendo transient ischemic attacks. This change is seen in the enlargement at the *bottom* of the picture At the *right* is the operative specimen

Fig. 2-57. Computerized tomogram with contrast material showing a spontaneous dissection of the internal carotid artery. The thrombus (*arrow*) is plainly seen

Fig. 2-58. Angiography in the same patient did not reveal an aneurysm

Figs. 2-59, 2-60. Spontaneous dissection of the internal carotid artery with development of an aneurysm in a 32 year woman. The angiograms show the carotid bifurcation with distal aneurysm formation just before the skull, both in *overview* and at the *right* in more detail. Because the patient had experienced multiple transient ischemic attacks, the aneurysm was resected and a vein graft inserted

Figs. 2-61, 2-62. Traumatic dissection of the internal carotid artery with aneurysm formation (*arrows*) in a 34 year old man whose neck was hyperextended in a skiing accident. The dissection extended to the base of skull, impinging on the bony canal

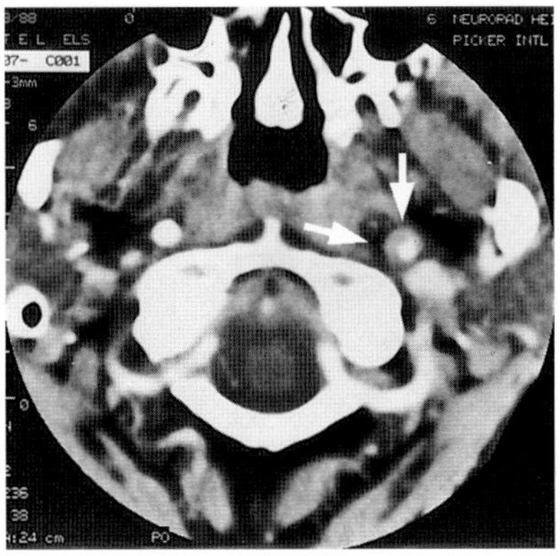

2-57

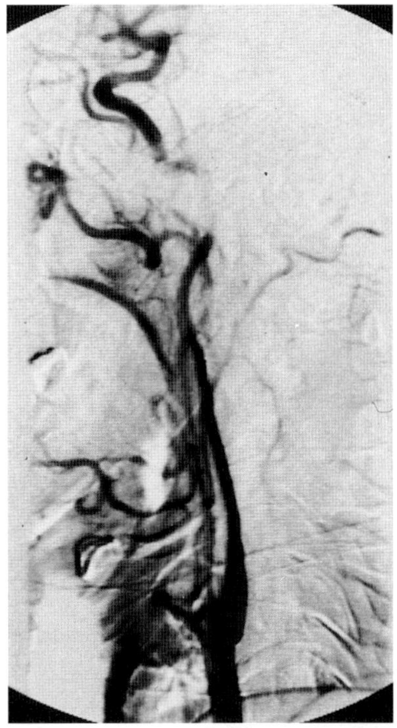

2-58

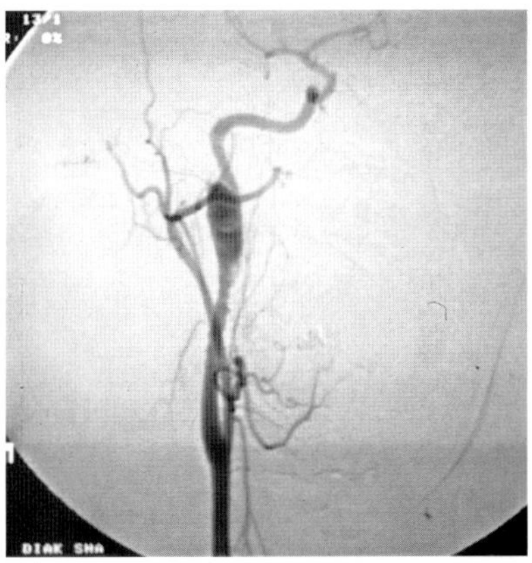

2-59

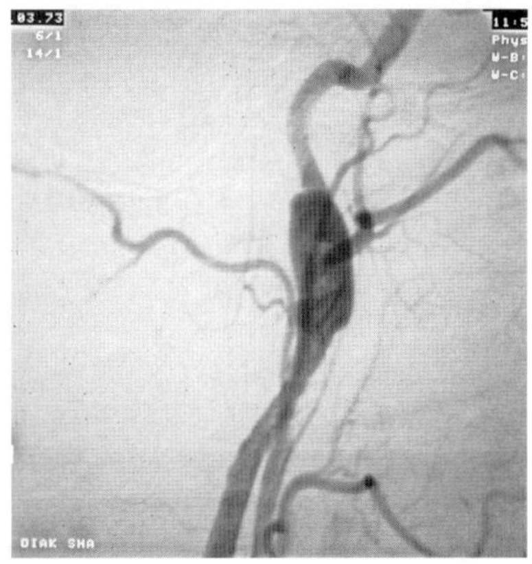

2-60

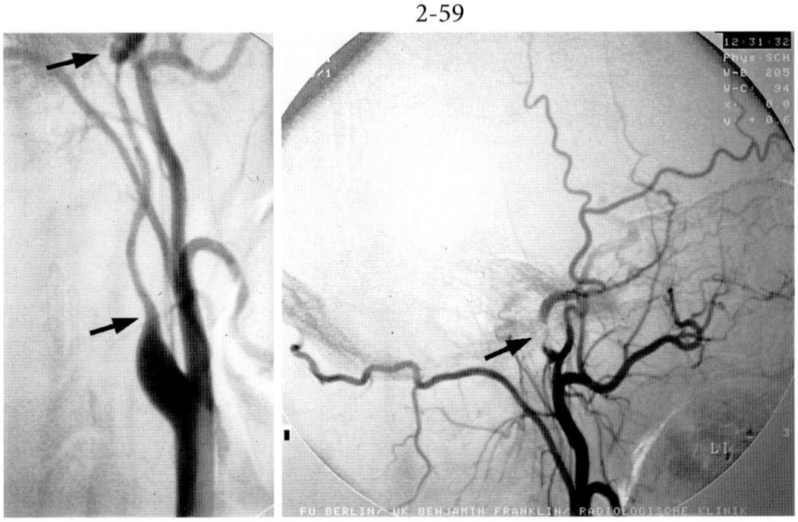

2-61

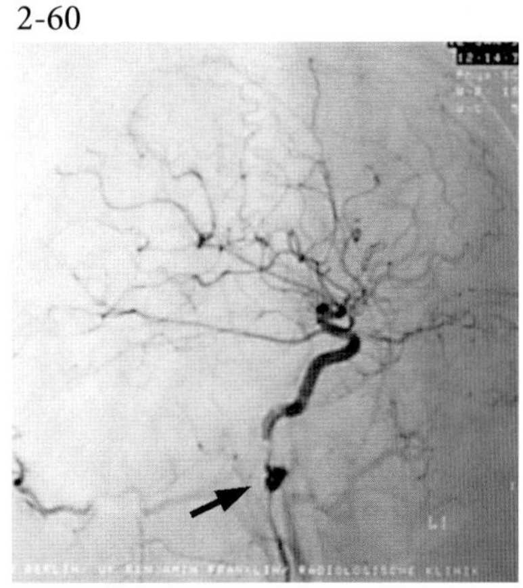

2-62

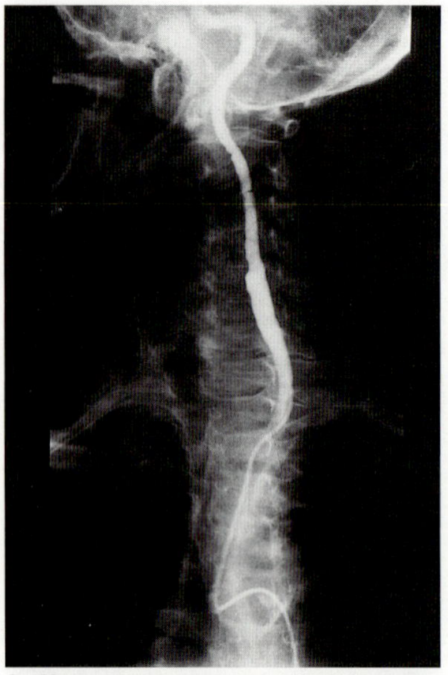

2-63

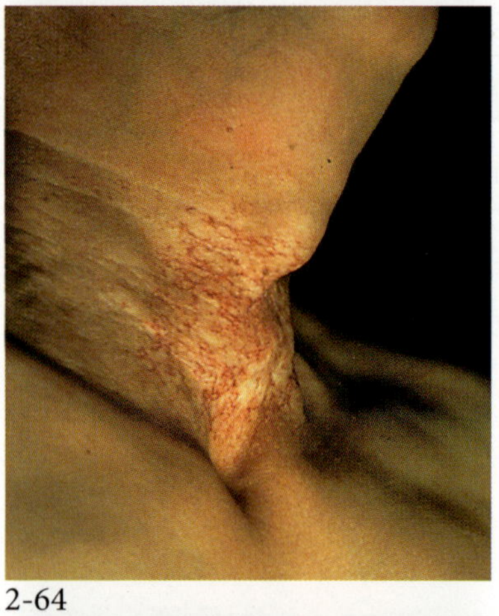

2-64

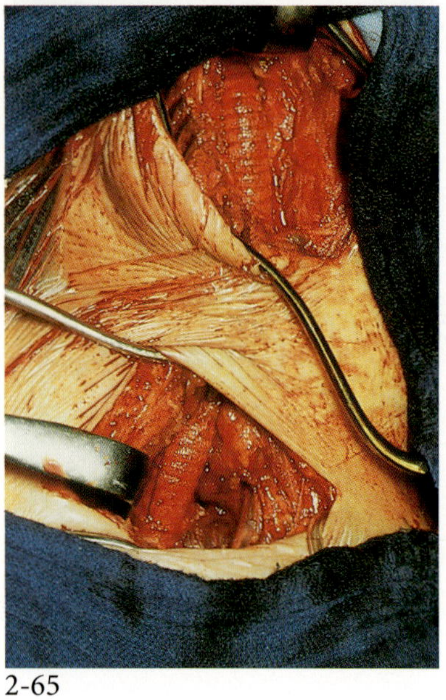

2-65

Figs. 2-63–2-65. The patient had been irradiated for non-Hodgkin lymphoma 15 years earlier. *Top*, signs of radiation damage involving the entire common carotid artery and the internal carotid artery with occlusion of the external carotid artery are seen. The skin shows extensive radiation damage including atrophy and telangiectases. *Bottom*, intraoperative view showing the use of a Dacron graft from the subclavian artery to the internal carotid artery bypassing the damaged tissue

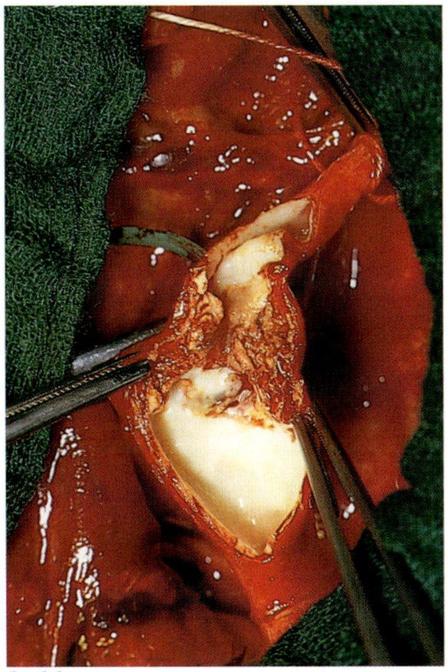

2-66

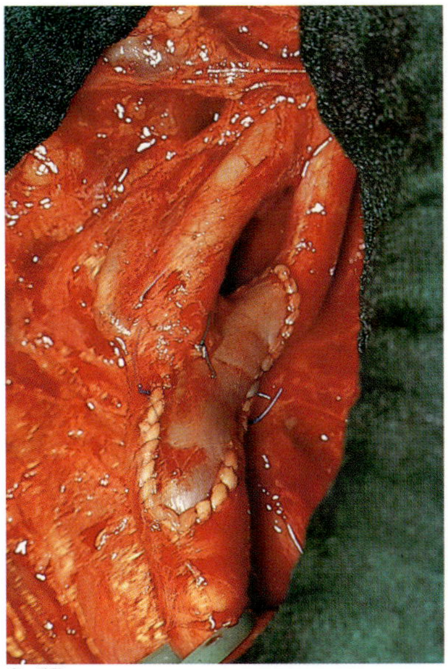

2-67

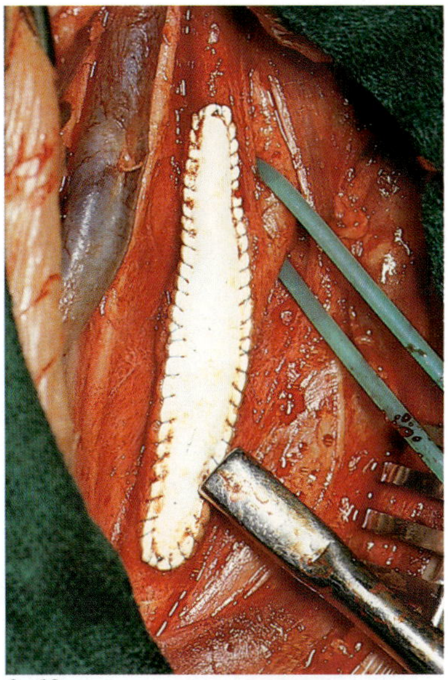

2-68

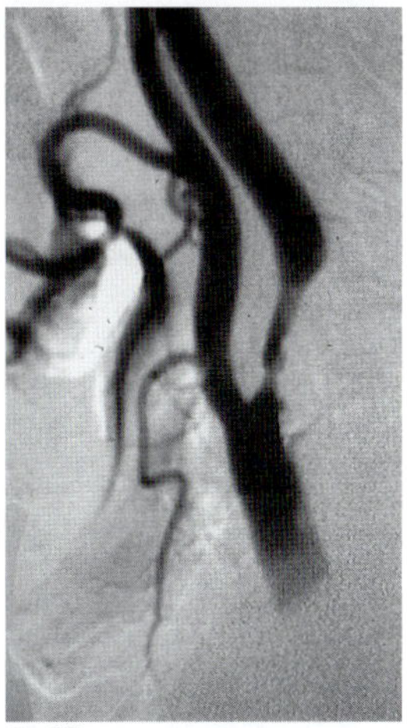

2-69

Fig. 2-66. Intraoperative view of the opened common and internal carotid arteries with a high-grade stenosis at the take-off of the internal carotid artery

Fig. 2-67. Postoperative appearance following thromboendarterectomy and insertion of a vein patch

Fig. 2-68. Similar case but with a synthetic patch. An eversion thromboendarterectomy is performed by diagonally cutting the internal carotid artery away at the bifurcation. The internal carotid artery is then everted over the arteriosclerotic plug at the level of the external elastic membrane. The eversion is carried out in a cranial direction until a normal intima is visua lized. The plug is removed and the internal carotid artery reattached

Fig. 2-69. Preoperative digital subtraction angiography showing high-grade internal carotid artery stenosis

Fig. 2-70. Intraoperative view following eversion thromboendarterectomy and reattachment of the internal carotid artery

Fig. 2-71. Intraoperative angiography showing unimpaired flow in the reimplanted internal carotid artery. No distal changes are seen

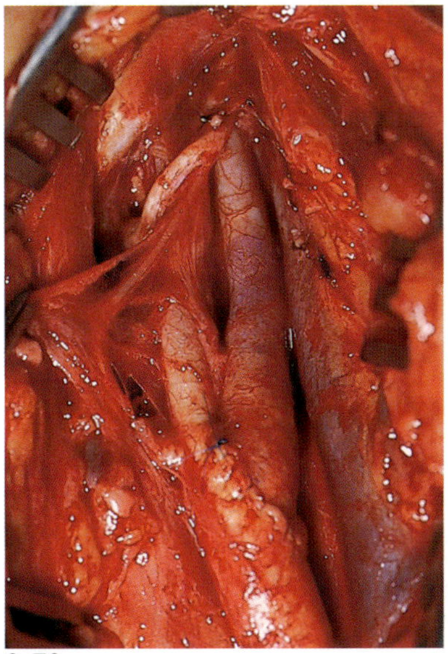

2-70

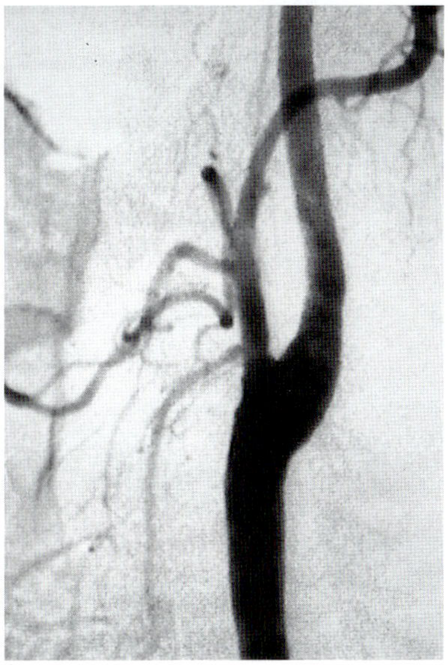

2-71

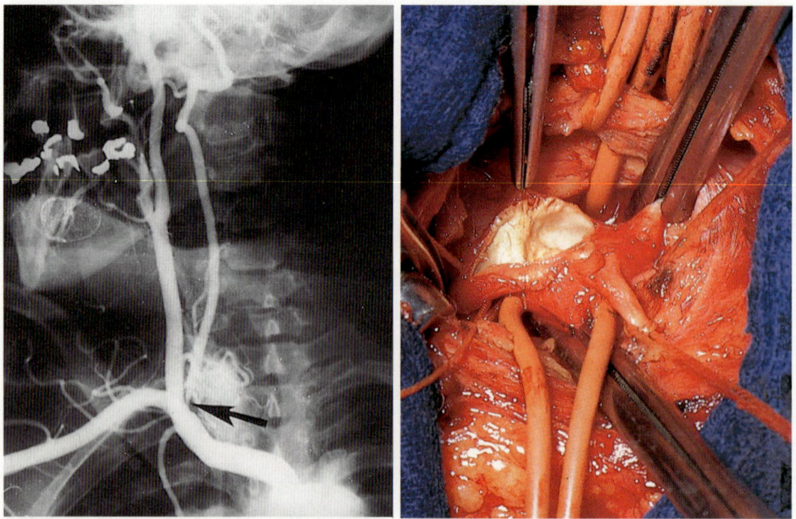

2-72

Fig. 2-72. Angiography showing a high-grade take-off stenosis of the right vertebral artery with occlusion of the left vertebral artery. Intraoperative view demonstrates the stenosis. The standard approach to such cases is the implantation of the vertebral artery into the common carotid artery. In this case, however, we chose to do a vein patch to widen the ostium

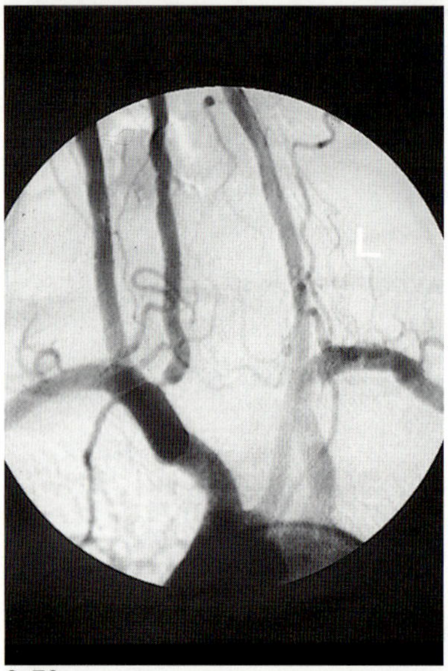

2-73

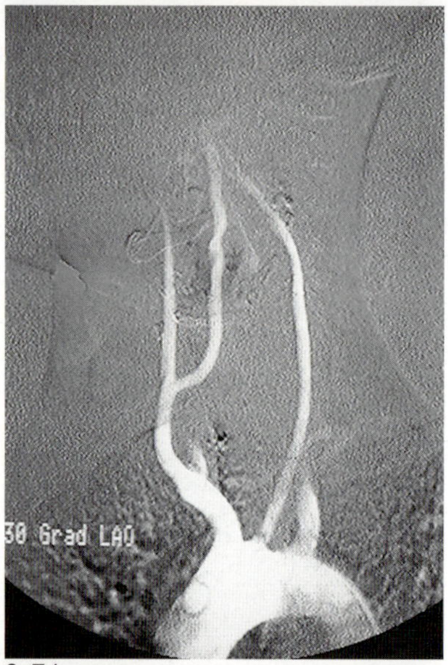

2-74

Fig. 2-73, 2-74. Angiography of the aortic arch in a 60 year old patient with vertebro-basiliar insufficiency. Filiform stenosis of the right vertebral artery with occlusion of the left. On the *right* the postoperative angiogram after successful transposition of the right vertebral artery into the right common carotid artery

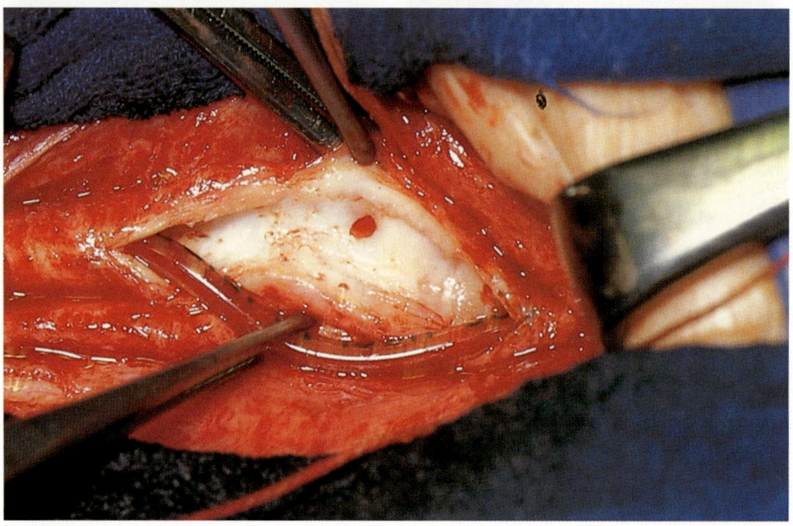

2-75

Fig. 2-75. An early postoperative complication is shown here. Because of neointimal hyperplasia, a stenosis of the internal carotid artery redeveloped soon after thromboendarterectomy

Fig. 2-76. Angiography showing a carotid bifurcation with venous patch. While the angiogram barely shows a thrombus (*arrow*) in the pseudoaneurysm, B-mode ultrasonography reveals it clearly (*arrow*)

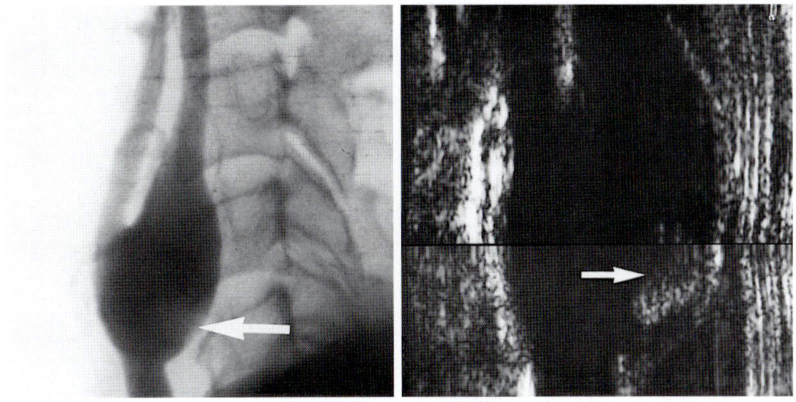

2-76

Fig. 2-77. On the left a recurrent stenosis with post-stenotic dilatation is shown. On the *right* the operative view of the same case is shown

Fig. 2-78. This patient had a carotid thromboendarterectomy a number of years ago. His hypoglossal nerve was injured resulting in paralysis and atrophy of the left half of his tongue, as shown in a picture taken at the time of a repeat operation

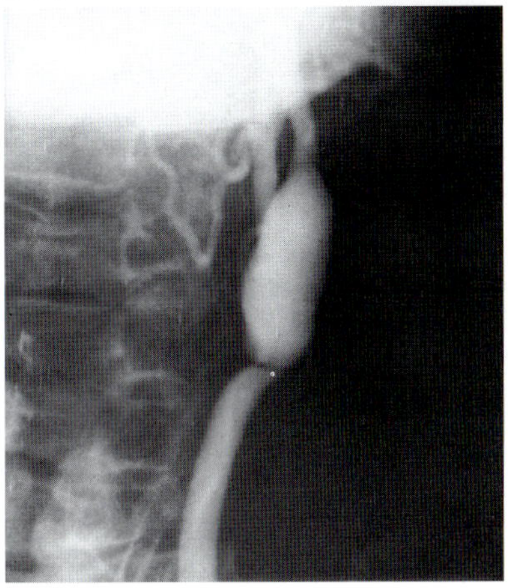

2-77

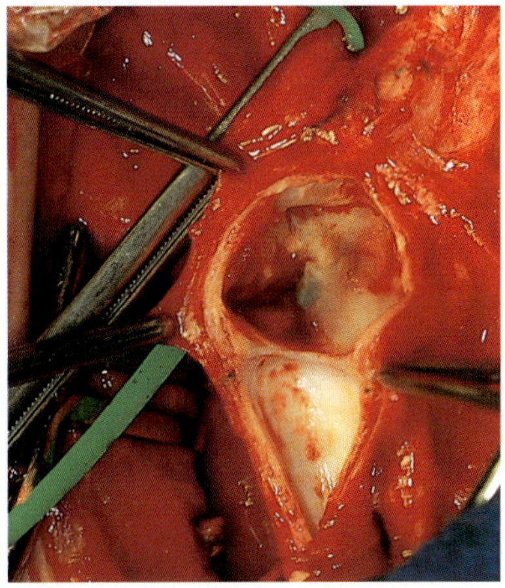

2-78

Fig. 2-79. Carotid body tumor. Angiography of the carotid bifurcation shows a tulip-like proliferation of vascular spaces with retention of the contrast material in the late phase of the procedure

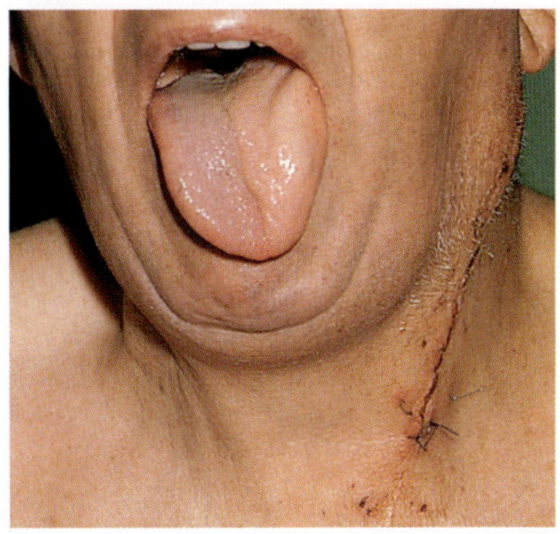

2-79

Fig. 2-80. Operative specimen. The carotid body tumor, also known as paraganglionoma or chemodectoma, is a slowly growing, usually asymptomatic but often pulsatile, tumor just below the angle of the jaw

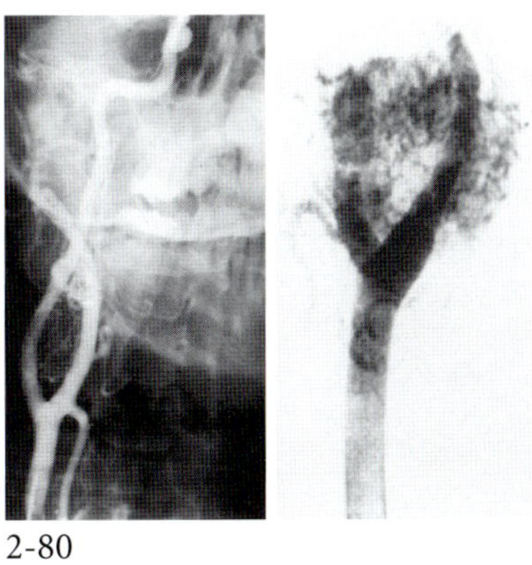

2-80

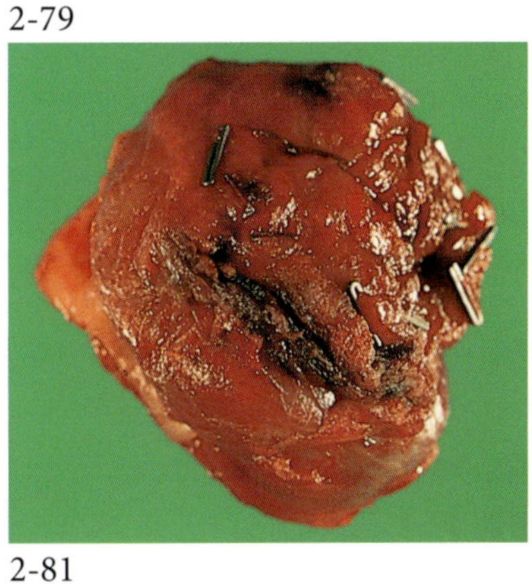

2-81

Chapter 3: Arteries of the Arm

Contents

A: Introduction

The subclavian artery supplies the arm. It arises on the left from the aortic arch and on the right from the brachiocephalic trunk (innominate artery). Both arteries pass in a curve through the thoracic outlet, behind the anterior scalene muscle and between the clavicle and first rib to reach the axilla.

In addition to the various compression syndromes, occlusive changes may also occur in the proximal segment of the subclavian artery. the usual cause is arteriosclerosis; less often inflammatory disease (Takayasu's disease), trauma or a dissection are responsible.

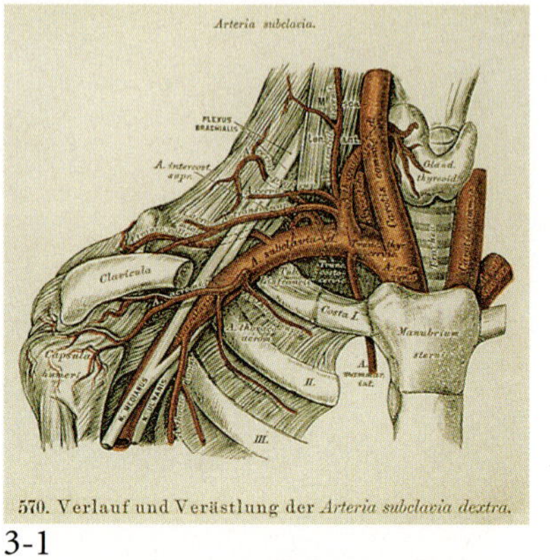

3-1

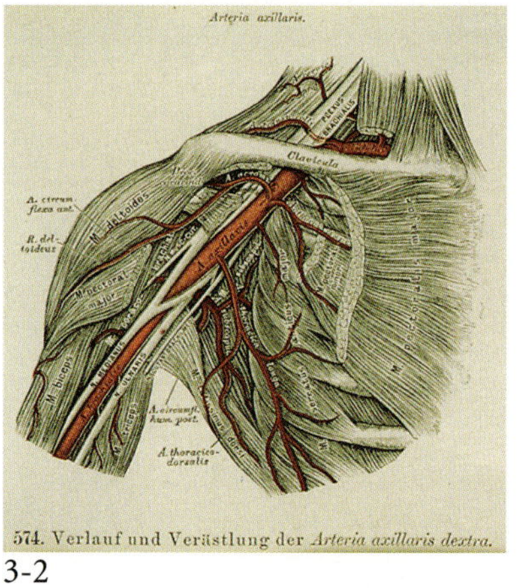

3-2

Figs. 3-1, 3-2. Anatomy of the region of the subclavian artery and the thoracic outlet. (From Descriptive und topographische Anatomie des Menschen, C. Heitzmann, 1893)

1. Neurovascular Shoulder Girdle Compression Syndromes

Synonym. Thoracic outlet syndrome (TOS), thoracic inlet syndrome (TIS)

Definition

Temporary or permanent compression of the subclavian artery, the subclavian vein or their accompanying nerves (the brachial plexus) with arterial and venous circulatory problems as well as neurological changes involving the arm, hand or fingers. TOS includes the cervical rib syndrome, the anterior scalene syndrome and the costoclavicular syndrome. One can also separate neurological changes from arterial obstruction (more limited TOS) and venous obstruction (TIS).

Etiology and Pathogenesis

Compression of the neurovascular bundle supplying the arm can be caused by different inherited or acquired narrowings of the thoracic outlet.

1. Structural abnormalities of the bones and fibrous bands which comprise the rim of the outlet. Examples include the cervical rib syndrome, first rib syndrome, anterior scalene syndrome, costoclavicular syndrome, pectoralis minor syndrome and Klippel-Feil syndrome (congenital vertebral anomalies).
2. Trauma in the shoulder and neck region. Examples include sport and whiplash injuries, as well as improper positioning of the arm during an operation.
3. Improper use or positioning of the arm, often related to repetitive occupational tasks.

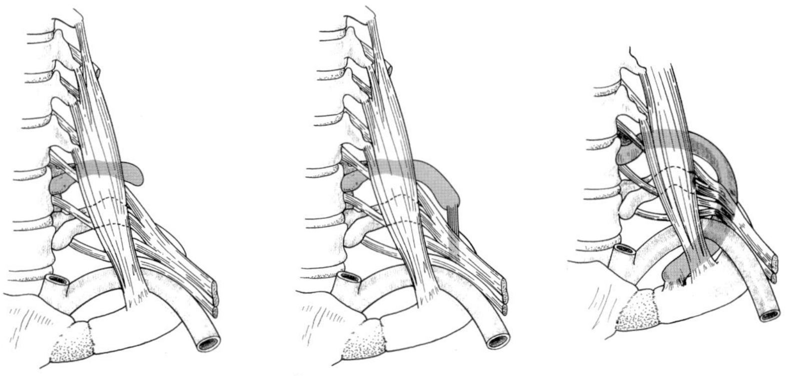

Fig. 3-3 a–c. Types of cervical ribs.
a Grade 1: Small stump
b Grade 2: Longer cervical rib with fibrous connection to first rib.
c Grade 3: Even longer cervical rib attaching directly to first rib

Clinical Features

- Arm tires quickly and hurts with activity, especially when working overhead (claudication of the arm).
- A variety of non-specific findings may be present including headache, neck pain, muscle atrophy, numbness and coolness of fingers and embolic occlusion of digital arteries. If the venous return is compromised, then the forearm and hand tend to be blue, have persistent venous filling and be swollen in the morning.
- Young and middle-aged adults are usually affected. The female: male ratio is 3 : 1.

Table 3-1. Major features of the different types of thoracic outlet syndrome

Neurological	Arterial	Venous
Pain	Usually associated with a cervical rib	Repeated venous stasis
Hypo- and paresthesias	Raynaud's phenomenon may with present with or without arterial occlusion in forearm and fingers	Subclavian or axillary vein thrombosis
Changing motor deficits	Finger tip necrosis	Paget-von Schrötter syndrome
Thenar atrophy	Necrosis of entire finger or even hand	Venous claudication

Diagnosis

Clinical evaluation:

- Inspection and palpation
- Provocative tests: costoclavicular and hyperadduction tests, or elevated arm stress (EAS) test.

Other diagnostic approaches:

- Roentgenologic examination of the thoracic outlet, looking for bony abnormalities
- Electromyography and measurement of nerve conduction rates
- Oscillography with and without exercise and positional changes
- Duplex ultrasonography
- Angiography in a variety of positions

Special clinical provocative tests for assessing TOS include the following tests.

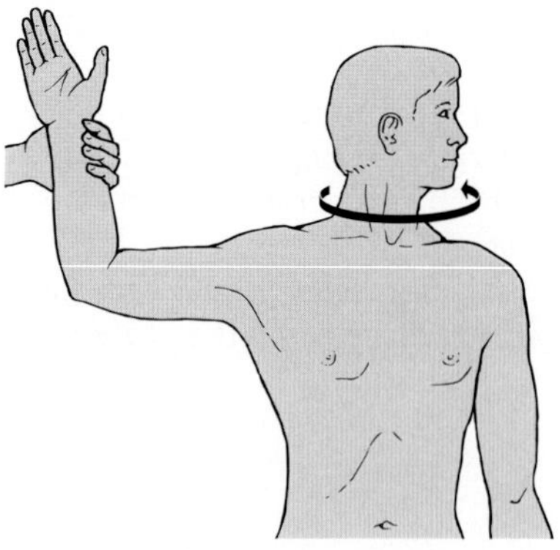

Fig. 3-4. Position of the body and head in Allen test II

Allen Test II (Fig. 3-4)

- The head is turned away and the arm is abducted, raised and supinated. If the radial pulse disappears, this suggests compression (Peter Dudley Allen, American surgeon, 1852–1915).

Adson Test

- When the head is maximally turned to the contralateral side, the anterior scalene muscle is placed under maximum tension and may cause loss of the radial pulse in the arm which is allowed to hang down (Alfred W. Adson, American surgeon, 1887–1951).

Elevated Arm Stress Test (after Roos)

- Both arms are held raised, flexed at the elbows and supinated. The shoulders are pushed dorsally. The patient clinches and relaxes his fists repeatedly for three minutes. This action usually reproduces the pain and makes the affected arm pale or livid blue with marked venous filling. To document this, a pressure cuff and oscilloscope can be employed (Fig 3-5).

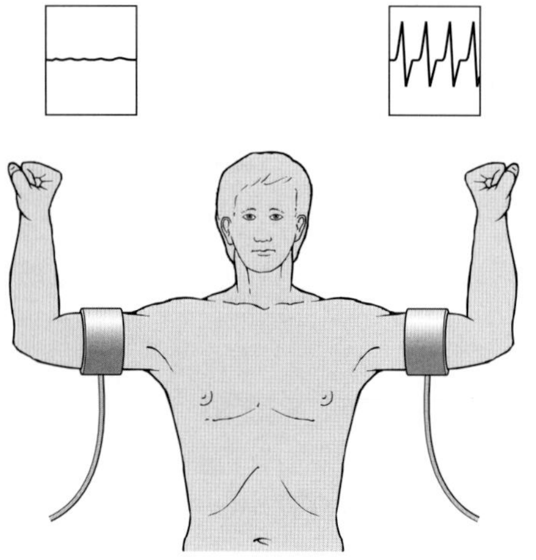

Fig. 3-5. Elevated arm stress test with oscillographic documentation in a patient with right-sided costoclavicular compression syndrome

Therapy

- Conservative
  - This approach is only warranted for mild to moderate cases. Local heat, short-wave or regular diathermy and careful massage may help. If the patient habitually carries their arm in the wrong position, physical therapy may be helpful.
- Surgical
  - For most patients the treatment of choice is resection of the first rib, combined with removal of the cervical rib and any fibrous bands.
  - If symptoms are not severe, conservative therapy should be tried first, unless arterial compression with poststenotic dilatation is present.

2. Subclavian Steal Syndrome

Definition

When the subclavian artery is blocked proximally, blood may flow in a retrograde fashion in the vertebral artery which becomes a collateral vessel for the arm. The subclavian steal syndrome can be congenital (atresia or stenosis of the subclavian artery) or acquired (usually arteriosclerosis). Only about 15% of the patients with an hemodynamically significant subclavian obstruction have clinical symptoms from the steal effect.

Clinical Features

The symptoms are the same as with vertebro-basilar insufficiency. There are cerebral and cerebellar problems because of inadequate blood supply. These symptoms include headache, impaired concentration, dizziness and visual problems. As the affected arm is used more, the cranial symptoms increase. The arm is also easily tired (dyspraxia intermittens, brachial claudication).

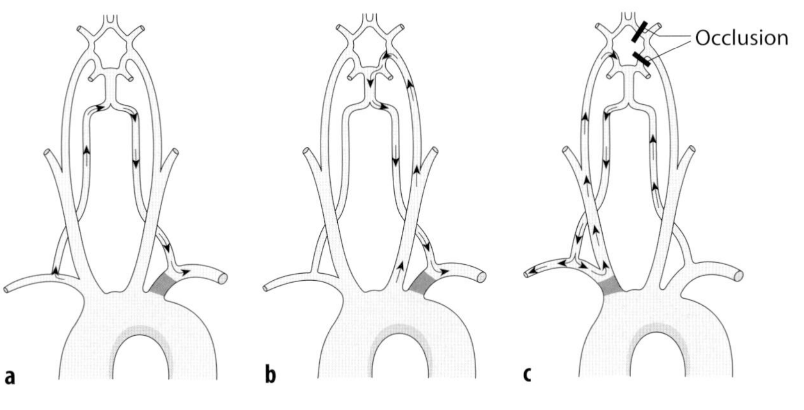

Fig. 3-6 a–c. The main forms of the subclavian steal syndrome are shown in (**a**) and (**b**). In the subclavian steal-carotid recovery syndrome (**c**), the brachiocephalic trunk and the circle of Willis are simultaneously occluded. In such a case the right subclavian artery is served by retrograde flow through the vertebral artery. At the same time, the right common carotid artery is provided with cranially flowing blood

Diagnosis

- Clinical evaluation: Palpation and auscultation of the subclavian artery reveal a supraclavicular bruit and sometimes a thrill. These findings can also be present in the infraclavicular region. Comparison of pulse and blood pressure on both sides; there may be a pressure difference of over 20 mg Hg
- Other diagnostic approaches: Oscillography, plethysmography, duplex ultrasonography, angiography and computerized tomography (spiral CT, CT angiography)

Therapy

In general one should be conservative; only if the symptoms are very disturbing should one attempt to correct the obstruction. Balloon dilatation via a transfemoral or retrograde brachial approach is possible, but stent placement may produce better results. Because the blood flow is cranio-brachial, the risk of cerebral emboli is small. Alternative treatments include a carotid-subclavian bypass operation or the transposition of the mid- or distal subclavian artery into the common carotid artery.

3. Distal Arteries of the Arm and Hand

While proximal subclavian artery occlusion is almost exclusively associated with arteriosclerosis, distal occlusion is usually caused by emboli, inflammation or trauma. Occlusion of individual arteries of the forearm is usually not compensated for by the collateral circulation of the palmar arch.

Clinical Features

Acute occlusion of an artery of the forearm or hand leads to a blue-livid, pale or marbled skin color coupled with pain and paresthesias.

Diagnosis

- Clinical evaluation
- History and inspection
- Palpation of pulses
- Other diagnostic approaches: Oscillography, Doppler- and duplex ultrasonography; if needed, angiography

Therapy

Medical

- Prostaglandin infusions – intra-arterial or intravenous
- Fibrinolytic regimens

Surgical

- Revascularization, often combined with medical measures

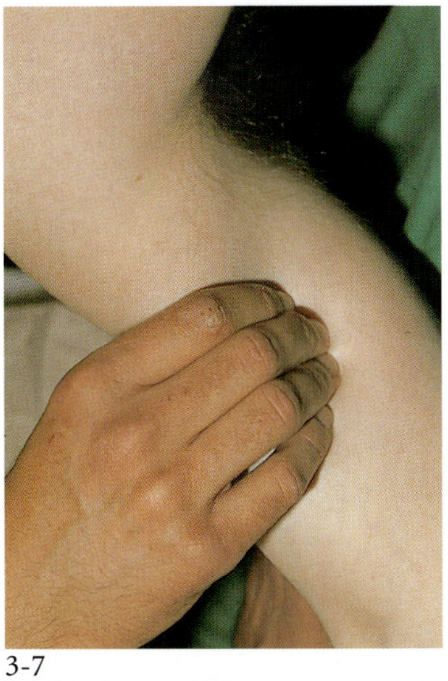

3-7

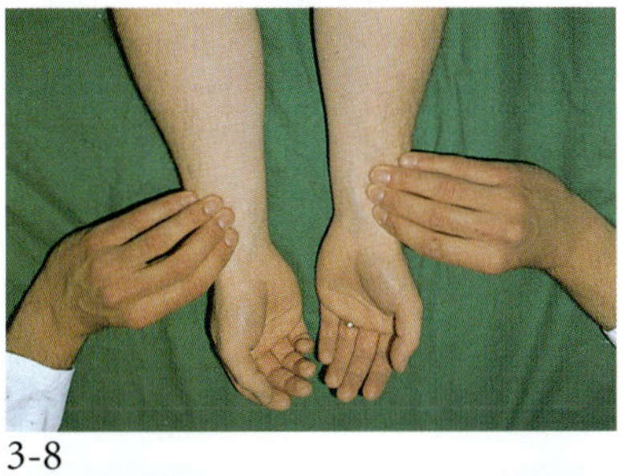

3-8

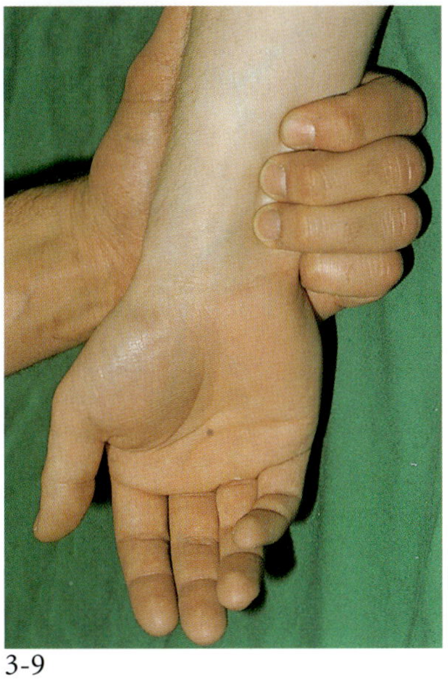

3-9

Fig. 3-7. Palpation of the brachial pulse

Fig. 3-8. Comparing the two radial pulses

Fig. 3-9. Palpation of the ulnar pulse

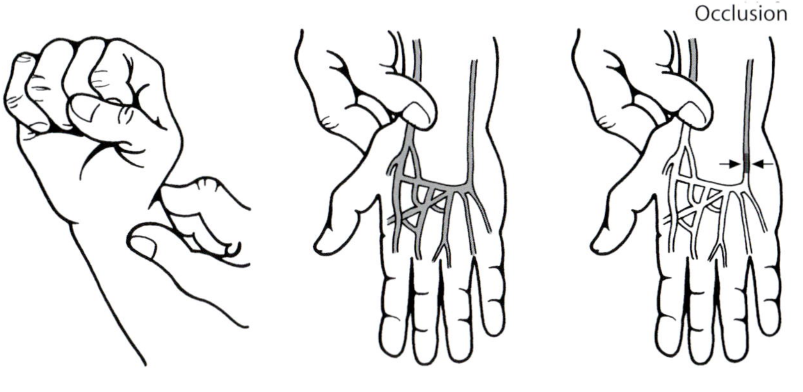

Fig. 3-10. Allen test I (special palmar provocative test). The radial artery is compressed and the patient opens and shuts his fist. If the ulnar artery is occluded, the hand will rapidly become pale and only become red when the compression is released. The same test is then done with the ulnar artery compressed. The two hands are compared. (From E.V. Allen, American internist)

B: Supplementary Figures and Legends

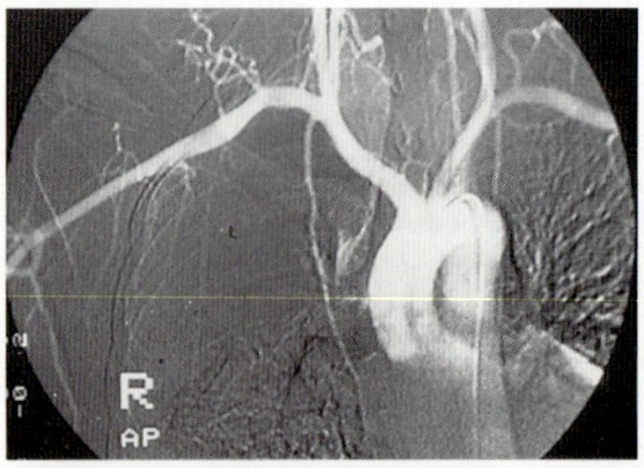

3-11

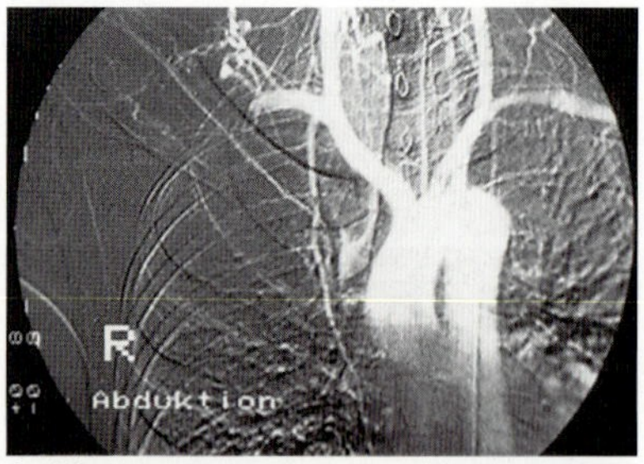

3-12

Figs. 3-11, 3-12. Angiography demonstrating a classic costoclavicular compression syndrome. When the right arm is elevated and abducted, there is obvious compression of the artery and abrupt stoppage of the contrast material where the clavicle and first rib meet

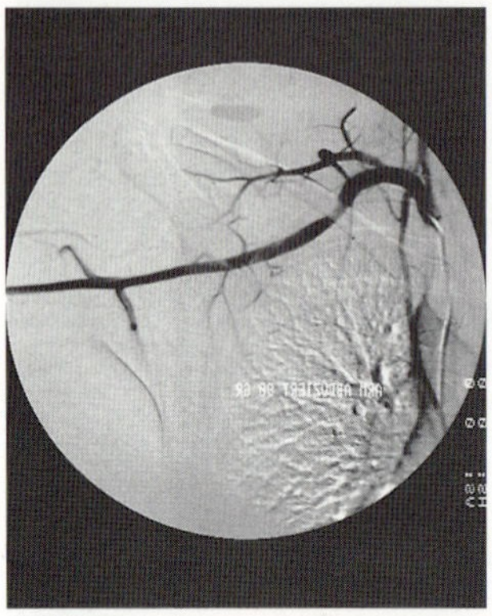
3-13

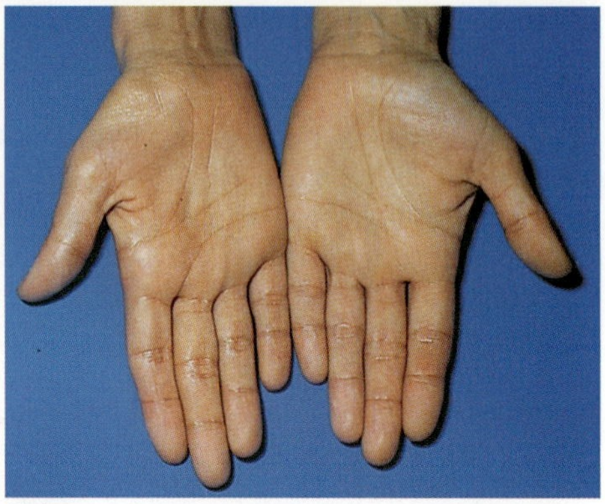
3-14

Figs. 3-13, 3-14. Another example of costoclavicular compression syndrome with angiographic evidence of the compression. In this patient, however, neural compression played a more important role. The atrophy of the right thenar eminence (ball of the thumb) is apparent. Even after resection of the first rib and restoration of the arterial flow, there was permanent nerve damage

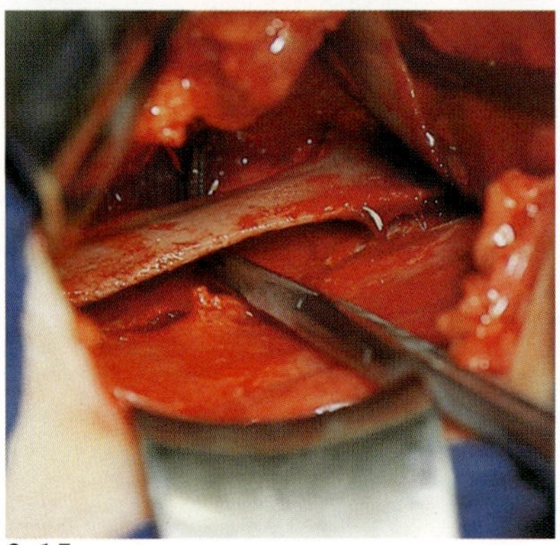
3-15

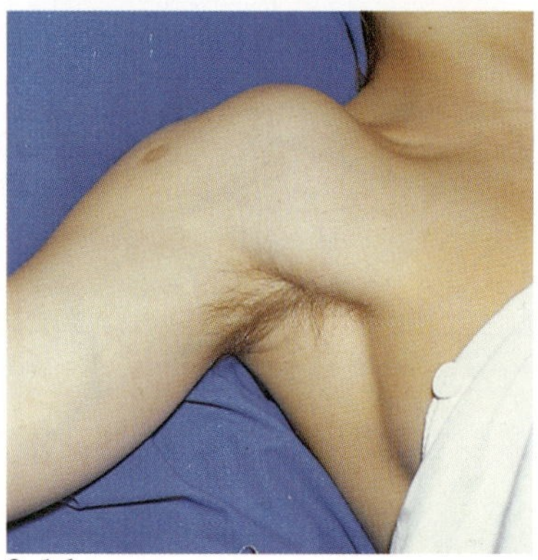
3-16

Figs. 3-15, 3-16. Operative view showing resection of the first rib in a patient with costoclavicular compression syndrome. On the *right*, the trans-axillary scar is difficult to see after 1 year

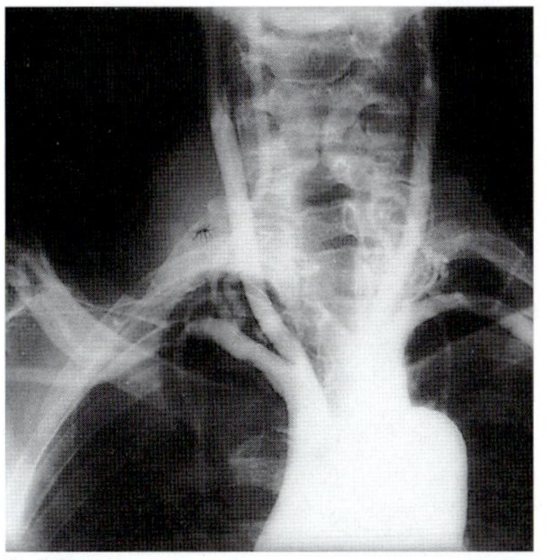

3-17

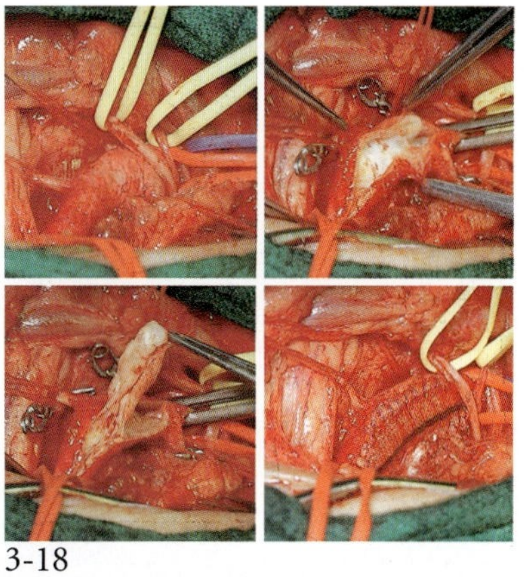

3-18

Figs. 3-17, 3-18. Subtotal subclavian stenosis because of compression by a cervical rib. The compression led to arteriosclerotic plaque formation. On the *right* a series of operative photographs show the artery (*red*), vein (*blue*) and nerve (*yellow*). After the artery was opened a thromboendarterectomy was performed and the defect closed with a patch

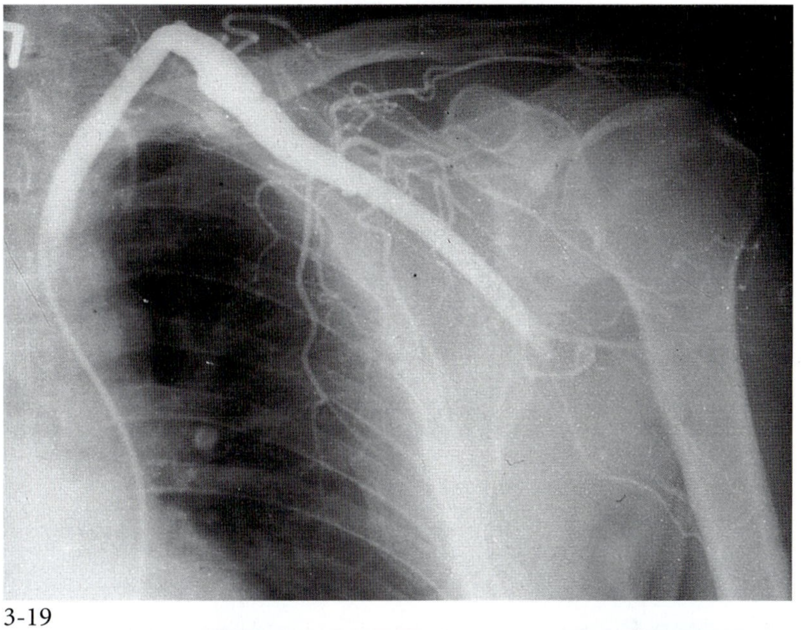

3-19

Fig. 3-19. Angiogram showing a grade III cervical rib extending quite far ventrally. The subclavian artery has been displaced cranially and clearly passes over the cervical rib. A post-stenotic dilation is present and can serve as a site for peripheral emboli. In addition an embolic occlusion of the axillary artery is shown

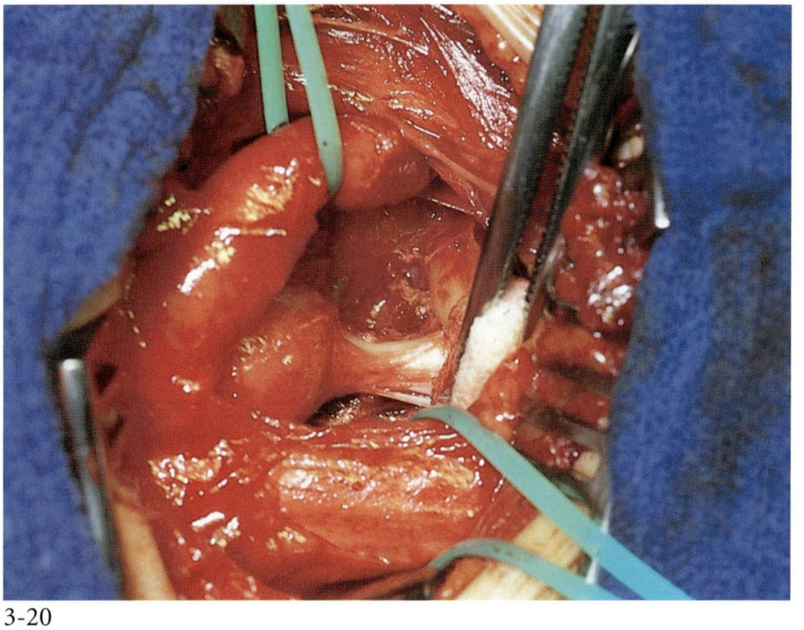

3-20

Fig. 3-20. The operative view of the same patient shows a supraclavicular approach to the subclavian artery (*green loops*) as it passes over the cervical rib to which it also has a fibrous band-like attachment

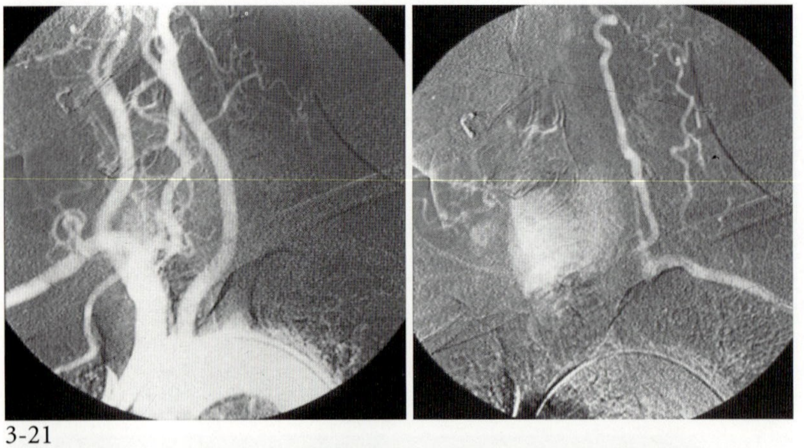

3-21

Fig. 3-21. Subclavian artery occlusion with subclavian steal syndrome. Two-phase angiographic demonstration of the left subclavian artery showing retrograde flow from the left vertebral artery into the subclavian artery

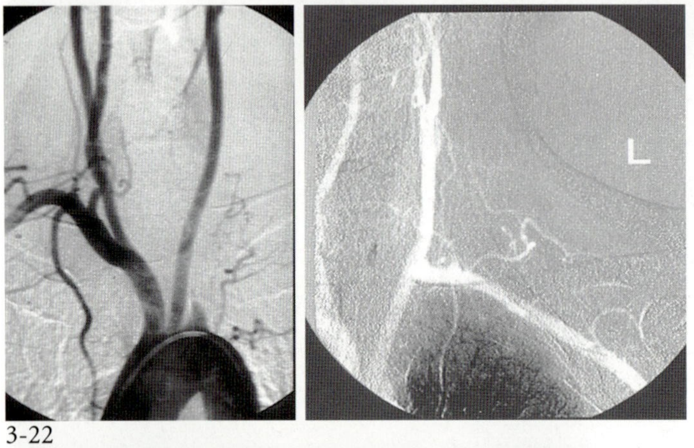

3-22

Fig. 3-22. Pre- and post-operative angiograms showing the transposition of the subclavian artery into the common carotid artery

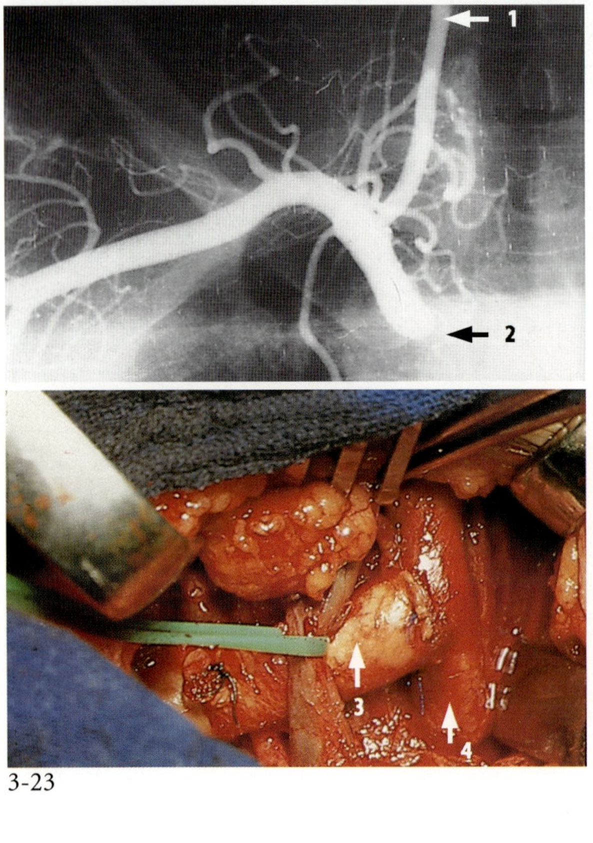

3-23

Fig. 3-23. Arteriosclerotic occlusion of the proximal part of the right subclavian artery with clinical features of the subclavian steal syndrome. *1*, vertebral artery; *2*, occlusion of the subclavian artery. The operative picture shows the transposition of the subclavian artery into the right common carotid artery. The *green loops* hold the internal jugular vein to the side; *3*, subclavian artery; *4*, common carotid artery

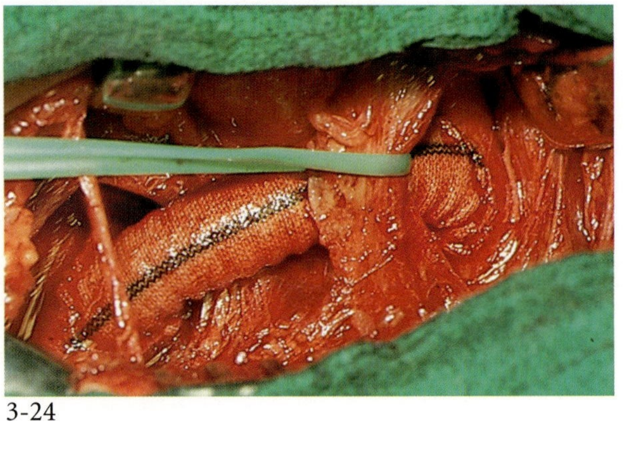

3-24

Fig. 3-24. The angiogram shows a typical occlusion of the right subclavian artery. In the operative view, a Dacron bypass connects the subclavian and common carotid arteries; this procedure is less frequently employed today

Fig. 3-25. Eight days after the acute blockage of the subclavian artery by a paraneoplastic thrombosis (metastatic gynecological tumor). A subclavian-common carotid artery bypass was performed and the vascular damage to the digits allowed to declare itself. A partial amputation of all fingers, but not the thumb, was required because of the necrosis and gangrene

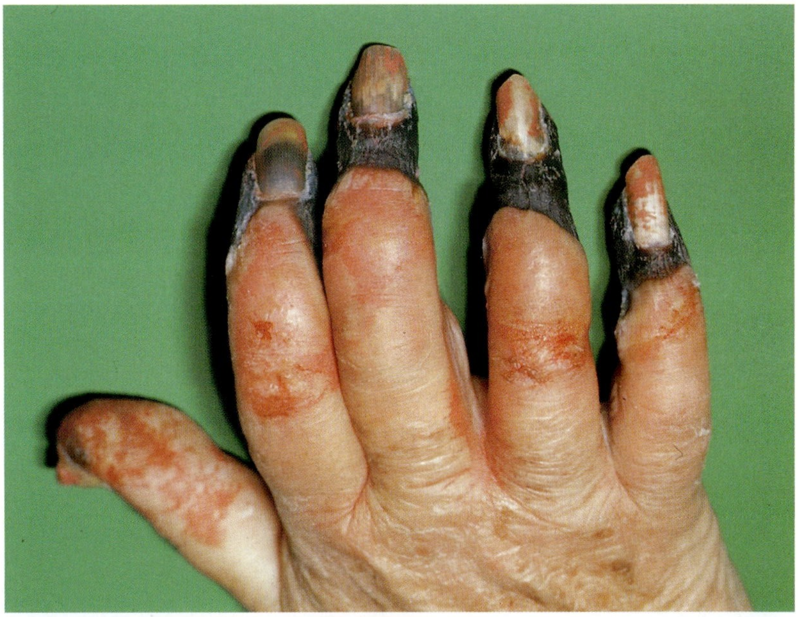

3-25

Fig. 3-26. Digital artery blockage (*arrow*) of the index finger via an embolus from a known subclavian stenosis

Fig. 3-27. Total occlusion of the subclavian artery because of a thrombus associated with arteriosclerotic plaque (*arrow*)

Fig. 3-28. Following urokinase thrombolysis, the responsible stenosis can be seen

Fig. 3-29. Following percutaneous dilatation, the residual stenosis is about 40%

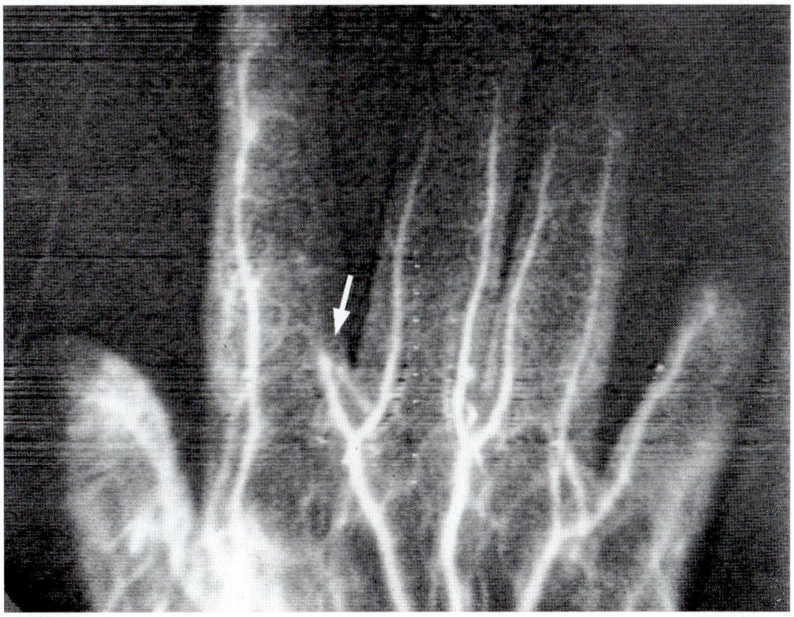

3-26

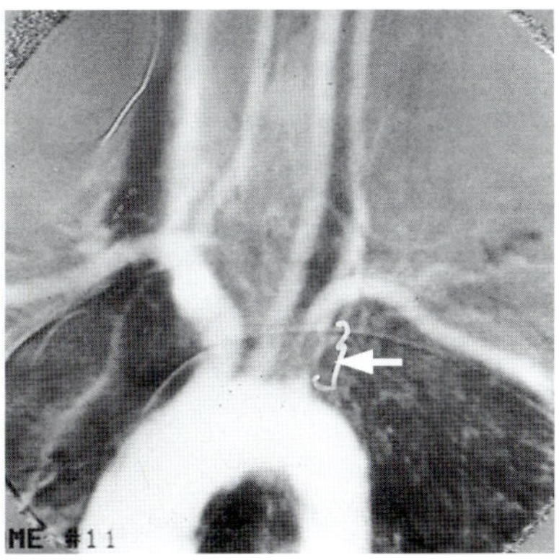

3-27

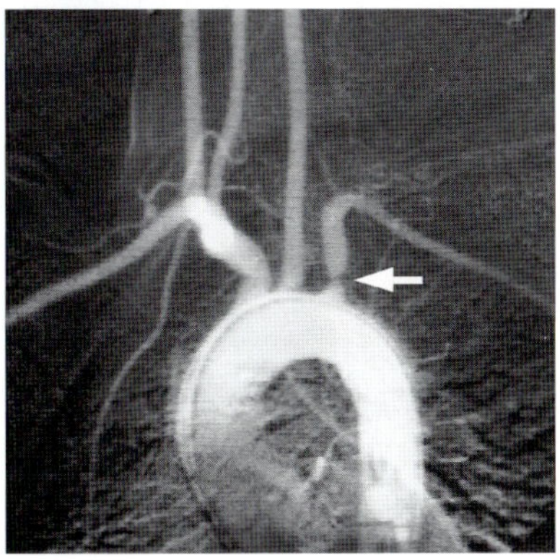

3-28

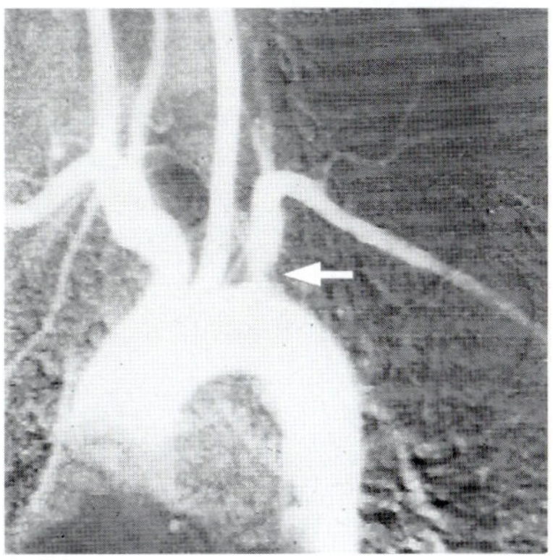

3-29

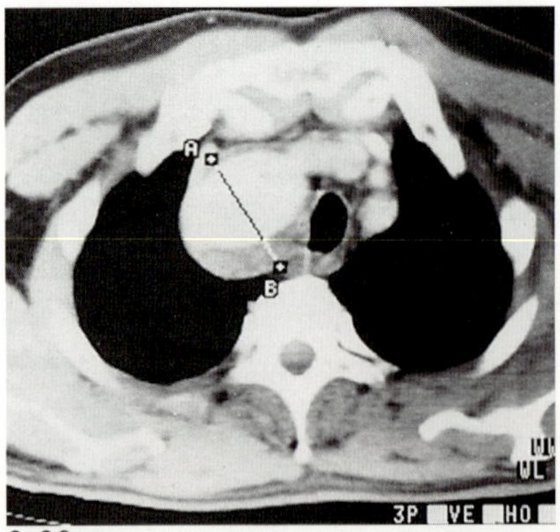

3-30

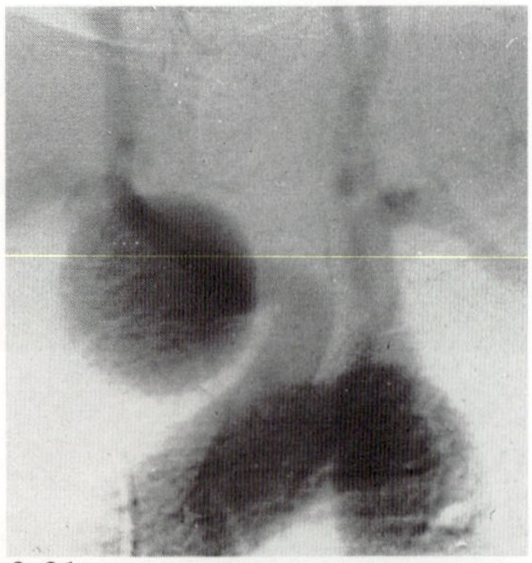

3-31

Figs. 3-30, 3-31. The computerized tomography shows a dramatic aneurysm of the subclavian artery. The lumen is made white by the contrast material while the thrombus is seen as a gray rim. The angiographic view shows the ball-shaped aneurysm of the proximal subclavian artery

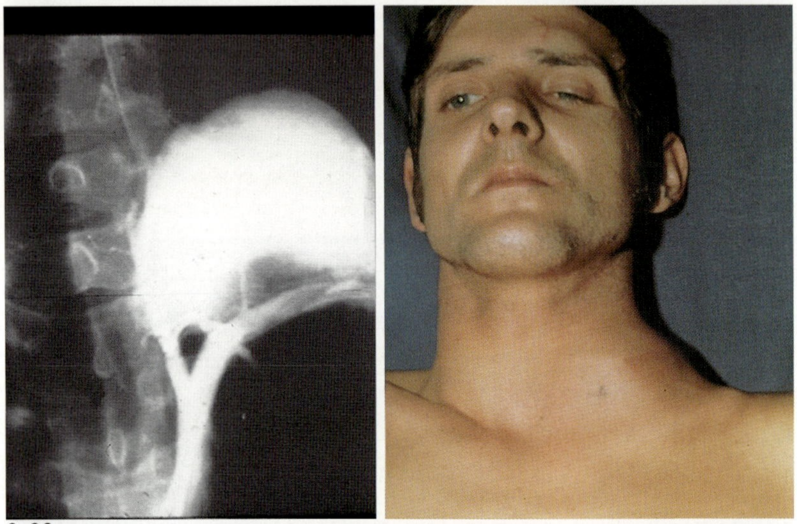

3-32

Fig. 3-32. The patient has a pulsating tumor in the left supraclavicular space. The dropping of the left upper lid indicated the presence of Horner syndrome as a result of compression of the stellate ganglion. The angiogram shows the filling of a left subclavian artery aneurysm about 1 cm distal to the take-off of the left vertebral artery. The lesion was a mycotic aneurysm

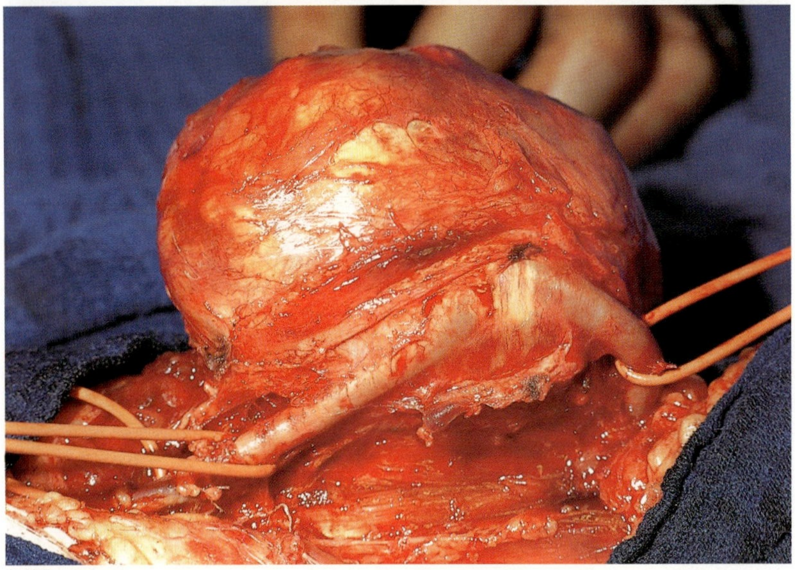

3-33

Fig. 3-33. Operative view of a saccular aneurysm of the brachial artery. There was no history of trauma and the etiology of this unusual aneurysm remained unknown

Fig. 3-34. Spontaneous or traumatic aneurysm of the radial artery in the proximal third of the forearm

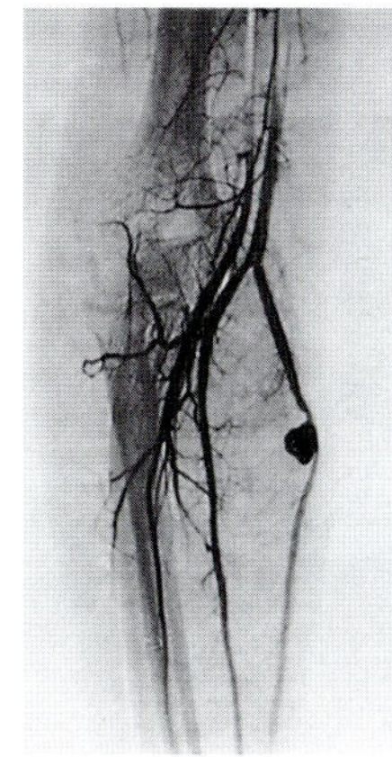

3-34

Figs. 3-35, 3-36. Brachial artery angiography showing an aneurysm of the carpal artery, shown in two planes and during the operation

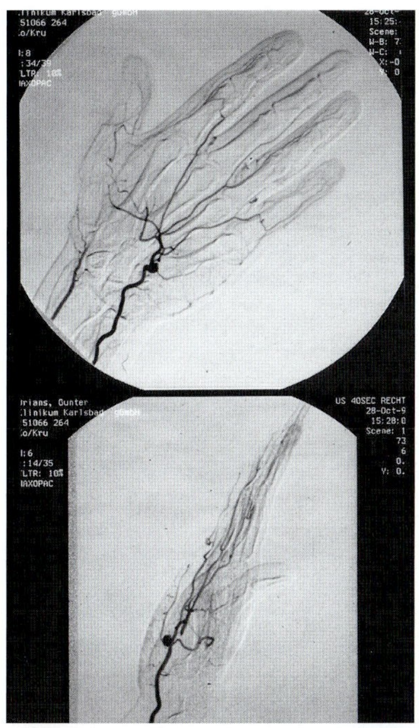

3-35

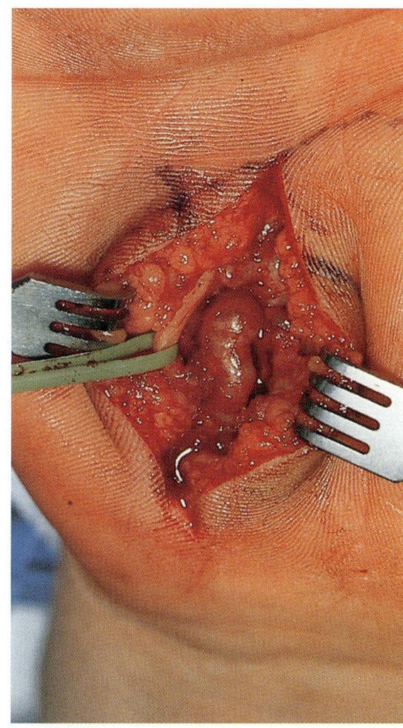

3-36

Fig. 3-37. Infected false aneurysm of the radial artery after arterial puncture to measure luminal pressure. If the palmar arch is sufficient, then the surgical approach is ligation of the radial artery above and below the aneurysm which is resected. If the collateral circulation is inadequate, then the aneurysm must be resected and the artery mobilized for an end-to-end anastomosis or interposition vein graft

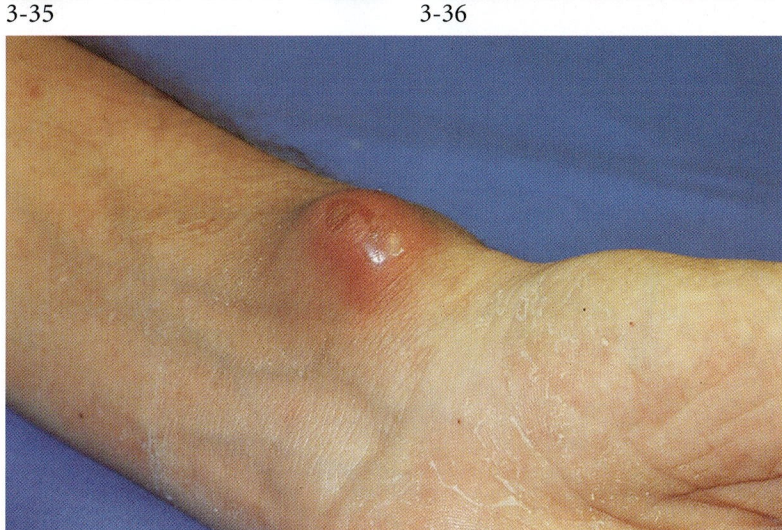

3-37

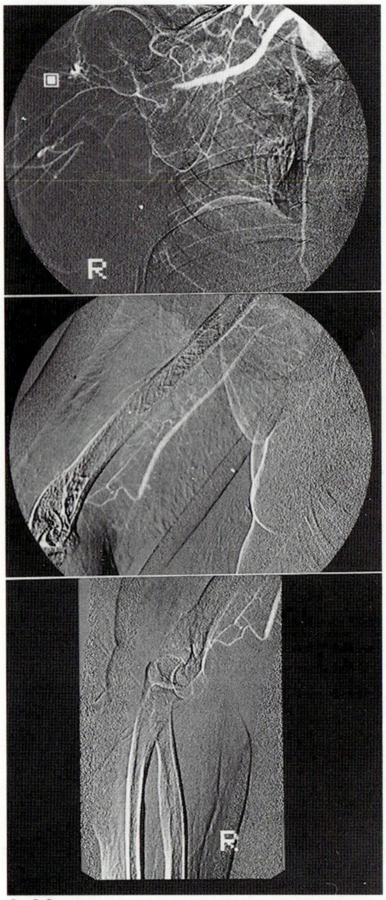

3-38

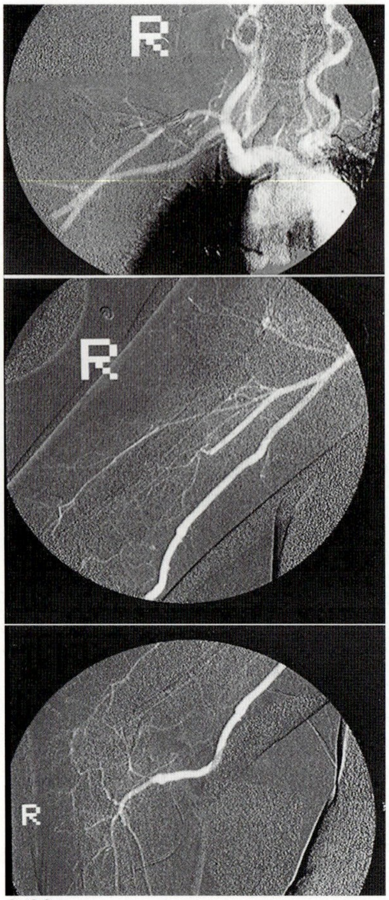

3-39

Fig. 3-38. Occlusion of the axillary artery. This 60 year old patient had radiation for carcinoma of the breast and developed a radiation-induced angiopathy, leading to acute ischemia of her hand. The series of angiographic pictures show the occlusion and absent refilling

Fig. 3-39. Follow-up angiography in the same patient after an axillo-to-brachial bypass with the antecubital vein

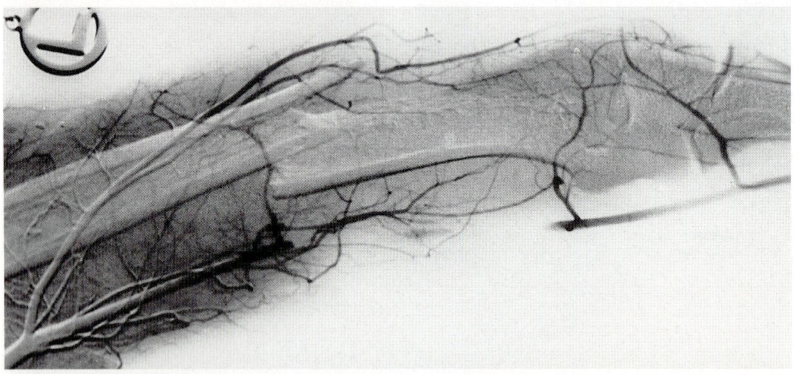

3-40

Fig. 3-40. Arterial occlusion associated with a fractured humerus. The angiogram shows the abrupt closure of the brachial artery at the level of the dislocated fracture. The closure can be the result of a stretch injury with unrolling of the intima and an associated thrombus, or it can represent a tear of the artery. Occasionally a false aneurysm follows such an injury. The fracture must be stabilized first and then the artery repaired

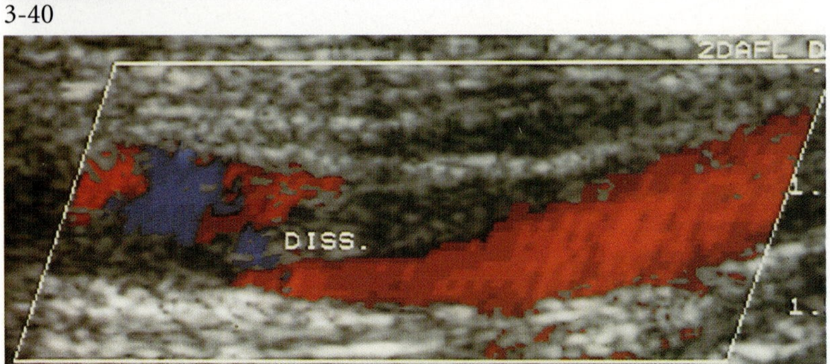

3-41

Fig. 3-41. Color duplex ultrasonography showing a dissection of the brachial artery following an injury to the arm

Fig. 3-42. Necrotic hand in a patient who over-indulged in alcohol and suffered compression of the arterial supply coupled with cold exposure

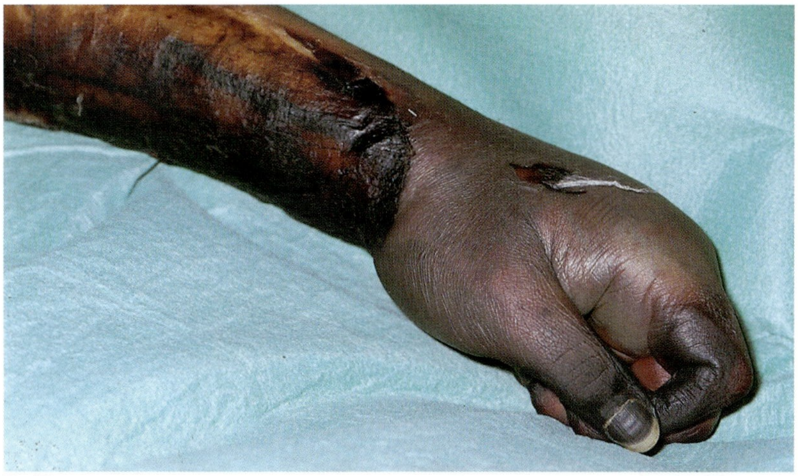

3-42

Figs. 3-43–3-46. Intra-arterial injection of promethazine in a 62 year old patient with asthma. The angiographic picture on the left shows fresh occlusion of the radial artery, as well as the 1st, 2nd and 3rd digital arteries and the deep palmar arch. The second angiogram shows the situation after thrombolysis with urokinase with a residual stenosis of the radial artery. The first clinical picture shows swelling and cyanosis just after the injection; the next shows demarcation of the necrotic areas and the third, the situation after debridement of the index finger

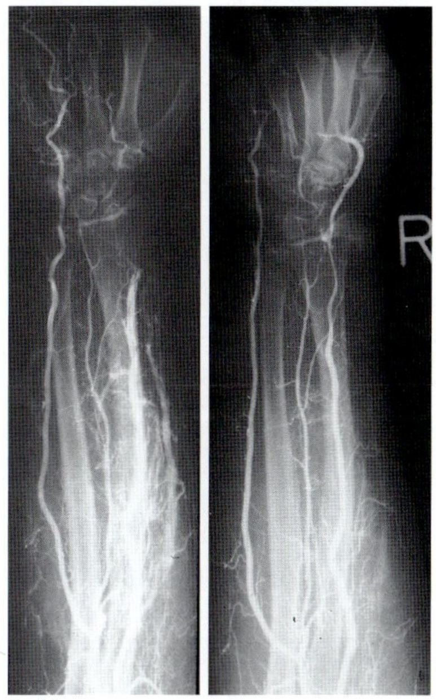

3-43

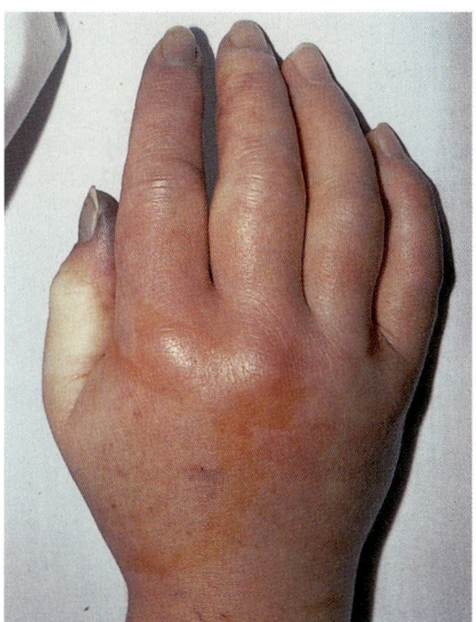

3-44

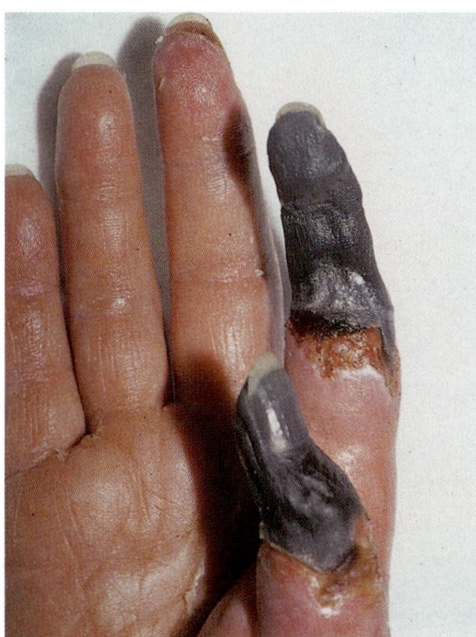

3-45

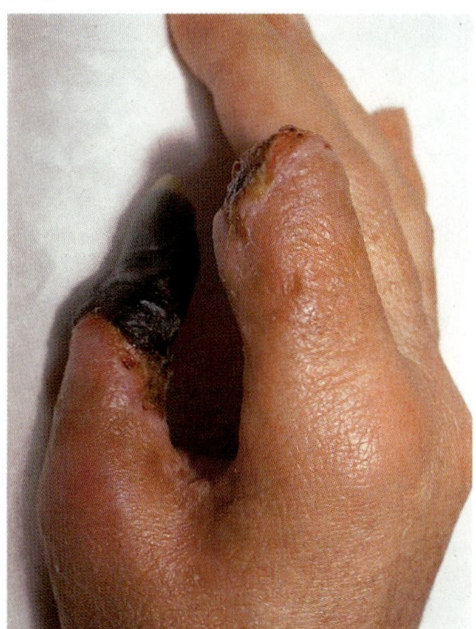

3-46

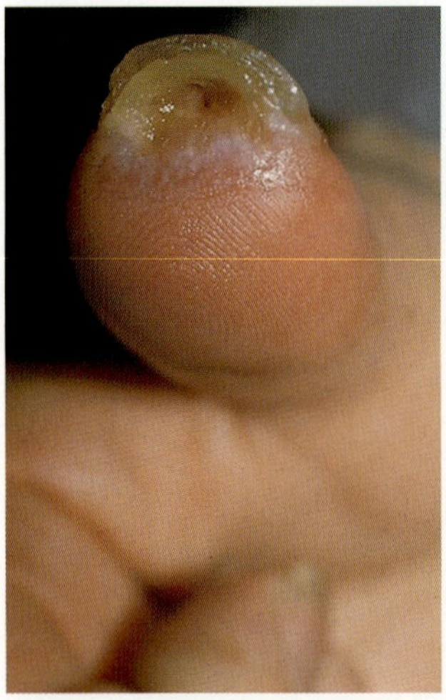

3-47

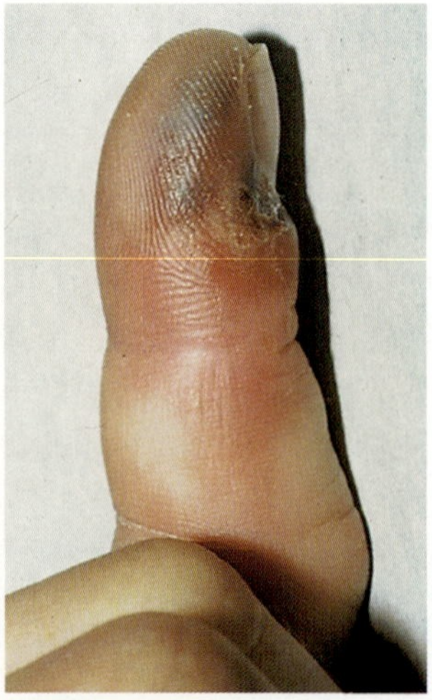

3-48

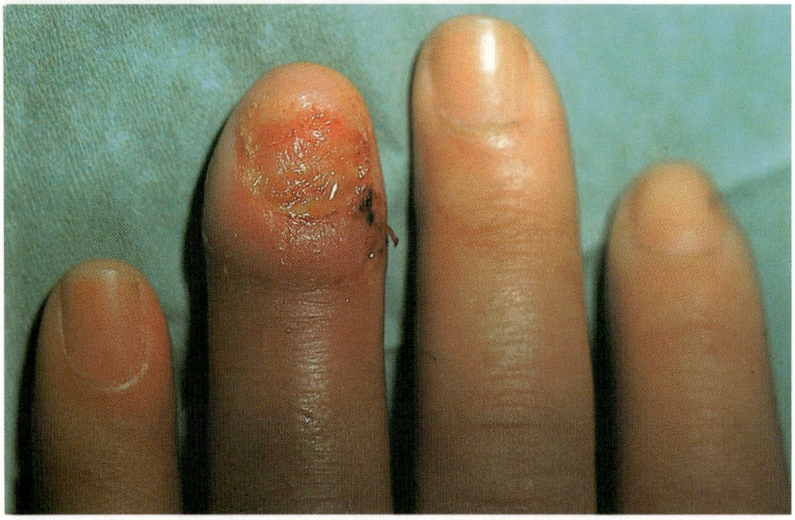

3-49

Figs. 3-47 – 3-49. Multiple views of the fingers in Buerger's disease showing painful digital tip ulcerations and subungual necrosis

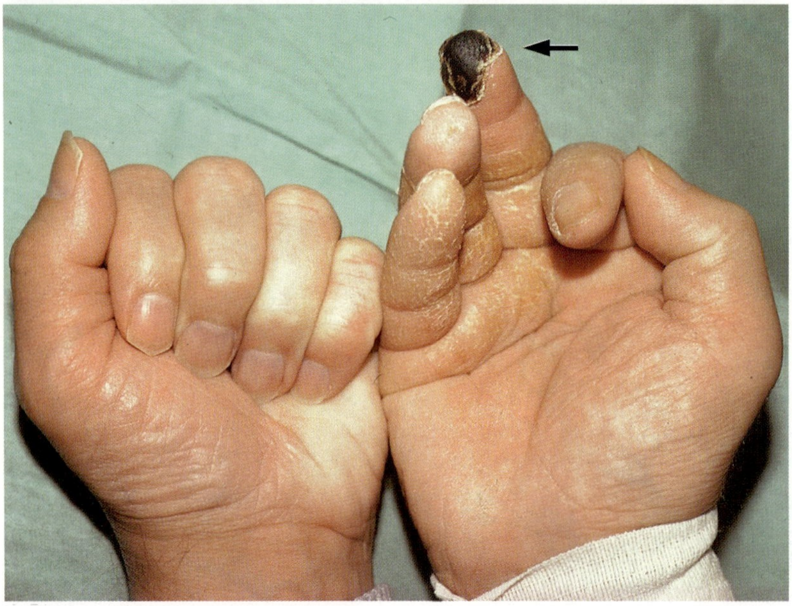

3-50

Case for Discussion

History: A 42 year old patient with asthma since age 4 years was treated with systemic corticosteroids in varying dosages for at least 8 years. A minor injury to the right hand led to the finger pad necrosis of the right middle finger.

Fig. 3-50. Clinical findings: appearance of the hands with a necrotic middle finger. Differential diagnostic possibilities:

1. Diabetic arteriopathy (corticosteroid-induced?)
2. Nicotine-induced angiitis (thromboangiitis obliterans?)
3. Corticosteroid-induced vasculitis
4. Collagen disease
5. Arteriosclerosis secondary to known hyperlipoproteinemia
6. Arteriosclerosis secondary to hypertension
7. Hyperparathyroidism/hyperkalemia
8. Trauma
9. Emboli
10. Paraneoplastic syndrome
11. Hematological disorder
12. Iatrogenic disease

Figs. 3-51, 3-52. Angiographic findings: The right arm shows marked arteriosclerotic changes in the proximal radial and ulnar arteries with complete occlusion of both vessels. Both palmar arches were blocked as were several digital arteries

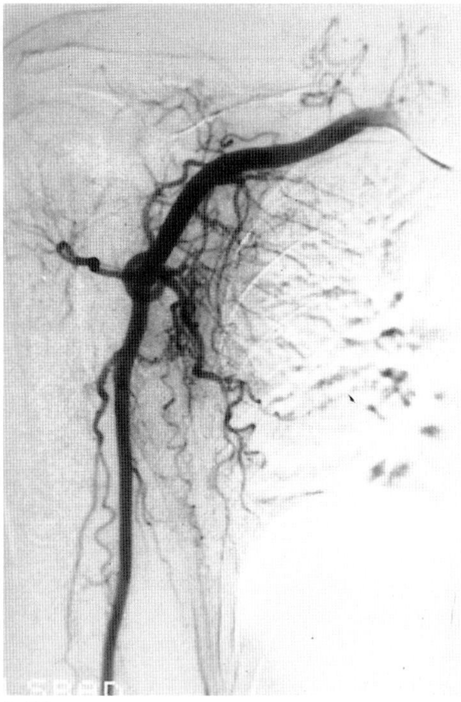

3-51

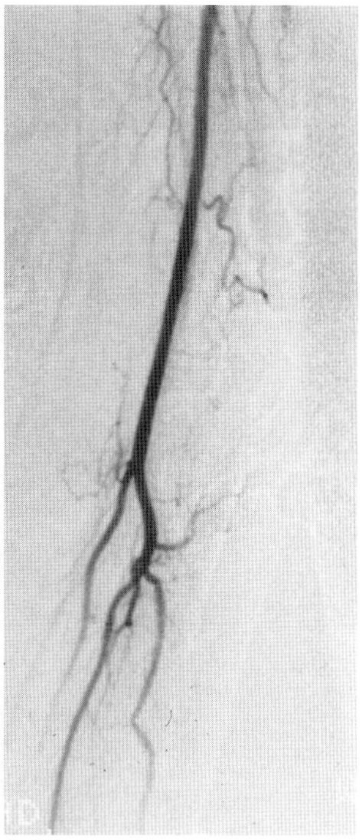

3-52

Fig. 3-53. Photo plethysmography of the finger circulation shows a null line for the right middle finger

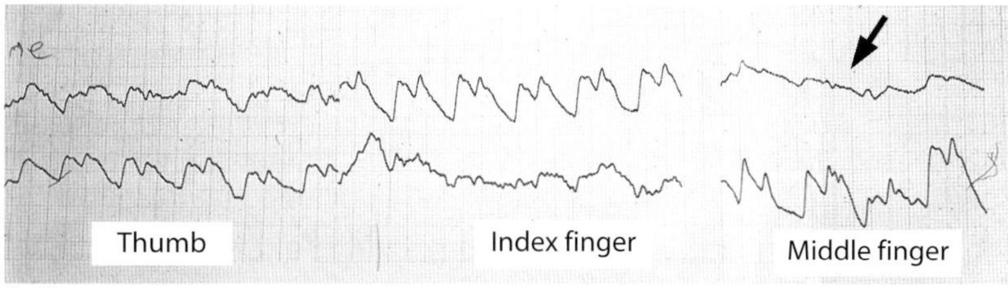

3-53

Fig. 3-54. X-ray examination shows massive calcification of the interdigital and digital arteries, confirming the diagnosis of medial calcinosis (medial sclerosis)

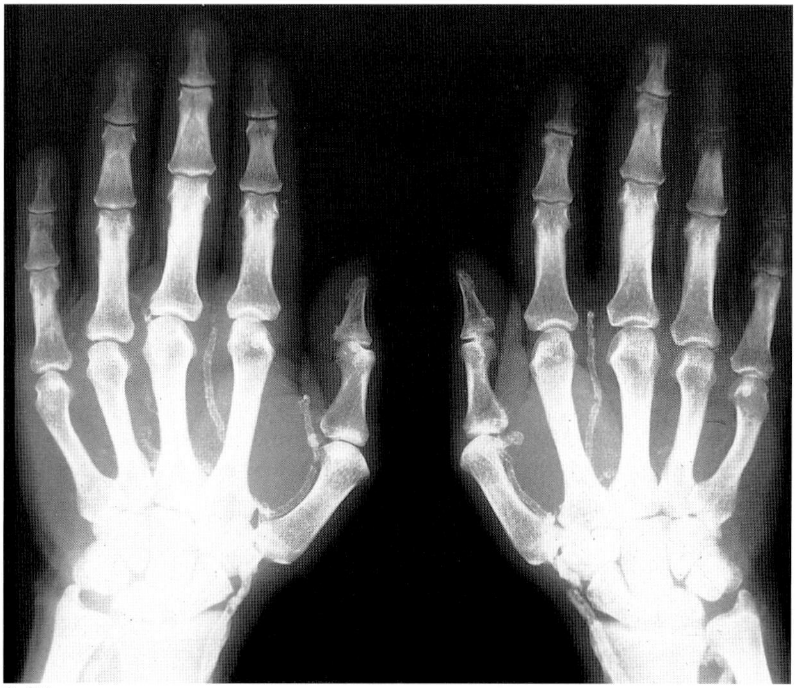

3-54

Chapter 4: Thoracic and Abdominal Aorta

Contents

A: Introduction

1. Arteriosclerotic Occlusion and Aneurysms

A. Arteriosclerotic Occlusion of the Distal Aorta

Epidemiology

Arteriosclerotic occlusions of the aorta account for 8%–28% of all arterial occlusions.

Morphology

The aorta is most often affected in its abdominal portion. Three types of occlusion can occur:

- Type I (segmental): Occlusion is limited to a small segment of the aorta or iliac arteries (37%).
- Type II (bifurcation or Leriche's syndrome): Occlusion occurs at the bifurcation (55%).
- Type III (high or juxtarenal): Blockage extends proximally to the ostia of the renal arteries (8%–12%).

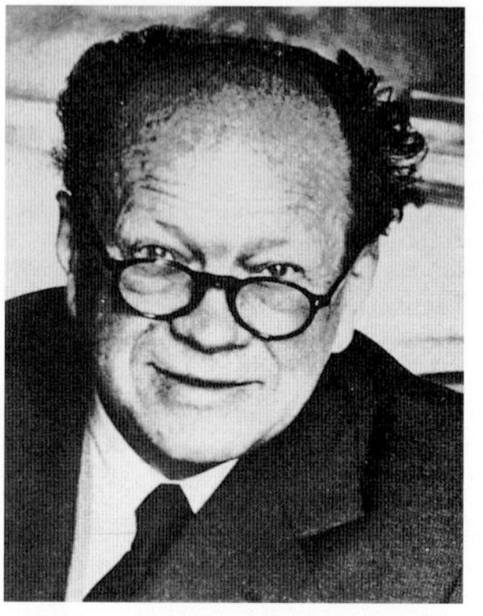

Fig. 4-2. René Leriche (1879–1555). In 1940 this French surgeon described the characteristic syndrome, with obliteration of the aorta and iliac arteries by plaque and thrombus

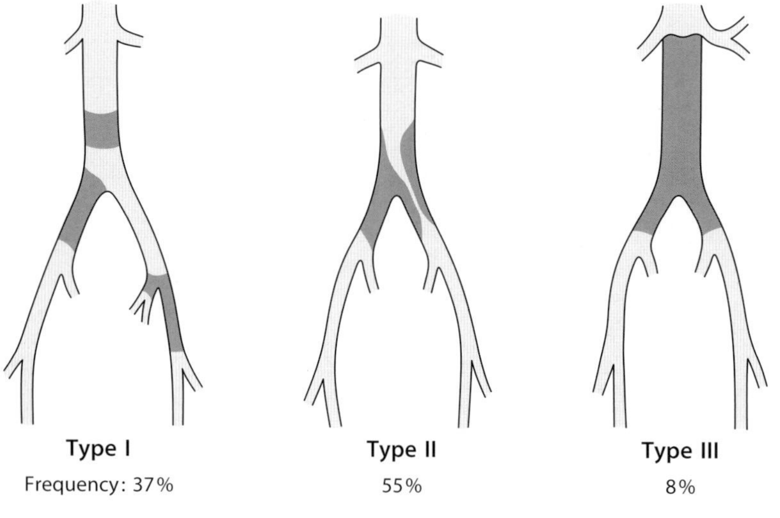

Fig. 4-1. Types of aortic occlusions. (After VOLLMAR 1965)

Clinical Features

The most common complaint is claudication of the muscles in the buttocks, thigh and calf. Often impotence is a problem. Isolated chronic aortic or iliac occlusion is usually well-compensated and produces no symptoms when the patient is at rest.

Diagnosis

The diagnosis of occlusion can usually be made on the basis of clinical criteria, as well as pulse examination, auscultation and oscillographic findings. The exact localization is determined with duplex ultrasonography and arteriography.

Therapy

- Conservative
  - The response to exercise training (walking) is less promising than in the case of more distal obstruction.
  - Balloon catheter dilatation with or without stenting is an effective way to treat high-grade stenoses or short occlusions of the aortic-iliac axis.
  - Thrombolytic therapy also may produce improvement with high-grade stenosis and segmental occlusion, if the blockage is only weeks to months old. The lesions may also be rendered more amenable to angioplasty or stenting.
- Surgical
  1. Thromboendarterectomy done with varying degrees of vessel exposure (open to partially closed)
  2. Replacement of the involved vessel with a bypass or interposition graft using either prosthetic or autologous material.

B. Aortic Aneurysm

Definition

Widening of the aorta in its abdominal (80%) or thoracic (15%) portion with the consequent dangers of life-threatening rupture, thrombosis or embolism.

Epidemiology

About 2% of people over 60 years of age are affected. The incidence increases with advancing age.

Etiology and Pathogenesis

Arteriosclerosis appears to be the major risk factor as damaged segments are more likely to form aneurysms, although some believe the association of aneurysmal disease and arteriosclerosis to be coincidental. Congenital aneurysms develop on a background of structural defects in the vessel wall. Other causes of wall weakness include trauma, inflammation and stenosis with altered pressures.

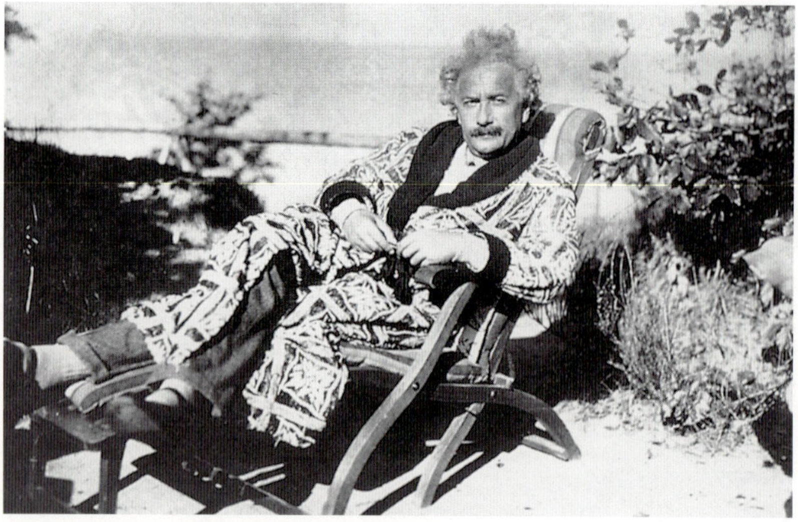

Fig. 4-3. Albert Einstein on vacation in 1928. Radiological images from this time showed cardiac enlargement and a large infrarenal abdominal aneurysm. Einstein was operated on in December 1948 by the famous surgeon Rudolf Nissen, who was a student of Sauerbruch; however, Einstein died April 18, 1955 from a ruptured aortic aneurysm

Morphology

Several different types of aneurysms can be identified:

- True aneurysms – all layers of the vessel wall are involved.
  1. Saccular (Fig. 4-4a)
  2. Fusiform (Fig. 4-4b)
  3. Dissecting (Fig. 4-4c)
- False or pseudo-aneurysms – a pulsating hematoma (Fig. 4-4d)

Clinical Features

Three clinical stages are seen:

- Asymptomatic (Stage I): This is the most common scenario. An aneurysm is identified during routine evaluation but it is totally asymptomatic.
- Symptomatic (Stage II): The pressure exerted by the expanding aneurysm on adjacent structures leads to a variety of problems. Thoracic aneurysms tend to cause persistent back pain, while those in the abdomen may lead to a ring-like constricting pain.

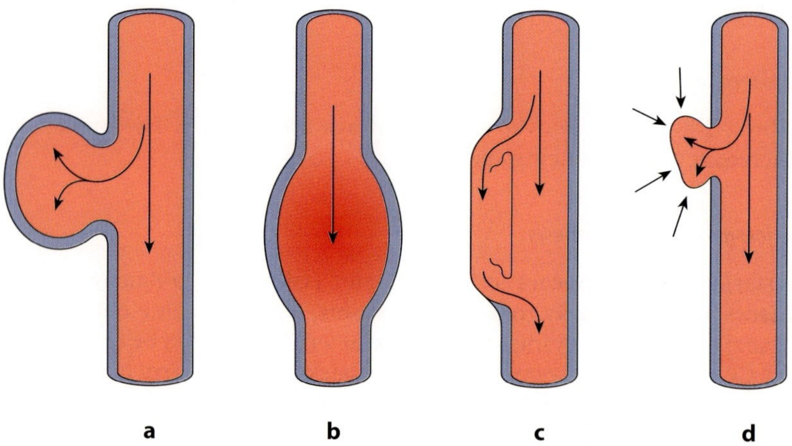

Fig. 4-4 a – d. Types of aneurysms (see text)

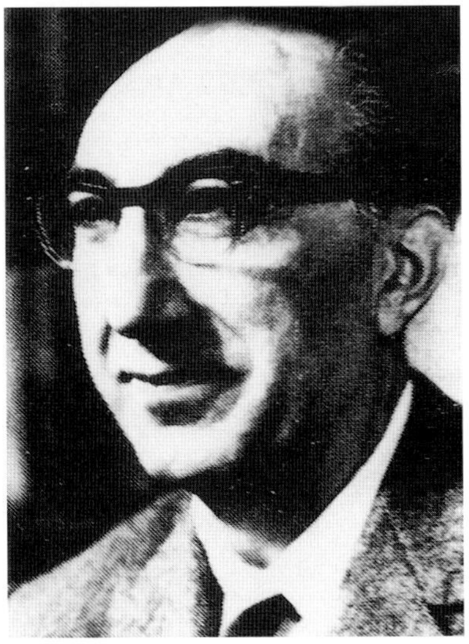

Fig. 4-5. Michael Ellis De Bakey, American surgeon, born 1908

- Ruptured (Stage III): Most ruptures occur in the retroperitoneal space. Patients present in hemorrhagic shock and often die, especially if the bleeding extends into the peritoneal cavity. Those with thoracic rupture have severe retrosternal pain, nausea, vomiting, shortness of breath and, with dissecting aneurysms, aortic valve insufficiency (20%–30%). The differential diagnosis includes myocardial infarction, pulmonary embolus and pneumothorax. If the rupture is more caudad, pain and shock dominate the picture.

Classification of Dissecting Aneurysms

Aortic dissection almost always starts in the thoracic portion of the vessel. De Bakey's classification is based on the point where the dissection begins.

- Type I: Dissection originates just superior to the aortic valve and spreads peripherally (60%).
- Type II: Dissection is limited to the ascending aorta (15%).
- Type III: Dissection begins after the take-off of the left subclavian artery. It can remain localized (type IIIa) or spread caudally (type IIIb) (25%).

In the Stanford classification type A includes De Bakey types I and II, while type B is equivalent to De Bakey types IIIa and IIIb.

Diagnosis

- Thoracic aneurysm
  - Chest X-ray
  - Transesophageal echocardiography
  - Computerized tomography
  - Arteriography
  - Magnetic resonance tomography
- Abdominal aneurysm
  - Palpation
  - Ultrasonography and duplex ultrasonography
  - Computerized tomography
  - Arteriography
  - Magnetic resonance tomography

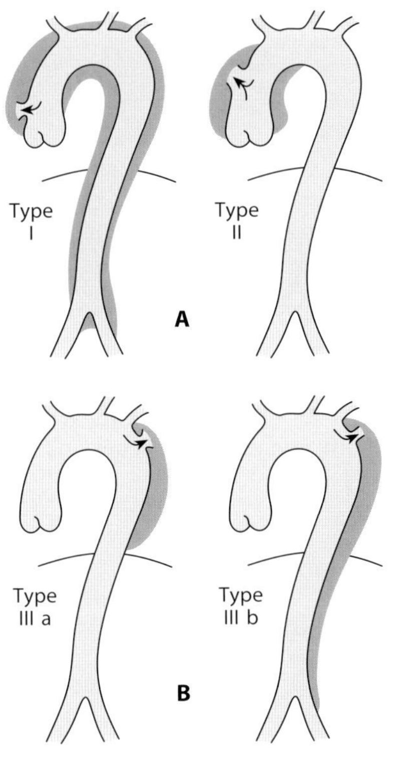

Fig. 4-6 A, B. Classification of aortic dissections (after De Bakey)

Therapy

- Conservative
  - The only medical management for dissecting aneurysms is to control the hypertension which is found in about 60% of patients.
- Surgical
  - Asymptomatic aneurysms with a diameter of greater than 5 cm are usually considered for surgical treatment. Smaller lesions which are highly irregular or not fusiform may also qualify. The usual procedure is the placement of an inlay graft with either a tubular or Y-shaped prosthetic conduit. The aneurysm is left in place and closed over the graft to separate it from the small bowel.

In the case of dissecting aneurysms, many type I and II (De Bakey) require surgery, while type III are usually followed, unless there are vascular complications (bleeding, impaired vascular supply to other organs, rupture).

Transluminally Placed Endovascular Grafts
In recent years transluminal insertion of stented vascular prostheses has become a possible approach for some patients. In the thoracic region, segmental saccular aneurysms are well suited to such treatment. In the infrarenal area, a morphological classification of aneurysms helps in deciding on the therapeutic approach.

Allenberg classification (Fig. 4-7)

- Type I features an intact subrenal segment and a healthy area before the bifurcation. An endoluminal straight tube prosthesis can be inserted.
- Type II also has a healthy subrenal segment but the aneurysm extends to (IIA) or past (IIB) the aortic bifurcation. In both instances a bifurcated endograft can be inserted.
- Type IIC aneurysms involve the iliac bifurcation so that an endoluminal prosthesis can only be used if the internal iliac artery is reimplanted or occluded by coils or ligation. In such cases, the endograft must be extended to the external iliac artery.
- Type III lacks an intact subrenal segment so that an endoluminal prosthesis can only be used if the renal arteries are sacrificed or bypassed.

The methods of treatment can be varied depending on the type of aneurysm and its location. As a simple example, the treatment of a saccular aneurysm of the ascending aorta is illustrated (Fig. 4-8).

2. Congenital Anomalies of the Aorta

There are many possible congenital anomalies of the aorta, usually arising in connection with abnormalities of the brachial arch arteries and other structures. Most are quite rare. The most common changes are congenital stenoses of the thoracic and abdominal aorta, as well as the common iliac artery.

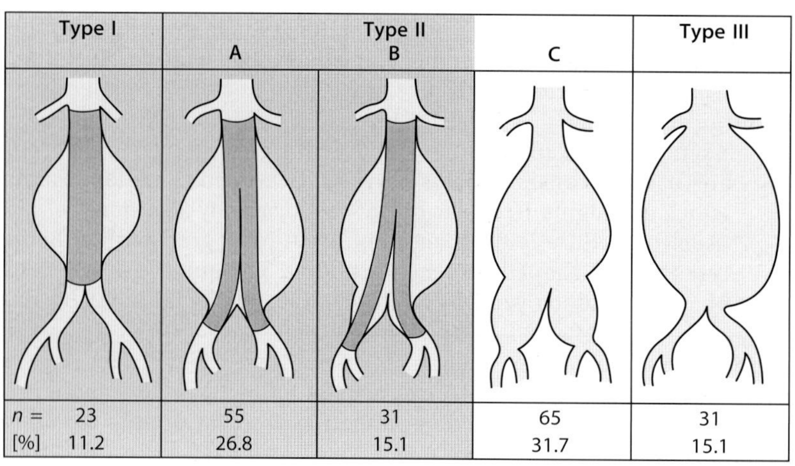

Fig. 4-7. Allenberg classification of infrarenal aortic aneurysms

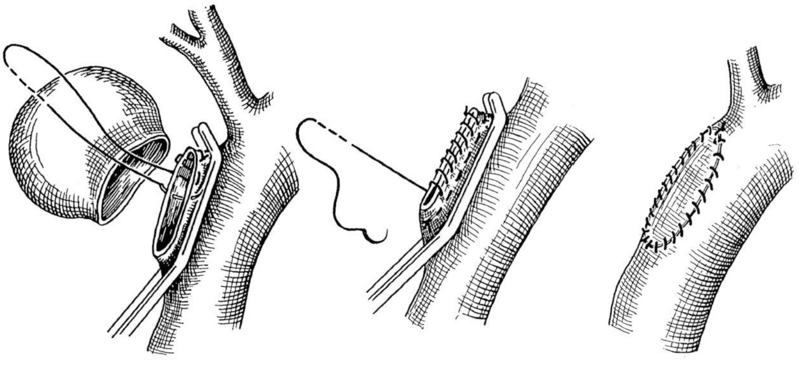

Fig. 4-8. Repair of a saccular aneurysm of the ascending aorta with tangential excision and then direct closure. If the aneurysm has a large neck or the aortic wall is damaged, then a patch graft can be used to close the vessel. (Figure and text from VOLLMAR 1965)

A. Aortic Coarctation

Synonym. Aortic isthmus stenosis

Definition

Stenosis of the aorta at the isthmus which is just distal to the origin of the left subclavian artery. Because similar changes can occur all along the aorta, the more general term of coarctation is preferred by many.

Morphology

Aortic isthmus stenosis was formerly divided into an adult form, with stenosis distal to the ductus arteriosus, and an infantile form, with the narrowing proximal to the ductus arteriosus. The aortic coarctation syndrome includes a patent ductus arteriosus and often various ventricular septal defects. It primarily involves infants.

Clinical Features

In infants the main problem is dyspnea. In adults there tends to be brachio-cephalic hypertension association with reduced to absent pedal pulses. Headaches and recurrent nose bleeds are common.

Diagnosis

Palpation and Doppler ultrasonography can compare the pressure differences bilaterally in the upper and lower extremities. Thoracic X-rays show pressure erosions of the ribs because of the collateral widening of the intercostal arteries.

Therapy

Early surgical excision of the stenotic section with either primary anastomosis or insertion of a graft prevents the development of the secondary problems.

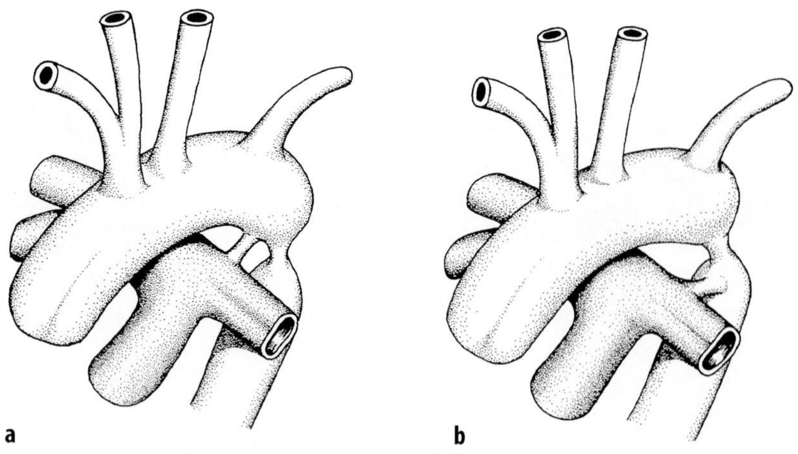

Fig. 4-9 a, b. Types of aortic isthmus stenosis:
a adult;
b infantile

B. Marfan's Syndrome

(Antoine Bernard Jean Marfan, French pediatrician 1858–1942)

Definition

Autosomal dominant, inherited, generalized connective tissue defect with characteristic changes in the cardiovascular system and eyes, as well as a distinctive habitus.

Epidemiology

The indigence is about 1:10,000 with no racial or sexual predilection. The average life expectancy is about 32–35 years if untreated.

Etiology and Pathogenesis

The genetic defect in Marfan's syndrome involves a mutation in the fibrillin-1 gene on chromosome 15. Fibrillin is a vital component of connective tissue.

Morphology

The fibrillin defect leads to medial necrosis of the aorta with degenerated elastic fibers. The fibers of the ciliary zonule supporting the lens are also abnormal.

Clinical Features

- Habitus: Patients tend to be tall with lower body length exceeding upper and with long limbs. Often their arm span is greater than their height. They tend to have long slender digits (arachnodactyly), a narrow, long head, pectus excavatum or pectus carinatum, kyphoscoliosis and frequent inguinal hernias.
- Ocular: About 70% of patients have a subluxated lens, usually with upward displacement.
- Cardiovascular: Over 95% of patents have a dilated ascending aorta, aortic valve insufficiency and dissecting aortic aneurysms.

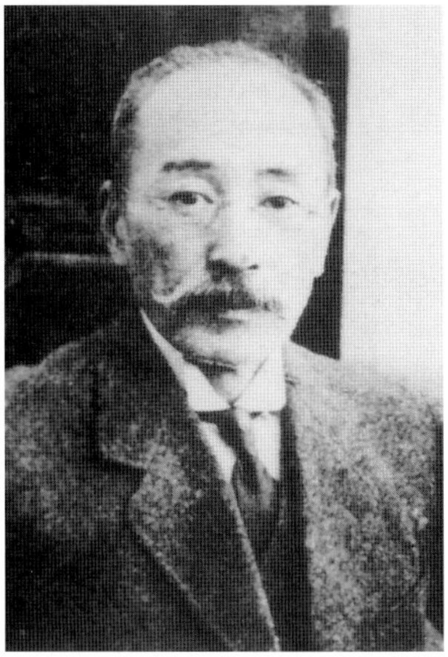

Fig. 4-10. Mikito Takayasu, Japanese ophthalmologist (1860–1939). "*I saw this unusual case in May 1906. The female patient had noted loss of vision with cloudiness and conjunctival hemorrhages in the previous fall. She improved with treatment, but relapsed again in the spring. The blood vessels of the retina showed a wreath-like circle of anastomoses that surrounded the optic disc at a distance of 2–3 mm. These structures were enclosed by additional circular anastomoses, representing arteriovenous shunts. The vessels about the disc were raised and most of the arterial segments showed segmental domed-shaped swellings. In some locations, blood clots were present but I saw no inflammation. Both eyes were involved, but the process was more striking on the left. I have no idea what disease the patient had.*" (M. Takayasu, 1908)

Diagnosis

The gene defect can be identified. The diagnosis can usually be made easily with transesophageal echocardiography, ultrasonography, duplex ultrasonography, computerized tomography or arteriography.

Several other congenital disorders also have marfanoid features including homocystinuria, some types of Ehlers-Danlos syndrome, congenital contractural acrachnodactyly, Klinefelter's syndrome and multiple endocrine neoplasia IIB.

Therapy

The use of β-blockers appears to slow the progression of disease. If dilatation is progressive, surgical repair is required.

3. Inflammatory Disease of the Aorta: Takayasu's Disease

Synonyms. Takayasu's aortitis, aortic arch syndrome, pulseless disease of young women, aortoarteriitis, Martorell-Fabre syndrome

Definition

The most common inflammatory aortic disease, with inflammation of the aortic arch associated with stenoses sometimes leading to thromboses and occlusion of the aortic arch vessels. The coronary, pulmonary and renal arteries can also be involved.

Epidemiology

Most patients are women under 40 years of age. The female:male ratio is 10:1. The usual onset of symptoms is between 15 and 30 years of age. The disorder is more common in Japan, India and Southeast Asia.

Etiology and Pathogenesis

The cause is unknown. Because of the sexual and racial predilections, both hormonal and genetic factors have been discussed. Mycobacterial infection has also been implicated. The inflammatory reaction is characterized by infiltration of all layers of the aorta by mononuclear and giant cells. Based on the localization, four anatomic types are identified (Fig. 4-11).

Clinical Features

- The symptoms depend on the localization and severity of the vascular inflammation.
- Loss of pulses involving the arms occurs in 95% of cases.
- During the acute inflammatory phase, complaints such as fatigue, malaise, fever, myalgias and arthralgias are common.
- Later, neurological problem dominate including aphasia, hemiparesis, seizures and cerebrovascular accidents. In addition, aortic valve insufficiency, aortic aneurysms and renovascular hypertension may be present.

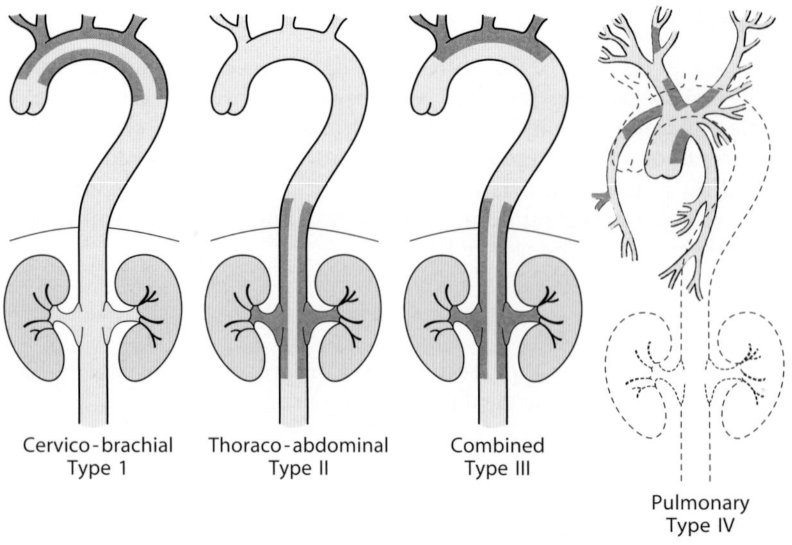

Fig. 4-11. Localization of the inflammatory changes in the aorta and pulmonary artery in Takayasu's disease

Diagnosis

The erythrocyte sedimentation rate and acute phase reactants (C-reactive protein) are elevated. There are no specific serological markers. Echocardiography, including that by the transesophageal approach, computerized tomography, duplex ultrasonography and arteriography help to confirm the diagnosis.

The differential diagnosis includes aortitis from rheumatoid arthritis, polymyalgia rheumatica, temporal arteritis, syphilitic aortitis, mycotic and idiopathic thoracic aortic aneurysms.

Therapy

- Conservative
  - Corticosteroids, usually prednisone 60 mg daily with gradual reduction to a maintenance dose of 5–10 mg. The erythrocyte sedimentation rate can be used to monitor therapy.
  - Sometimes cyclophosphamide is employed.
  - The effectiveness of platelet inhibitors is not well-proven.
- Surgical
  - Surgery is reserved for the later phases when aneurysms may be repaired or organ ischemia corrected by bypass procedures.

B: Supplementary Figures and Legends

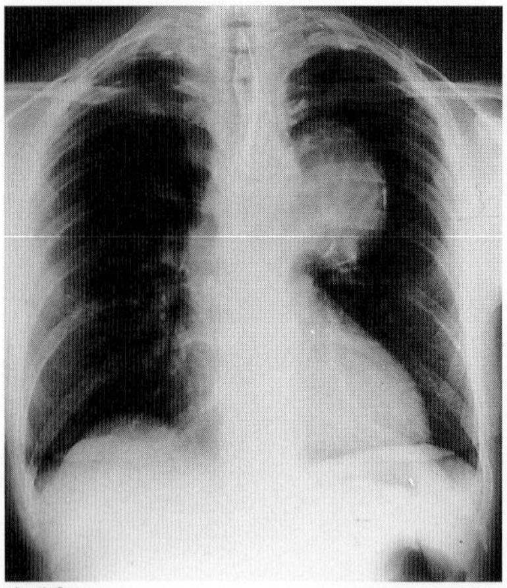

4-12

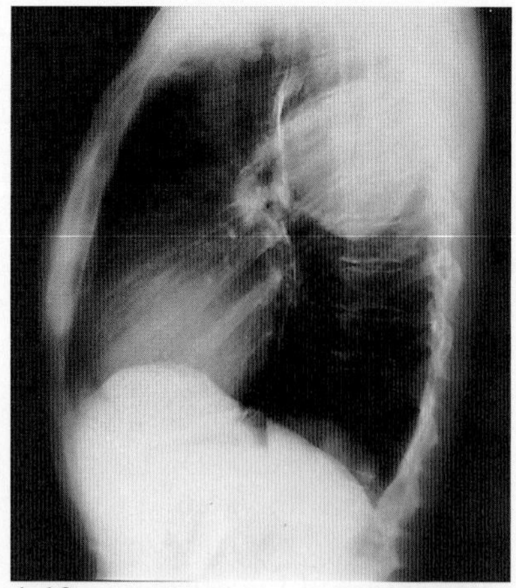

4-13

Figs. 4-12, 4-13. Saccular thoracic aortic aneurysm, antero-posterior and lateral views. This aneurysm was discovered during routine radiological evaluation. Such lesions are often asymptomatic until they rupture

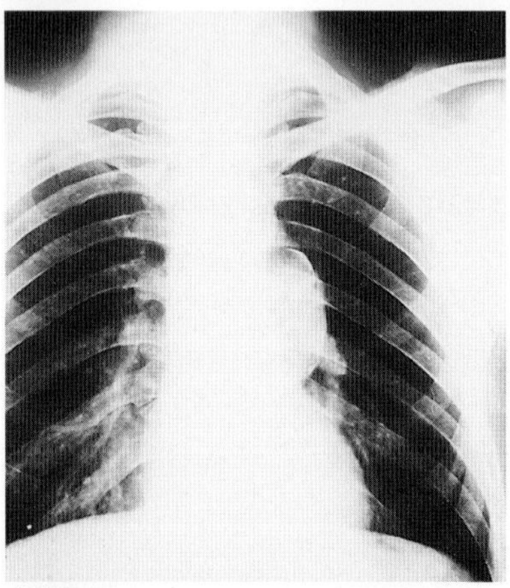

4-14

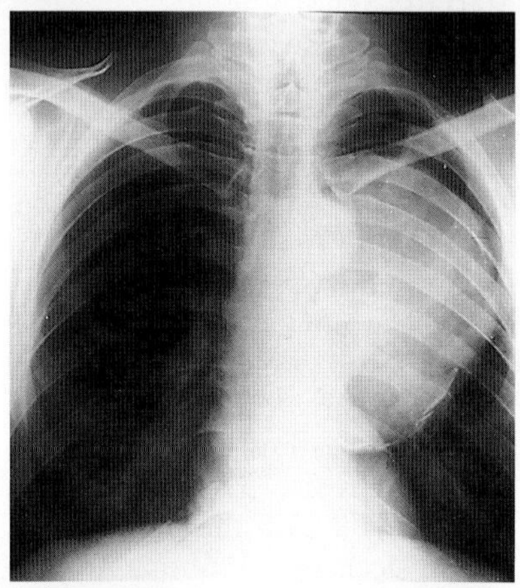

4-15

Fig. 4-14. Aneurysm of the descending aorta secondary to arteriosclerosis in a 42 year old patient. The X-ray shows a distinctly widened aorta without other abnormalities

Fig. 4-15. Follow-up evaluation 6 years later shows a enormous aneurysm

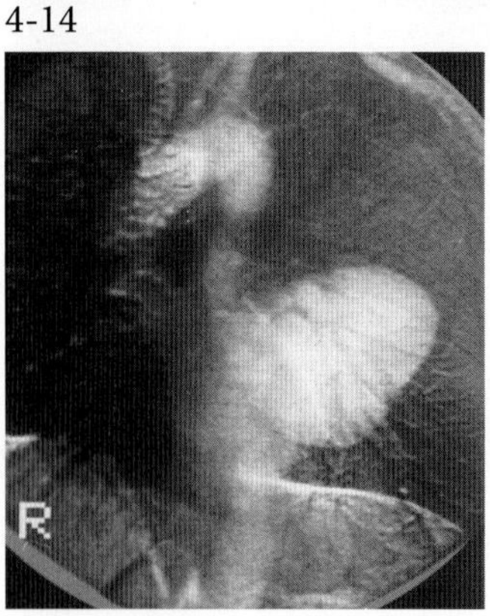

4-16

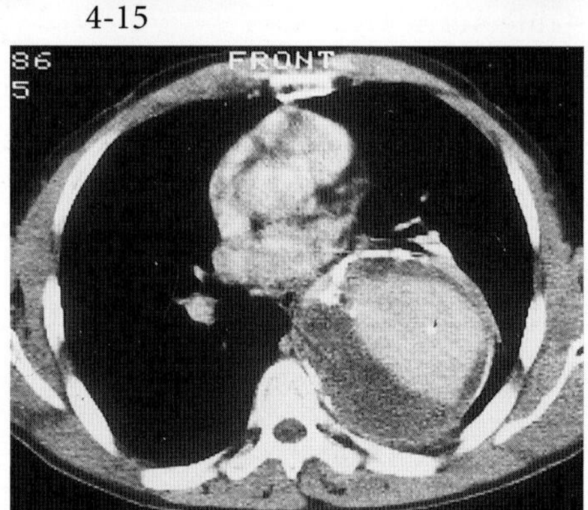

4-17

Figs. 4-16, 4-17. Angiogram and computerized tomography of the same patient. The computerized tomography shows a massive thrombus surrounding the still patent lumen

Fig. 4-18. Typical aneurysm of the descending thoracic aorta shown on angiography and intraoperatively with a Dacron prosthesis in place

Fig. 4-19. Magnetic resonance image in sagittal section showing the thoracic component of a thoraco-abdominal aneurysm (*arrows*)

Fig. 4-20. Chest roentgenograms of a patient with a thoracic aneurysm. Antero-posterior and lateral views show the aneurysm overshadowing the silhouette of the heart

Fig. 4-21. The two-dimensional spiral computerized tomography shows the saccular aneurysm in the mid-portion of the descending aorta

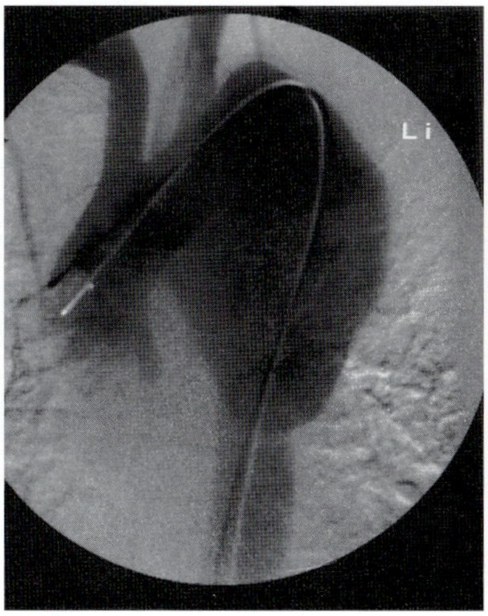

4-18

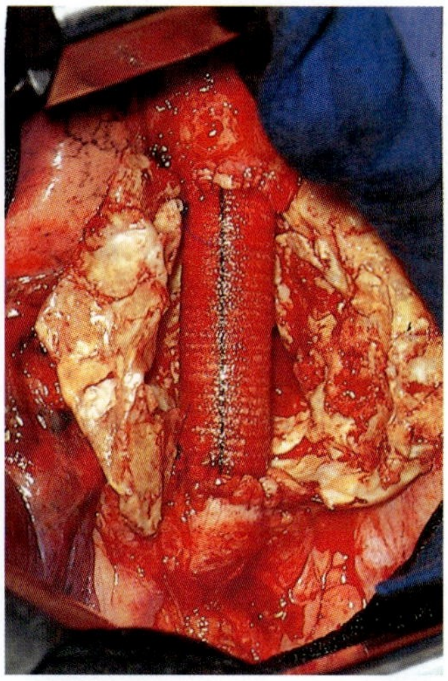

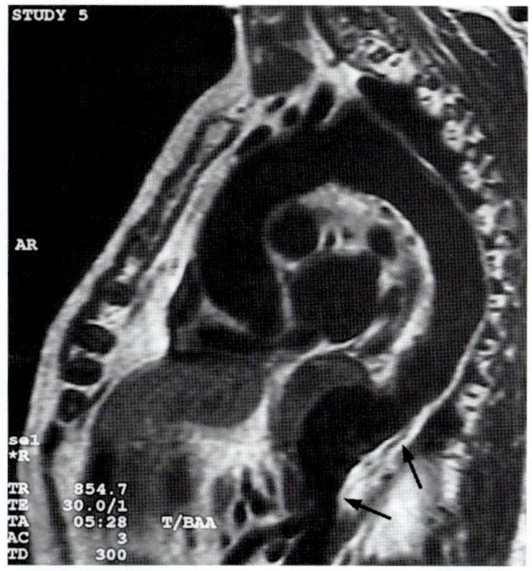

4-19

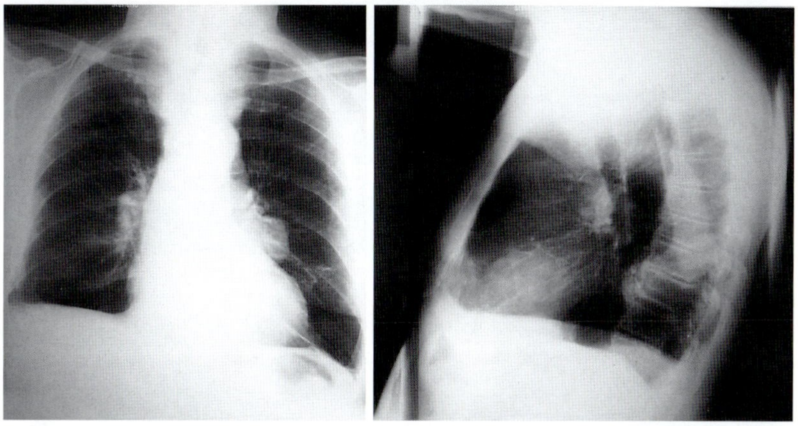

4-20

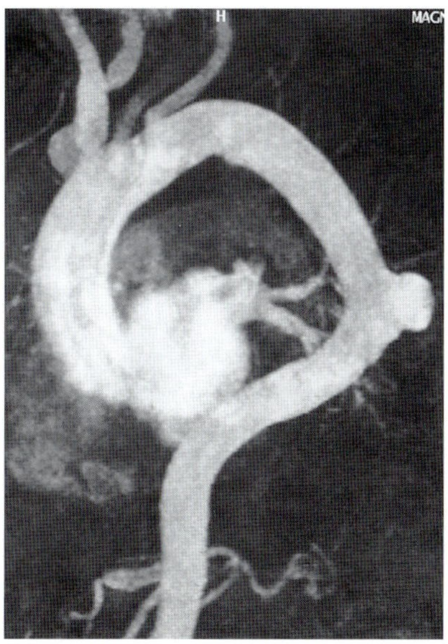

4-21

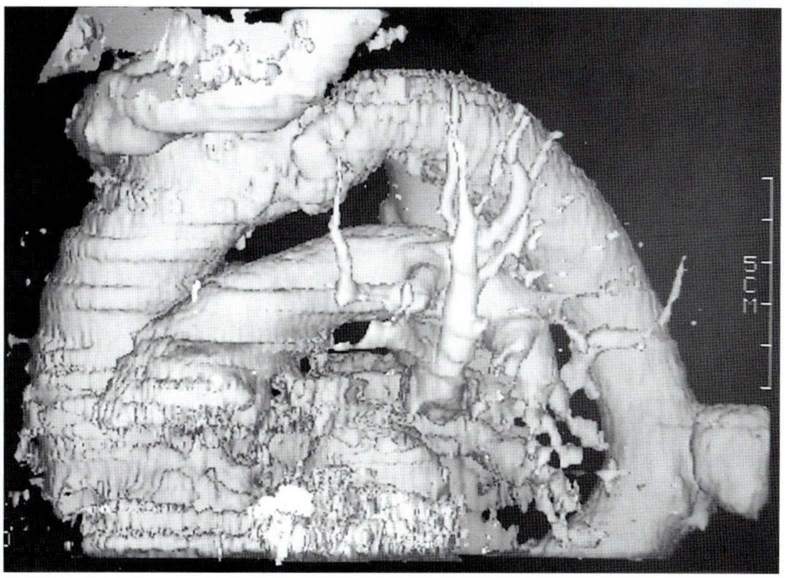

4-22

Fig. 4-22. In the spiral three-dimensional image the aneurysm is better seen

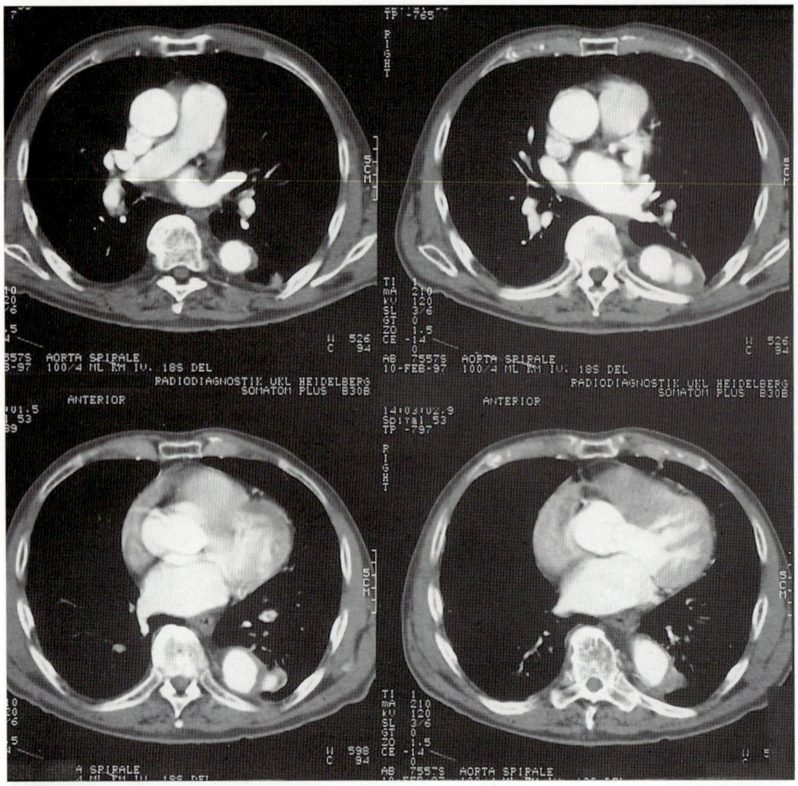

4-23

Fig. 4-23. Computerized tomography of the same patient shows the thrombotic and luminal components of the aneurysm

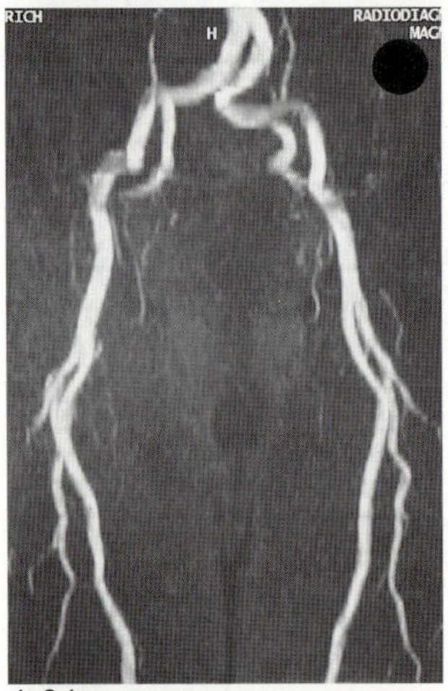

4-24

Fig. 4-24. Magnetic resonance angiography of the iliac arteries shows marked kinking. For this reason it would be difficult to place a thoracic stent-graft from below

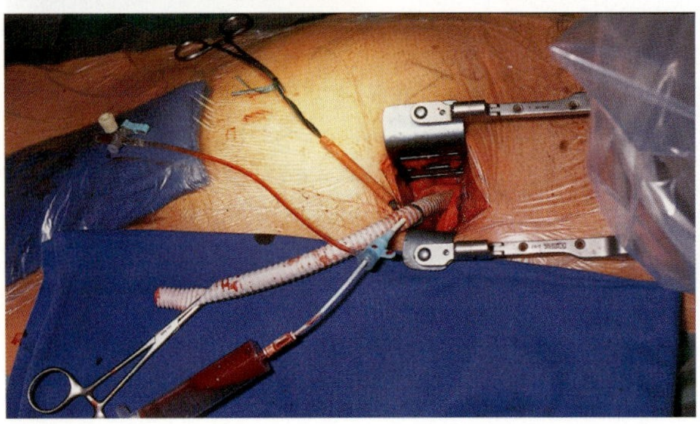

4-25

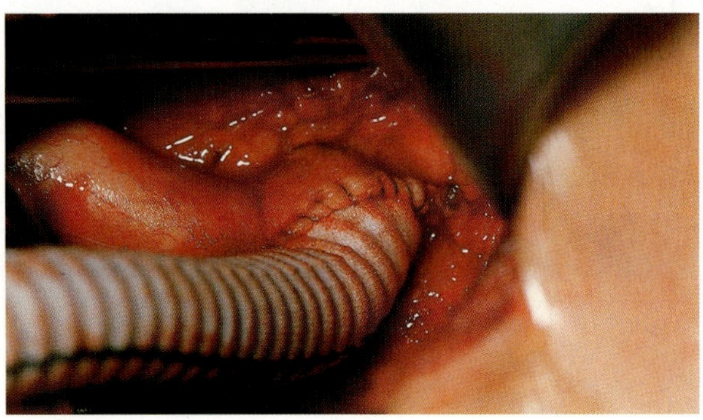

4-26

Figs. 4-25, 4-26. Small flank incision to expose the distal aorta at the level of the bifurcation. A Dacron prosthesis is attached here and can serve as a site for the introduction of the stent-graft-carrying catheter

Fig. 4-27. X-rays of the chest following implantation of a stent-graft in the descending aorta with compete exclusion of the saccular aneurysm

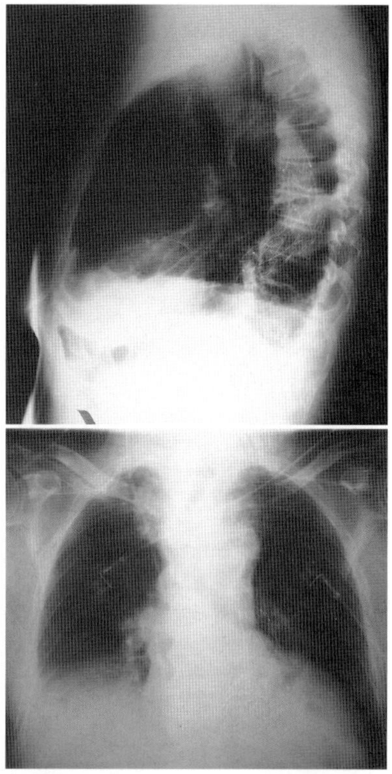

4-27

Fig. 4-28. Magnetic resonance control evaluation 6 months after insertion of the stent-graft

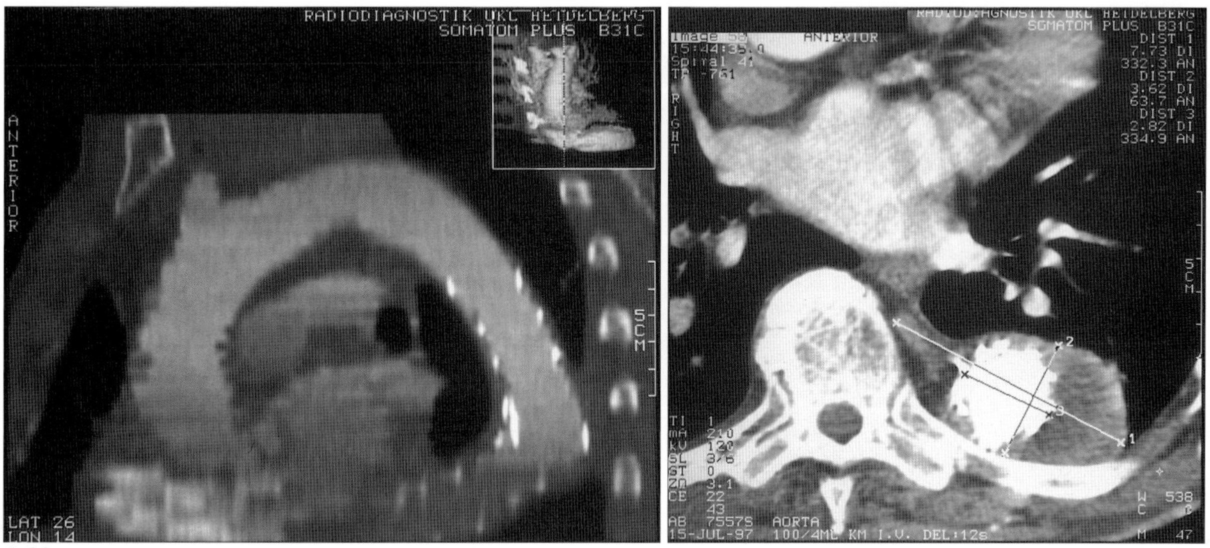

4-28

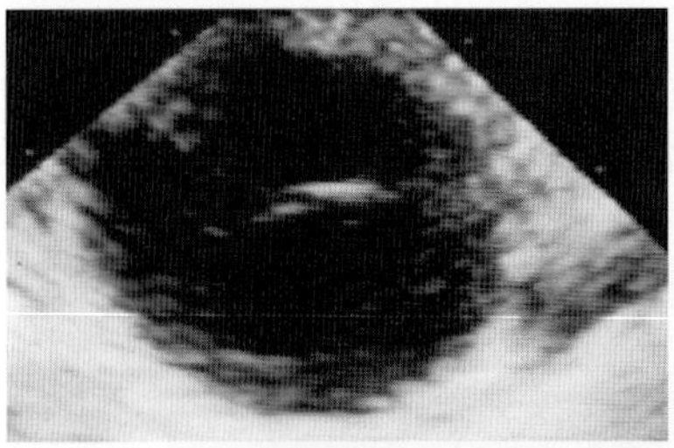
4-29

Fig. 4-29. Transesophageal echocardiography (TEE) almost always allows diagnosis of a dissecting aneurysm

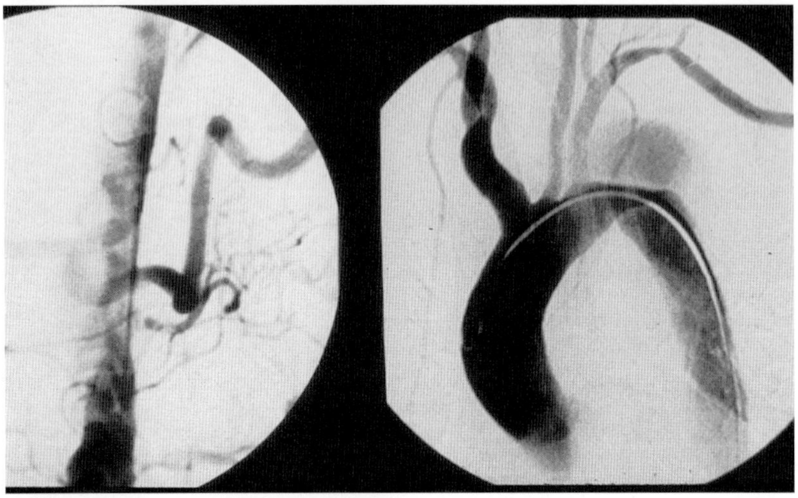
4-30

Fig. 4-30. Intra-arterial digital subtraction angiography (DSA) demonstrating a type B aortic dissection. The start of the dissection just after the left subclavian artery is well shown, but the true and false lumens are poorly demonstrated in the course of the procedure

Fig. 4-31. Three-dimensional spiral computerized tomography of the aortic arch and descending aorta; the dissection membrane is clearly indicated as a line within the vessel

Fig. 4-32. Three-dimensional spiral computerized tomography with dorsal view of the aortic arch showing a sharp increase in caliber just distal to the subclavian artery

Fig. 4-33. Cross-sectional view with three-dimensional spiral computerized tomography at the level of the visceral arteries clearly demonstrating the dissection membrane

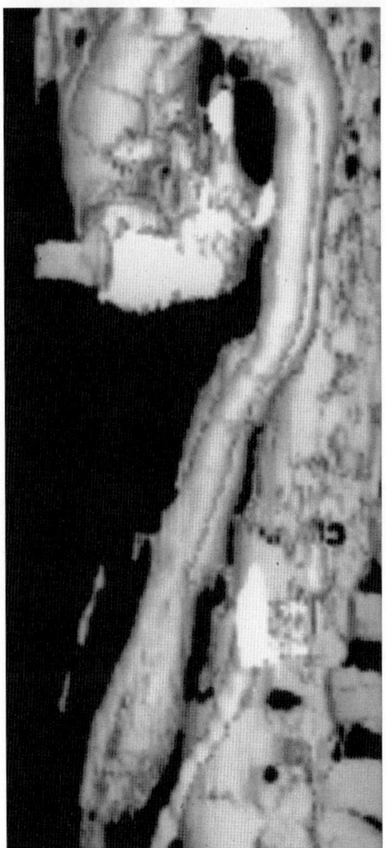
4-31

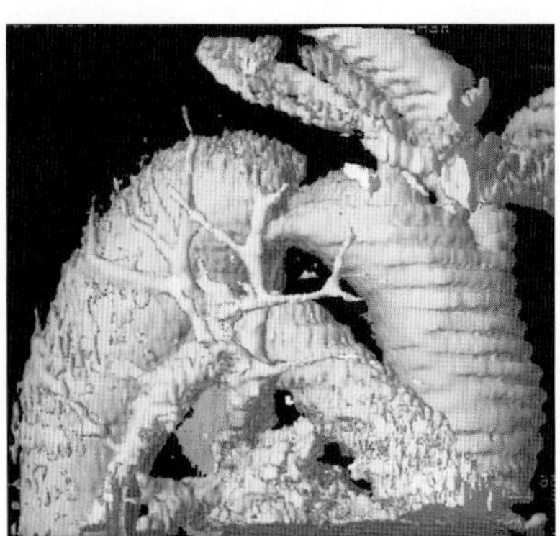
4-32

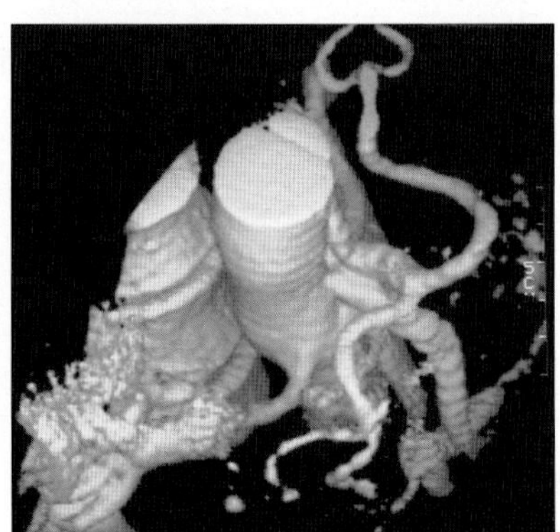
4-33

Fig. 4-34. Dissection of the aorta. A gadolinium magnetic resonance image shows the entire aortic arch, the descending thoracic and abdominal aorta. The visceral arteries can be seen arising from the true lumen; the dissection membrane and the false lumen are also easily seen

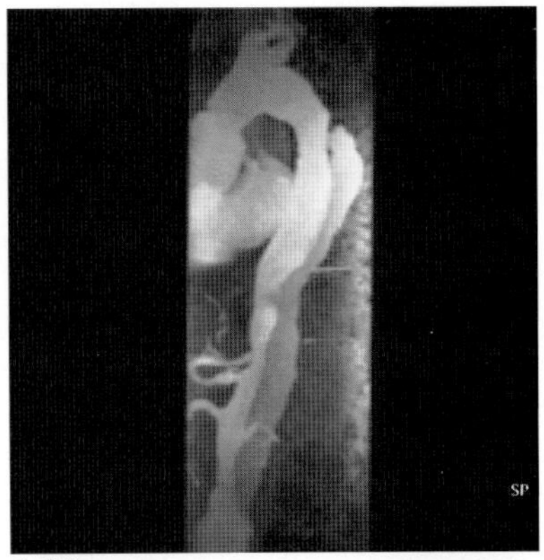

4-34

Fig. 4-35. In an antero-posterior view the celiac trunk and the right renal artery are seen leaving the true lumen, while the left renal artery appears to be connected to the false lumen

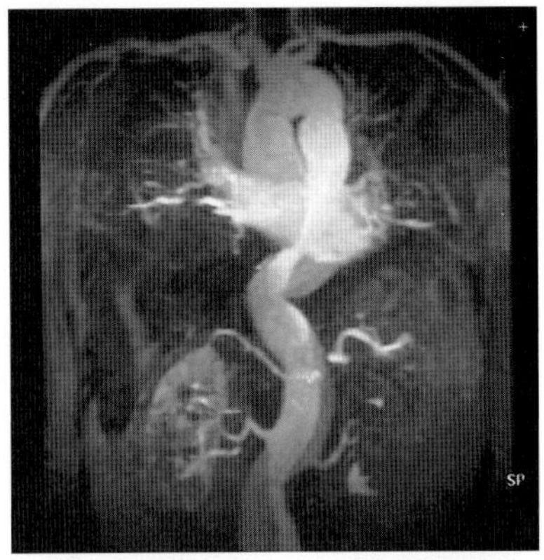

4-35

Fig. 4-36. At the level of the renal arteries it is possible to clearly demonstrate the origin of both renal vessels

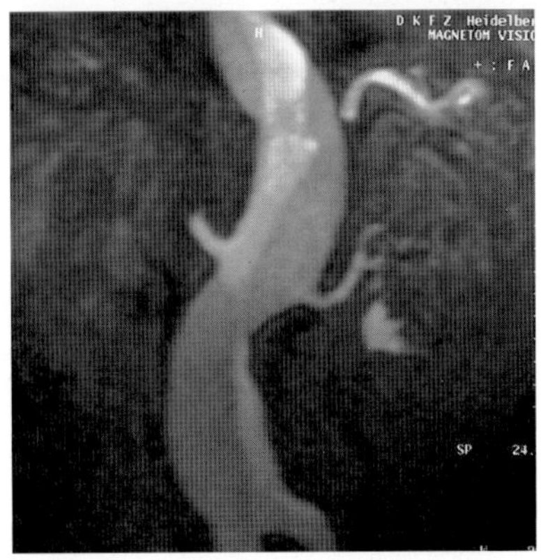

4-36

Fig. 4-37. By turning the image, it is possible to even better demonstrate the renal and visceral arteries and their connection with the true or false lumen. Here an infrarenal aortic aneurysm with associated right-sided high-grade renal artery stenosis is shown

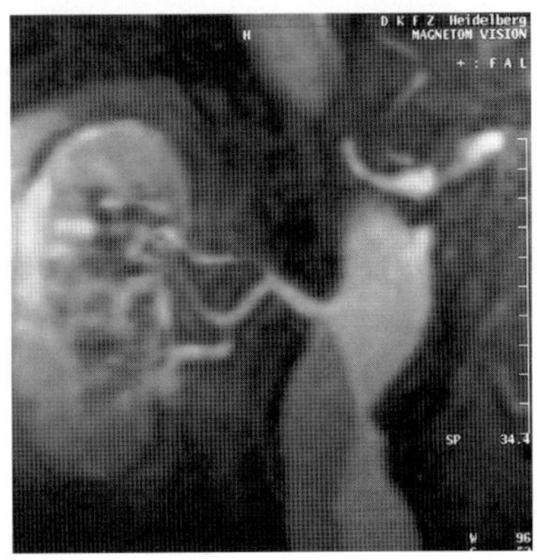

4-37

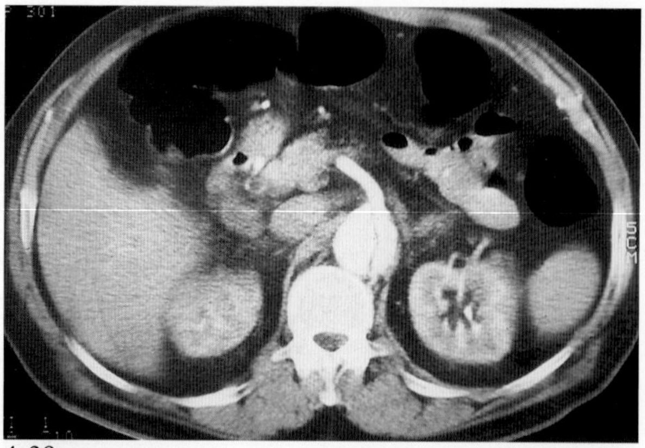

4-38

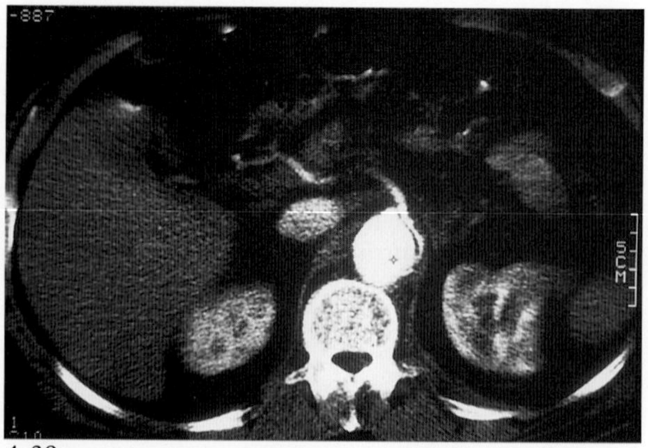

4-39

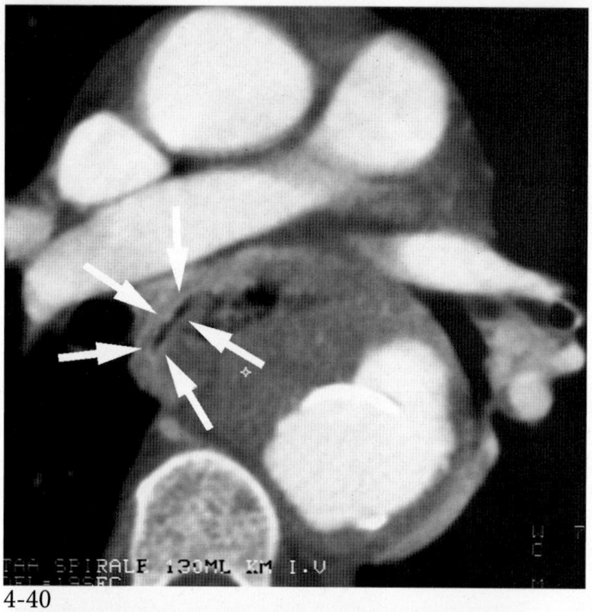

4-40

Fig. 4-38. Dissecting aneurysm (Stanford type B) with vascular complication: residual perfusion of the celiac trunk from the true lumen

Fig. 4-39. After 24 h nearly complete loss of perfusion of the celiac trunk

Fig. 4-40. Computerized tomography of an arteriosclerotic aneurysm which has ruptured into the esophagus (*arrows*). A Dacron prosthesis was inserted, coupled with an omental wrap

Figs. 4-41, 4-42. Two computerized tomography images of a 75 year old patient with both thoracic and abdominal aneurysms. The thoracic lesion has ruptured but the infrarenal aneurysm is still intact

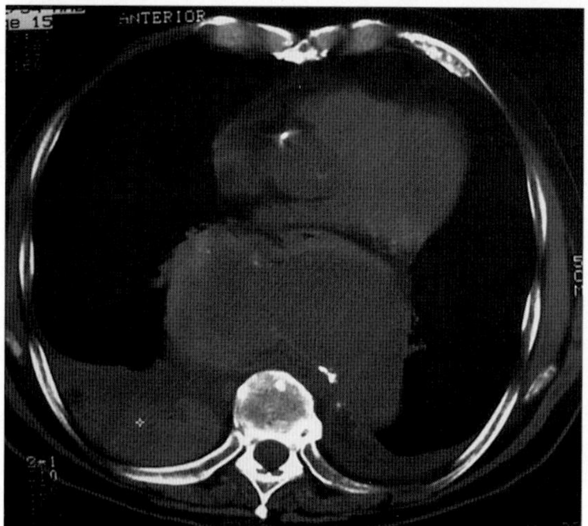

4-41

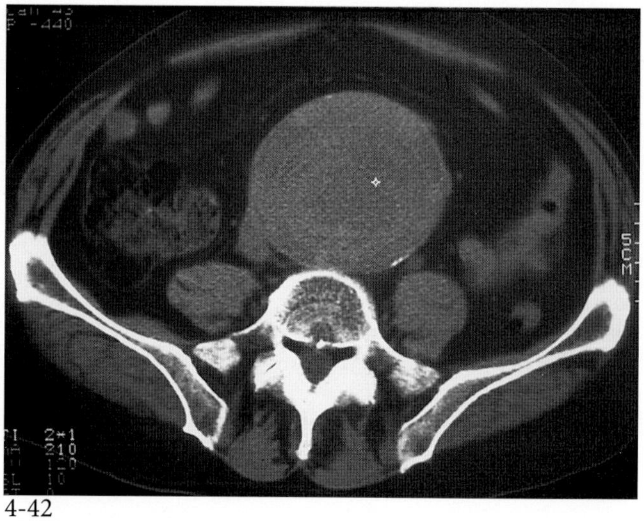

4-42

Fig. 4-43. Initial thoracic view of an acute aortic rupture in a 52 year old patient. The mediastinum is widened and the left apical cap is depressed by a hematoma (apical cap sign)

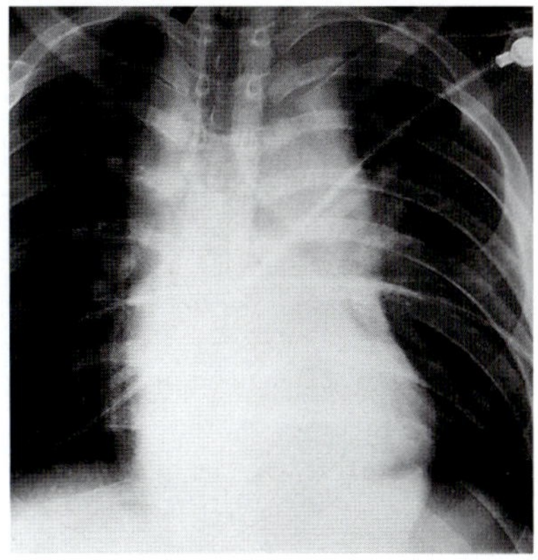

4-43

Fig. 4-44. The same patient 11 years later with a remarkable aortic arch (*arrows*) as the result of an aneurysm arising from the original trauma

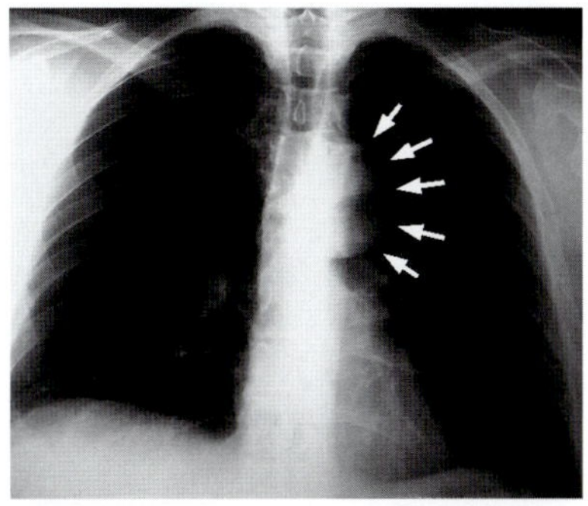

4-44

Figs. 4-45, 4-46. Computerized tomography and three-dimensional spiral computerized tomography both demonstrate the aneurysm

Fig. 4-47. Operative view of the same patient with insertion of a Dacron graft

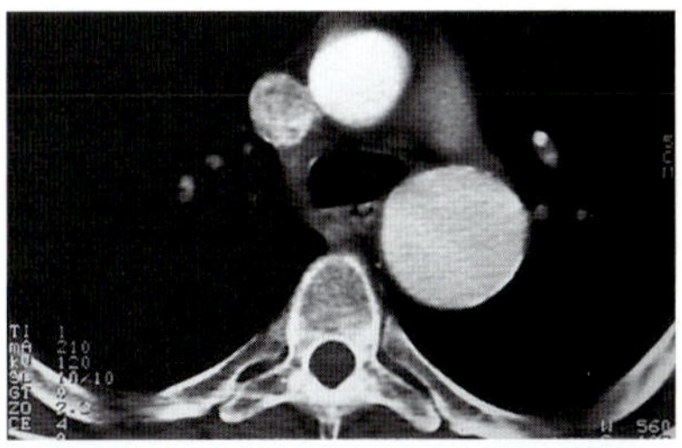

4-45

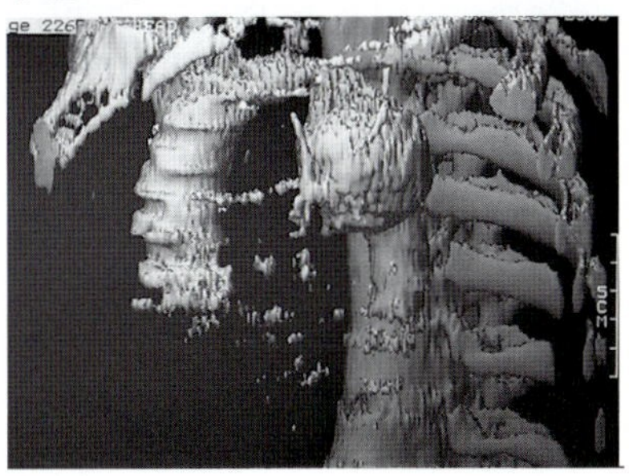

4-46

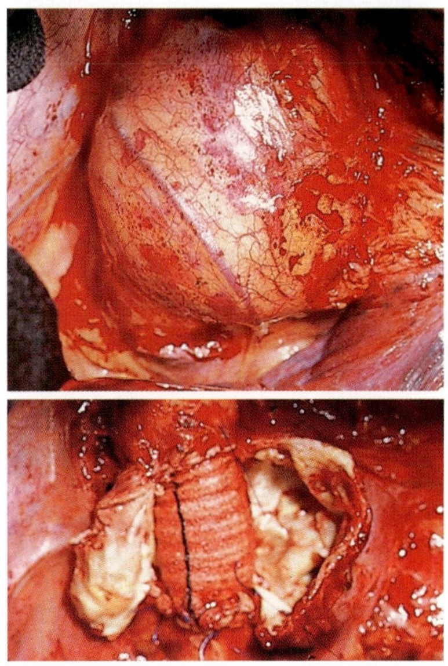

4-47

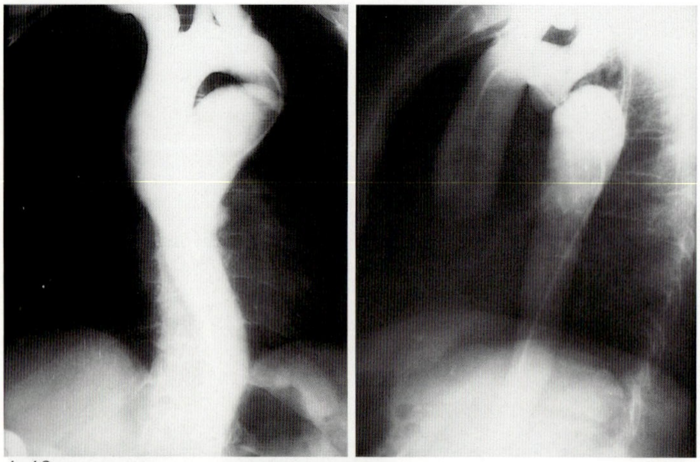

4-48

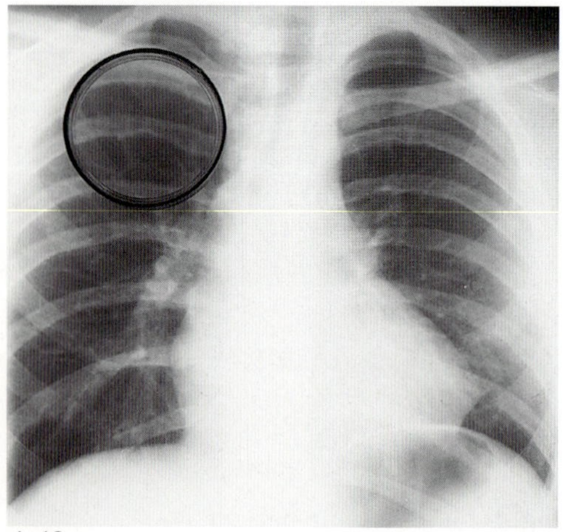

4-49

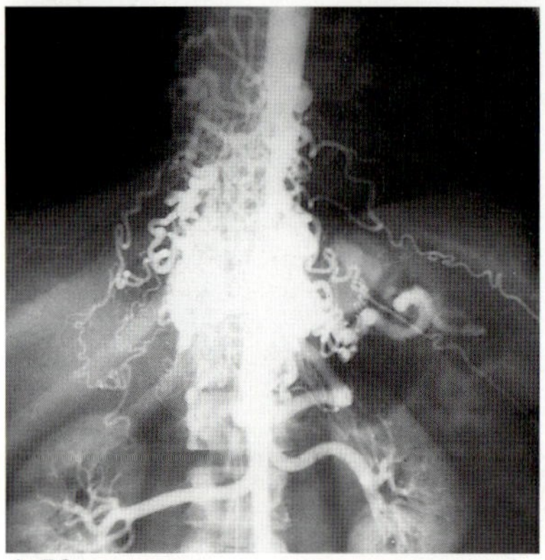

4-50

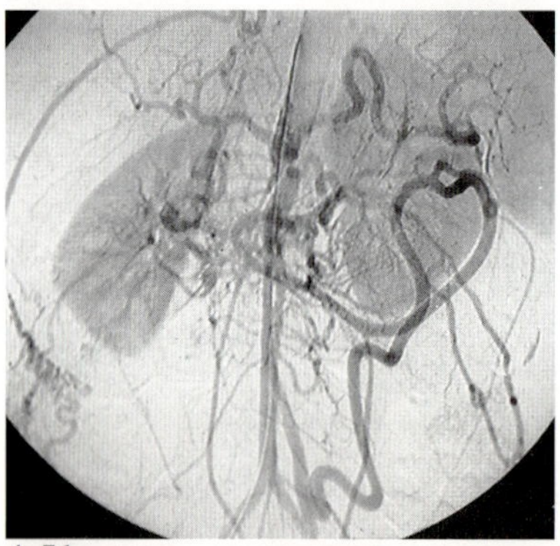

4-51

Fig. 4-48. Angiographic views of congenital aortic coarctation

Fig. 4-49. Chest X-ray shows the characteristic erosions (*magnified view*) on the inferior surfaces of the ribs caused by the enlarged intercostal arteries from collateral circulation

Fig. 4-50. Atypical coarctation of the thoraco-abdominal aorta with marked formation of collaterals. This 26 year old patient had uncontrolled hypertension with systolic blood pressure values approaching 300 mg Hg and presented with intermittent claudication. The narrowing was successfully repaired with a Dacron tube bypass

Fig. 4-51. Atypical coarctation in the infrarenal aortic segment reaching to the inferior mesenteric artery in a 36 year old women. The aortic lumen is about the thickness of a pencil

Fig. 4-52. The operative field shows the massive Riolan anastomosis of the inferior and superior mesenteric arteries providing collateral circulation for the legs

Fig. 4-53. The patient was treated with a thoraco-abdominal bypass. This was connected via a shunt to the part of the aorta where the renal arteries arose

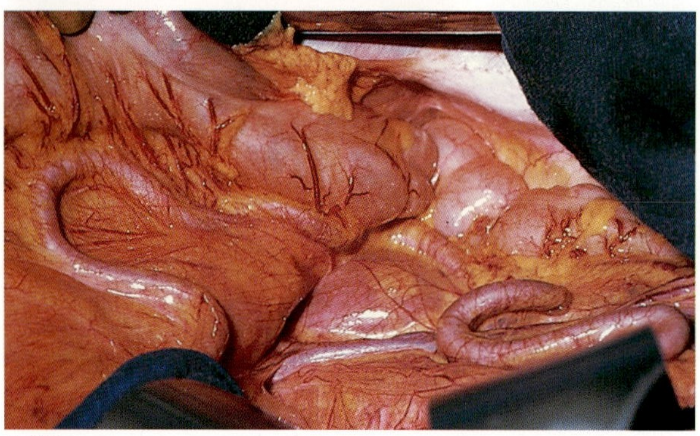

4-52

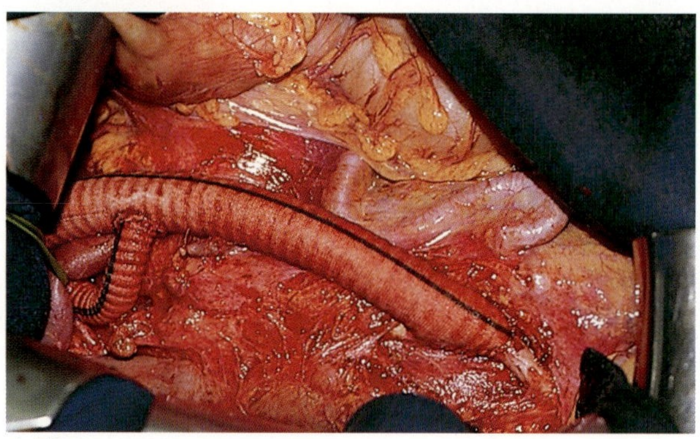

4-53

Case Presentation of a 46 Year Old Patient with Marfan's Syndrome

Fig. 4-54. Clinical view of patient, with long, thin fingers (arachnodactily), long arms (whose span often exceeds the patient's considerable height) and pectus carinatum

Fig. 4-55. Angiographic image following two operations. In the first procedure, a conduit operation was done replacing the aortic valve and the ascending aorta. In the second, the aortic arch was replaced and the supra-aortic vessels re-implanted. Nonetheless there was rapid progression of a thoracic aneurysm with prominent dissection. After the thoracic aneurysm reached 7 cm, and the infrarenal aneurysm 6 cm, a third operation was needed

Fig. 4-56. Angiogram after the third operation. Replacement of the thoracic aorta with a Dacron tube, aortoplasty with resection of the dissection membrane in the lower segments and an infrarenal bifurcation prosthesis with re-implantation of the inferior mesenteric artery. Both the visceral and renal arteries are shown to be patent

Figs. 4-57, 4-58. Operative view of the third operation with diagram on the *right*. The thoracic prosthesis can be seen, as can the bifurcation prosthesis with re-implantation of the inferior mesenteric artery and the repaired segment with the left renal artery

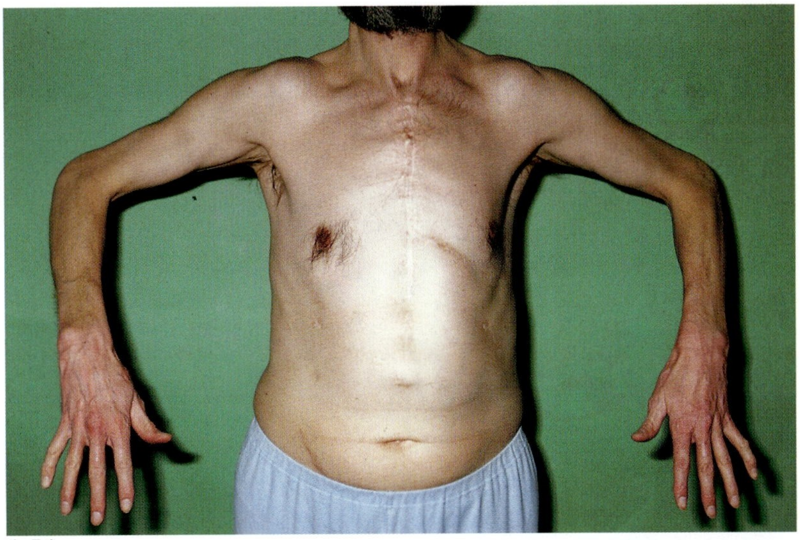

4-54

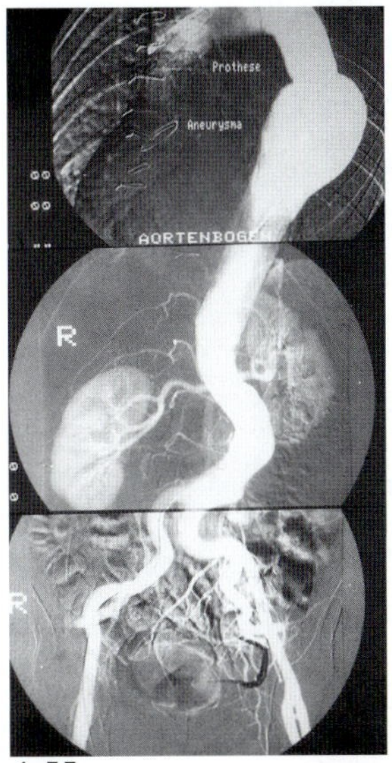

4-55

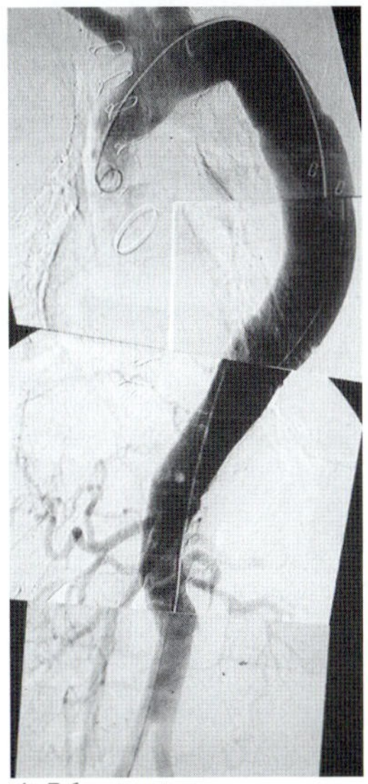

4-56

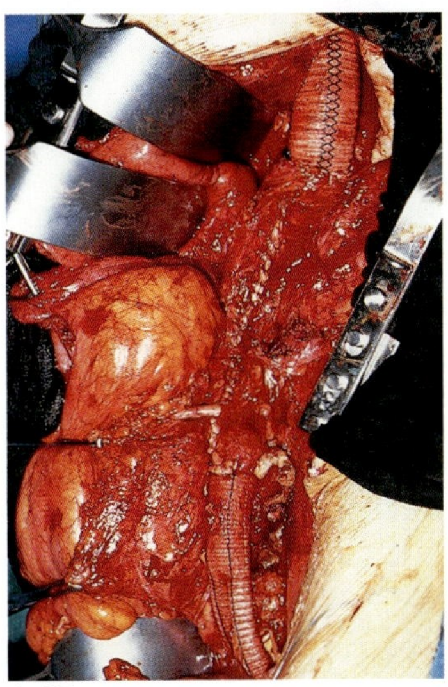

4-57

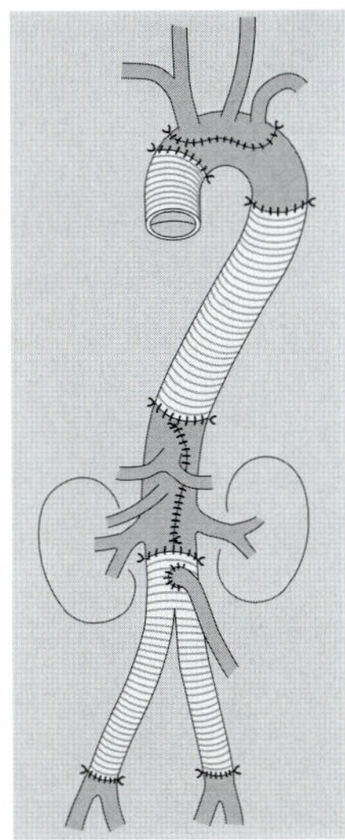

4-58

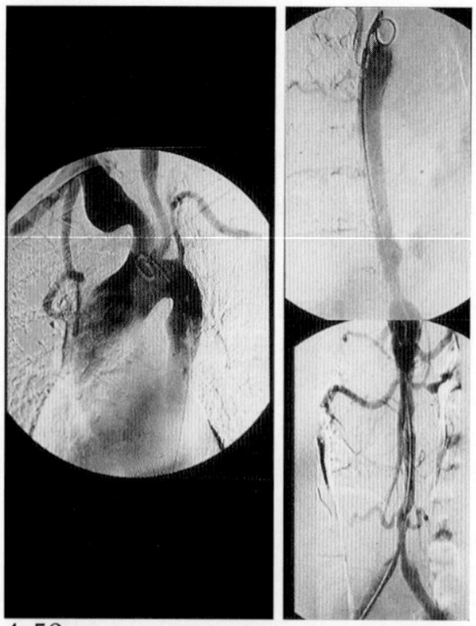

4-59

Fig. 4-59. Takayasu's disease showing the aortic arch, the thoracic aorta and the infrarenal aorta. The most prominent inflammation involves the supra-aortic vessels, as shown by dramatic changes in caliber, but there are signs of inflammation in all segments

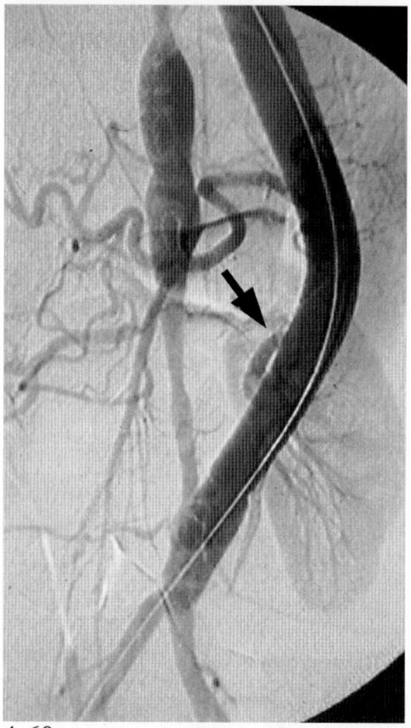

4-60

Fig. 4-60. Follow-up angiogram in the same patient showing the renal arteries implanted into the bypass (*arrow*)

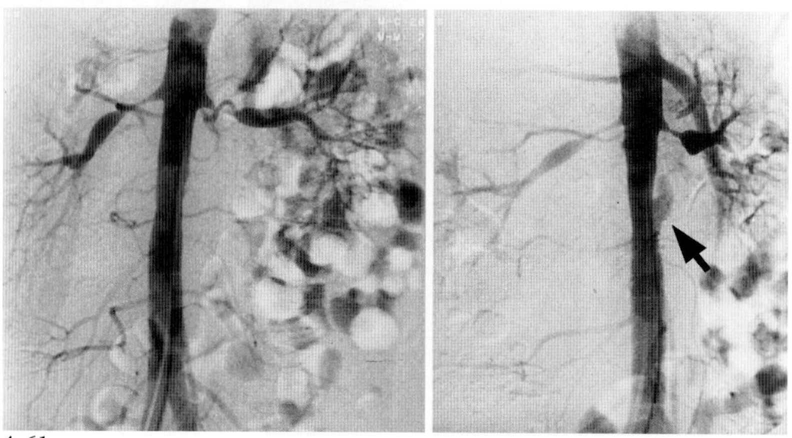

4-61

Fig. 4-61. A 26 year old man with Takayasu's disease. Involvement of the abdominal aorta with dissection (*arrow*) and of both renal arteries. Surgical repair consisted of placing a Dacron interposition aortic graft with vein bypasses to connect the prosthesis to both kidneys

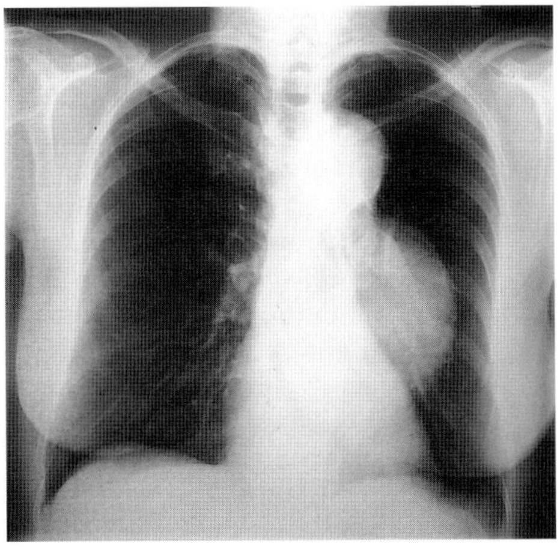

4-62

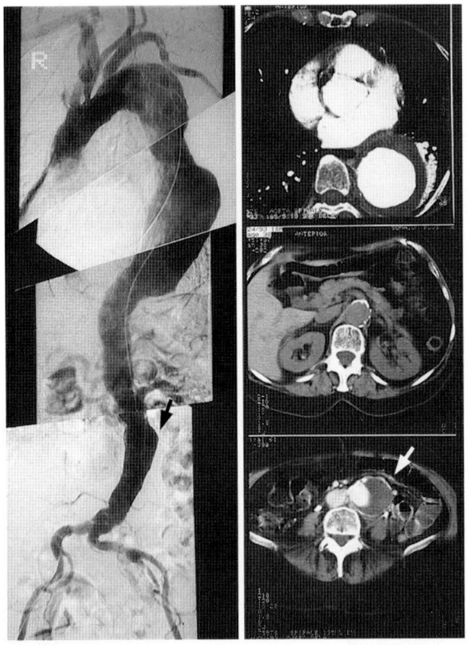

4-63

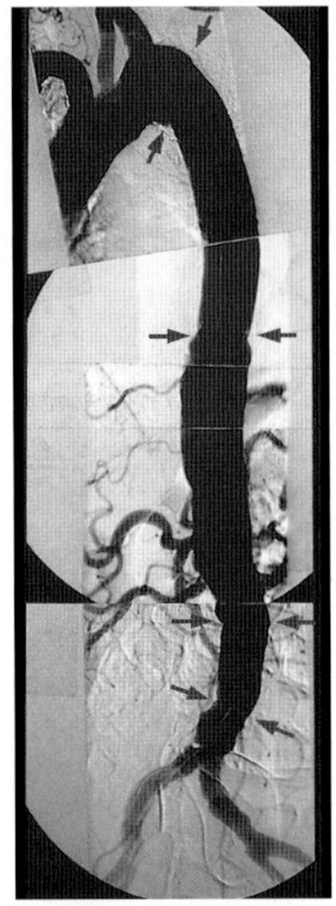

4-64

Arteriosclerotic Thoraco-abdominal Aneurysm

Fig. 4-62. Thoracic view of a patient with thoraco-abdominal aortic aneurysm

Fig. 4-63. In the angiogram only the thoracic component can be appreciated. The small infrarenal aneurysm is first seen in the computerized tomography (*arrow*)

Fig. 4-64. Angiographic follow-up view after the operation (*arrows*)

Fig. 4-65. Kinking of the aorta with aneurysmal outpouching, as shown with computerized tomography

Fig. 4-66. Lateral view of same patient with magnetic resonance imaging of the aorta showing the superior mesenteric artery

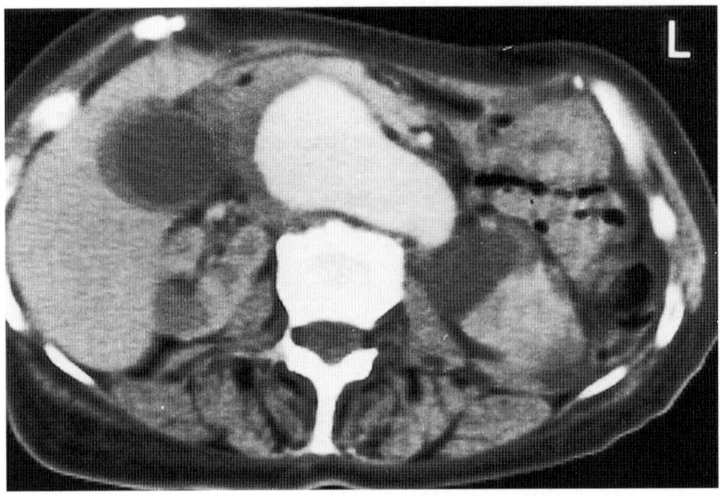

4-65

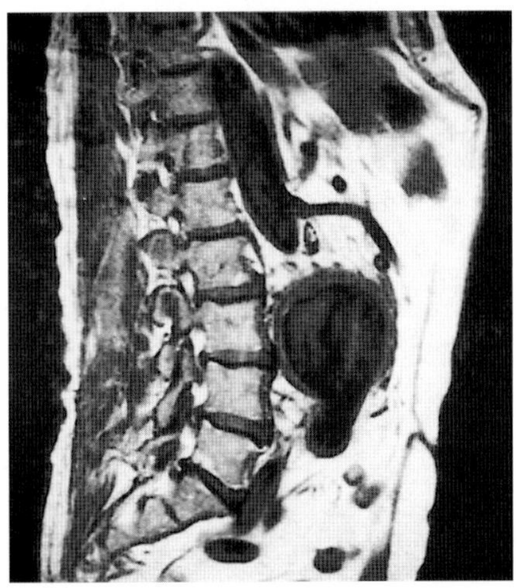

4-66

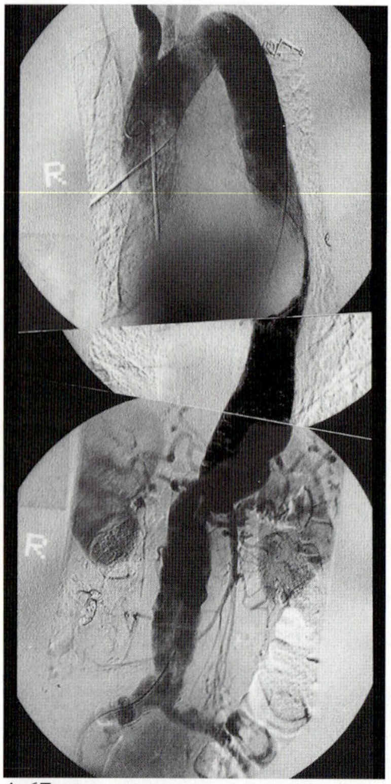

4-67

Fig. 4-67. Thoraco-abdominal aneurysm in a 53 year old man. Angiography from the aortic arch to the bifurcation only partially shows the aneurysms

Fig. 4-68. Computerized tomography at the appropriate levels shows both the thoracic and the thoraco-abdominal aneurysms

Fig. 4-69. Clinical appearance following reconstruction of a thoraco-abdominal aortic aneurysm using the Crawford approach (combined abdominal and thoracic approach with division of the diaphragm)

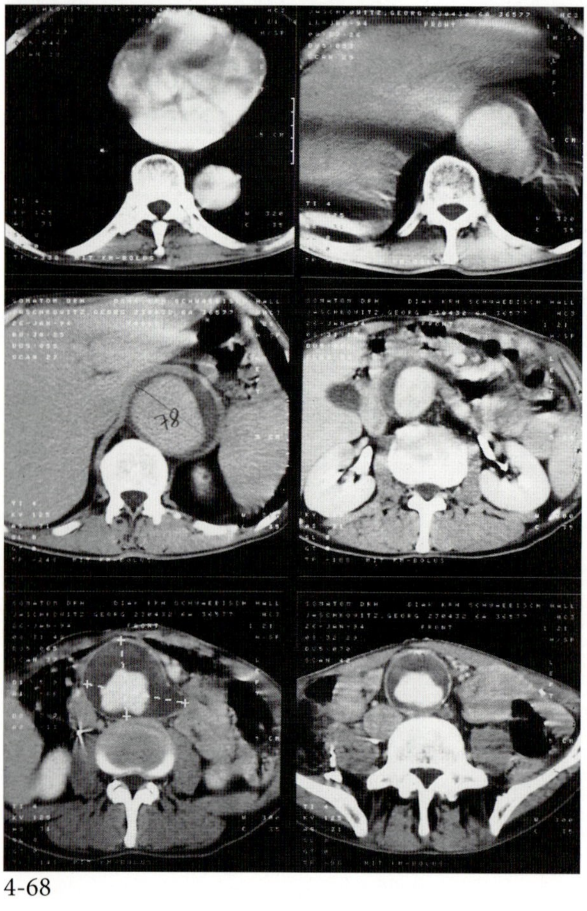

4-68

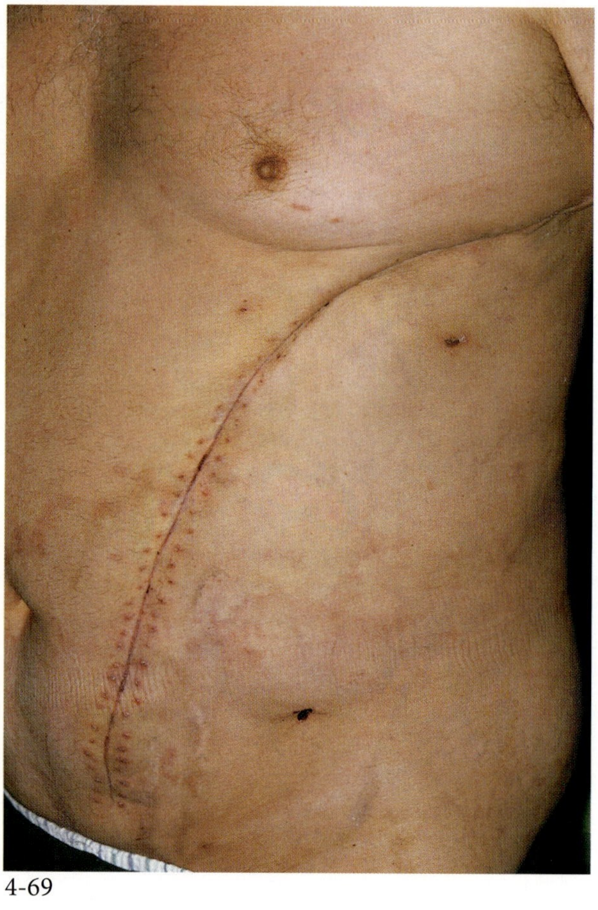

4-69

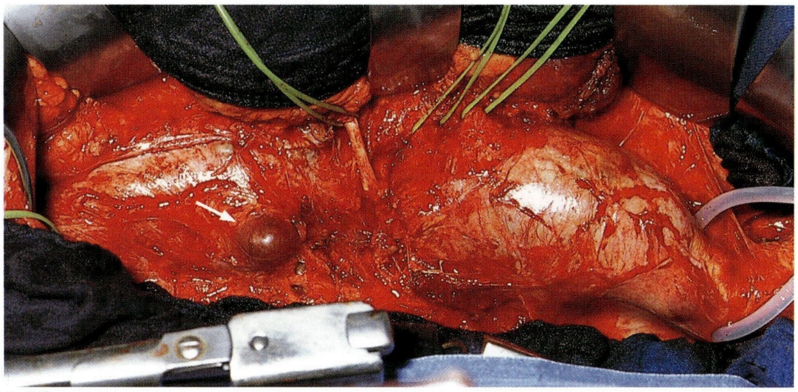

4-70

Fig. 4-70. Operative view of the Crawford procedure showing the thoraco-abdominal aneurysm. The visceral arteries are marked with green vessel ties while a saccular bulge in the wall is also present (*arrow*)

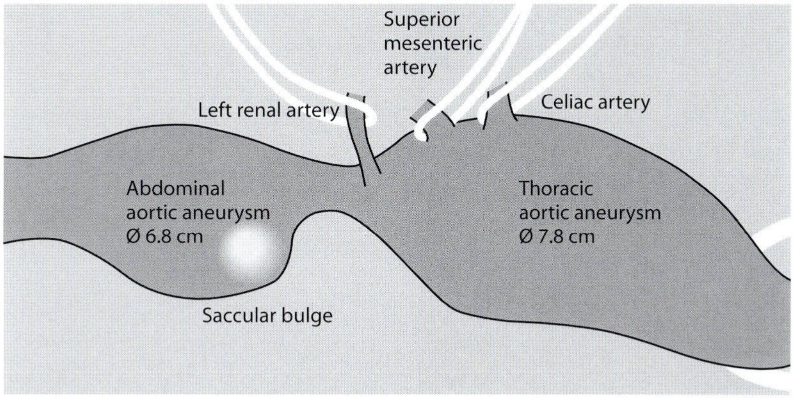

4-71

Fig. 4-71. Schematic drawing of the operative field

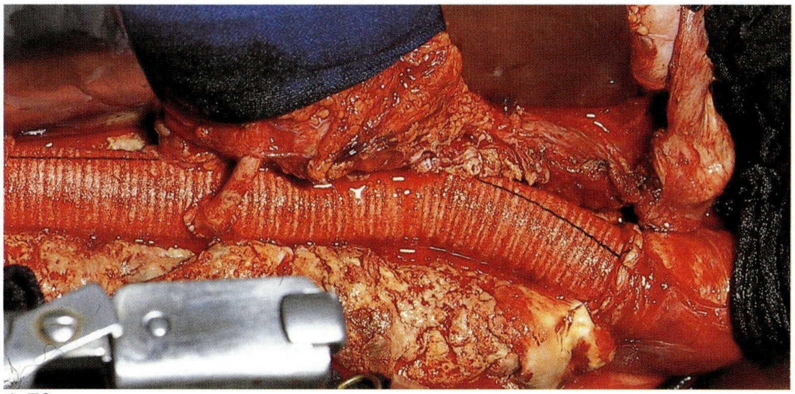

4-72

Fig. 4-72. Appearance following placement of Dacron prosthesis within the aneurysm with reconstruction of the visceral arteries and re-implantation of the left renal artery

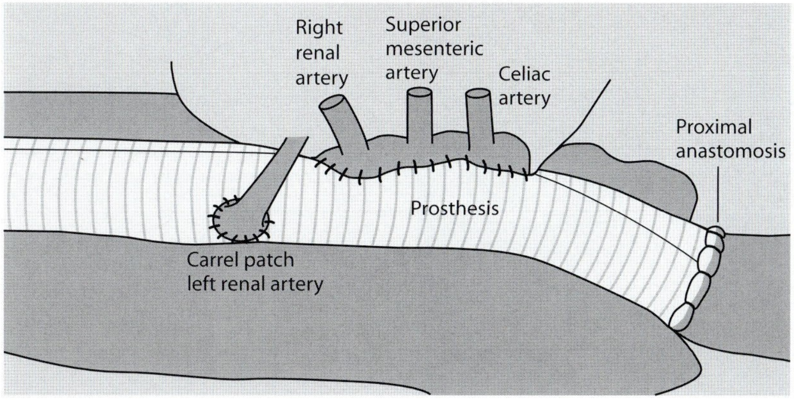

4-73

Fig. 4-73. Schematic drawing of the operative procedure

Supra-aortic Saccular Arteriosclerotic Aortic Aneurysm

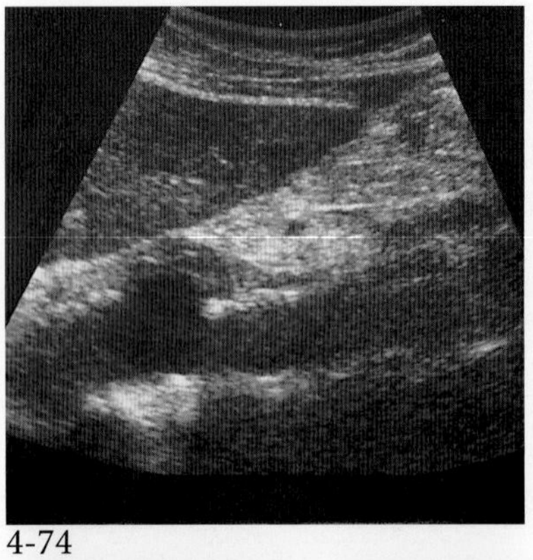

4-74

Fig. 4-74. Conventional view with ultrasonography

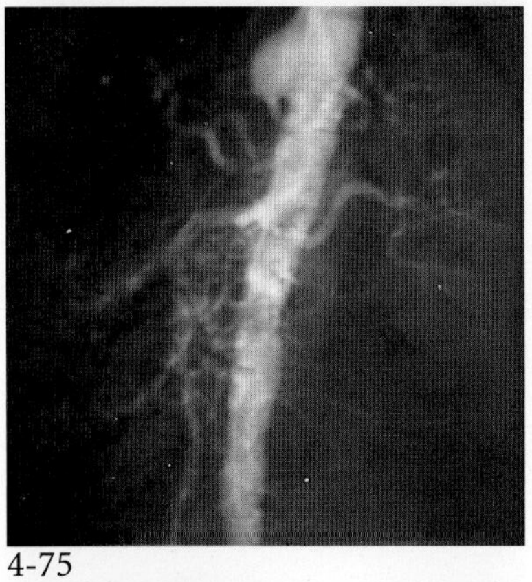

4-75

Fig. 4-75. Angiographic view

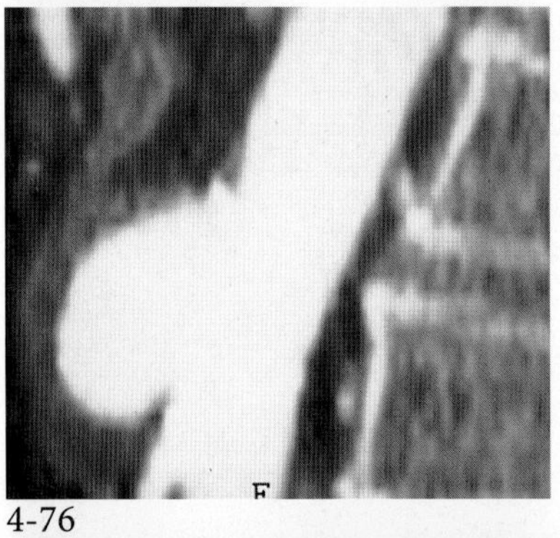

4-76

Fig. 4-76. Two-dimensional spiral computerized tomographic view

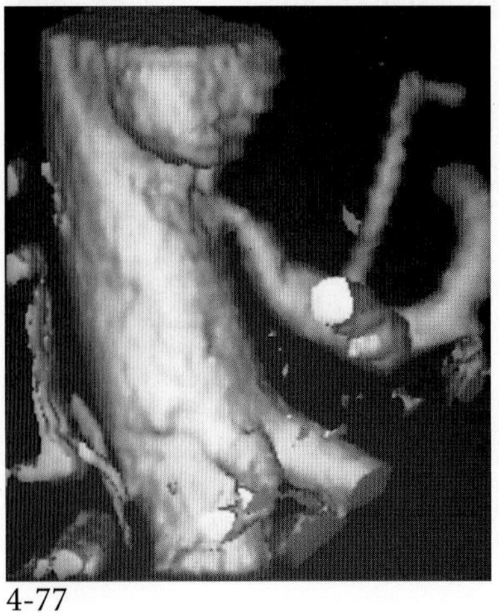

4-77

Fig. 4-77. Three-dimensional spiral computerized tomographic appearance, which offers the most detail

Figs. 4-78, 4-79. Infrarenal saccular arteriosclerotic aneurysm shown via angiogram and three-dimensional spiral computerized tomography

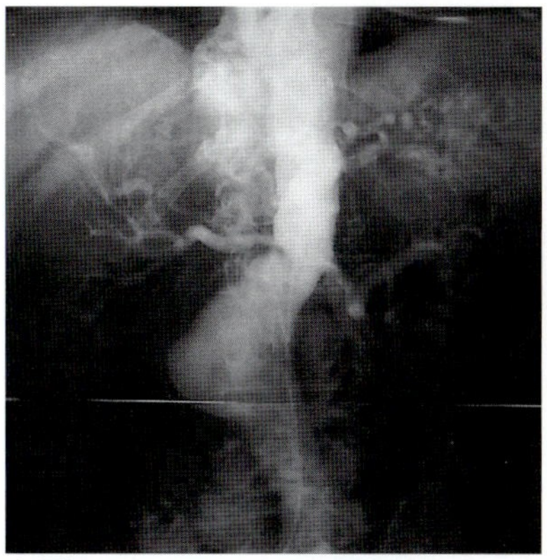

4-78

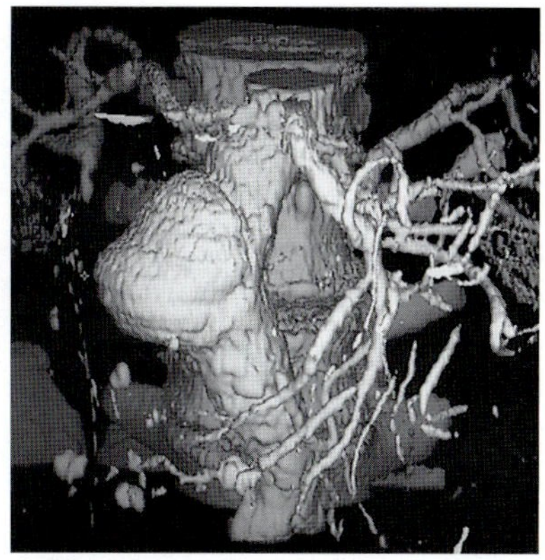

4-79

Fig. 4-80. Operative view of the aneurysm

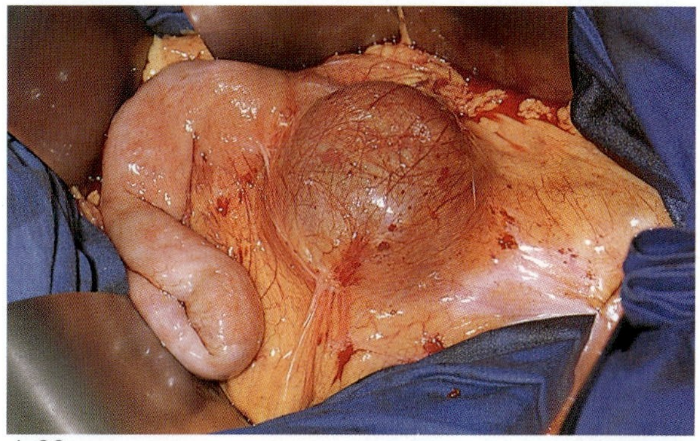

4-80

Fig. 4-81. Extremely large infrarenal aortic aneurysm with proximal kinking of the aorta as shown by three-dimensional spiral computerized tomography. The aneurysm is clearly lifted away from the vertebral column. Such an aneurysm may not be suited for endovascular stent-grafts; the best approach is an open surgical repair

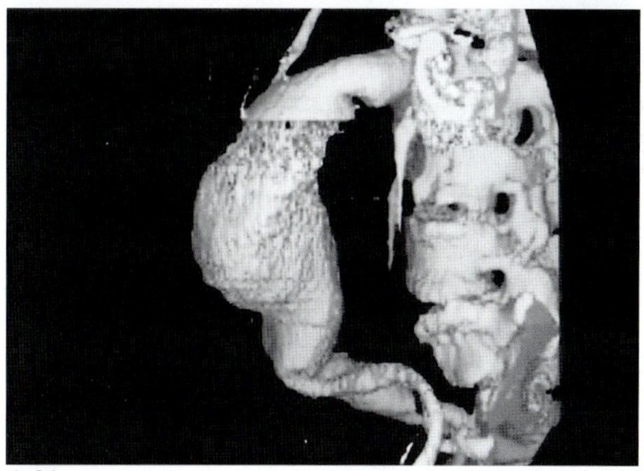

4-81

Fig. 4-82. Spiral computerized tomographic angiography of the lower aorta showing the visceral arteries, renal arteries and an infrarenal aneurysm, as viewed both from the side and from above

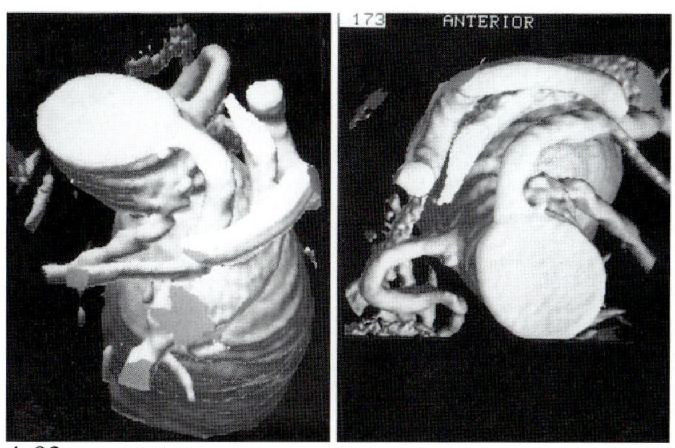

4-82

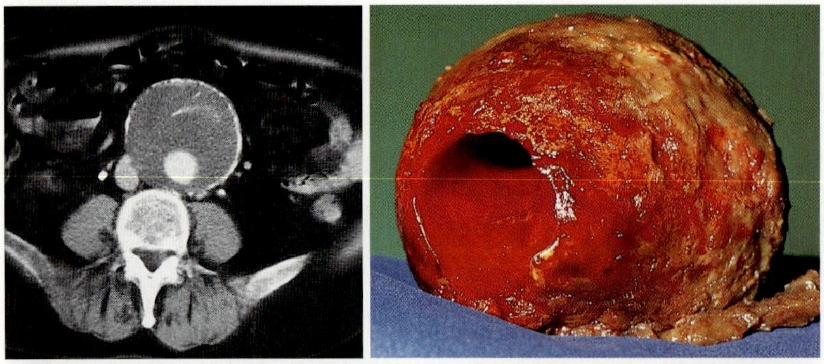

4-83

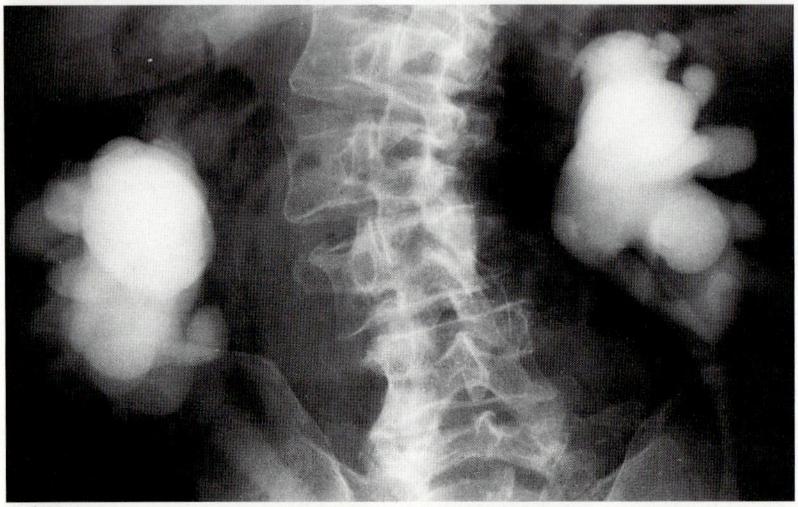

4-84

Fig. 4-83. Computerized tomography showing an infrarenal aortic aneurysm with marked thrombus. At the right is the surgical specimen showing the thrombus with a patent lumen

Fig. 4-84. Large abdominal aortic aneurysm with compression of both ureters, dilatation of the renal pelvises and cupping of the renal calyces

Fig. 4-85. Typical operative view of an infrarenal aortic aneurysm prior to opening

Figs. 4-86, 4-87. The same lesion after opening the aneurysm and implanting a Y-shaped Dacron graft replacing the aorta and part of both common iliac arteries. At the end of the operation the aneurysmal sack is closed over the graft

Fig. 4-88. Pre- and post-operative angiograms following placement of Y-shaped graft with bypass to right renal artery

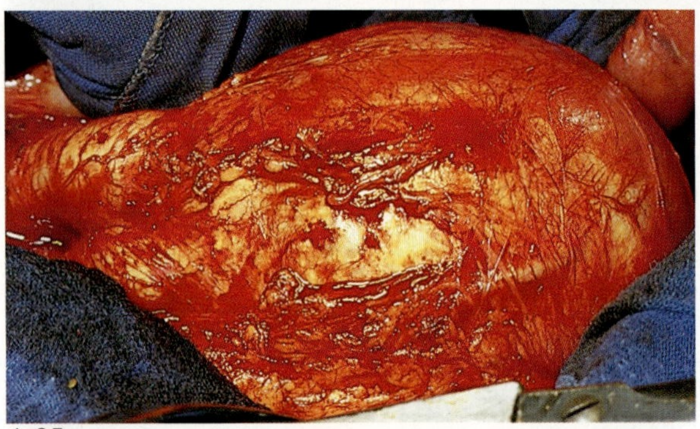

4-85

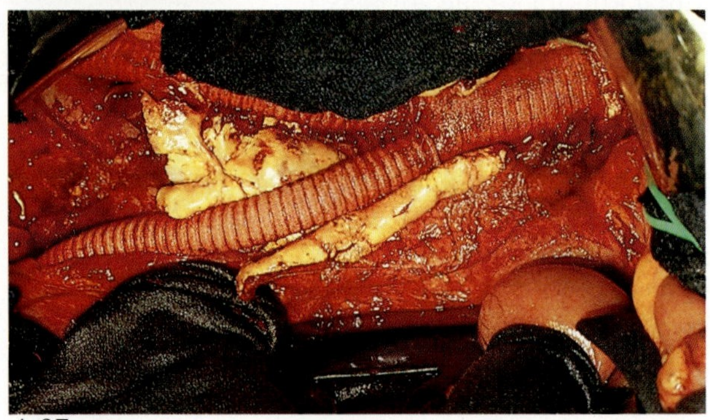

4-87

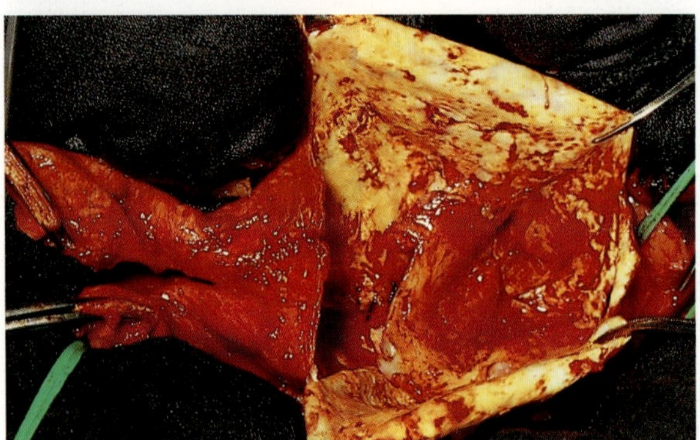

4-86

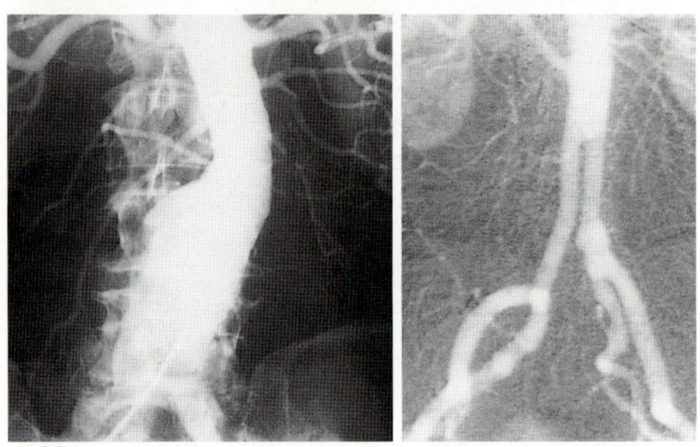

4-88

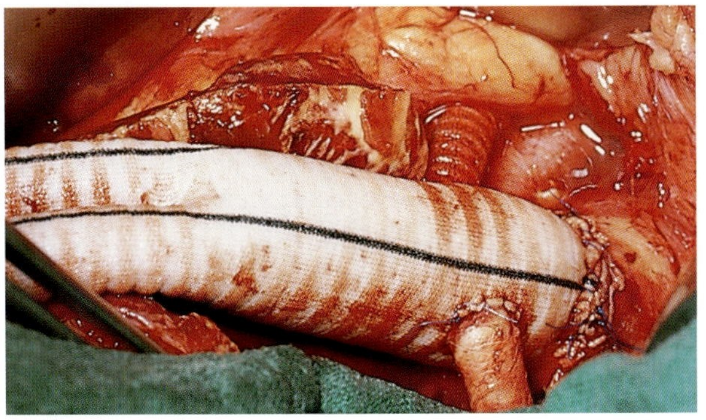

4-89

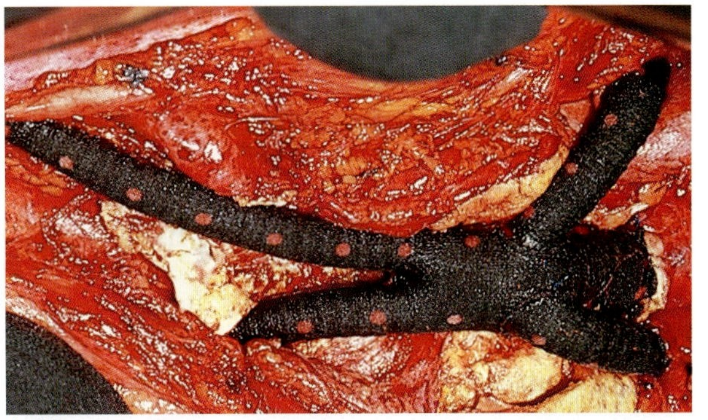

4-90

Fig. 4-89. Appearance following repair of an infrarenal aortic aneurysm. A Dacron graft is in place with the left renal artery re-implanted and the right kidney connected via a graft

Fig. 4-90. Operative view after repair of an aortic aneurysm with aorto-renal bypass grafts bilaterally

Legend to **Fig. 4-91 – 4-94** s. p. 98.

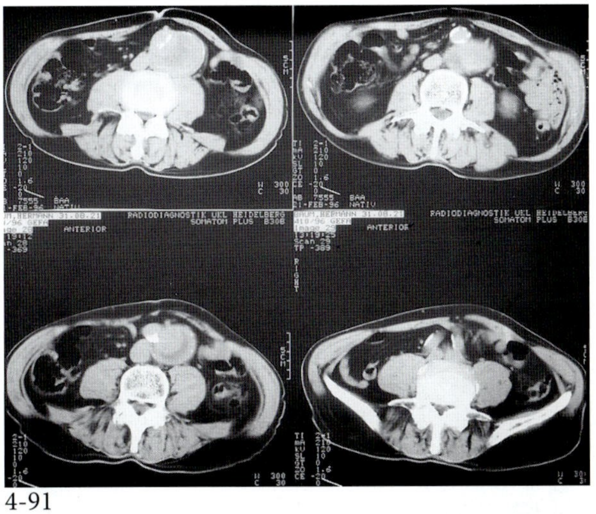

4-91

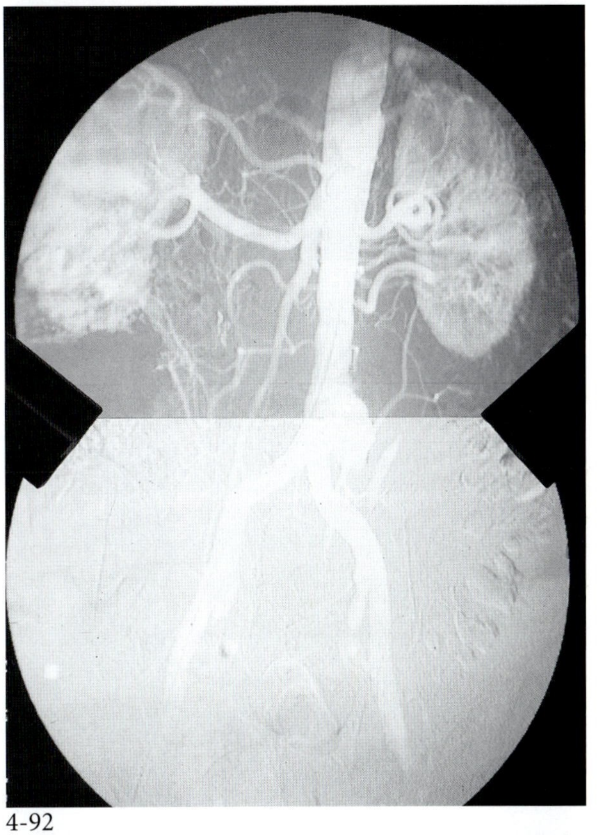

4-92

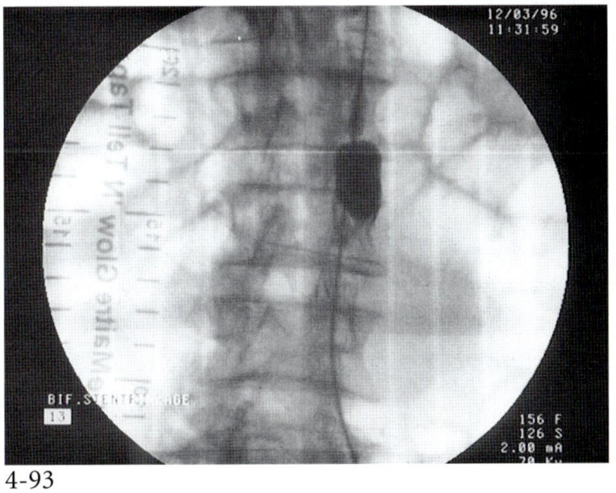

4-93

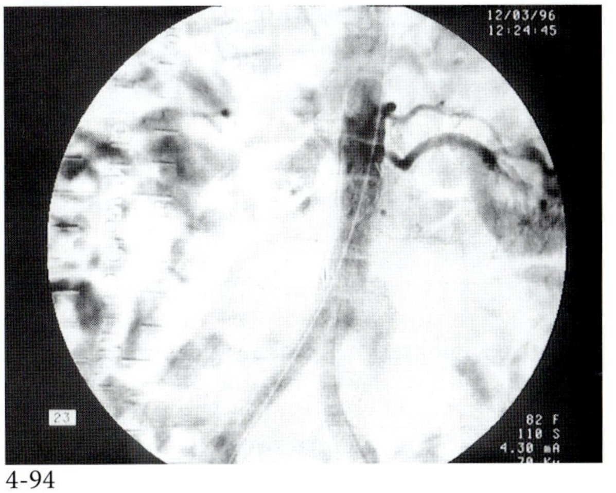

4-94

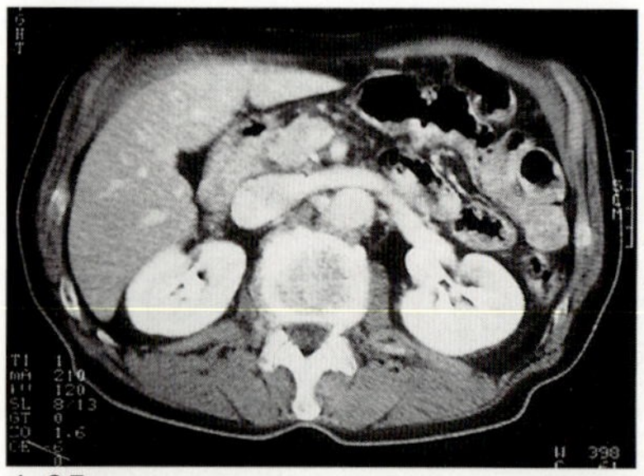

4-95

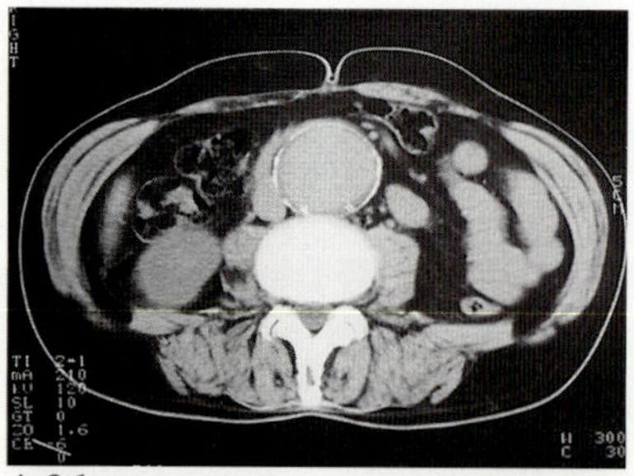

4-96

Figs. 4-95, 4-96. A 72 year old patient with an infrarenal aortic aneurysm. The proximal neck just below the take-off of the renal arteries is healthy so an endovascular stent-graft can be employed

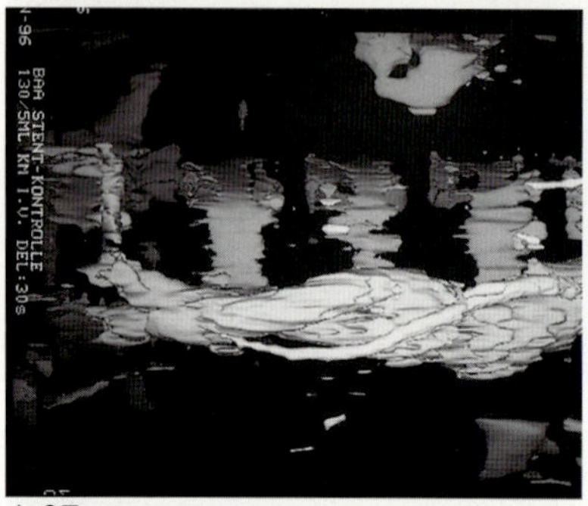

4-97

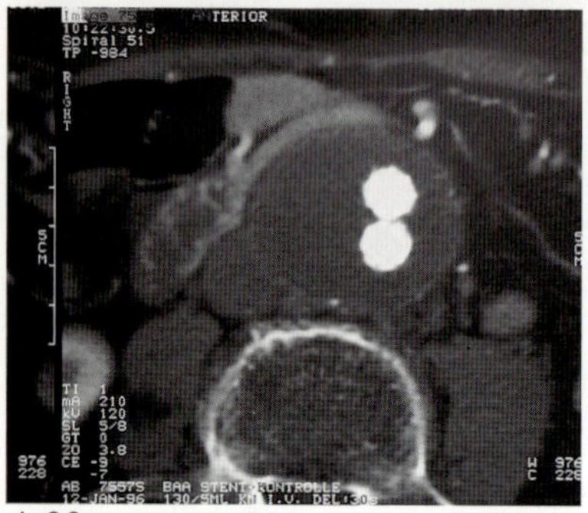

4-98

Figs. 4-97, 4-98. The same patient with a Y-shaped stent-graft in place. Three-dimensional spiral computerized tomography shows the patency of the stent-graft without any signs of leakage

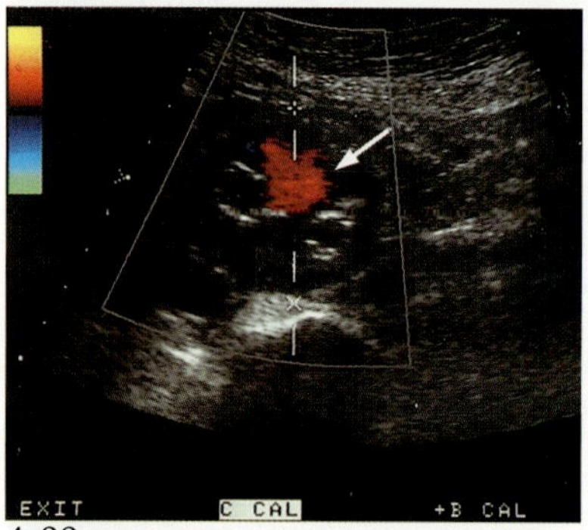

4-99

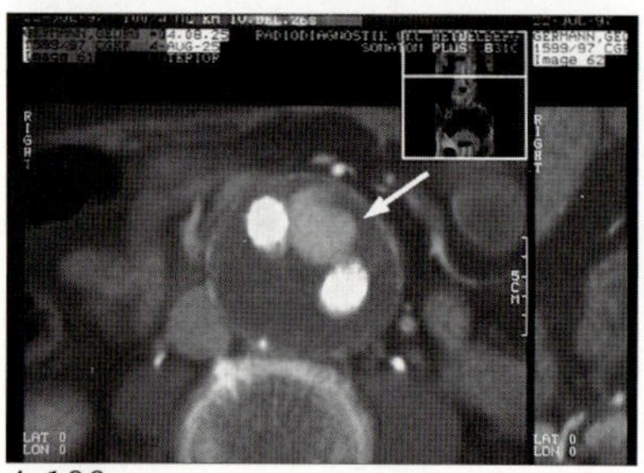

4-100

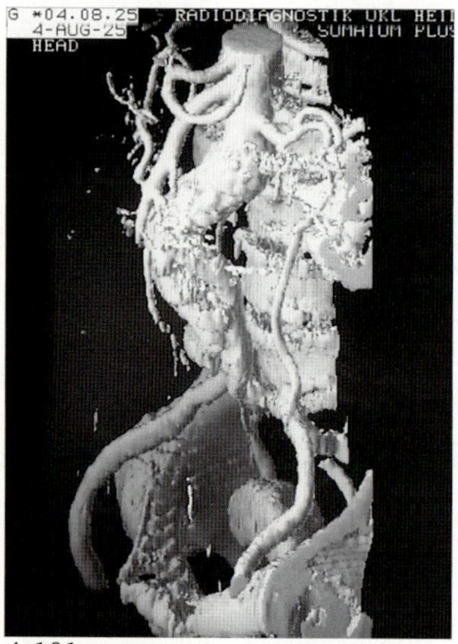

4-101

Figs. 4-99–4-101. In the same patient, ultrasonography shows leakage at the bifurcation of the stent-graft with the flowing blood color-coded in *red*. Computerized tomography also shows leakage of contrast material out of the right arm of the graft. Three-dimensional spiral computerized tomography demonstrates the blood exiting at the level of the stent-graft bifurcation with a bulge above the contour of the graft. Another endovascular stent-graft was placed on the right side but failed to seal the leak. Yet another stent-graft was inserted from the left side, producing so-called kissing stents. Despite these two measures, the endovascular stent-grafts continued to leak

Figs. 4-91 – 4-94. Case description: A 70 year old patient with an infrarenal saccular aortic aneurysm (Allenberg type A). In the preoperative angiogram only the residual lumen is shown. The computerized tomography shows the true extent of the aneurysm. The first intraoperative angiogram shows the positioning of the endoluminal stent-graft; the final angiogram shows the exclusion of the aneurysm by the stent-graft

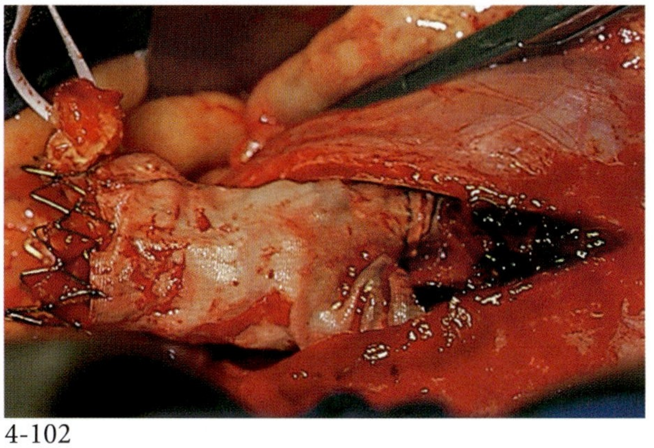
4-102

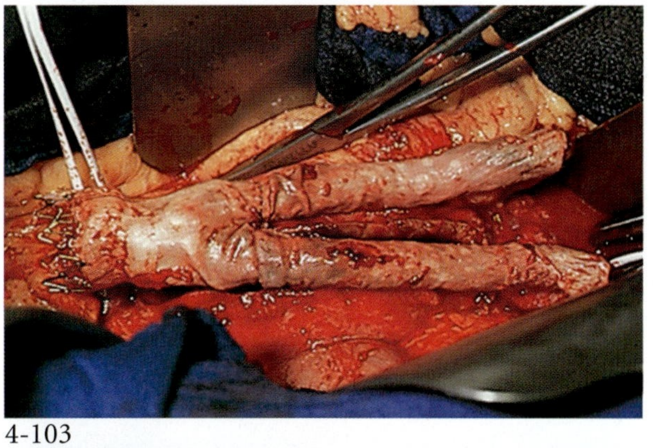
4-103

Figs. 4-102 – 4-106. Because of the persistent leakage and the failure of the aneurysm to shrink, an operation was performed 2 and 1/2 years after the stent-graft placement. In the operative field one can see the opened aneurysm with thrombi and the Dacron graft with the caged wire stents at the proximal end. In the next view the entire prosthesis is shown on top of the aneurysm. A cranial view shows the two kissing stents that were introduced to stop leakage. The actual defect was in the seam of the Dacron prosthesis just at the bifurcation. The final figure shows the appearance following removal of the old graft and interposition of a Dacron tube graft

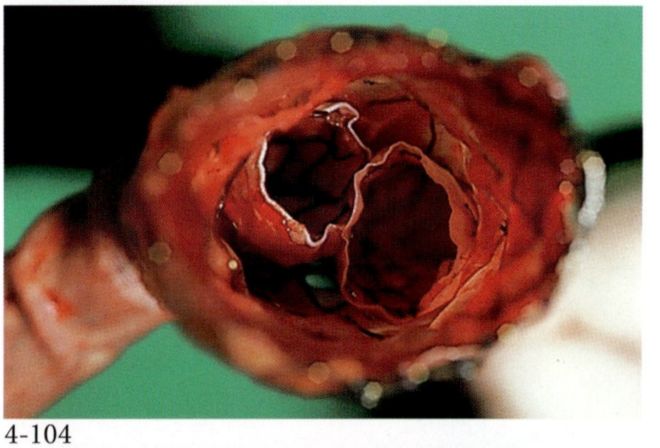
4-104

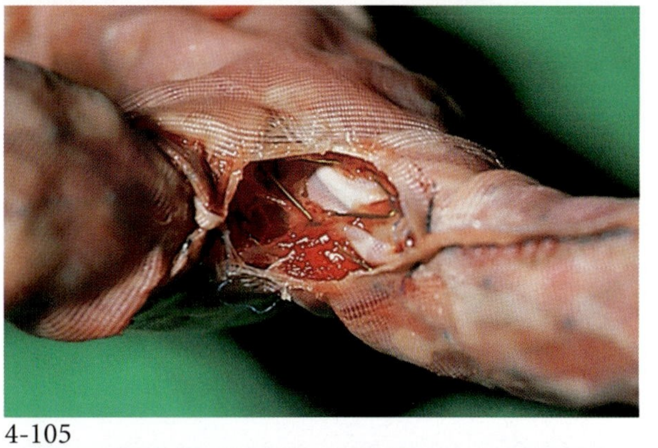
4-105

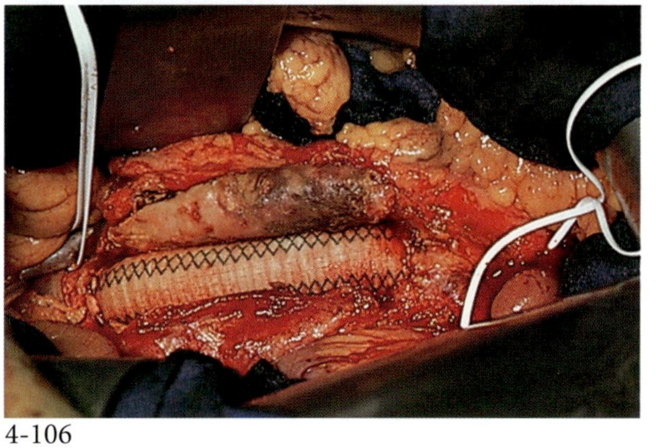
4-106

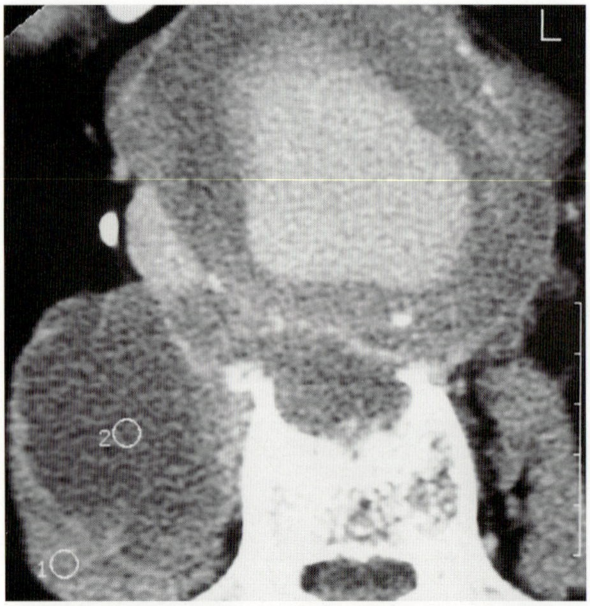

4-107

Fig. 4-107. Computerized tomography of aortic aneurysm showing erosion of the vertebral body and a contained paravertebral rupture. Numbers *1* and *2* show the thickness of the contained rupture

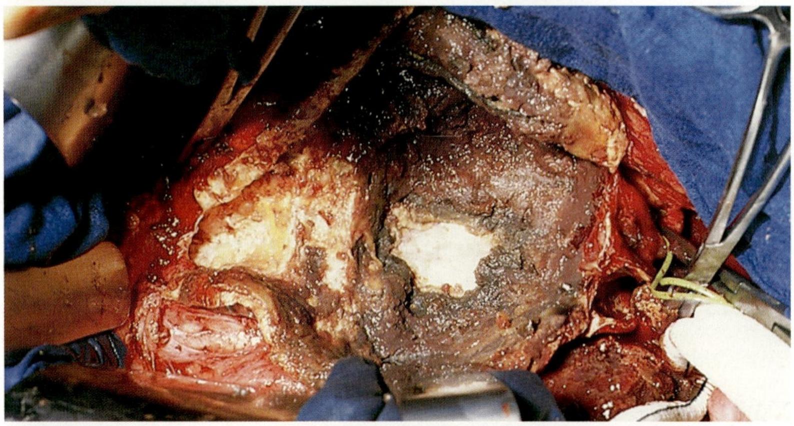

4-108

Fig. 4-108. Operative view with opened aortic aneurysm and view of the spine. The dorsolateral aortic wall is completely destroyed

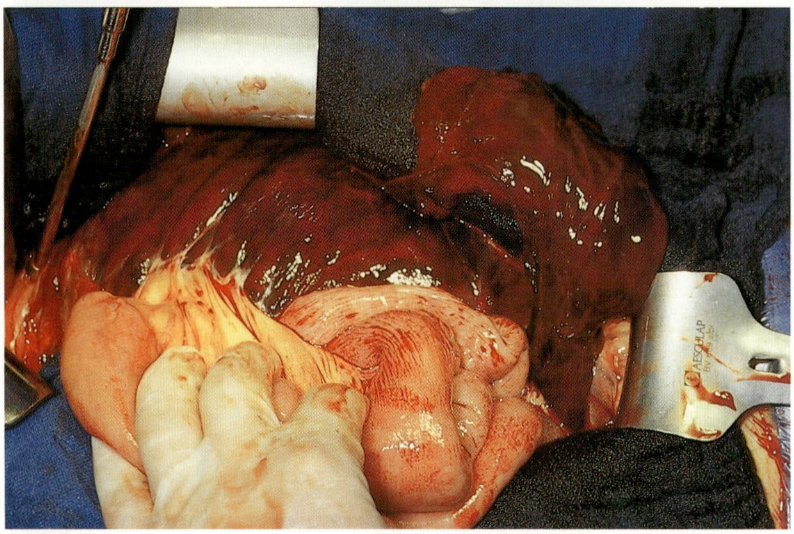

4-109

Fig. 4-109. A 42 year old man with spontaneous rupture of an aortic aneurysm with a retroperitoneal hematoma and clots in the abdominal cavity

Figs. 4-110, 4-111. Ruptured aortic aneurysm with contained retroperitoneal hematoma as shown with computerized tomography and in the operative field

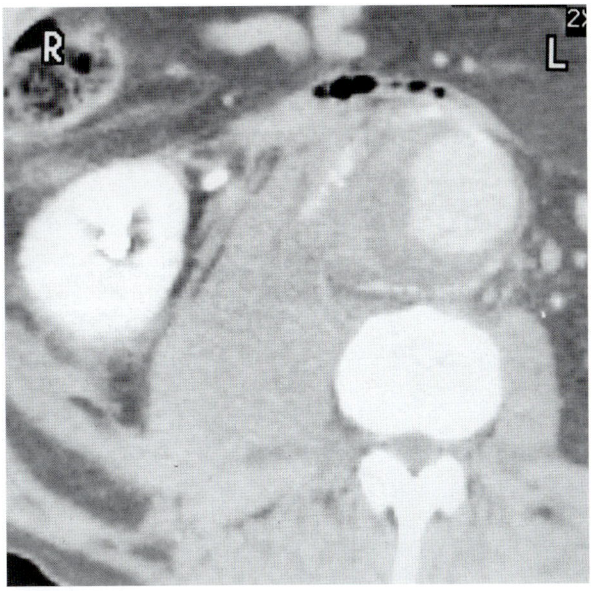

4-110

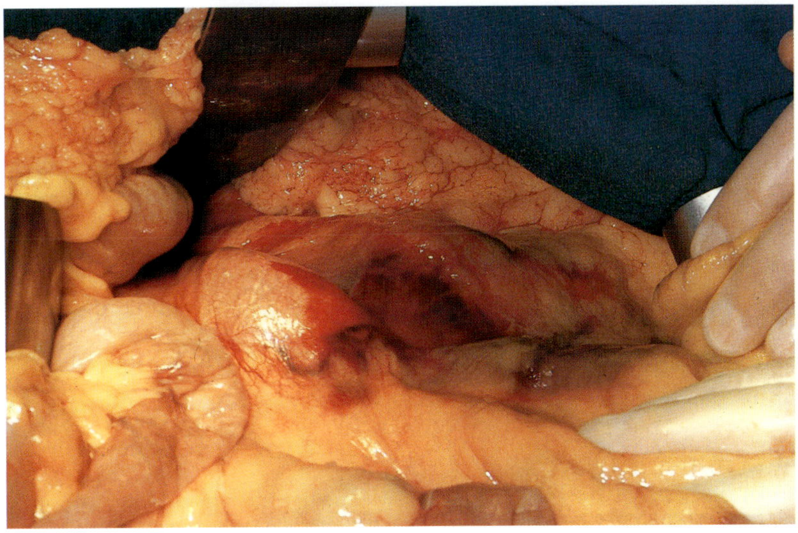

4-111

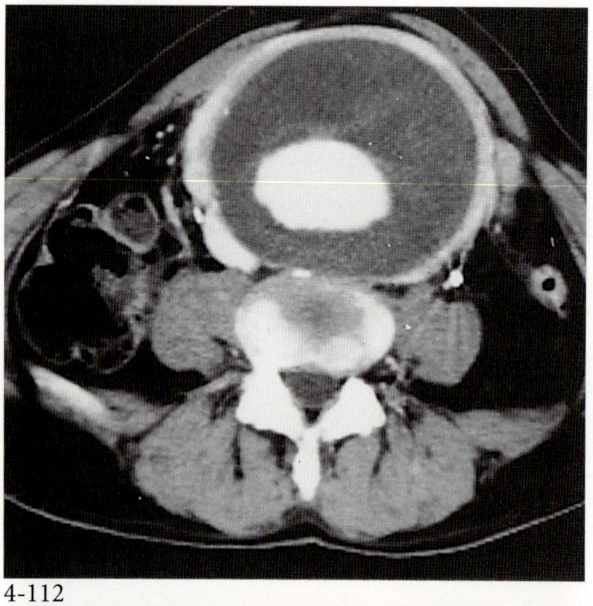

4-112

Fig. 4-112. Computerized tomography showing an inflammatory aneurysm. The inflamed wall shows marked enhancement from uptake of contrast material. During the operation, this part of the aortic wall was porcelain-like. The horseshoe shape is also typical, as often inflammatory aneurysms fail to involve the dorsal wall

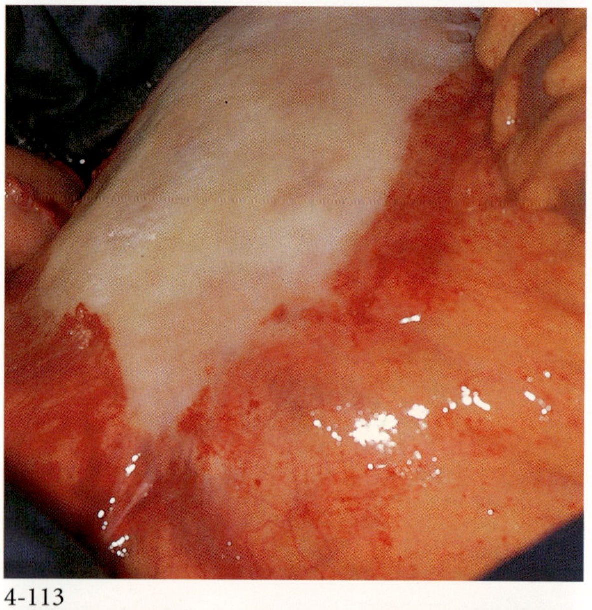

4-113

Figs. 4-113, 4-114. Classic infrarenal inflammatory aneurysm with porcelain-like anterior wall

Fig. 4-115. Histological view of the aneurysmal wall with two multinucleated giant cells and chronic inflammation

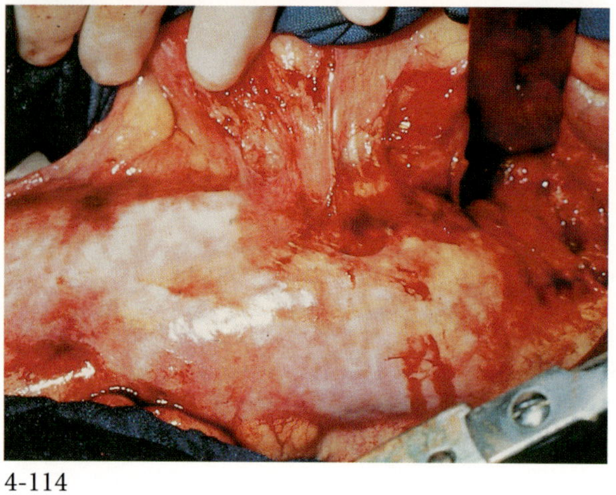

4-114

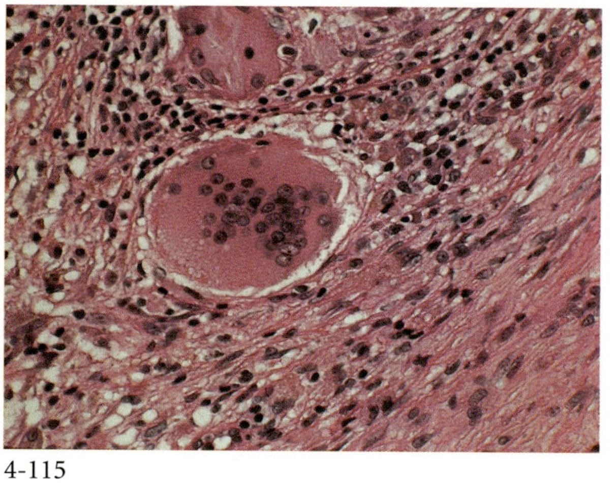

4-115

Fig. 4-116. False aneurysm at the proximal anastomosis 10 years after placement of an aorto-bifemoral Dacron bypass. The patient complained of marked back pain and had developed a fist-sized, paravertebral false aneurysm which was pressing against his vertebrae

Fig. 4-117. Post-operative angiography in the same patient following excision of the aneurysm and insertion of a new tubular graft with end-to-end attachment

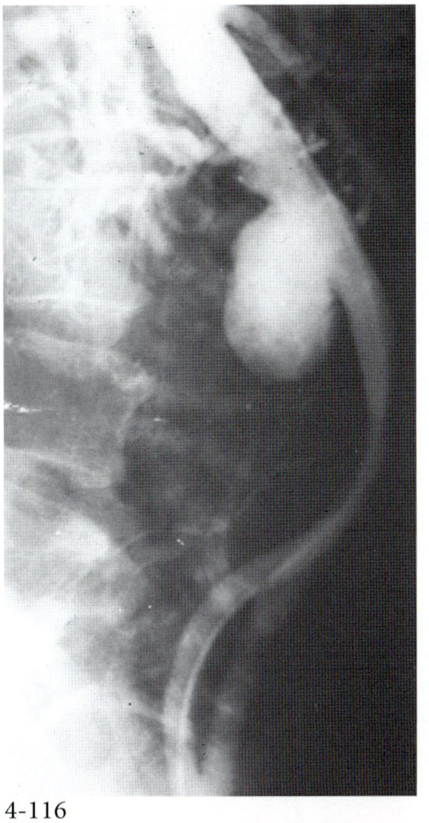

4-116

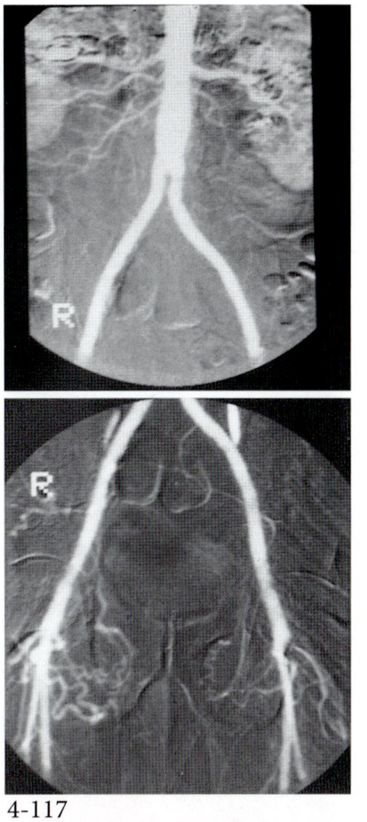

4-117

Fig. 4-118. Intraoperative view in the same patient. The Dacron prosthesis has been separated and one is looking directly into the false aneurysm. The base of the aneurysm is formed by the spinal column with the longitudinal anterior fascia clearly seen

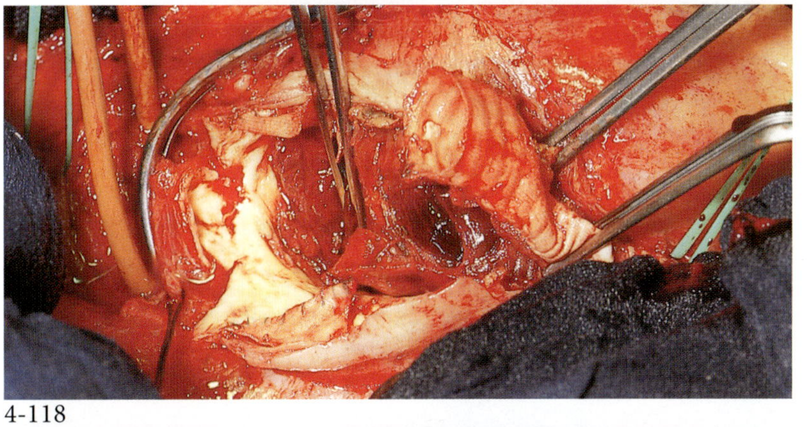

4-118

Fig. 4-119. Appearance following insertion of the Dacron tube between the infrarenal aorta and the original bifurcated prosthesis

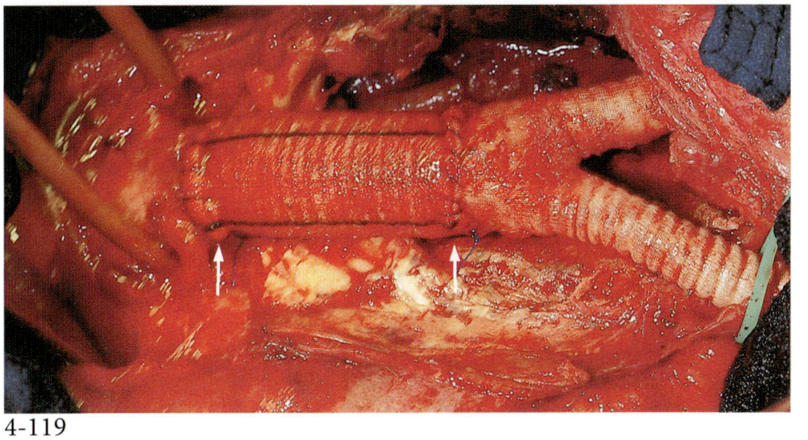

4-119

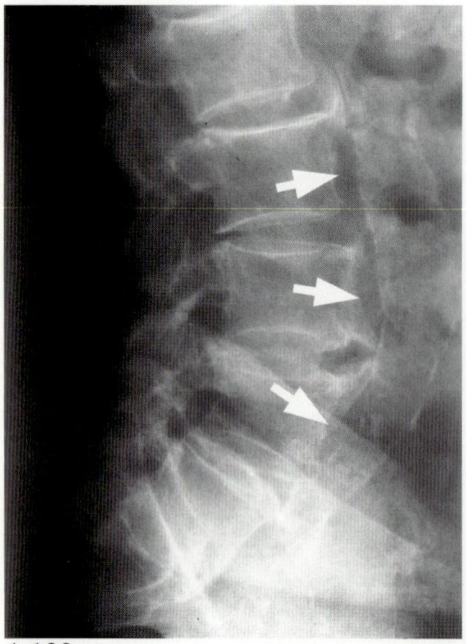

4-120

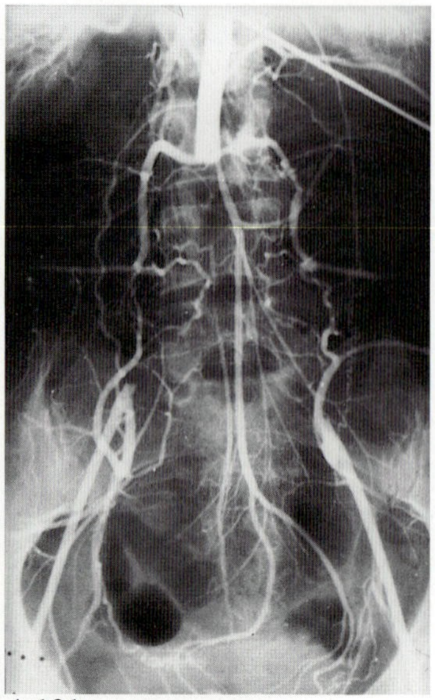

4-121

Fig. 4-120. Extensive calcification of the abdominal aorta (*arrows*) in routine X-ray

Fig. 4-121. Chronic occlusion of the abdominal aorta with good collateral supply and filling of both iliac arteries

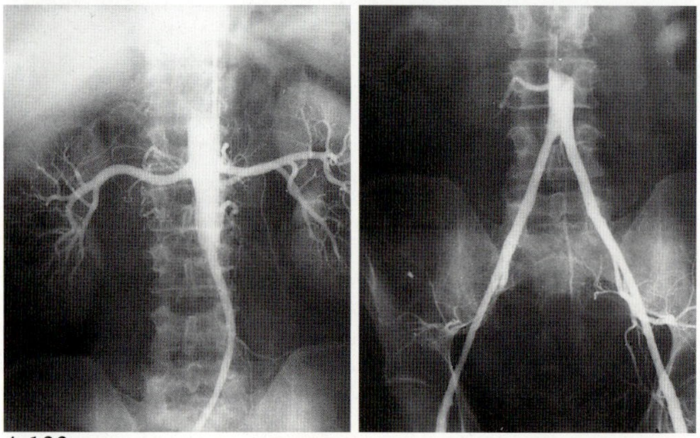

4-122

Fig. 4-122. Infrarenal arteriosclerotic aortic occlusion.
On the *left* a transbrachial angiogram is shown while on the *right* retrograde transfemoral angioplasty has been performed

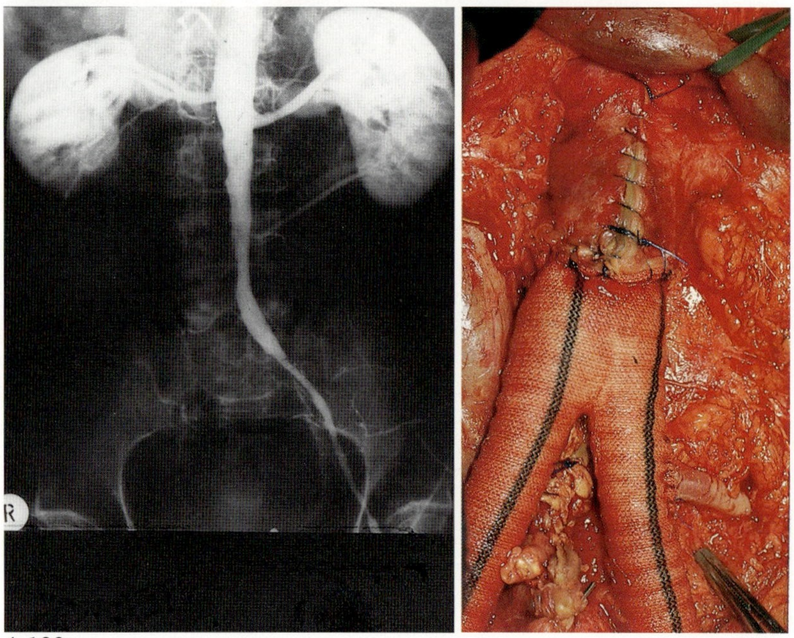

4-123

Fig. 4-123. Partial aortic stenosis with complete occlusion of the left iliac artery. Surgical repair included an infrarenal thromboendarterectomy and interposition of a Dacron bifurcation bypass

Fig. 4-124. Green prosthesis syndrome: development of a fistula between the graft and the duodenum. The endoscopic picture shows a green-tinged vascular graft. The dark stripe is part of the graft (*arrow*)

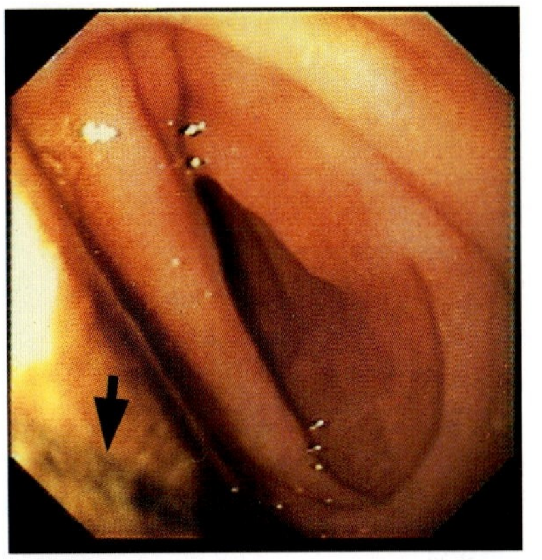

4-124

Fig. 4-125. In the operative view, one can see the repaired duodenal erosion (*two arrows*) and the green spots on the graft (*one arrow*) caused by bile salts

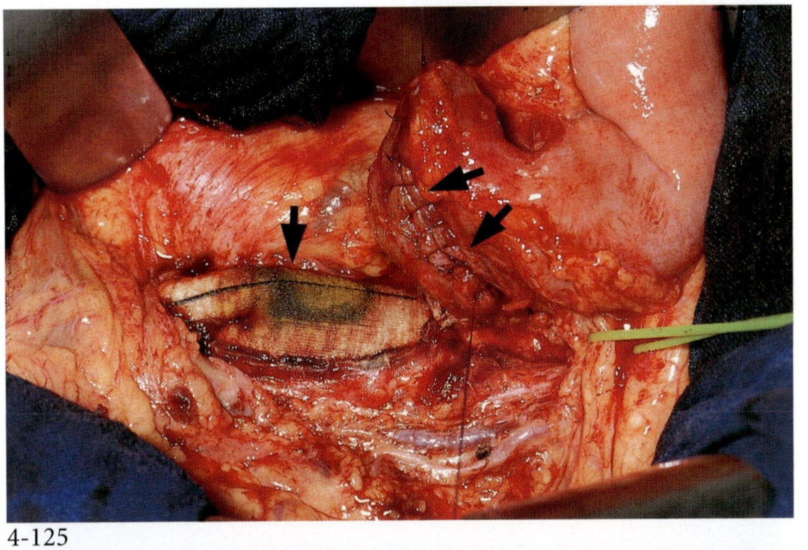

4-125

Fig. 4-126. To repair the defect, the graft was removed and an axillary-bifemoral bypass was performed, as shown in the angiographic image. Another approach would be to replace the graft with a new orthoptic one and do an omental wrap

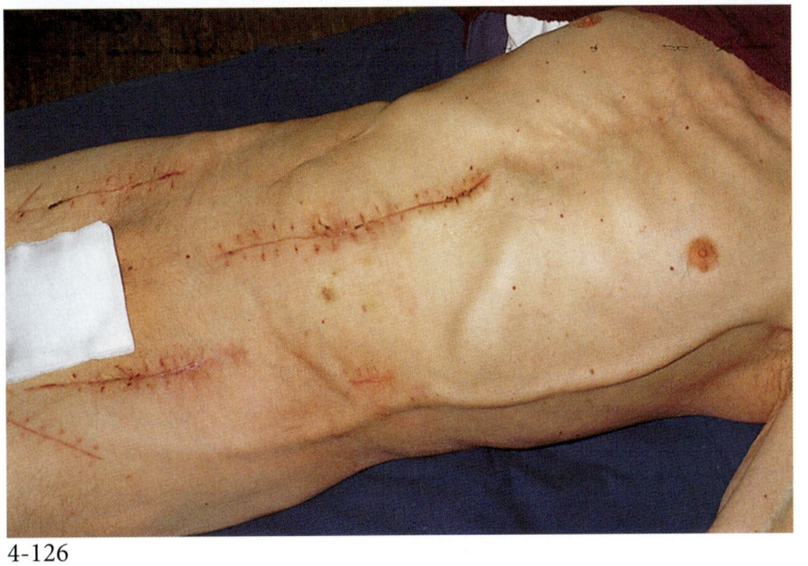

4-126

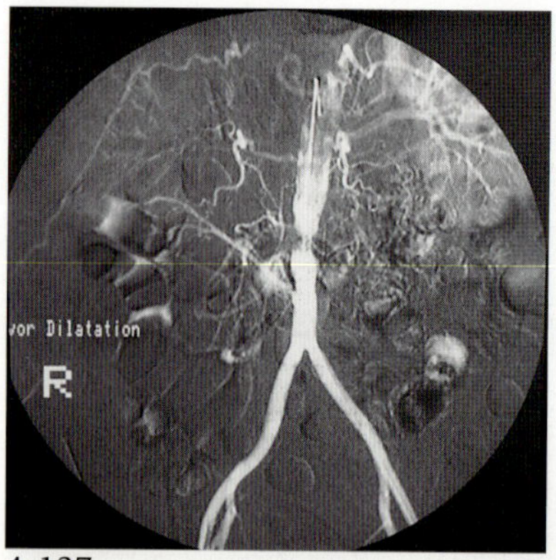

4-127

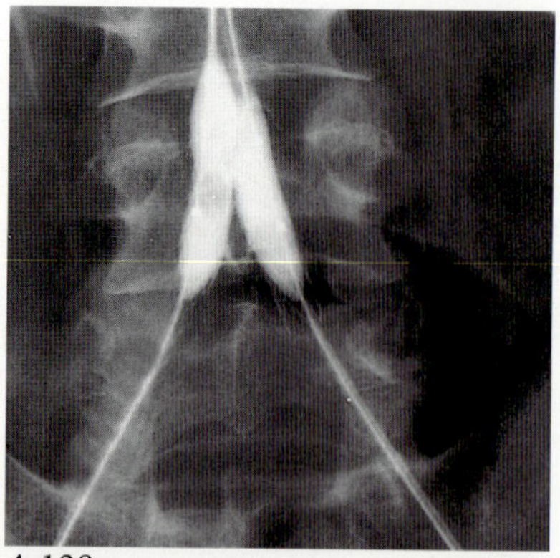

4-128

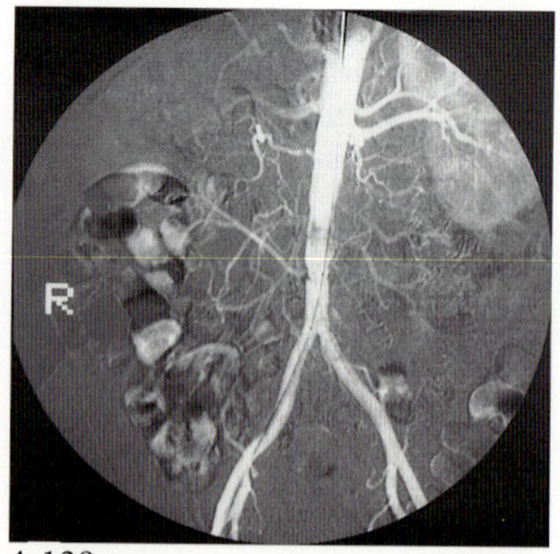

4-129

Figs. 4-127 – 4-129. A 51 year old patient with high-grade short infrarenal aortic stenosis with normal distal arterial pattern. Treatment was percutaneous transluminal angioplasty (PTA) using two balloons in the so-called kissing balloon technique. The final figure shows the appearance after the first PTA with slight residual stenosis

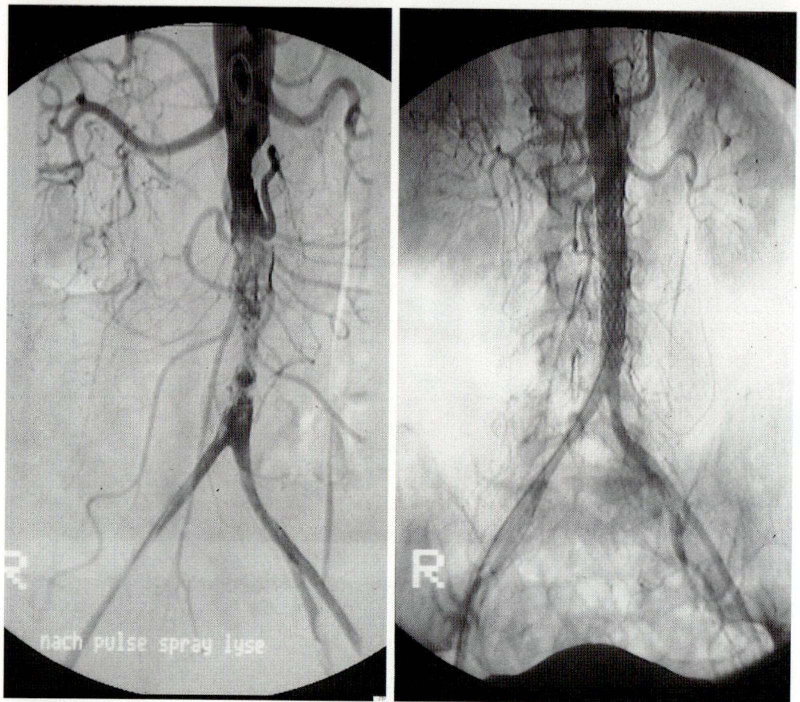

4-130

Fig. 4-130. Severe arteriosclerosis of the infrarenal aorta in a 76 year old woman. After dilation with a balloon catheter, the entire infrarenal aorta was braced with a Palmaz stent. The pre- and post-operative angiograms speak for themselves

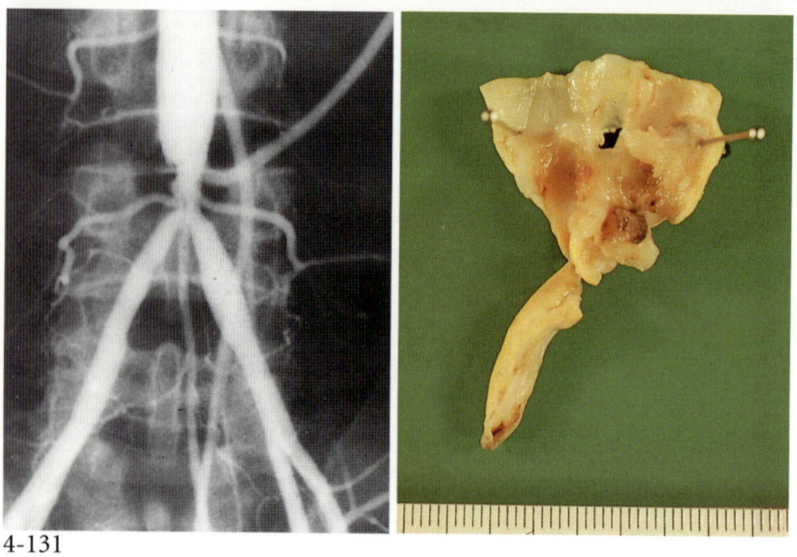

4-131

Fig. 4-131. Angiogram showing a short aortic stenosis, and the operative specimen following thromboendarterectomy (TEA)

Figs. 4-132, 4-133. Localized arteriosclerosis at the transition between thoracic and abdominal aorta with coral reef-like, hard calcifications in a 52 year old female. Computerized tomography without contrast material shows the circular aortic stenosis

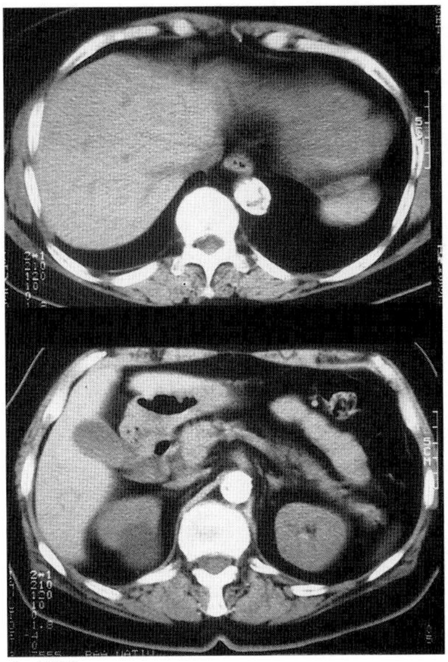

4-132

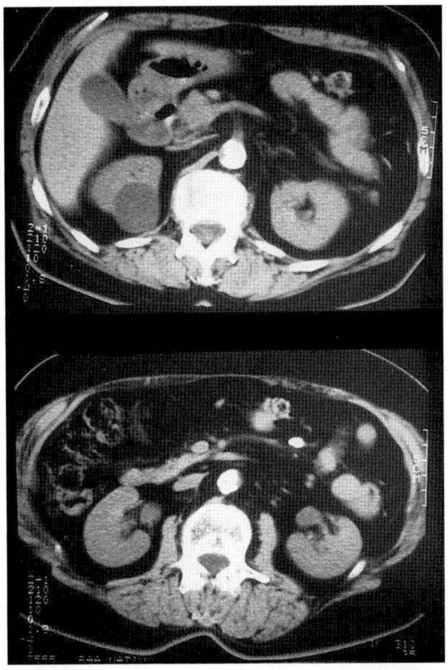

4-133

Fig. 4-134. Pre-operative angiogram from the same patient showing perfusion defect but failing to reveal the marked calcification

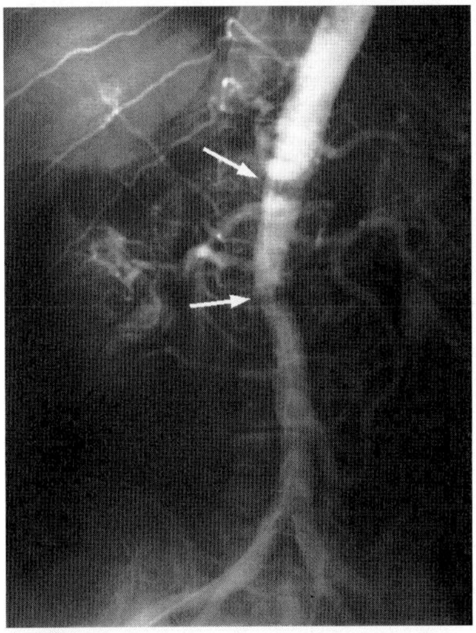

4-134

Fig. 4-135. Post-operative angiogram with aortic graft and re-implantation of both renal arteries in the graft. In the second angiogram the Riolan anastomoses are seen, including the connection between the inferior mesenteric artery on the upper left and the common hepatic and splenic arteries on the right

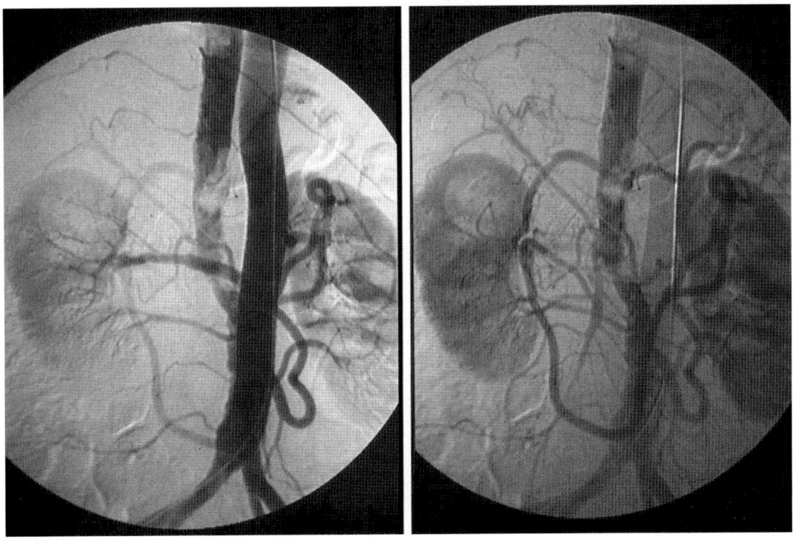

4-135

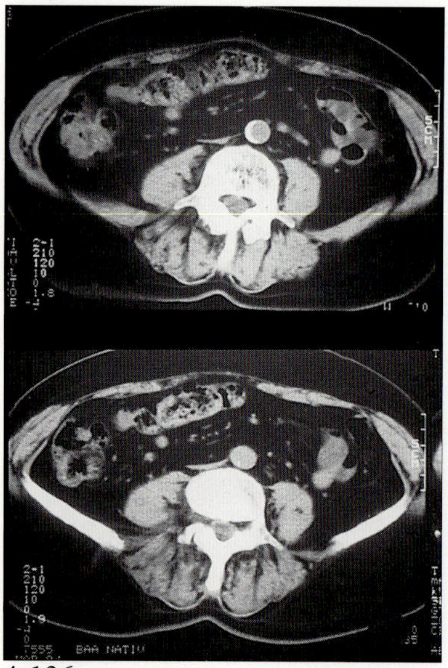
4-136

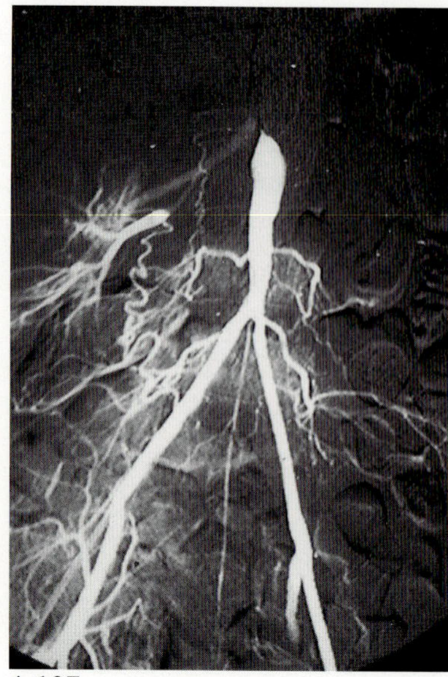
4-137

Fig. 4-136. Computerized tomography without contrast material of a 37 year old patient; the aorta is so calcified that it is contrast-rich. The abdominal arteries are heavily calcified, as in the coral reef syndrome. This patient had a motorcycle accident 15 years ago which left him partially paralyzed

Fig. 4-137. Retrograde angiography shows complete aortic occlusion at the level of the renal arteries with blockage of both renal arteries (filling was retrograde)

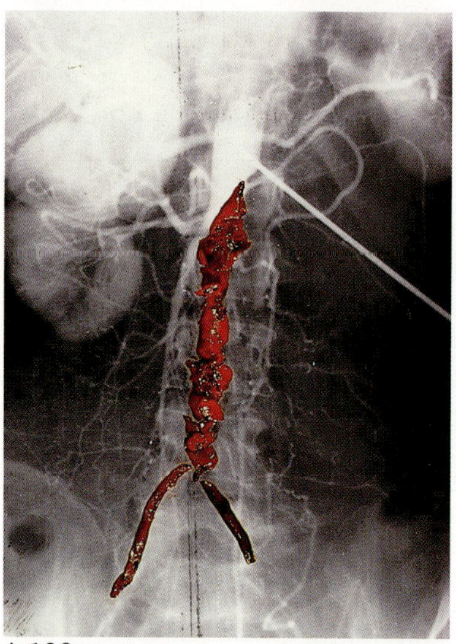
4-138

Fig. 4-138. Complete infrarenal aortic occlusion following a cardiac embolus in a 52 year old women

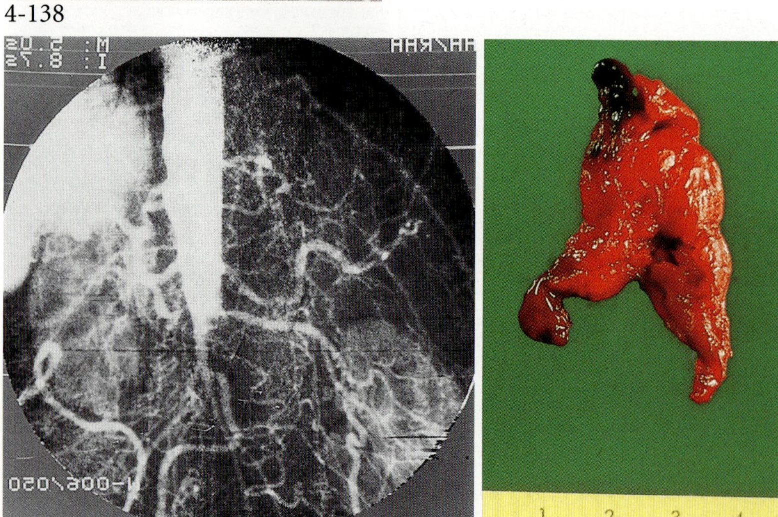
4-139

Fig. 4-139. Embolic occlusion of the aortic bifurcation –a so-called saddle embolus. Pre-operative angiogram and the removed embolus

Figs. 4-140–4-142. With acute aortic occlusion, initially the skin of the abdomen and legs becomes pale. As the circulation become stagnant, mottled or livedo changes develop

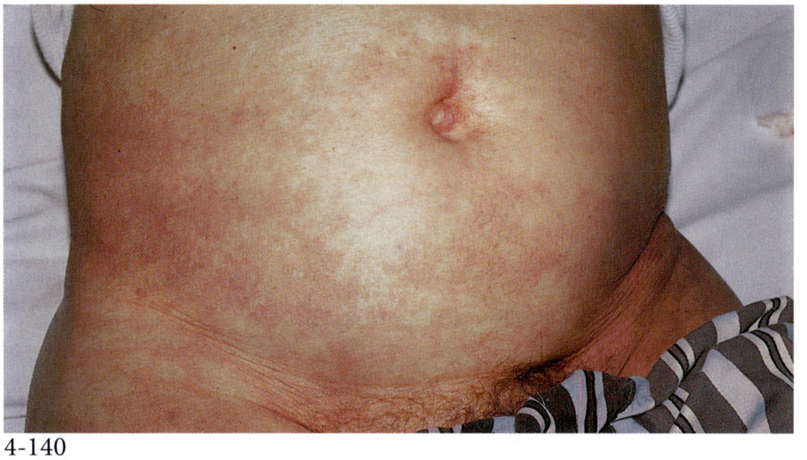

4-140

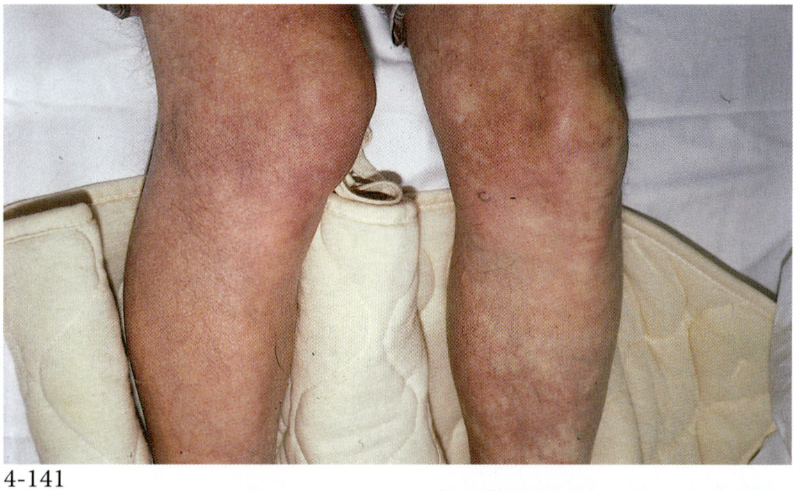

4-141

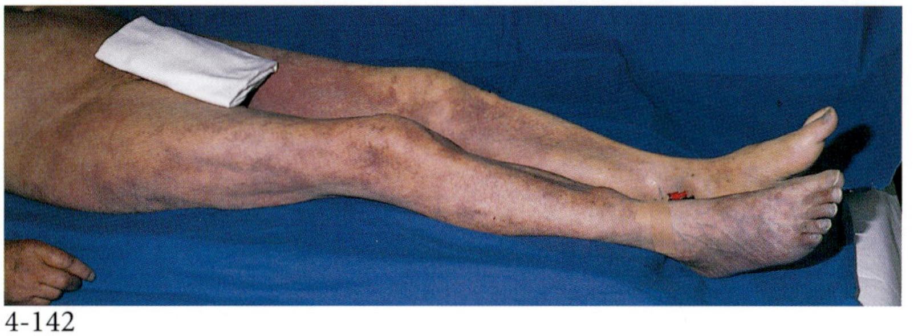

4-142

Fig. 4-143. Gangrene of the buttocks following acute occlusion of the aorta and iliac arteries

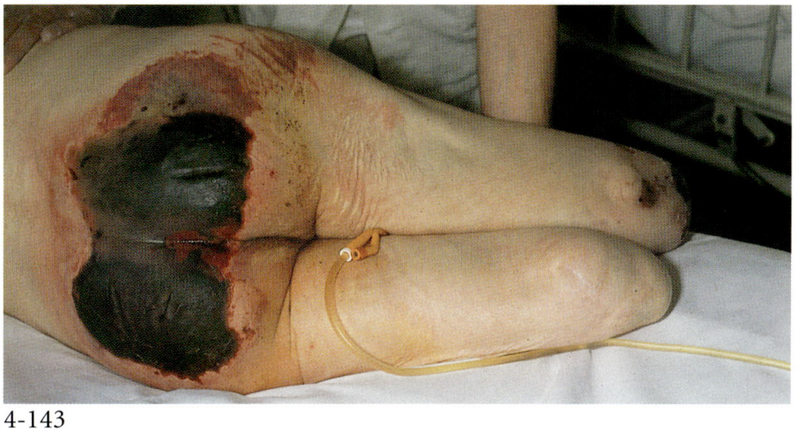

4-143

Chapter 5:
Arteries of the Abdominal Organs

CONTENTS

A: Introduction

1. Chronic Renal Artery Occlusion

History

J.H. Respinger first described renal artery stenosis in 1777. In 1836 Richard Bright, in London, first associated renal disease with hypertension. Tigerstedt and Bergmann discovered the renal substance which raised blood pressure in rabbits and named it renin. In 1934, the American physiologist Harry G. Goldblatt, in his classic experiments, showed that restricting renal artery flow leads to renal atrophy and hypertension. In the following two decades a number of patients with hypertension underwent nephrectomy. In the beginning of the 1950s, reconstruction of the renal artery was undertaken; Thompson and Smithwick, in 1952, performed the first repair of a renal artery stenosis, using a spleno-renal shunt. Freeman and colleagues did the first renal thrombendarterectomy in 1952, while later De Bakey and associates helped perfect the techniques of renal artery repair.

Epidemiology

Stenosis and occlusion of the renal artery lead to two major problems:

1. Development of renovascular hypertension
2. Progressive renal failure

Stenosis of one or both arteries is found in about 2%–5% of patients with hypertension (renal hypertension). In over 70% of patients greater than 60 years of age, autopsies show arteriosclerosis of the renal arterioles and smaller arteries (arteriolar nephrosclerosis), especially in patients with diabetes mellitus and hypertension.

- Some 75% of renal artery stenoses are arteriosclerotic.
- In 15%–20% of cases fibromuscular hyperplasia is found.
- Of the patients with arteriosclerotic renal artery stenosis, 60% are men.
- Of those with fibromuscular hyperplasia, 80% are women.
- In 25% of patients bilateral stenosis is present.

Clinical Features

Renal artery stenosis causes no subjective complaints, other than those associated with hypertension or decreased renal function.

Diagnosis

Non-invasive imaging is usually successful in clarifying the diagnosis.

- Sometimes bruits can be heard in the periumbilical region.
- Measurement of the kidneys with ultrasonography is helpful; if a kidney is 1.5 cm or more shorter than its partner, impaired circulation should be suspected.
- Color duplex ultrasonography allows visualization of the renal arteries (sensitivity 95%, specificity 90%).
- Intravenous urography.
- Isotope nephrography.
- Angiography: Either conventional or intra-arterial digital subtraction angiography allows a definitive diagnosis and a consideration of the therapeutic possibilities, including surgery, balloon dilatation and or conservative measures.
- Spiral computerized tomography.
- Magnetic resonance angiography and flow measurements.

Therapy

The localization and nature of the stenosis determines the surgical approach. If the renal artery is involved, but neither the ostium or the branches are affected, percutaneous transluminal angioplasty is reasonable. If the ostium or distal branches are involved, direct surgery is usually favored, although the introduction of stents may change this preference. The reconstruction techniques range from thrombendarterectomy with or without patch graft, resection with end-to-end anastomosis, re-implantation of the renal arteries in the aorta or aorto-renal bypass. Usually the patient's leg veins are used as bypass material, although synthetic grafts can also be employed. With extremely complex peripheral stenoses of the renal artery, occasionally the kidney is removed, the repair made outside the body and the kidney re-implanted.

2. Acute Renal Artery Occlusion

Etiology and Pathogenesis

The causes of acute occlusion include:

- Cardiac emboli associated with myocardial infarction, atrial fibrillation or endocarditis.
- Atherosclerosis of the renal artery.
- Iatrogenic following a balloon catheter angioplasty.
- Dissection following blunt abdominal trauma.
- Occlusion of the ostia because of aortic dissection.

Clinical Features

Small wedge-shaped renal infarcts are usually clinically silent. Larger infarcts may be associated with acute pain in the flank or abdomen, fever, leukocytosis, micro- or macrohematuria and elevated BUN or creatinine. If the occlusion is bilateral, oligo- or anuria can develop suddenly.

Diagnosis

The differential diagnosis includes pyelonephritis, nephrolithiasis, bleeding into a renal tumor, pancreatitis, abdominal aortic aneurysm and aortic dissection. Angiography is the quickest way to clarify the diagnsosis.

Therapy

The non-perfused kidney can tolerate ischemia for 20–40 min at body temperature. If the occlusion blocks an already stenotic area, there may be collateral circulation lengthening the survival time to days or even weeks. Suspicion of acute thrombotic closure of the renal artery mandates angiography and revascularization, even when the collateral circulation makes visualization of the peripheral branches difficult. Following repair, long-term coumarin therapy is indicated.

3. Visceral Artery Ischemia

Synonyms. Abdominal angina, ORTNER disease, visceral intestinal ischemia, acute intestinal ischemia, mesenteric artery insufficiency

History

Occlusion of the visceral arteries was first noted on autopsies. J.W. ELLIOTT, in 1895, first described acute mesenteric artery infarcts. Until about 1950, the only treatment was bowel resection, which had a mortality of 85%. At that time the first successful superior mesenteric artery embolectomies were performed.

"Cases of infarction and gangrene of the intestine due to thrombosis or embolism of the mesenteric vessels are not often seen... it is distinctly stated by certain authorities that such cases are beyond the help of surgery" (J.W. ELLIOTT, 1895)

Etiology and Pathogenesis

In 90% of the cases arteriosclerotic changes are responsible. In younger patients rarely TAKAYASU's disease or fibromuscular dysplasia may be found. The commonest cause of occlusion is a cardiac embolus. The ischemic tolerance of the intestines is about 120–180 min. In about 1%–2% of cases of acute abdominal pain, a mesenteric artery occlusion is found.

Clinical Features

- Acute onset
  - Severe abdominal pain, then a 24 h break and then once again severe pain as peritonitis sets in secondary to intestinal gangrene.
- Chronic disease
  - About 50% of patients have abdominal angina. The pain typically starts 30 min after eating, is usually periumbilical and can be colicky.

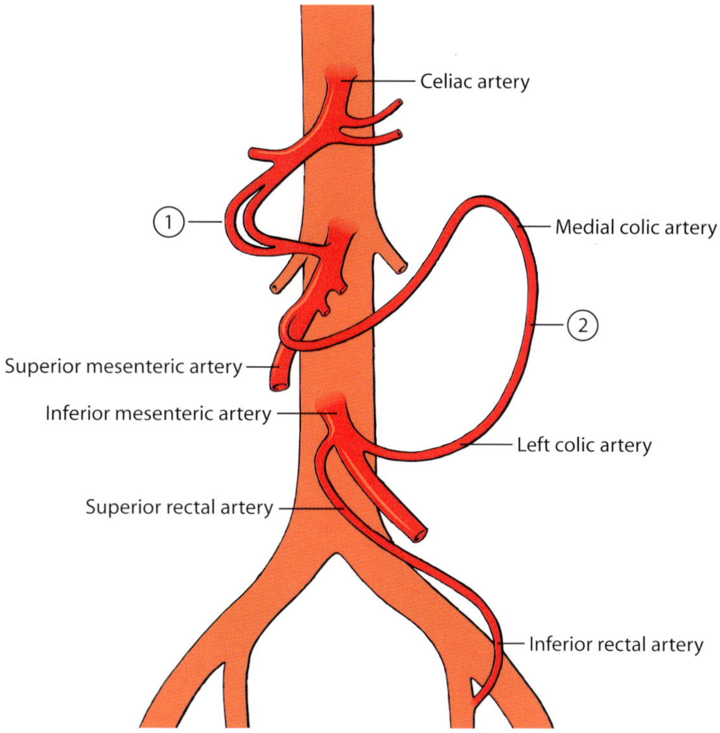

Fig. 5-1. Arterial supply of the abdominal organs with collaterals.

- Celiac artery (liver, stomach, duodenum, spleen)
- Superior mesenteric artery (pancreas, jejunum, ileum, colon)
- Inferior mesenteric artery (colon, rectum)

Collaterals exist between the celiac artery and the superior mesenteric artery (pancreatico-duodenal anastomosis, ①), between the superior and inferior mesenteric arteries (arc of Riolan, ②), and between inferior mesenteric artery and the internal iliac artery. (After Koller)

- Weight loss is very common (90%) as the pain discourages patients from eating. Often a gastrointestinal malignancy is suspected.
- Abdominal bruits (75%)

Diagnosis

The diagnosis is best confirmed by selective abdominal angiography. Endoscopic evaluation, computerized tomography and laboratory investigations can help exclude a malignancy.

Therapy

A timely operation is potentially life-saving in acute embolic mesenteric artery occlusion. Often this diagnosis is made too late, as the brief pain-free interval misleads the physician. About 65% of the usually older patients, who often have multiple associated diseases and are poor operative risks, die prior to or during the operation. Usually the surgical procedure is an embolectomy via either a transverse or vertical incision in the artery and simple closure. Only rarely are reconstructive procedures such as a thrombendarterectomy or a bypass needed. They may be required in individuals with severe arteriosclerotic disease and abdominal angina.

B: Supplementary Figures and Legends

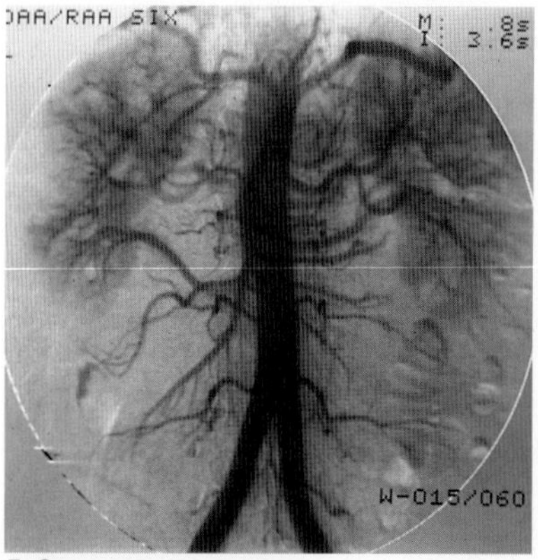

5-2

Fig. 5-2. Multiple renal arteries arising from aorta. The frequency of anomalies in the renal arteries is about 30%, including multiple arteries and early division. In 70% of individuals there is a single renal artery on each side

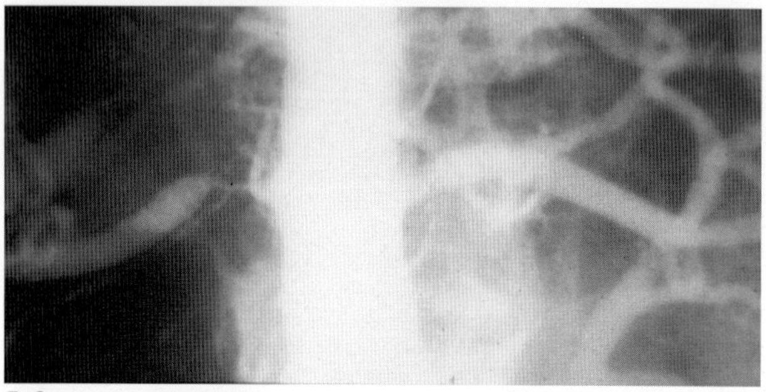

5-3

Fig. 5-3. Angiography showing a right-sided renal artery stenosis. It is difficult to determine if the ostium or post-ostial segment is involved

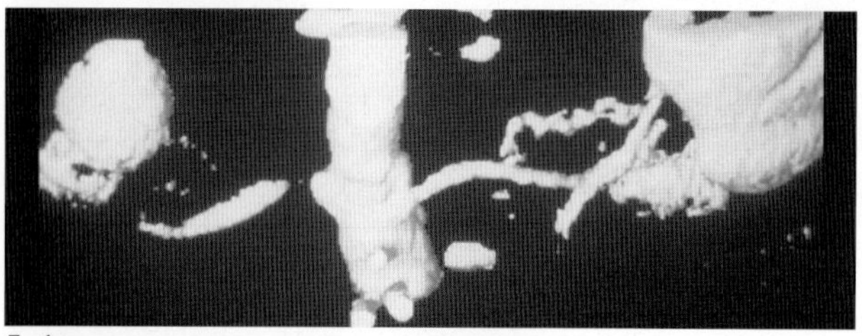

5-4

Fig. 5-4. The same stenosis viewed with spiral computerized tomography is clearly post-ostial

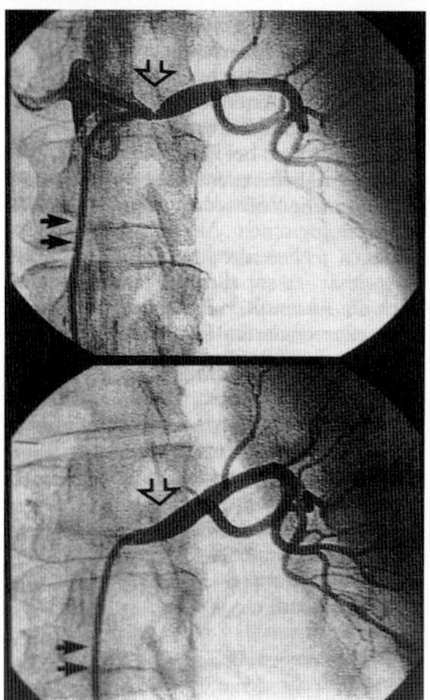

5-5

Fig. 5-5. Percutaneous transluminal angioplasty of a renal artery stenosis (*arrow*). *Above*, the pre-operative angiogram; *below*, following balloon dilatation

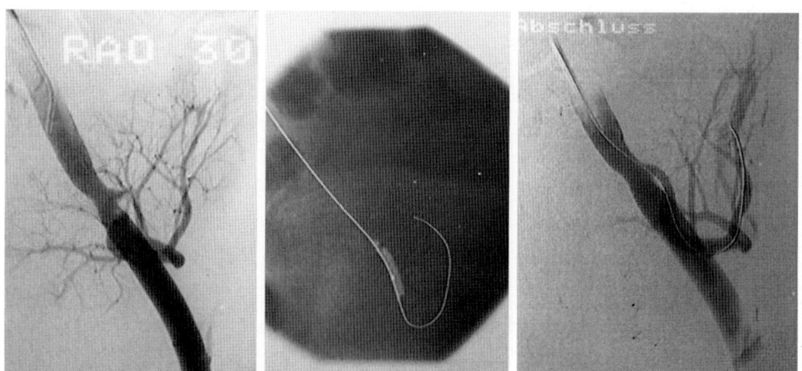

5-6

Fig. 5-6. A transplanted kidney with proximal stenosis of the renal artery. At *left*, the pre-operative angiogram; in the *middle*, the dilatation catheter is in place; at *right*, following balloon dilatation

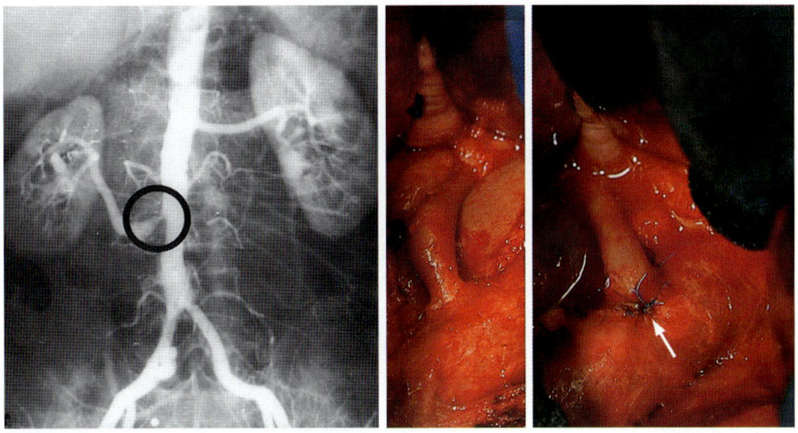

5-7

Fig. 5-7. High-grade renal artery stenosis at the ostium of an anomalous artery running in front of the vena cava. At *right*, the operative field following resection of the stenosis and reimplantation (*arrow*)

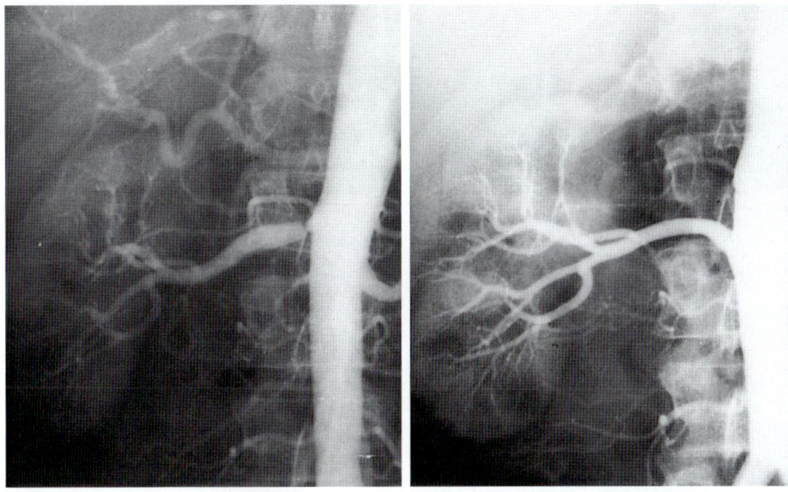

5-8

Fig. 5-8. Typical stenosis near the ostium before and after excision and re-implantation of the renal artery

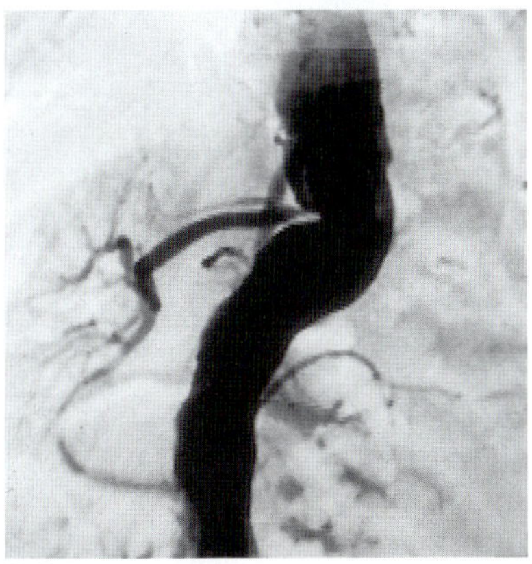

5-9

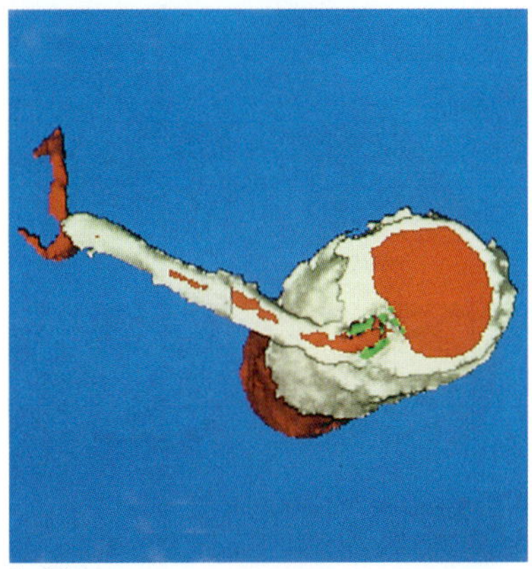

5-10

Fig. 5-9. An angiogram from a patient with severe athero-sclerosis of the aorta. There is occlusion of the left renal artery and high-grade stenosis of the right. A renal artery stent was placed in the right ostium

Fig. 5-10. The color three-dimensional spiral computerized tomography shows that the plaque is in the aorta and extends into the ostium of the renal artery; *simple* dilatation of such a stenosis can be expected to fail

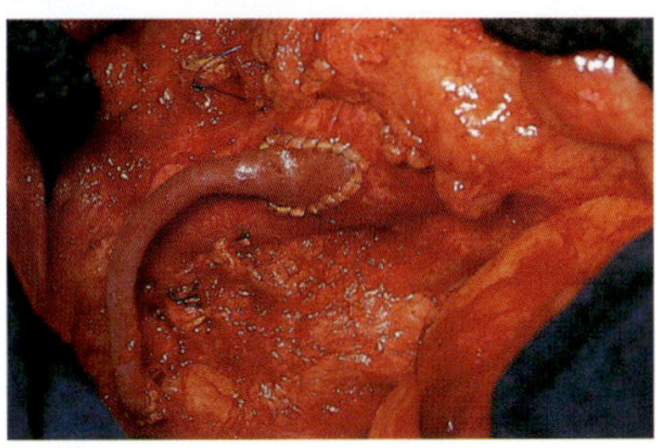

5-11

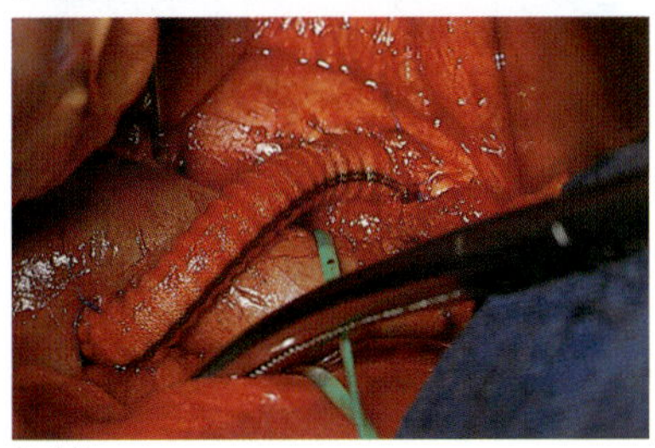

5-12

Fig. 5-11. An aorto-renal vein bypass

Fig. 5-12. An aorto-renal Dacron bypass, placed in front of the vena cava

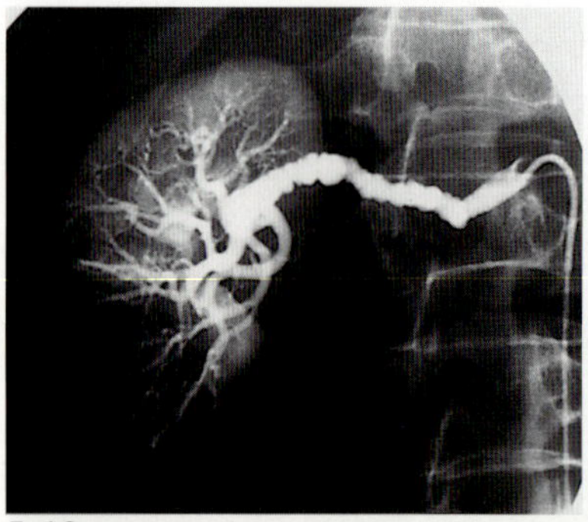

5-13

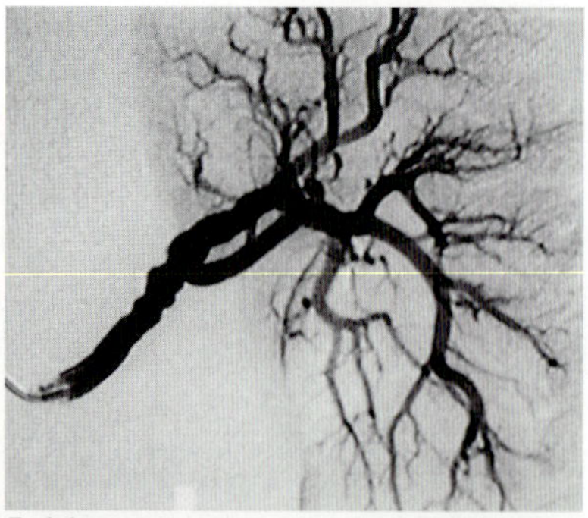

5-14

Fig. 5-13. Typical fibromuscular dysplasia with a "storing of pearls" appearance to the main trunk and saccular aneurysms at the periphery

Fig. 5-14. Fibromuscular dysplasia with a similar appearance on the left side

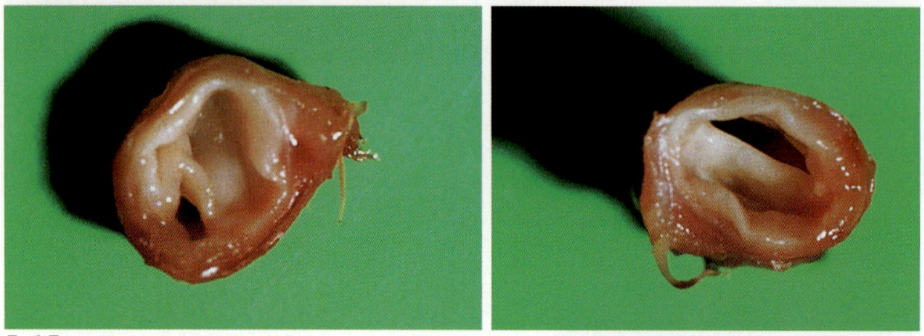

5-15

Fig. 5-15. Two operative specimens following resection of fibromuscular dysplasia with septum-like stenosis

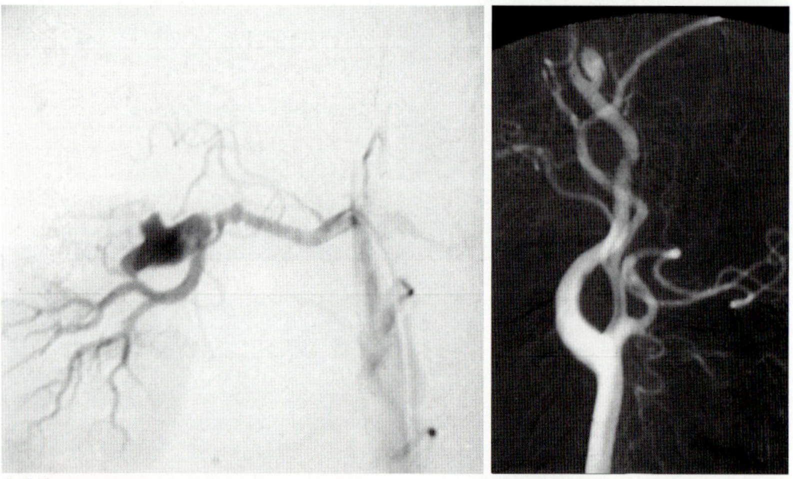

5-16

Fig. 5-16. Case description: fibromuscular dysplasia with changes in the main trunk and aneurysm formation. The same patient had fibromuscular dysplasia of the internal carotid artery with formation of a peripheral aneurysm

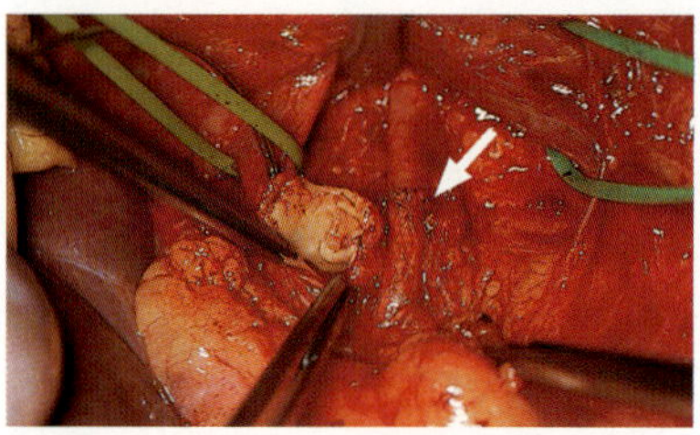

5-17

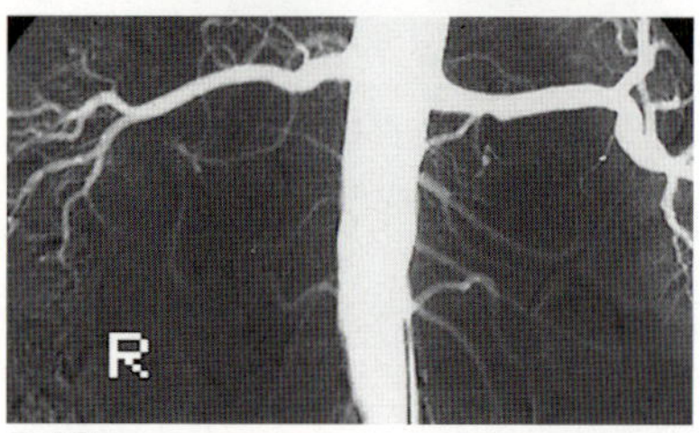

5-18

Fig. 5-17. Operative view of same patient, looking into the aneurysm of the renal artery. Following resection of the aneurysm, the artery was closed in an end-to-end fashion with individual sutures (*arrows*)

Fig. 5-18. Post-operative view shows that the renal artery is fully patent and the anastomosis is not identifiable

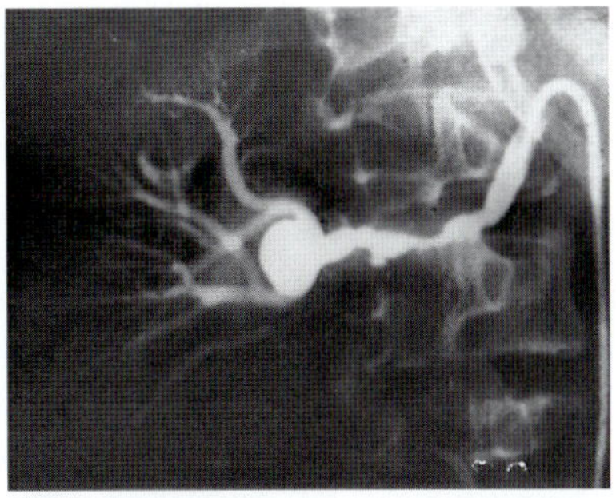

5-19

Fig. 5-19. Case description: Fibromuscular dysplasia in a 14 year old boy with peripheral aneurysm

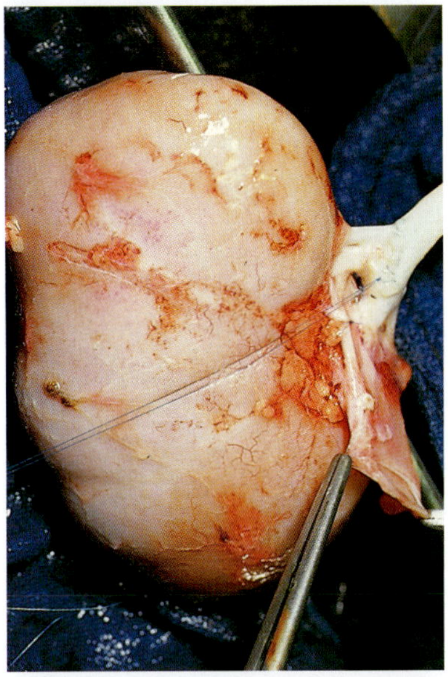

5-20

Fig. 5-20. Extracorporeal reconstruction. The segmental arteries are brought into a common ostium and connected to a large saphenous vein used for a bypass

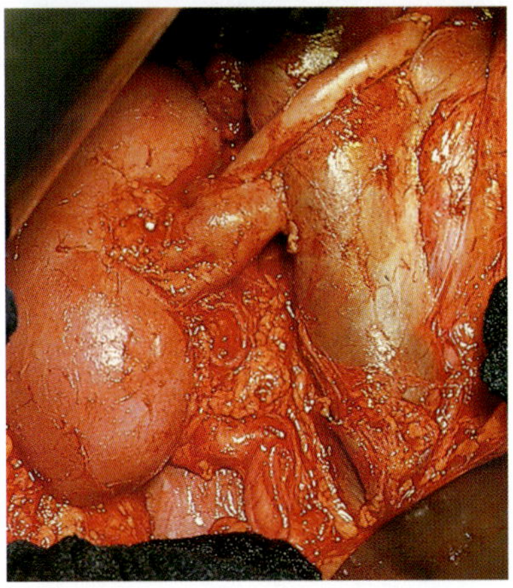

5-21

Fig. 5-21. Operative view with the re-implanted kidney and the bypass running in an antecaval manner from the aorta to the kidney

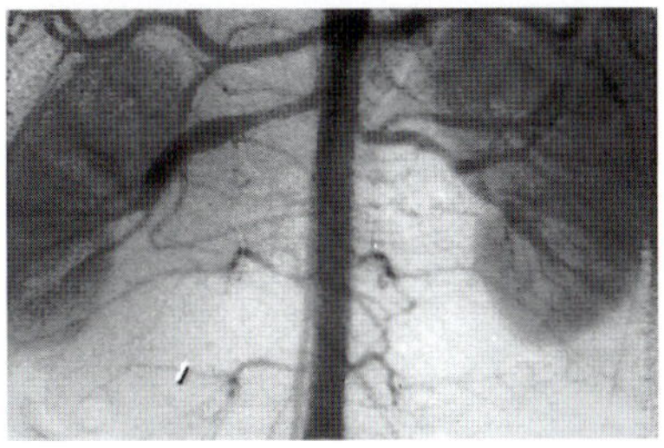

5-22

Fig. 5-22. Follow-up angiogram 2 years later showing slight dilatation of the vein graft

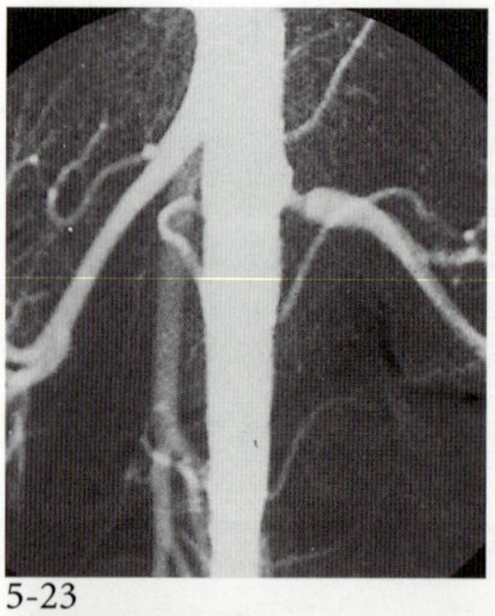

5-23

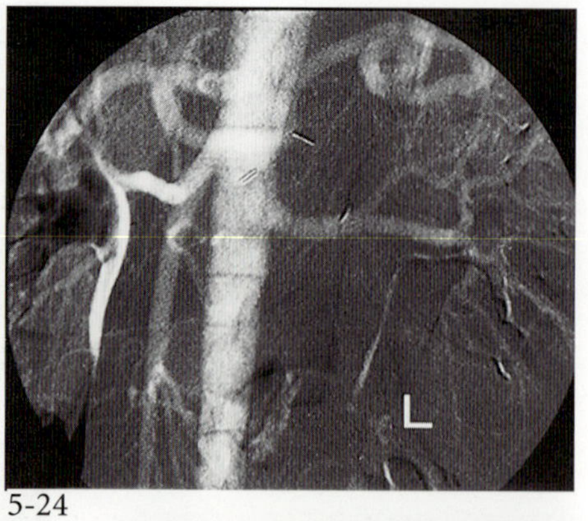

5-24

Fig. 5-23. Case description: 42 year old patient with stenosis of left renal artery close to the ostium

Fig. 5-24. Post-operative angiogram after 5 days shows no sign of stenosis

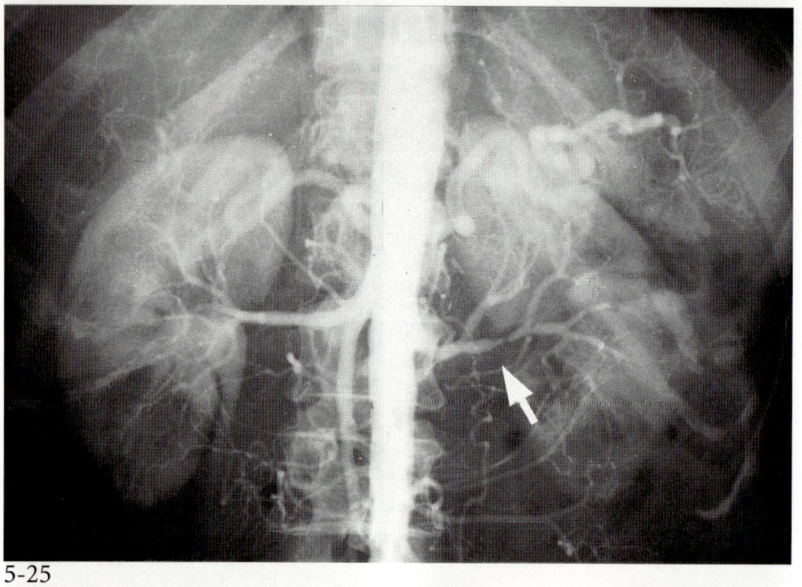

5-25

Fig. 5-25. The patient re-developed hypertension after 6 weeks. Another angiogram showed spasm of the left renal artery (*arrow*) which had been triggered by ergot alkaloids.
The patient underwent a percutaneous transluminal angioplasty and was treated with nifedipine

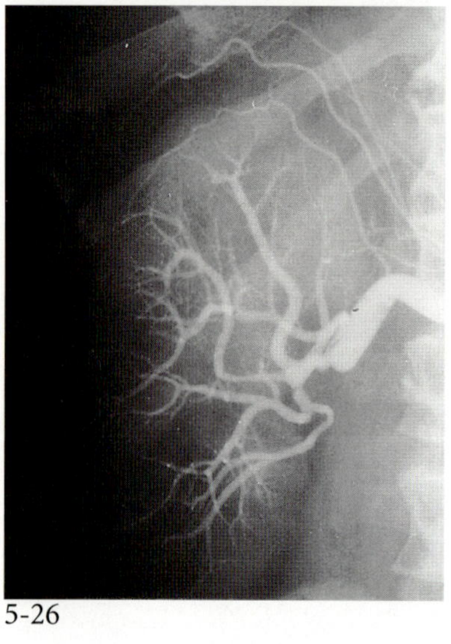

5-26

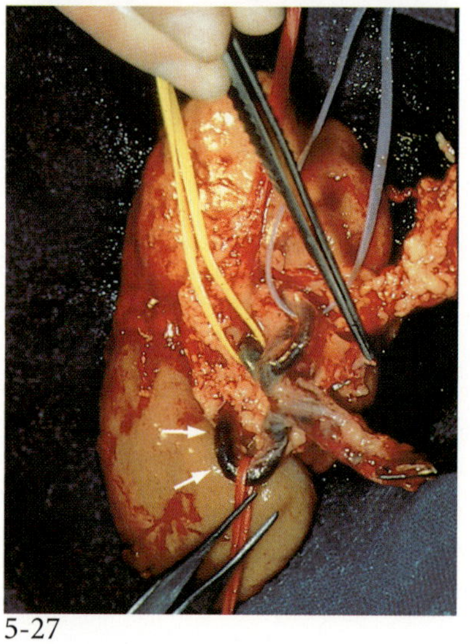

5-27

Fig. 5-26. Angiography showing spontaneous right renal artery dissection in a 52 year old patient with Gsell-Erdheim disease (median cystic necrosis of the aorta) who had undergone a left nephrectomy 4 years previously for the same problem

Fig. 5-27. The operative view shows subadventitial dissection in the renal artery (*arrow*)

Figs. 5-28, 5-29. Case description: 36 year old women with reno-vascular hypertension. The four angiograms were taken over a 5-year period. There is a saccular aneurysm of the right renal artery along with agenesis of the left kidney. The aneurysm appears to have disappeared spontaneously because of increasing thrombosis. Unfortunately reno-vascular hypertension still resulted from persisting microembolization arising from the thrombosed aneurysm

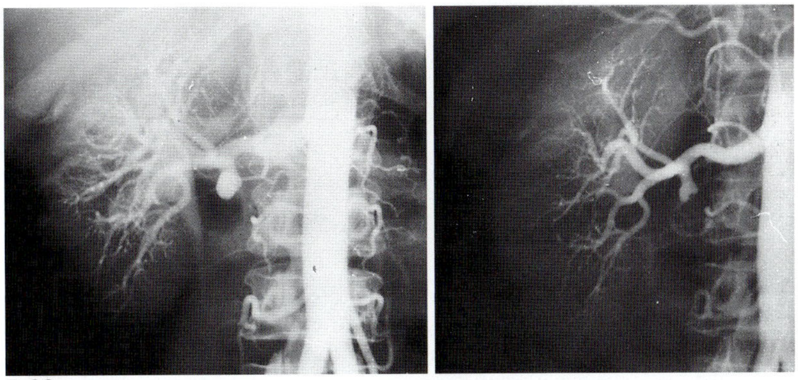

5-28

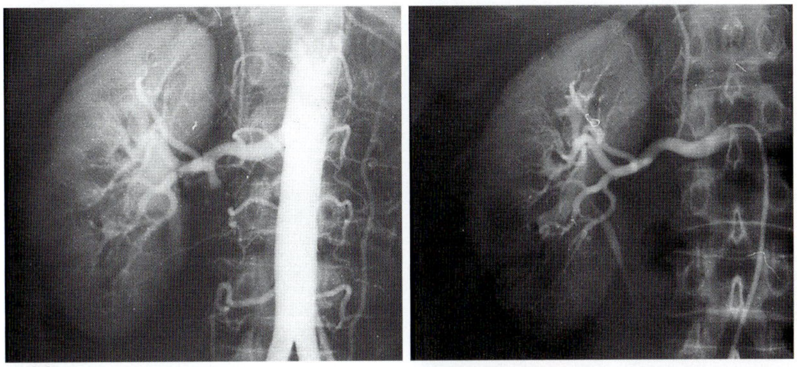

5-29

Fig. 5-30. Arteriosclerotic saccular aneurysms at the trifurcation of the right renal artery. The operative view shows main trunk with the segmental arteries arising from the aneurysms (*black threads*)

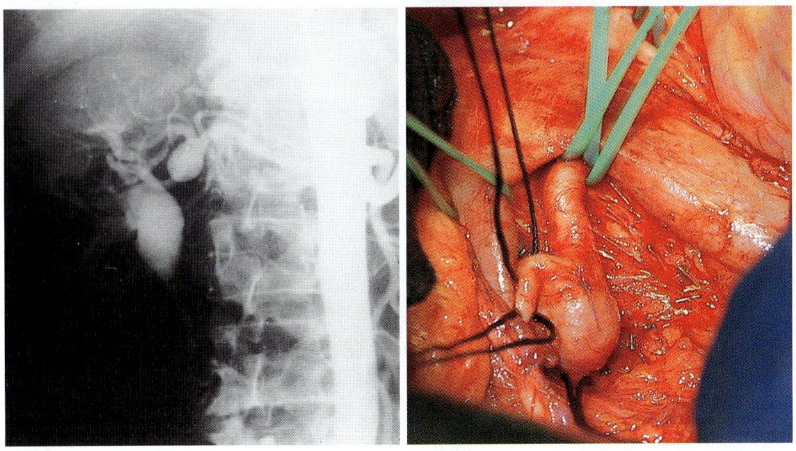

5-30

Fig. 5-31. A 50 year old man with a left renal artery aneurysm which completely compressed and destroyed the left kidney. The aorta has been distorted in a saber-shaped fashion to the right. Therapy consisted of resection of the left kidney with a patch graft to close the left renal artery ostium

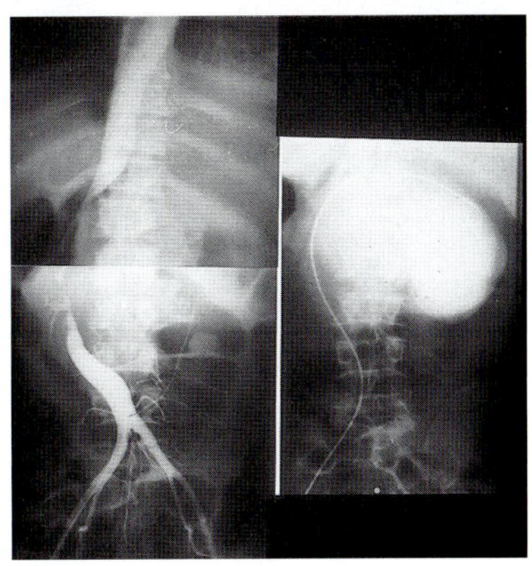

5-31

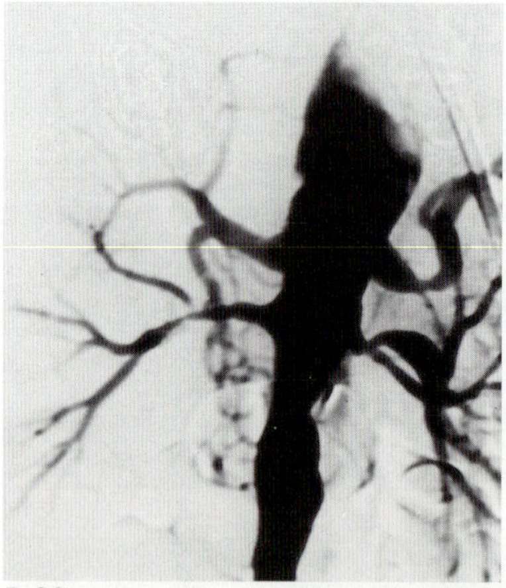

5-32

Fig. 5-32. Angiogram of a 14 year old patient with TAKAYASU arteritis and hypertension who has bilateral renal artery stenosis

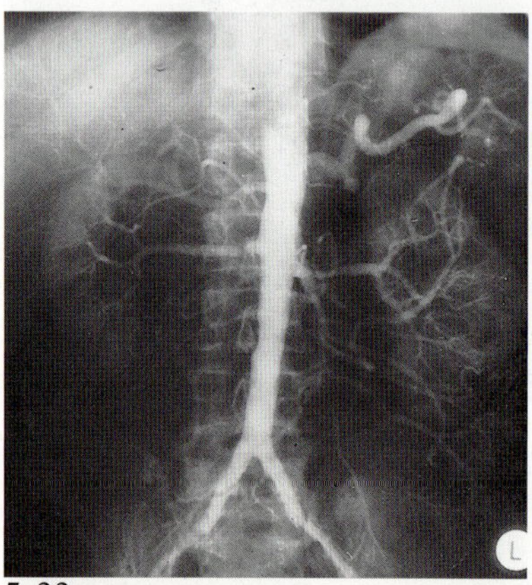

5-33

Fig. 5-33. Even though the angiogram looks like arteriosclerotic damage, this case of bilateral renal artery stenosis was caused by therapeutic ionizing radiation

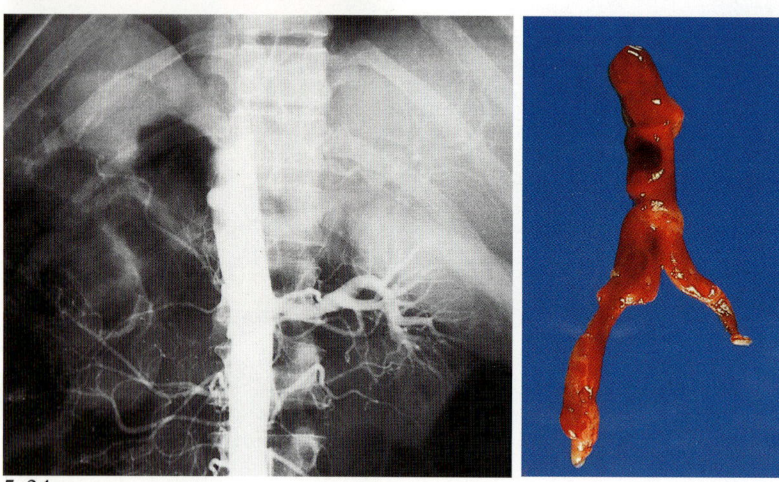

5-34

Fig. 5-34. Acute renal artery thrombosis in a 42 year old patient with atherosclerosis and sudden right flank pain

Fig. 5-35. Aortic angiogram in a patient with acute abdominal pain. Complete embolic occlusion of the superior mesenteric artery

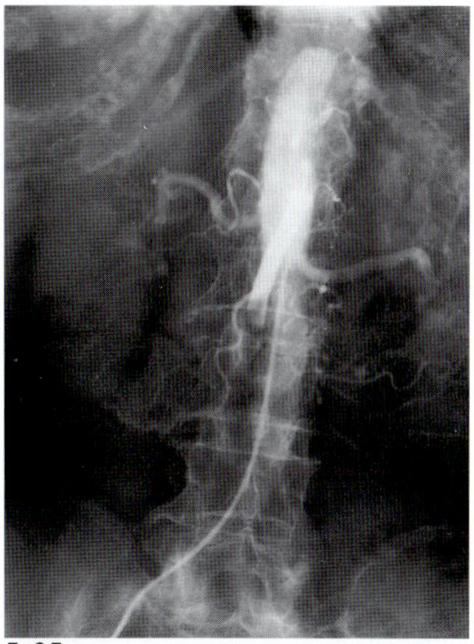

5-35

Fig. 5-36. Segmental perfusion defect in isolated intestinal loops in a patient with an embolus in the superior mesenteric artery

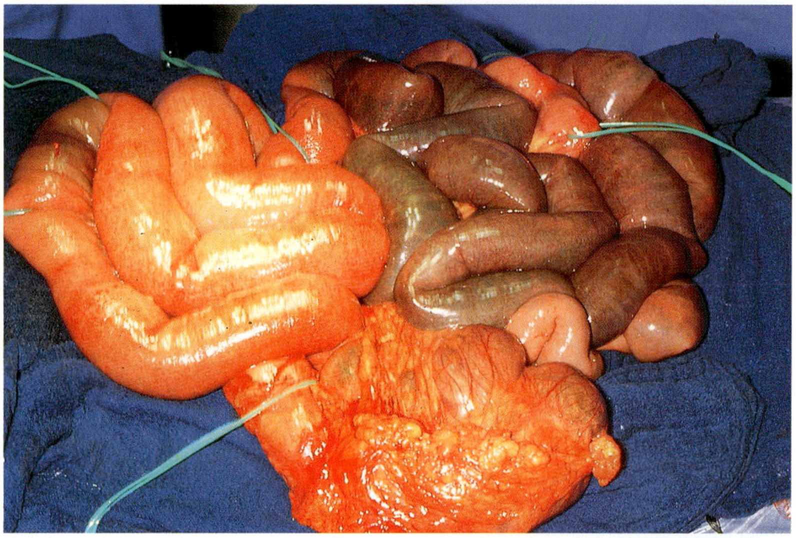

5-36

Fig. 5-37. Resection of the small intestine because of advanced gangrene following embolic occlusion of the superior mesenteric artery

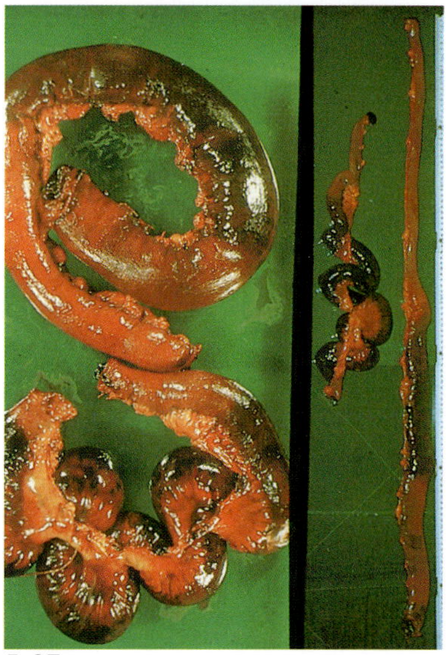

5-37

Chapter 6:
Arteries of the Leg

Contents

A: Introduction

1. Peripheral Arterial Occlusive Disease

Synonym. Peripheral arterial disease (PAD)

Definition

Circulatory impairment of legs due to stenosis and occlusion of the large and intermediate-sized limb arteries. Typical is leg pain on exercise, which is relieved by rest.

History

The phenomenon of intermittent claudication was apparently first described in 1831 in a mare by M. Boullay, a member of the Académie de Médecine in Paris.

"Tant que l'animal était en repos, e sang pouvait arriver aux membres par les collatérales, mais dès qu'il trottait, les collatérales comprimées ne fournissaient plus assez de sang et les membres étaient frappés d'un engourdissement et d'une douleur profonde."

The first description of claudication in a human was offered in 1846 by Benjamin Brodie, a physician to the British royal family.

"Such patients walk a very short distance very well, but when they attempt more than this the muscles seem to be unequal to the task and they can walk no further."

In 1885, Jean Charcot (Hôpital Salpetrière, Paris) described precisely the typical features of intermittent claudication.

Epidemiology

Many epidemiological studies show a 5-year incidence for peripheral occlusive arterial disease (PAD) of 60–80 per 1000; thus it is about as common as coronary artery disease.

- Two thirds of all PAD patients are asymptomatic.
- The prevalence of intermittent claudication varies with age between 2% and 11%; for 50 year old individuals, it is 5%.
- Men are twice as often affected as women, who generally experience the onset of vascular problems about 10 years later (hormonal protection).
- In less than 10% of patients with claudication, the limb ischemia will become severe enough that amputation must be considered.

Association of Arteriosclerotic Vascular Diseases

The association of PAD and coronary artery disease (CAD) is much higher than previously thought.

Table 6-1. Clinical features of different levels of occlusion

	Aorto-iliac	Femoro-popliteal	Crural (tibial/peroneal)	Combined
Age (years)	<55	>65	No age factors	>70
Main risk factors	Nicotine, hyper-tension, lipids	Nicotine, hyper-tension	Diabetes mellitus, hyper-tension	Many
Frequency (%)	8–28	41–75	17–30	20–25
Claudication	Buttocks, hips, back	Calf or more distal	Sole (instep claudication)	Varied
Condition of distal tissue	Good	Fair to good	Clearly reduced	Poor, pain at rest, ulcers, gangrene
Loss of pulses	Complete, sometimes weak femoral pulse	Distal to inguinal ligament	Absent foot pulses	Complete

- Every second PAD patient has the symptoms of coronary or cerebral ischemia; every fourth suffers a myocardial infarction.
- Various studies show that PAD patients have a 1.7- to 3.3-fold increased risk of dying from CAD.
- The life expectancy of individuals with intermittent claudication is almost 10 years less than the norm.

Etiology and Pathogenesis

Arteriosclerotic disease is responsible for well over 90% of PAD. In younger patients (<40 years of age) one should also think of BUERGER's

Table 6-2. Risk factors for peripheral arterial occlusion

Classical	New, well-established	Possible
Smoking	Hyperfibrinogenemia	Lipoprotein (a)
Hypertension	Glucose intolerance	Apolipoprotein B
Hypercholesterolemia	Lack of activity	Vitamin A, E deficiencies
Diabetes mellitus	Hyperhomocystinemia	Essential fatty acid deficiency
Genetic factors	Isolated systolic hypertension	Hypertriglyceridemia Hyperviscosity/Hypercoaguability Elevated levels of factor VIII, XIII and plasminogen Hyperuricemia Marked alcohol consumption

disease and mechanical factors such as entrapment. Based on localization, M. Ratschow divided arterial diseases of the legs into three types:

- Pelvic: aorto-iliac arteries
- Thigh: femoro-popliteal arteries
- Calf: infrapopliteal or more distal arteries

Many patients have disease in more than one location producing the more severe degrees of lower limb ischemia.

Clinical Features

René Fontaine (French surgeon in Strasbourg, 1899–1979) divided PAD into four degrees of severity Fontaine classification. A second well-known classification is the Rutherford classification:

Table 6-3. Classification of peripheral arterial disease: Fontaine's stages and Rutherford's categories

Fontaine		Rutherford		
Stage	Clinical	Grade	Category	Clinical
I	Asymptomatic	0	0	Asymptomatic
IIa	Mild claudication	0	1	Mild claudication
IIb	Moderate-severe claudication	1	2	Moderate claudication
		1	3	Severe claudication
III	Ischemic rest pain	II	4	Ischemic rest pain
		III	5	Minor tissue loos
IV	Ulceration or gangrene	III	6	Major tissue loss

In the Anglo-American literature, Fontaine's stages are often not used. Instead one distinguishes between intermittent claudication and critical leg ischemia. Initially this latter term was defined in 1991, at a consensus conference, as a sufficient reduction in blood supply to an extremity that the leg or at least the toes and foot are threatened with the need for amputation. Later, two more exact criteria were added:

1. Persistent pain at rest so that analgesics are needed for more than 2 weeks, along with a systolic blood pressure at the ankle of <50 mm Hg or at the toes of <30 mm Hg.
2. Ulceration or gangrene of the foot or toes, along with a systolic blood pressure at the ankle of <50 mm Hg or at the toes of <30 mm Hg.

Diagnosis

- History
- Inspection, palpation and auscultation (bruits)
- Ratschow's Test (see Fig. 6-6) checking for dependent rubor
- Oscillography before and after activity, to localize the occlusions
- Ergometry
  - Walking on a level surface at 80 steps/min
  - Treadmill: standardized at 3.0 km/h and 12% grade (constant lood) or graded exercise test

- Doppler and duplex ultrasonography
  - Doppler pressure measurements at rest and after exercise
  - Visualization of the flow curve
  - Color-coded representation of the vessels
- Venous occlusion plethysmography
  - Measurement of blood flow at rest and with reactive hyperemia (arterial tourniquet)
- Thermography
- Arteriography
  - Transfemoral conventional arteriography, occasionally translumbar or transbrachial, if femoral pulses are absent
  - Digital subtraction arteriography
- Angioscopy
- Special evaluation of microcirculatory disease
  - Transcutaneous partial pressure of O_2 ($tcPO_2$)
  - Laser duplex flow measurements

Therapy

A. Basic Therapy

Medical treatment of intermittent claudication

General measures
Correct care of feet and toenails
Avoid trauma
Normalize body weight

Exercise programme
Avoid tobacco products
Treatment of risk factors
Hyperepidemia
Diabetes mellitus
Hypertension

Vasoactive drugs
Pentoxifylline
Naftidrofuryl
Cirostazole

Antiplatelet Drugs
Aspirin, Ticlopidin,
Clopidogrel

Prostanoids in CLI
Prostaglandin E_1 (Alprostadie)
Prostaglandin I_2 (Ilomedin)

L-Carnitine

- Eliminate or treat the risk factors (smoking, elevated lipids, hypertension, diabetes mellitus)
- Treat cardiac failure or arrhythmias
- Alterations in life style (avoid cold and wet feet, professional foot care)

B. Additional Possibilities

- Walking and exercise therapy for stages II (and III)
- Secondary prevention with anticoagulants and platelet aggregation inhibitors
- Prophylactic measures following revascularization procedures
- Defibrinogenization with snake venom proteases or low-dose intermittent urokinase therapy
- Tetanus prophylaxis
- Antimycotic therapy for dermatophyte infections which offer entry sites for other problems
- Analgesics for stages III and IV
- Epidural anesthesia and spinal cord stimulation

Many alternative therapies have not been proven effective and may have considerable side effects. Included in this group are ozone therapy, ultraviolet irradiation of the blood, oxidation therapy of the blood, O_2-step therapy (increasing the amount of O_2 in inhaled air incrementally), chelation therapy, hyperbaric oxygen chambers and acupuncture.

C. Revascularization Procedures

C-1. Systemic Fibrinolysis
Systemic fibrinolysis may be helpful for acute arterial thromboses, although it is rarely used in the United States. Some current studies are seeking to learn which protocol and which fibrinolytic agents are most appropriate in different clinical settings.

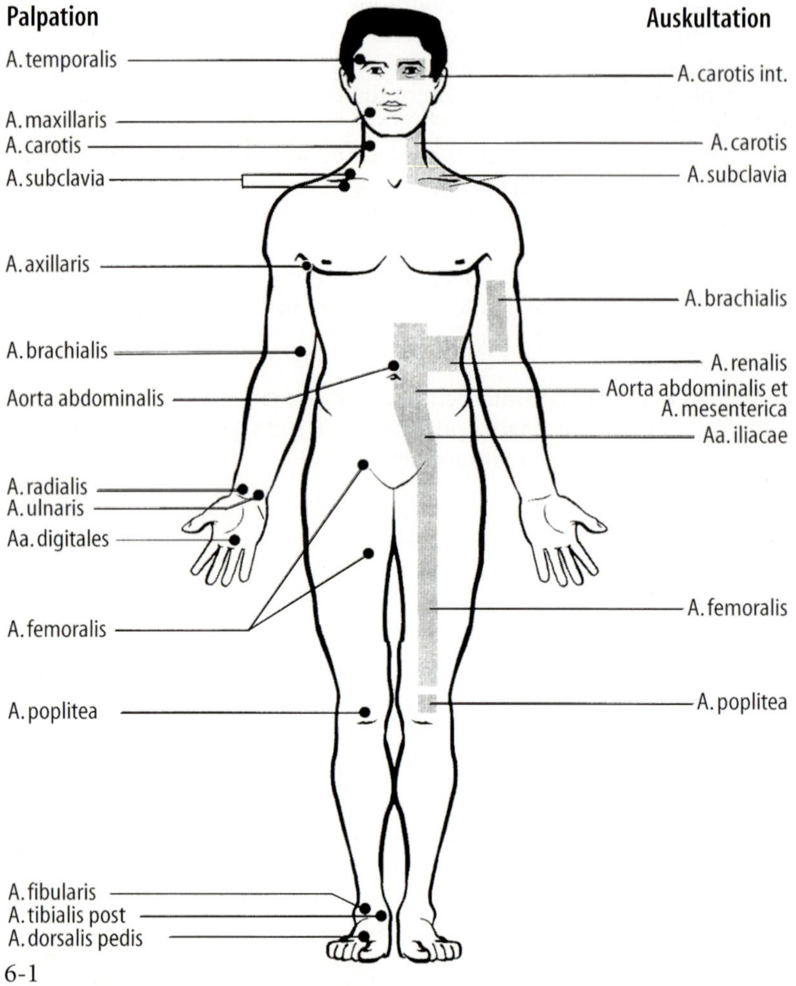

6-1

Fig. 6-1. The main sites for palpation and auscultation of arteries. Palpating pulses, interpreted in light of claudication distance and location of pain, usually indicates the location and severity of the responsible arterial lesion(s). Auscultation of bruits may give additional useful information

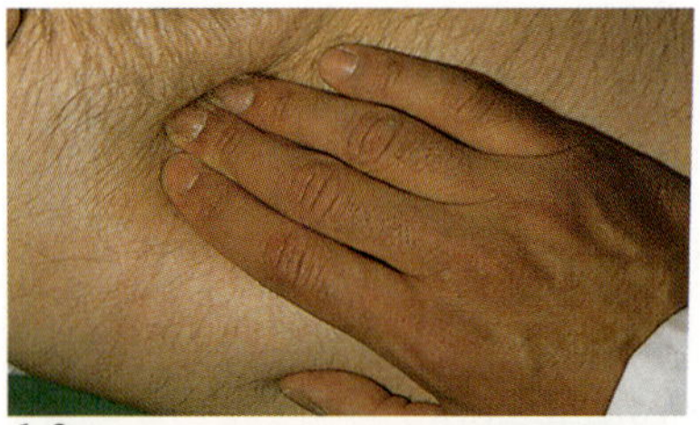
6-2

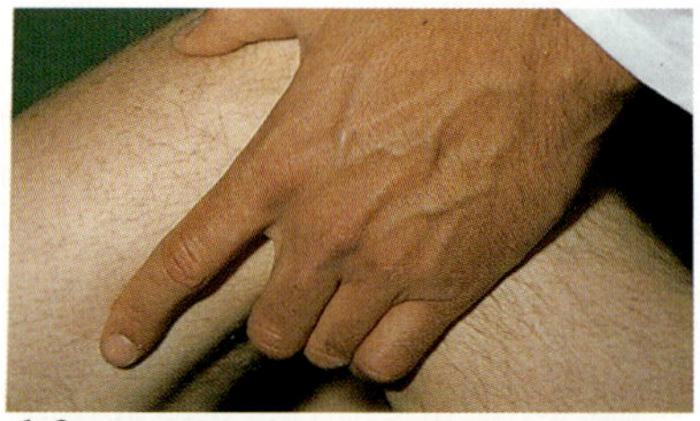
6-3

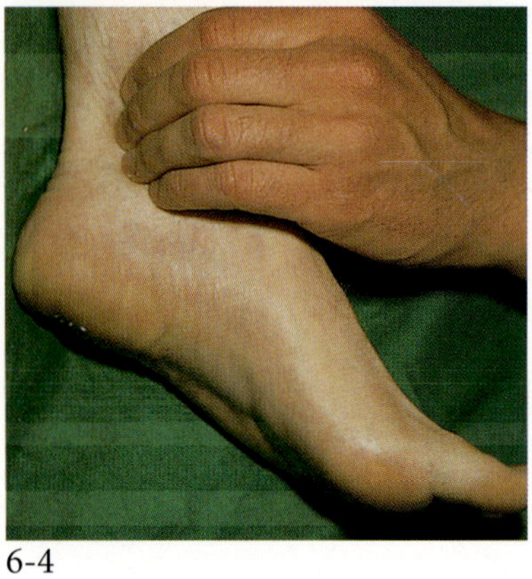
6-4

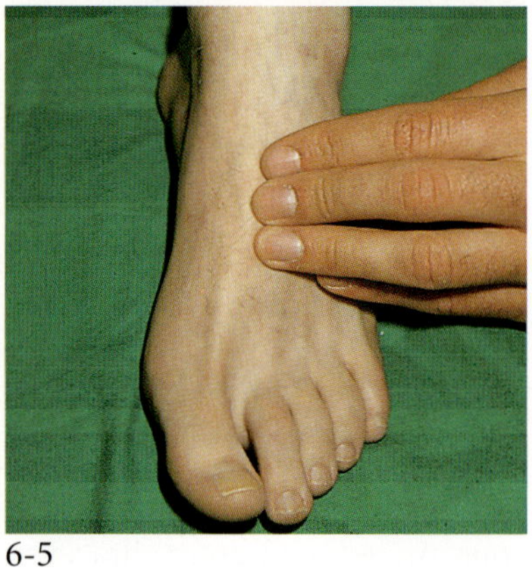
6-5

Figs. 6-2 – 6-5. Palpation sites on the lower extremity (femoral artery, popliteal artery, posterior tibial artery and dorsalis pedis artery)

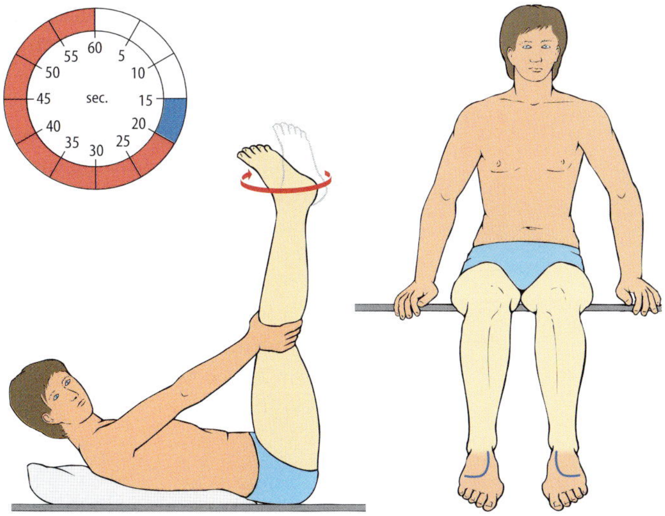

6-6

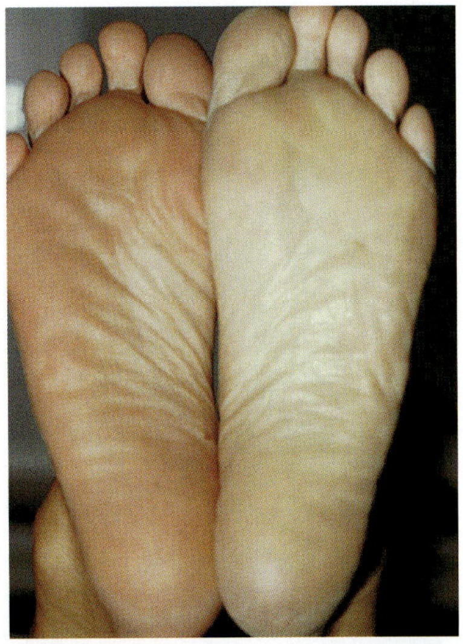

6-7

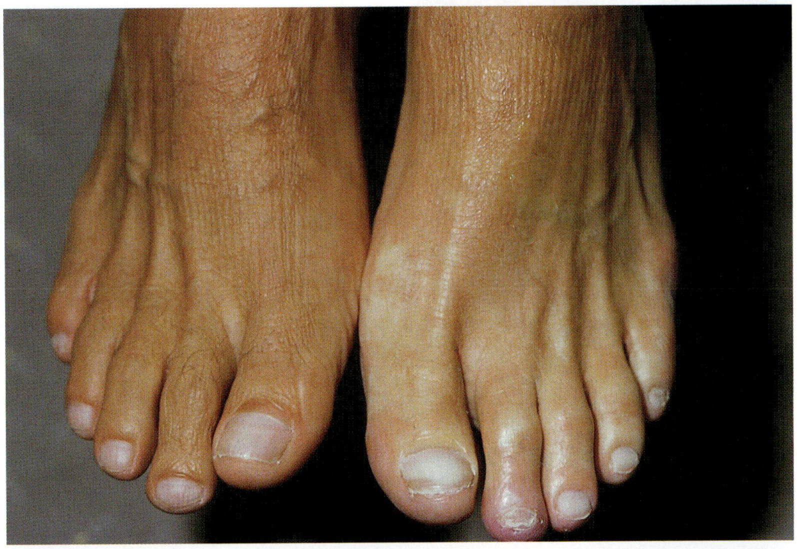

6-8

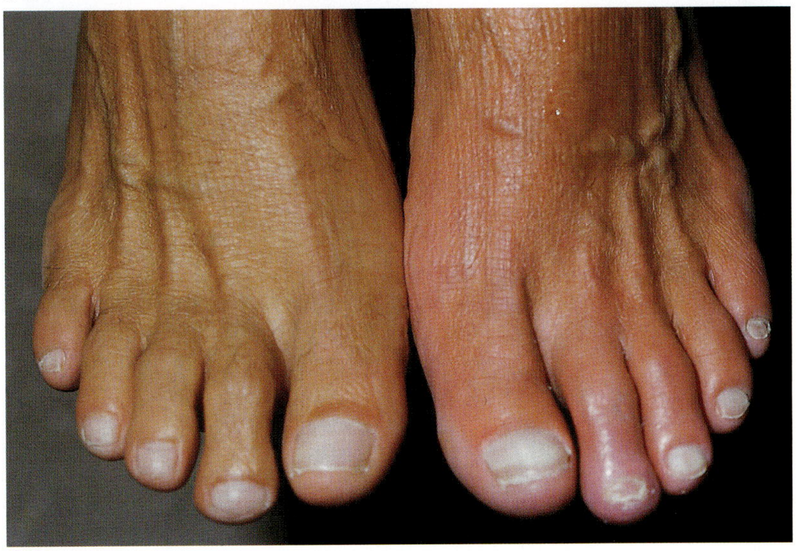

6-9

Fig. 6-6. The Ratschow test is a reliable clinical way to evaluate the peripheral arterial circulation of the limb. First, the patient holds his or her feet vertically in the air and moves them in a circular pattern. Then the patient assumes a sitting position and the paleness of the skin, the vein filling and the reactive hyperemia are evaluated. If the arteries are normal, the skin becomes diffusely red within 5–10 s. Increased venous filling on the back of the foot is seen with 8–12 s. If arterial occlusion is present, the skin will have a pale, often mottled, color. The venous filling occurs later and is then followed by a reactive hyperemia with livid tones, representing stasis

Fig. 6-7. Following repeated plantar and dorsal flexion, the sole of the left foot became pale in this patient with occlusion at multiple levels

Fig. 6-8. After the patient put his feet down, the right foot quickly developed physiologic hyperemia. On the *left*, the process is delayed and the vein filling is also less prominent

Fig. 6-9. After a few minutes the pathological hyperemia (rubor) of the diseased leg is easily appreciated

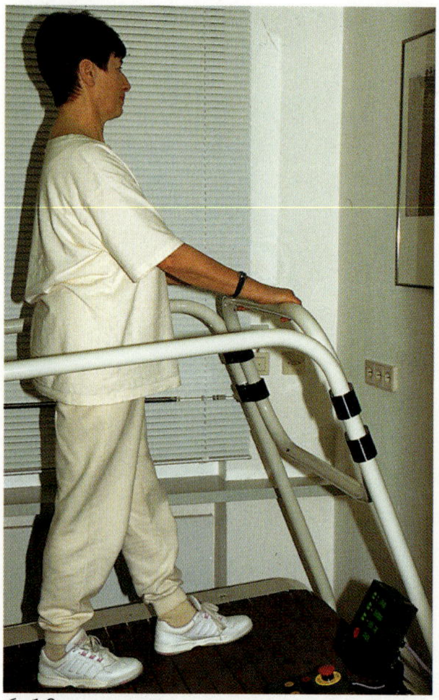

6-10

Fig. 6-10. Standardized treadmill test with a speed of 3.0 km/h and a grade of 12%. Usually two values are measured: S1, the time to initial claudication, and S2, the time to inability to continue the test. The localization of the pain and the reason why the patient stopped are noted. A conventional walking or exercise test can be done in a hallway; in this case, the patient should walk at 80–120 steps/min and a metronome is often required

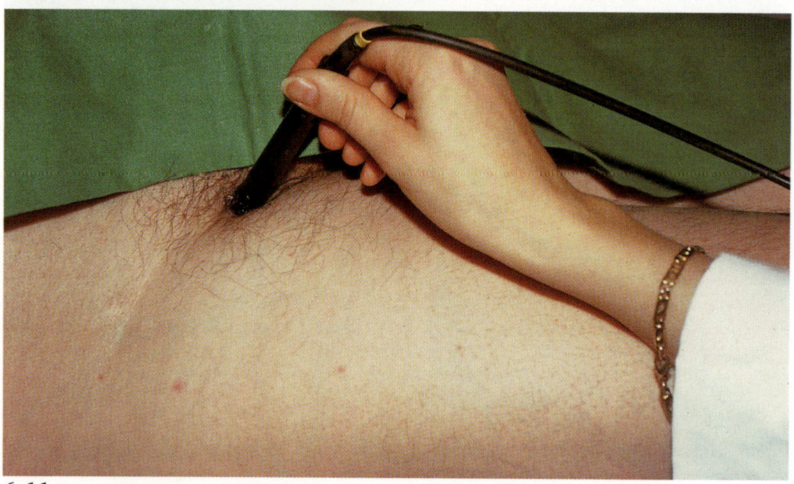

6-11

Fig. 6-11. Doppler Velocity Wave Form (VWF) analysis is used in some Vascular Diagnostic Laboratories (continuous wave Doppler)

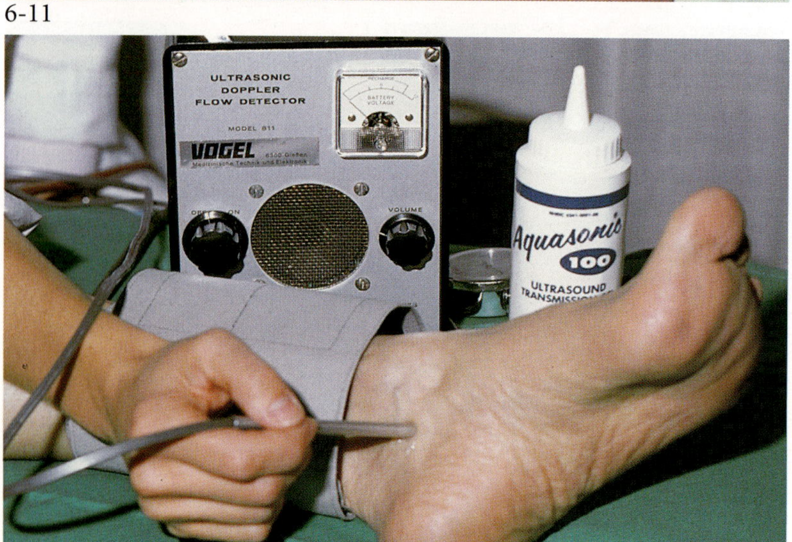

6-12

Fig. 6-12. Measurement of the systolic blood pressure in the posterior tibial artery using Doppler ultrasonography. The test is done with the patient supine. The blood pressure cuff is placed as distal as possible on the calf and the pressure measured in the posterior tibial artery and dorsalis pedis artery. In healthy individuals the values are about 20 mm Hg higher than in the radial artery (ankle: arm ratio>1). If the ankle and arm pressures are about equal, the test is regarded as borderline, and an exercise test should be done. Here the same measurement are made

Figs. 6-13 – 6-15. Color duplex imaging. The most important measuring sites in the groin, popliteal fossa and on the calf are shown. The simultaneous demonstration of the B-mode picture, the color-coded blood flow and the Doppler signal allows a relatively simple evaluation of vessel wall changes and their influence on blood flow. Color Duplex imaging is an attractive alternative to angiography. Duplex scanning, in expert hands, can provide most of the essential anatomical informations plus some functional information, for instance velocity gradients over stenoses. The lower extremities arterial tree can be visualized

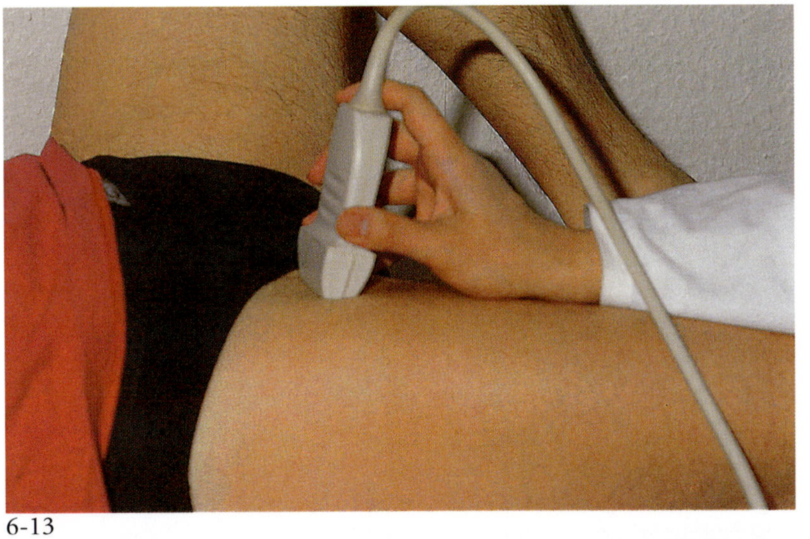

6-13

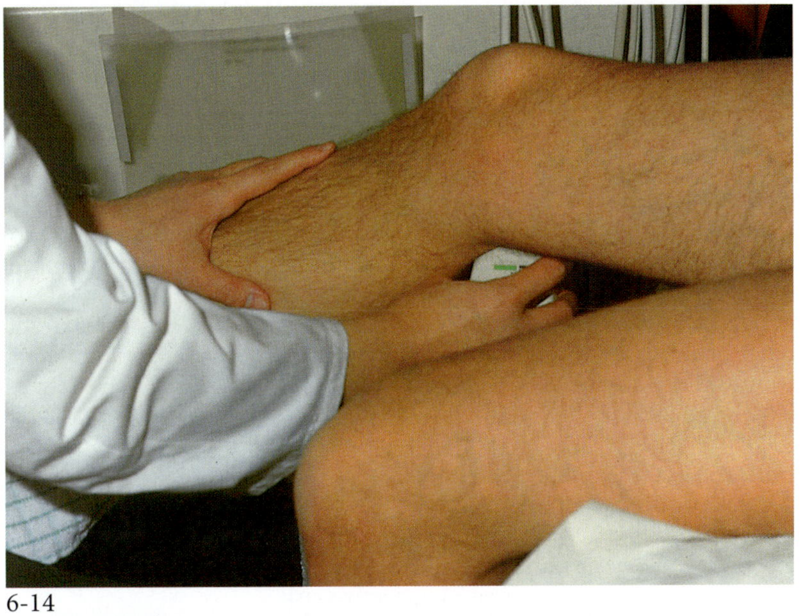

6-14

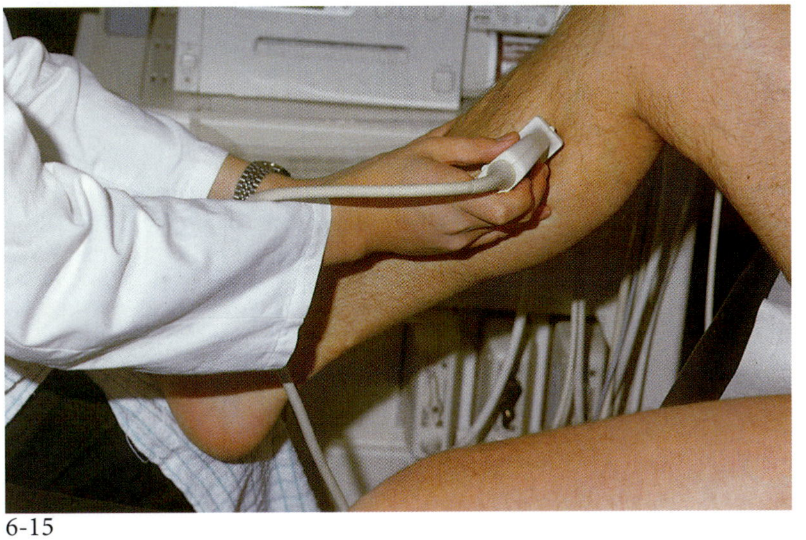

6-15

after 10–20 deep knee bends or repeated standing on tip toes. The Ankle: Brachial Pressure Index (ABPI) should be measured in all patients with intermittent claudication and critical leg ischemia, in both legs

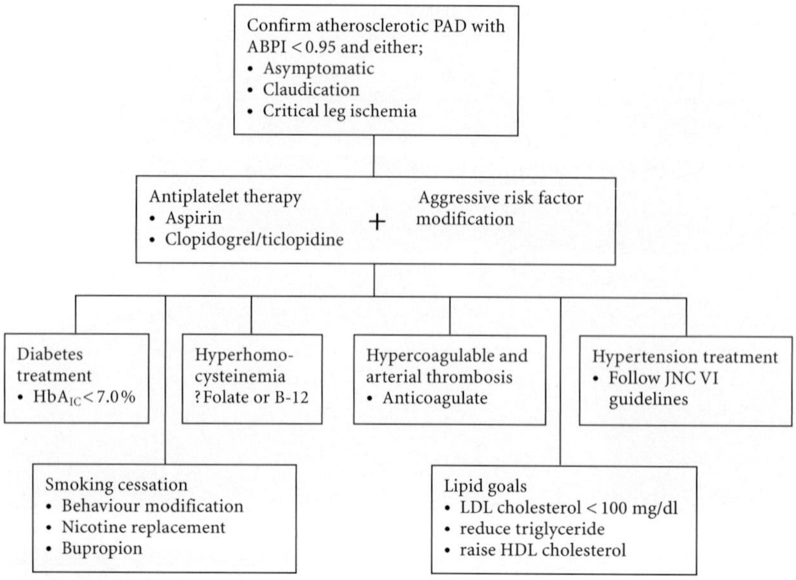

? = insufficient data to support treatment at this time
JNC = Joint National Commission

Fig. 6-16. Treatment algorithm for intermittent claudication (from TASC CONSENSUS DOCUMENT 2000). Treatment to alter natural history and reduce systemic risk

C-2. Catheter or Local Fibrinolysis

Arterial catheters can be used to deliver the thrombolytic agent directly to the occluding clot. Urokinase, streptokinase or rTPA can be used to lyse fresh or partially organized arterial thrombi. The main theoretical advantages are the reduced systemic effects and the ability to extract parts of the lysed thrombi. During the same procedure, percutaneous transluminal angioplasty (PTA) can be used to treat discovered arteriosclerotic lesions.

Indications for Catheter Fibrinolysis

- Lack of suitable alternatives.
- Fresh occlusions of the femoro-popliteal and popliteal-crural regions involving either native vessels or bypasses.
- Older patients with increased operative risk.
- Older occlusions are not suitable for treatment by operation or PTA.
- Recurrent occlusion following PTA or distal emboli resulting from PTA.

C-3. Percutaneous Transluminal Angioplasty

The technique of percutaneous transluminal angioplasty, as introduced by Charles Dotter, has established itself as a low-risk method to recanalize some arterial occlusions. A significant improvement in the procedure was the development of the double lumen balloon catheter by Grüntzig.

C-4. Stenting

In 1984 Dotter proposed the concept of using an intravascular stent or support to keep a dilated vessel open. The stents or endovascular prostheses are balloon-expandable or self-expanding wire mesh tubes made of different alloys. They are delivered to the lesion site with a balloon catheter or sheath and deployed under fluoroscopic guidance often with the help of road mapping techniques. The expansion of the delivery balloon opens the stent and imbeds the wire mesh into the vessel wall. In this way the elastic recoil of the artery wall is reduced but it is also possible to induce a dissection. During healing, the stent is covered by a neointima; occasionally this process is too exuberant producing intimal hyperplasia and restenosis within the stent.

The use of stents in small infrainguinal arteries is limited by the likelihood of intimal hyperplasia. In addition, in the small vessels anticoagulation and platelet inhibition may help to prevent thrombosis. In larger vessels such as the iliac arteries only a short period of heparinization is required. Thus far, the long term results are promising. The next few years will show which stents work best in different locations and with which types of lesions.

C-5. Operative Methods

Orthotopic Reconstruction

Long stenoses and occlusions in the suprainguinal arteries still often require surgery, despite the many advances in endovascular treatment. Generally unilateral or bilateral aorto-femoral prosthetic grafts are used.

Extra-anatomic Reconstruction

Axillo-femoral bypasses to one or both femoral arteries are reserved for patients with increased operative risks. When there is an occlusion of the femoro-popliteal axis, one should lean towards the simpler lesser procedures rather than extensive vascular reconstruction. Standard procedures include:

(a) Profundaplasty, in which normal flow is provided to the deep femoral artery and its collaterals in the first segment of the popliteal artery, circumventing an occlusion of the superficial femoral artery
(b) Above-knee femoro-popliteal bypass using vein or synthetic graft
(c) Below-knee femoro-popliteal bypass, preferably using a vein graft

An operation is indicated for calf (crural) artery occlusion only when stage III-IV disease is present. At least one of the leg arteries should be shown on angiography to be patent to the sole of the foot. The use of foot artery bypasses in patients with diabetes mellitus can reduce the number of major amputations. Most bypasses to foot and leg arteries are performed in specialized centers.

Anticoagulation following operation: Long-term oral anticoagulants are not needed following procedures involving the aorta and iliac arteries. Short-term intraoperative heparinization suffices. The large vessels have such high flow rates that thrombi are unlikely. On the other hand, following procedures to the smaller vessels of the leg and foot, particularly if a prosthetic graft is used, long-term oral anticoagulation is usually indicated.

2. Inguinal Region

Vascular Anatomy

The femoral triangle is bordered by the inguinal ligament, the sartorius muscle and the long adductor muscle. The main structures moving from lateral to medial are the femoral nerve, the common femoral artery and the femoral vein. In addition numerous lymphatics are present.

Atherosclerosis

Common femoral artery: Chronic occlusion is uncommon in this short section. But when arteriosclerotic disease is present, the effects are usually severe as the origin of the deep femoral artery is almost always involved. Since this is the most important collateral vessel of the leg, not only claudication but also pain at rest and necrosis with a risk of amputation can be expected.

Deep femoral artery: Isolated occlusion of the deep femoral artery is also rare. If the superficial femoral artery is occluded, the deep femoral is the usual source of collateral circulation. The diameter of the vessel may increase by two- to threefold in this setting. The effectiveness of the deep femoral collateral circulation is sharply reduced when the peripheral arterial segments also have occlusive changes.

Emboli

Most leg emboli come from a cardiac source. Only rarely do peripheral emboli arise from a stenosis or aneurysm of the aorta. The bifurcation of the femoral artery is a high-risk point for emboli, as are most areas where branching occurs.

Aneurysms

Almost all degenerative aneurysms are associated with some atherosclerosis. They can involve the groin, where the common femoral artery is involved. Aneurysms may be bilateral. In addition to the degenerative true aneurysms, false aneurysms may develop following invasive diagnostic or therapeutic catheterization procedures. These are also called iatrogenic aneurysms, since they usually result from inadequate compression at the site of a puncture of the common femoral artery. They can sometimes by treated by ultrasonographically guided compression; in other instances, they must be surgically repaired.

Another unique entity is the anastomotic aneurysm, which develops following the placement of an aorto-femoral bypass. Mechanical or flow factors are one cause of dilatation and the development of an aneurysm in the inguinal region.

A-V Fistulas

Most A-V fistulas in the lower extremity are acquired. Usually a penetrating injury involves both an artery and a vein. During the healing process a fistula develops. Iatrogenic A-V fistulas can develop following a variety of procedures including venipuncture, minor operative damage, and ligatures that catch an additional vessel.

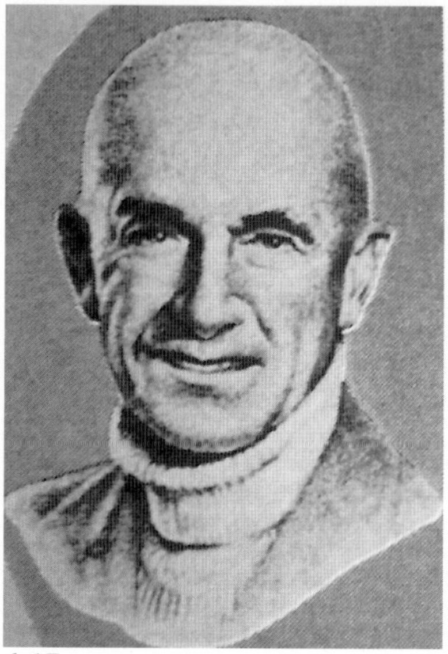

6-17

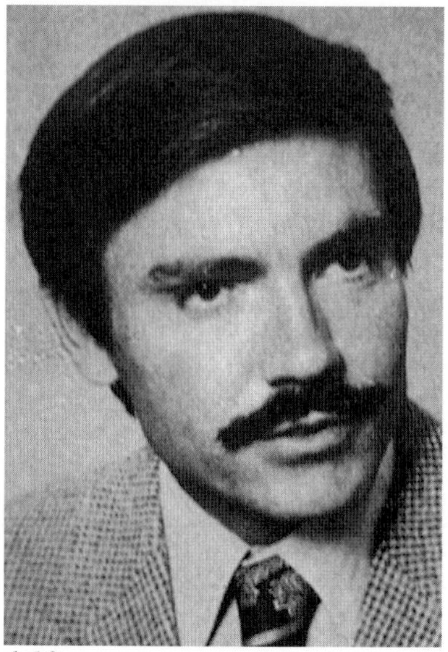

6-18

Fig. 6-17. Charles Theodore Dotter (1920–1985), US radiologist. The first intraluminal vessel dilatation was performed by Dotter and Judkins, in 1964, in a patient with occlusion of the leg arteries

Fig. 6-18. Andreas Roland Grüntzig (1939–1985), German cardiologist and angiologist. He developed a special balloon catheter for percutaneous angioplasty and performed the first successful angioplasty in Zürich, in 1977

3. Popliteal Region

Vascular Anatomy

The popliteal artery starts at the adductor canal as a continuation of the femoral artery. It is divided into three segments:

1. The proximal segment extends from the adductor canal to the gastrocnemius tunnel (Pars I)
2. The middle segment extends from the gastrocnemius tunnel to the middle of the knee joint (Pars II)
3. The distal segment extends from the middle of knee joint to the origin of the anterior tibial artery (Pars III)

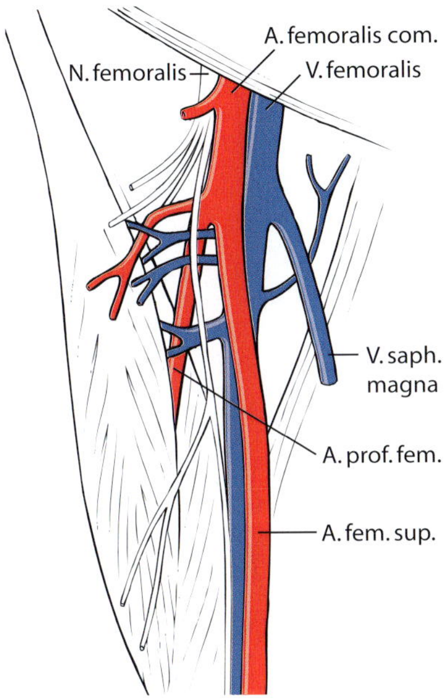

Fig. 6-19. Anatomy of the inguinal region

Atherosclerosis

The physiologic narrowing in the adductor canal and the gastrocnemius tunnel favor the formation of arteriosclerotic plaques in the vessel wall. At the transition from the femoral artery to the popliteal arty, isolated stenoses and occlusions are common; at the same site, thrombi with retrograde propagation may develop. Isolated arteriosclerotic occlusion in the third part of the popliteal artery is unusual.

Stenoses and occlusions of the popliteal artery can cause severe ischemic problems. This is probably due to the limited potential for collaterals in the soft tissues about the knee.

Popliteal Aneurysms (with secondary thromboembolism)

Aneurysms of the popliteal artery are the most common peripheral aneurysm. They are usually asymptomatic for many years. Usually the first clinical clue is recurrent thromboemboli in the leg or an acute thromboembolic occlusion. Acute closure of the popliteal artery carries a high risk of amputation because of the limited compensatory ability of the collaterals.

Inflammatory Diseases

In patients under the age of 40 years, one must consider the possibility of Buerger's disease.

Emboli

The most likely sites of embolic occlusion in the leg are the common femoral artery (at the femoral bifurcation), the adductor canal and the trifurcation of the popliteal artery.

Popliteal Artery Entrapment Syndrome

The entrapment, or compression, syndrome involving the popliteal artery results from aberrant anatomic coursing of the vessel or because of variation in the attachment sites of muscles. Typically the tendinous

Differential diagnosis of intermittent claudication

Vascular causes
Arterosclerosis obliterans
Thromboangiitis obliterans
Arterial embolus
Advential cyst of popliteal artery
Popliteal artery entropment syndrome
Ileofemoral venous obstruction

Non vascular causes
Neurogenic claudication
Lumbar disc disease
Artheritis
McArdle's syndrome
Painful calf muscle spasms

insertion of the medial aspect of the gastrocnemius head or an intracondylar fibrous band compress the popliteal artery. The repeated trauma damages the vessel wall and its intima until finally a local stenosis or occlusion develops. In more advanced stages, the changes appear identical to atherosclerosis. The clinical symptoms vary from progressive claudication to severe ischemia. At rest the pulses may be intact and the Doppler ultrasonography normal. Duplex ultrasonography allows good visualization of the compression during plantar flexion of the foot, a provocative test. Preoperative angiography, also during provocative testing, is recommended.

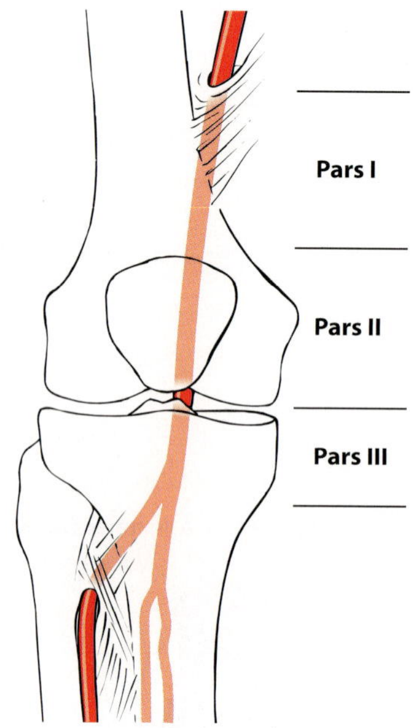

Fig. 6-20. Three segments of the popliteal artery

Cystic Degeneration (Advential Cysts of Popliteal Artery)

Mucoid degeneration of the adventitial connective tissue leads to intramural cyst formation outside the media. The cyst secondarily compresses the arterial lumen. The etiology is unknown. It is speculated that during embryological development mucin-secreting fibroblasts erroneously wander from the nearby joint structures into the vessel wall.

Duplex ultrasonography and angiography should be performed prior to operation. On angiography, a smooth, sharply bordered, curved indentation is seen in the vessel lumen.

Vascular Syndromes with Tumors of the Popliteal Space

A variety of tumors in the region of the knee can impinge on vessels and cause vascular problems. The tumors may arise from bone, cartilage or synovium.

Benign tumors include:

- Exostosis
- Osteoma
- Baker's cyst

Malignant tumors include:

- Ewing sarcoma
- Chondrosarcoma
- Synovial sarcoma (from the joint capsule)

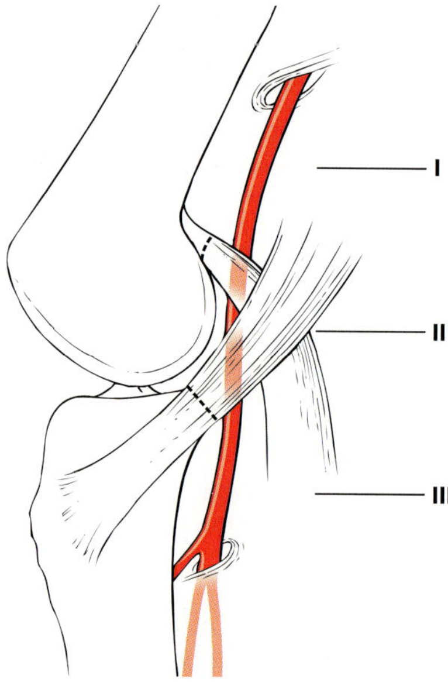

Fig. 6-21. Surgical anatomy of the popliteal artery. The best surgical method to expose the artery is the tibial approach. If the occlusion is in the second part, the crossing tendons of pes anserinus and the medial insertion of the gastrocnemius must be divided. (From VOLLMAR J. et al. 1963, Langenbecks Arch Clin Chir 302:588)

Vascular Injury of the Popliteal Artery

Blunt trauma to the second part of the popliteal artery is the most common type of injury. The vessel is typically stretched and squeezed by a knee joint injury. The cause of the high rate of amputation is once again the lack of collateral circulation to the lower leg once the popliteal artery is suddenly interrupted. Neurovascular complications are also common.

Injury of the popliteal artery carries the highest amputation rate of all arterial injuries to the lower extremity. As a small vessel the popliteal artery is harder to repair than the more proximal vessels. As this vessel does not have collateral supply it is functionally and "end artery".

B: Supplementary Figures and Legends

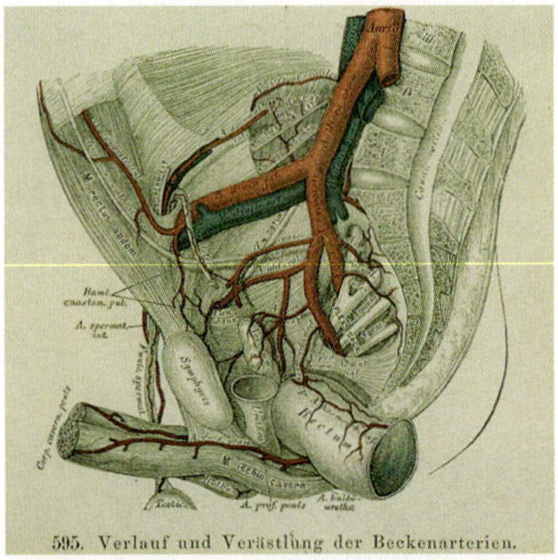

6-22

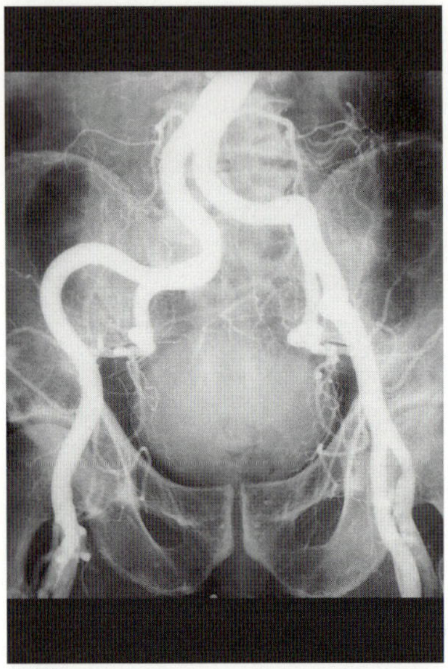
6-23

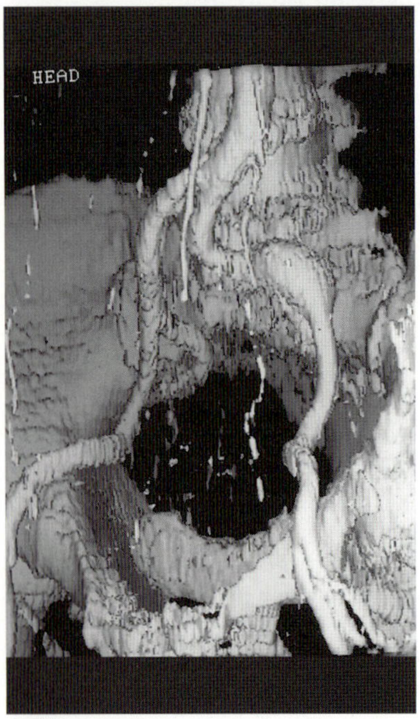

6-24

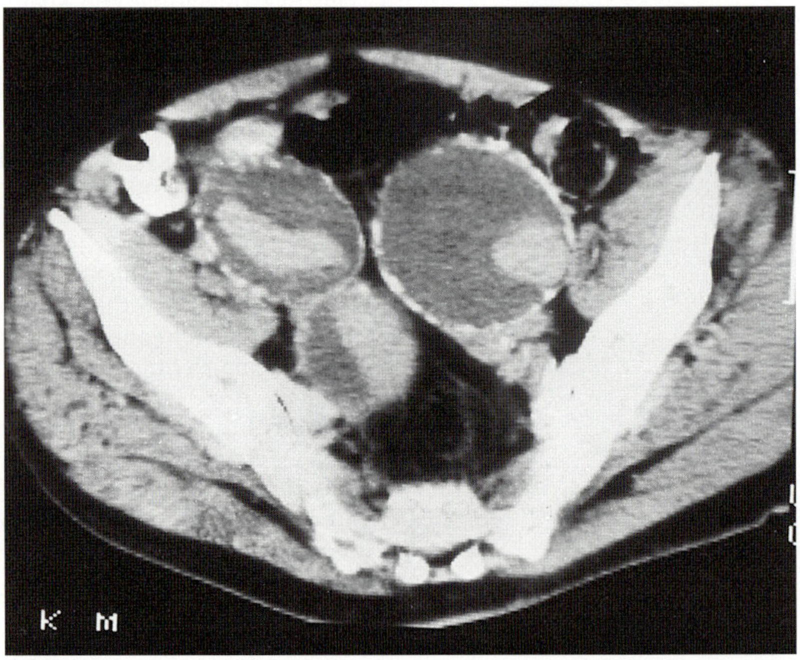

6-25

Fig. 6-22. Anatomy of the pelvic arteries. (From: Descriptive and Topographic Anatomy of Man, C. Heitzmann, 1893)

Fig. 6-23. Elongation of the aorta and the entire pelvic axis without aneurysms or signs of an occlusive arteriosclerotic process; a phenomenon which can occur in some elderly patients

Fig. 6-24. Reconstructed three-dimensional spiral computerized tomography scan showing the elongated pelvic arteries with aneurysms

Fig. 6-25. Computerized tomography with contrast material shows bilateral aneurysms of the common iliac artery, as well as aneurysmal dilatation of the right internal iliac artery

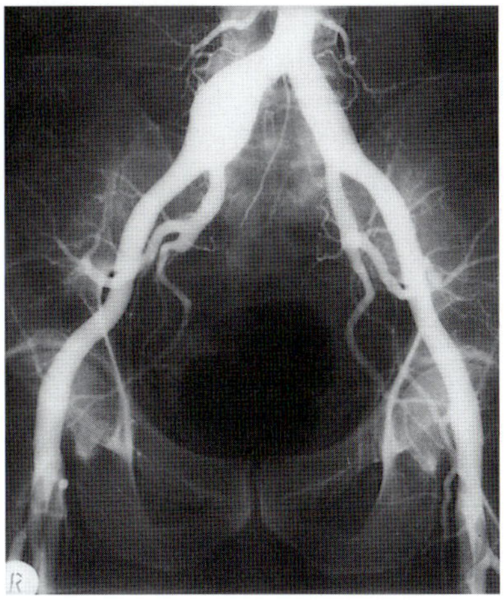

6-26

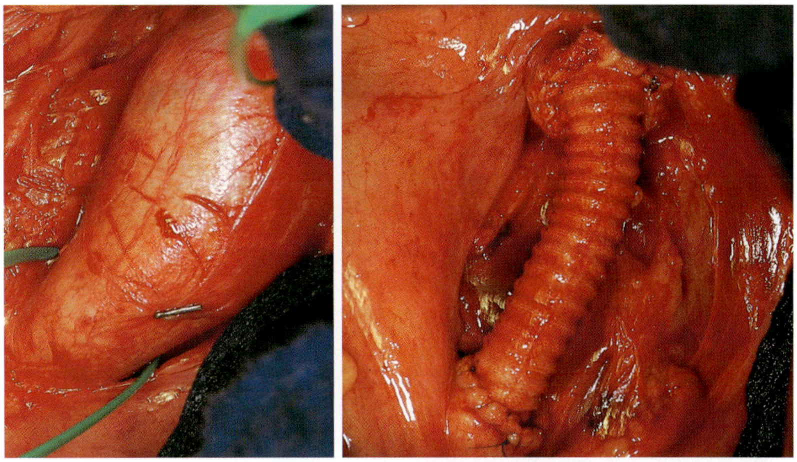

6-27

Fig. 6-26. Angiographic picture of an isolated, spindle-shaped aneurysm of the right common iliac artery

Fig. 6-27. Operative views demonstrating the aneurysm; *right*, a Dacron graft between the origin of the common iliac artery and the iliac bifurcation

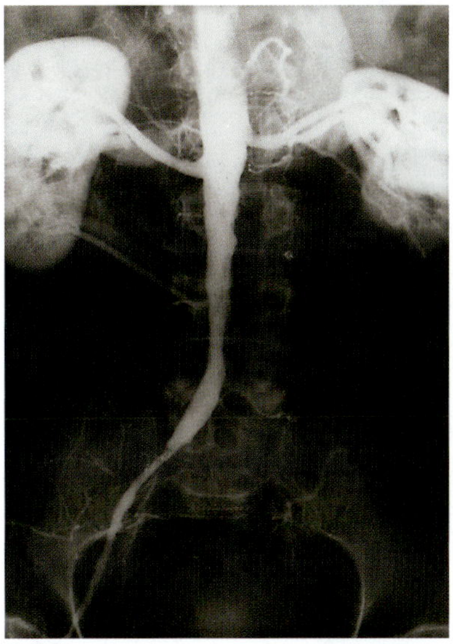

6-28

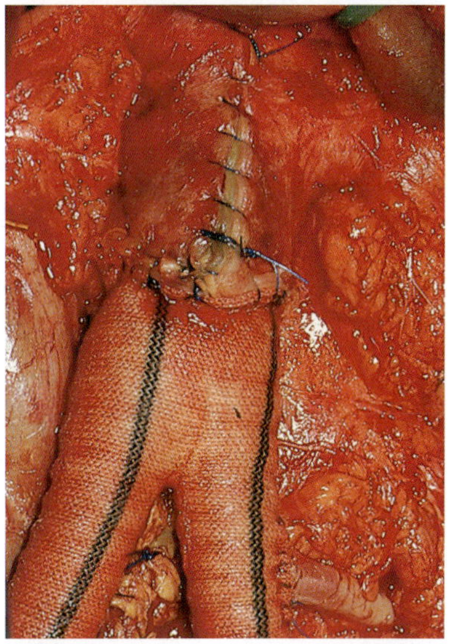

6-29

Fig. 6-28. The angiogram shows atherosclerosis and thrombus within the infrarenal aorta with occlusion of the left common and external iliac arteries, as well as bilateral occlusion of the internal iliac arteries

Fig. 6-29. The surgical approach involved a thromboendarterectomy of the aorta up to the level of the renal arteries. In this case the aorta was closed in a longitudinal manner below the renal arteries and attached to a Y-shaped Dacron prosthesis in an end-to-end fashion. The two arms of the Y were joined to the femoral arteries, bypassing the long occlusion

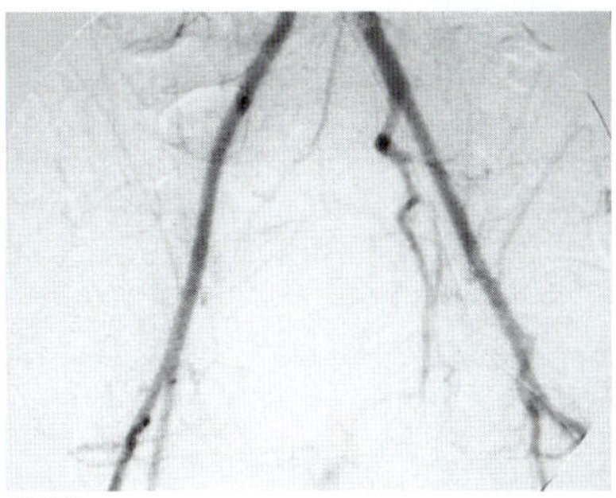

6-30

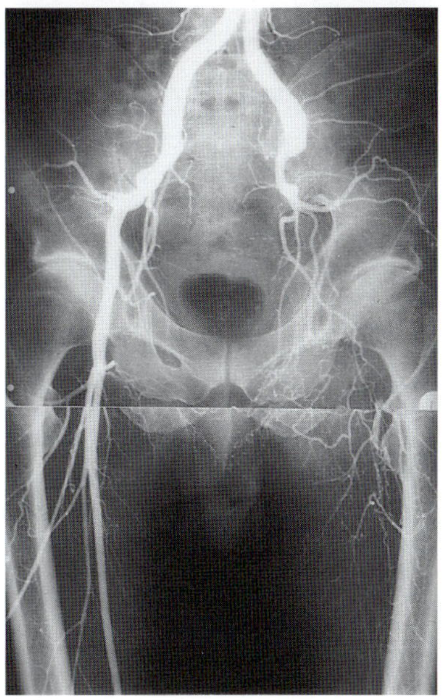

6-31

Fig. 6-30. Isolated occlusion of the right internal iliac artery in a 38 year old patient with BUERGER's disease. In addition there is a bilateral occlusion of the calf arteries with chronic ischemia and gangrene

Fig. 6-31. Embolic occlusion of the left external iliac artery and femoral arteries in an otherwise healthy patient with atrial fibrillation

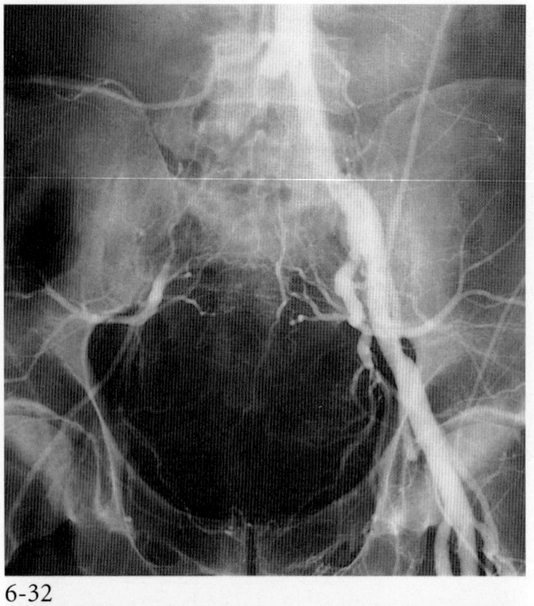

6-32

Fig. 6-32. Right-sided occlusion of the common and external iliac arteries following thrombosis in an area already threatened by artherosclerotic stenosis

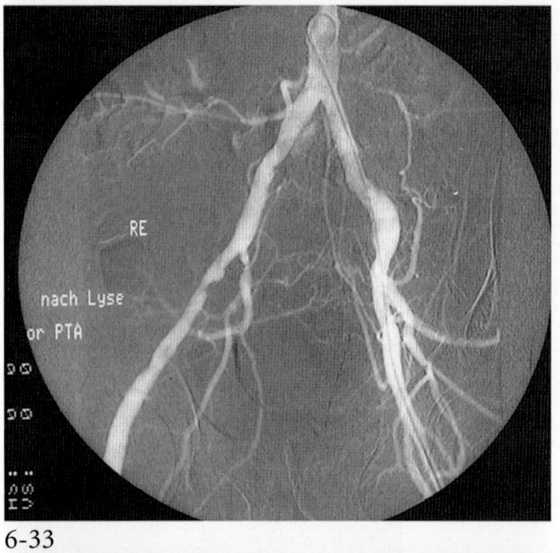

6-33

Fig. 6-33. Unmasking of the chronic stenosis through fibrinolytic therapy in the area of the right common and external iliac arteries

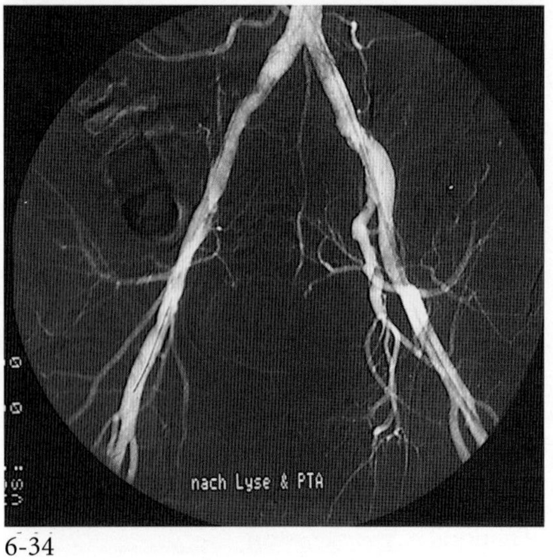

6-34

Fig. 6-34. Appearance after balloon catheter dilatation of the artherosclerotic stenosis with restoration of the entire right iliac system

Fig. 6-35. Older thrombotic occlusion of the right common iliac artery with marked collateral circulation via the lumbar arteries. Systemic fibrinolysis revealed the arteriosclerotic stenoses which were treated by percutaneous transluminal angioplasty (PTA)

Fig. 6-36. Appearance following percutaneous transluminal angioplasty (PTA)

Fig. 6-37. Color duplex ultrasonography showing dissection of the external iliac artery with two channels separated by a septum

Fig. 6-38. Severe artherosclerosis of the left pelvic arteries in the region of the common and external iliac arteries

Fig. 6-39. Following percutaneous transluminal angioplasty (PTA), a dissection of the external iliac artery developed coupled with thrombotic occlusion

Fig. 6-40. Re-opening of the occlusion with fibrinolysis

Fig. 6-41. Fixing the dissection plane to the true wall by a stent after the successful lysis of the thrombus

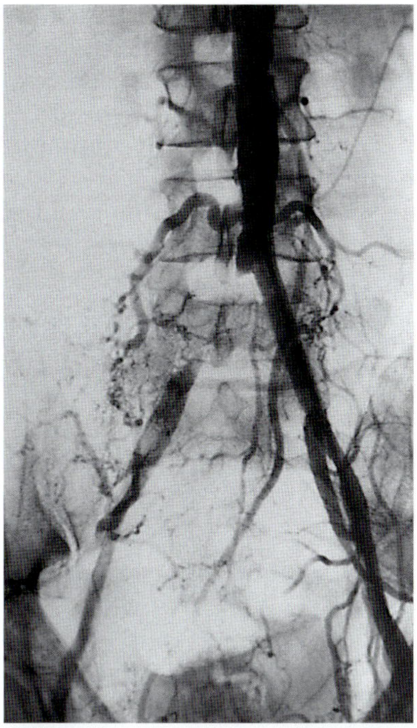

6-35

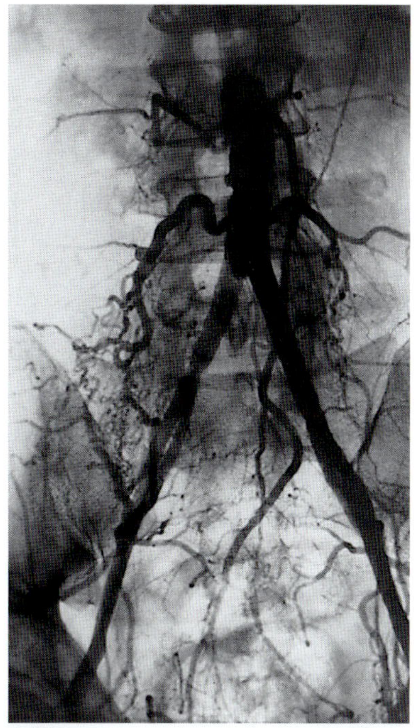

6-36

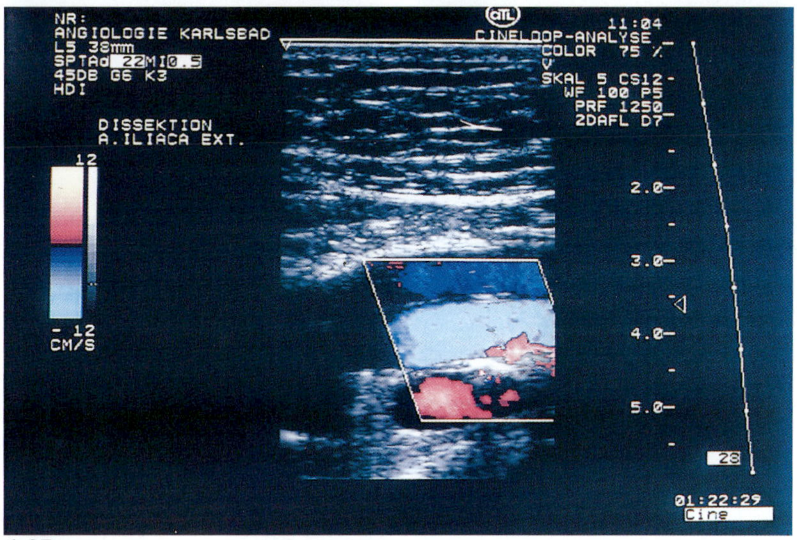

6-37

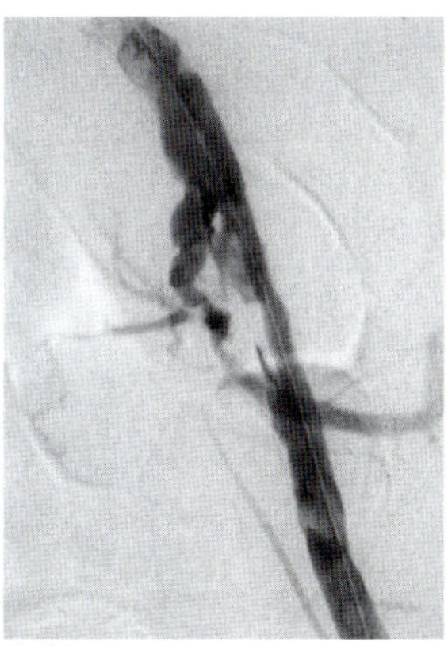

6-38

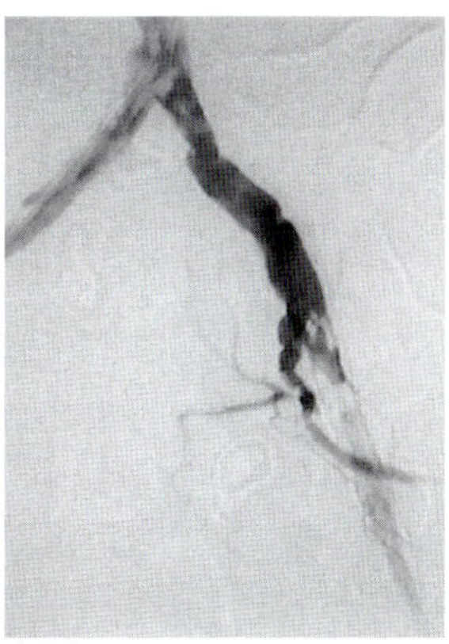

6-39

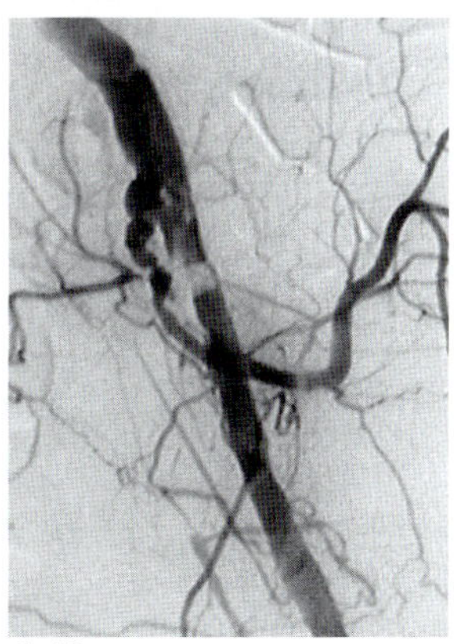

6-40

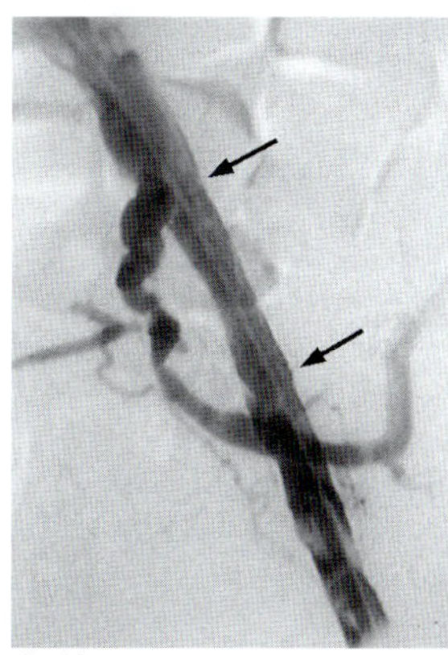

6-41

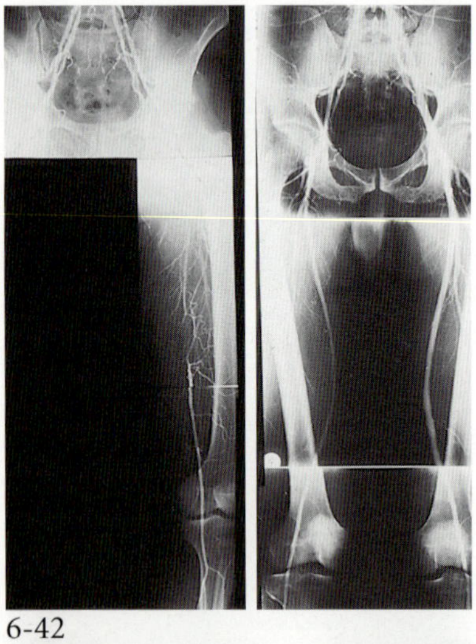

6-42

Fig. 6-42. A 52 year old patient with arteriosclerotic occlusion of the pelvic and thigh arteries, shown pre-preoperatively and then following extensive thromboendarterectomy of the pelvic axis involving the common and superficial femoral arteries as well as the first part of the popliteal artery

Fig. 6-43. An 80 year old patient with multiple lesions in the infrarenal aorta and both iliac systems with filling of the femoral arteries after an aorto-bifemoral Dacron Y-shaped graft was performed with end-to-side anastomoses

Fig. 6-44. Dacron Y-bypass in a patient with bilateral occlusion of the iliac vessels. The operative view shows the retroperitoneal aortic anastomosis with a short main body of the graft

Fig. 6-45. Angiogram of an aorto-femoral bypass. A 65 year old woman with a left-sided iliac artery occlusion with femoral filling. An iliac-to-femoral bypass(unilateral bypass) was performed with the proximal anastomosis placed near the aortic bifurcation

Figs. 6-46, 6-47. Operative view of the same patient. The proximal anastomosis extends onto the aorta, while the distal one connects to the common femoral artery. The ostia of the deep and superficial femoral arteries are widened by a Y-shaped patch angioplasty using the distal end of the graft at the anastomotic site

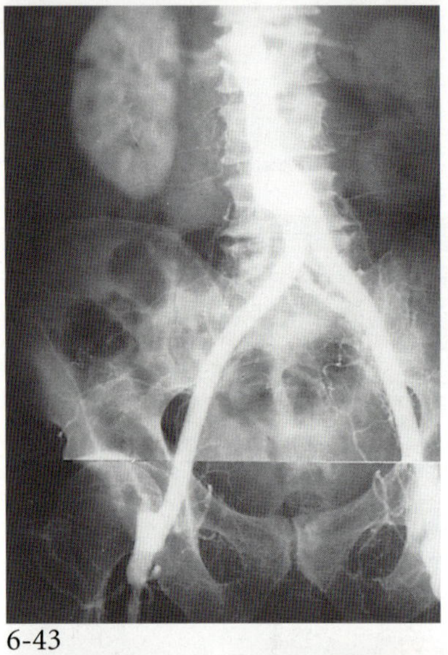

6-43

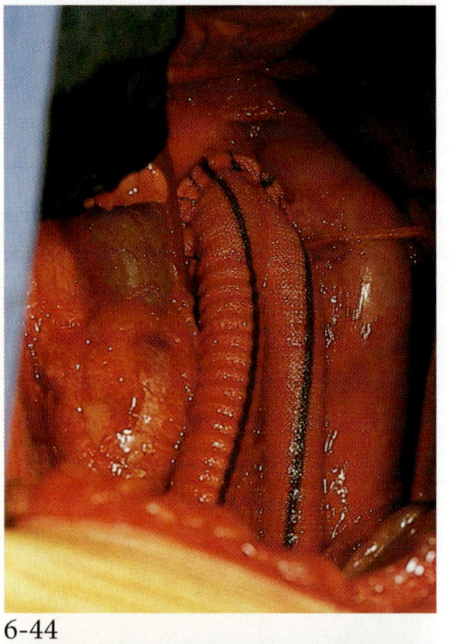

6-44

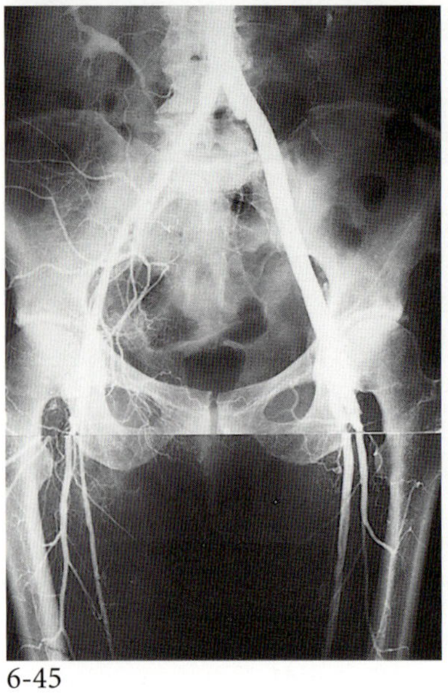

6-45

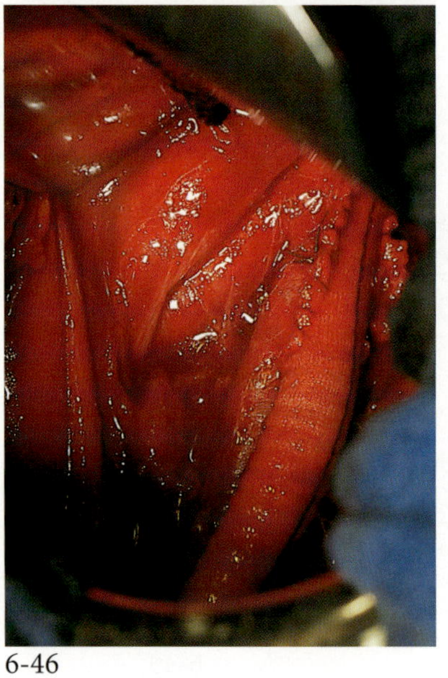

6-46

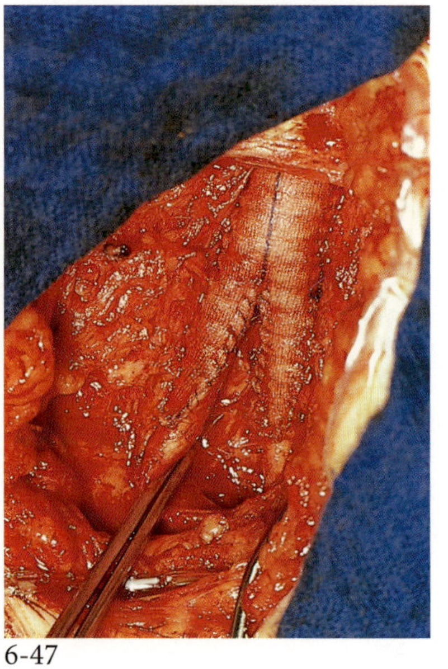

6-47

Fig. 6-48. A 73 year old patient with severe obliterative arthero-sclerosis of the right iliac arteries and a stenosis in the left femoral artery bifurcation. At *right*, angiogram following iliac-to-femoral crossover bypass from left to right, and a simultaneous profundaplasty on the left

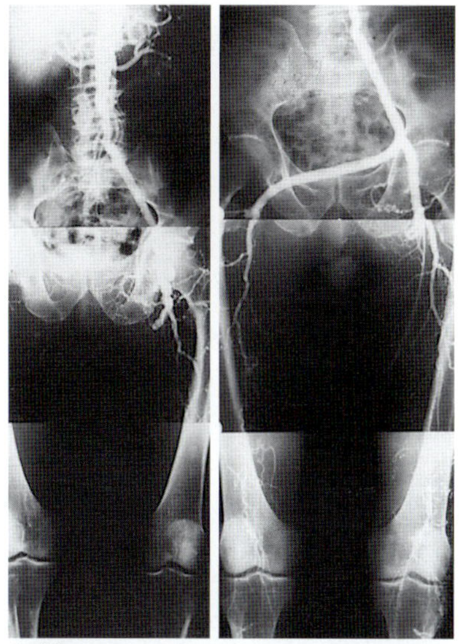

6-48

Fig. 6-49. Axillo-bifemoral bypass. Occlusion of the infrarenal aorta and both iliac systems in a 70 year old women with high medical risks. A Dacron bypass graft was placed from the right axillary artery to both common femoral arteries

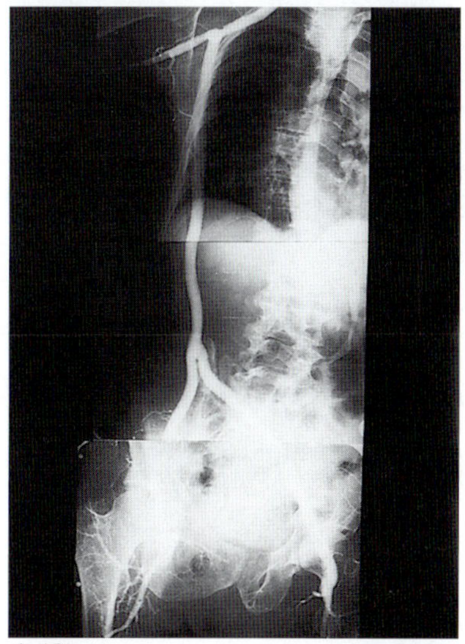

6-49

Fig. 6-50. Radiation-induced arteriopathy in the pelvis. The skin shows typical poikiloderma 17 years after ionizing radiation was used to treat a gynecological tumor. Angiography shows narrowing of the left common iliac artery and occlusion of the left external iliac artery and common femoral artery without any suggestion of arteriosclerotic lesions in other vessels

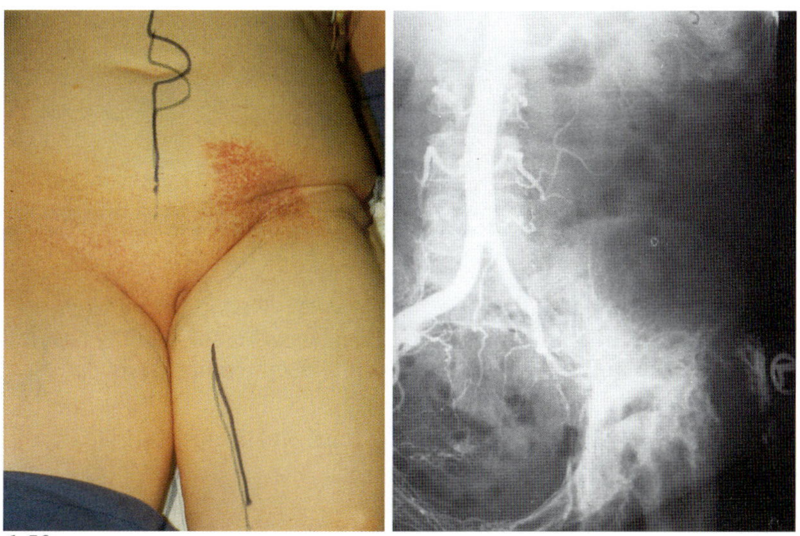

6-50

Fig. 6-51. Appearance after a high iliac-to-femoral crossover bypass using a prosthetic bypass graft. The incision sites, as drawn in Fig. 6-50, were designed to avoid the radiation dermatitis

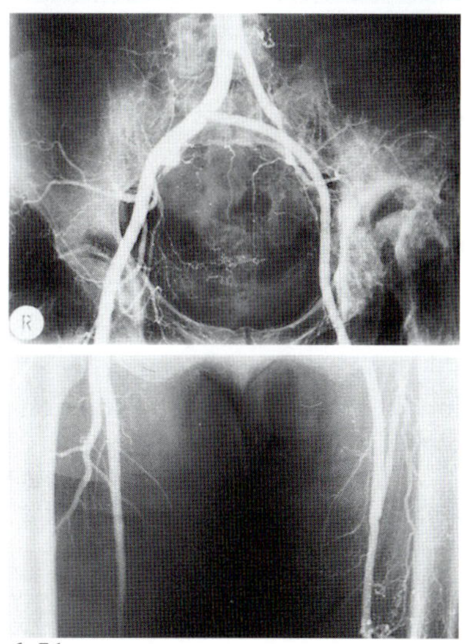

6-51

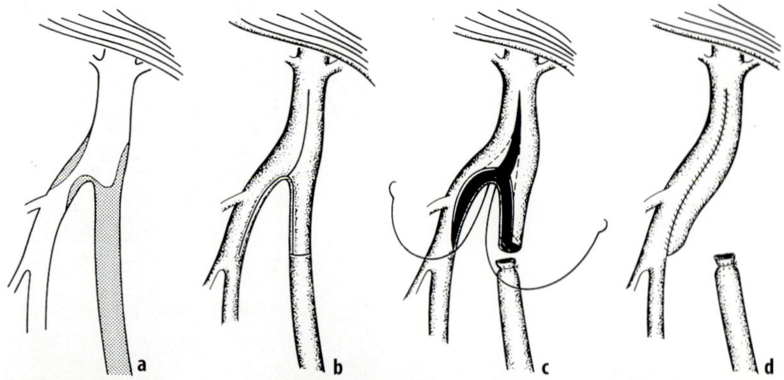

6-52

Fig. 6-52. Schematic drawing of a profundaplasty with stenoses in the common and deep femoral arteries with occlusion of the superficial femoral artery. The drawing shows the steps in reconstruction of the take-off of the deep femoral artery with an arterial patch made from the proximal superficial femoral artery. The corresponding incisions in the deep and superficial femoral arteries allow the artery to be used without torsion to enlarge the proximal part of the deep femoral artery

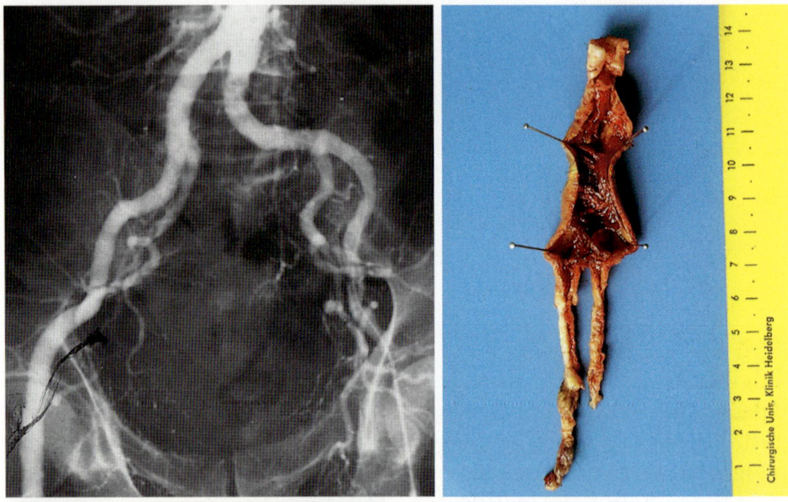

6-53

Fig. 6-53. Preoperative angiogram showing occlusion of the common, deep and superficial femoral arteries, as well as the surgical specimen after thromboendarterectomy of the femoral bifurcation addressing the occlusions in all three arteries

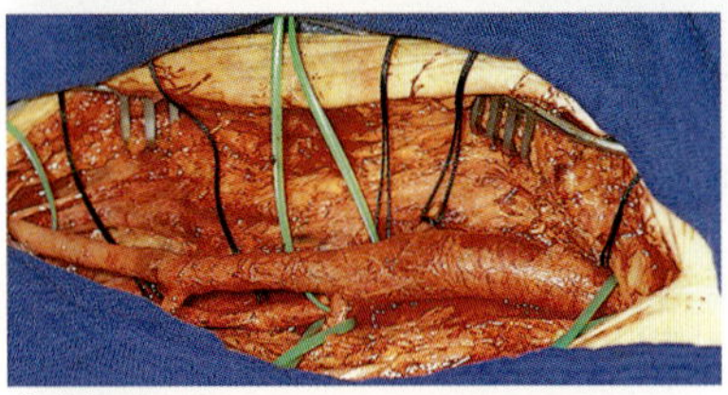

6-54

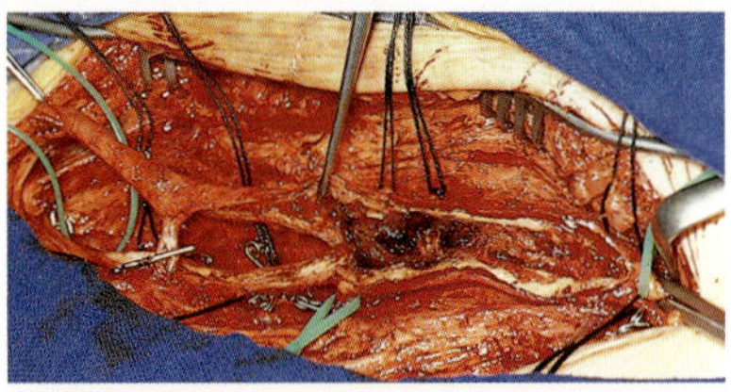

6-55

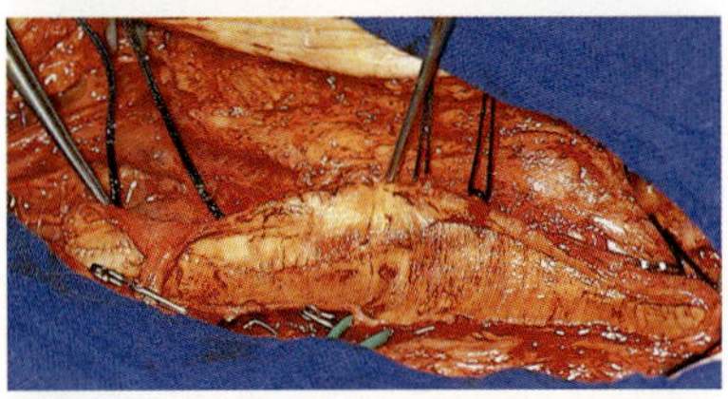

6-56

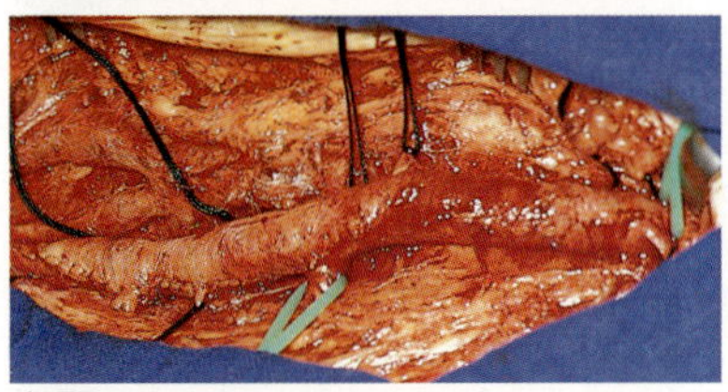

6-57

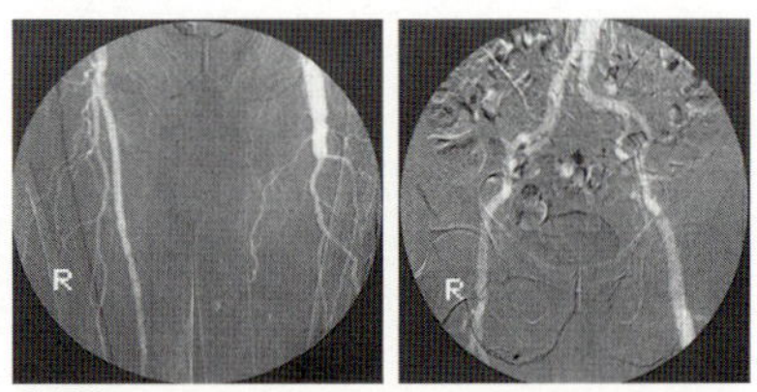

6-58

Fig. 6-54. Operative field showing the entire femoral bifurcation with the various branches

Fig. 6-55. Longitudinal arteriotomy involving all the femoral arteries. The occlusive cylinder with focal fresh thrombi is easily seen

Fig. 6-56. Appearance following thromboendarterectomy of the common, deep and superficial femoral arteries

Fig. 6-57. Operative site following preparation of the artery patch to widen the proximal part of the deep femoral artery

Fig. 6-58. Postoperative angiogram showing the lengthy repair of the deep femoral artery

Fig. 6-59. High-grade proximal stenosis of the deep femoral artery with lengthy occlusion of the superficial femoral artery

Fig. 6-60. Condition following crossover balloon dilatation (PTA) of the proximal deep femoral artery without any residual stenosis. The calcified wall of the superficial femoral artery is seen

Fig. 6-61. A 40 year old patient with partial occlusion of the deep femoral artery because of a femoral aneurysm. Preoperative angiogram showing occlusion of the main trunk of the deep femoral artery (*arrows*)

Fig. 6-62. Operative view showing a small aneurysm (*arrow*) 2.5 cm distal to the take-off of the deep femoral artery

Fig. 6-63. Operative view with open aneurysm

Fig. 6-64. The specimen shows the organized thrombus attached the aneurysm; this caused the occlusion of the deep femoral artery

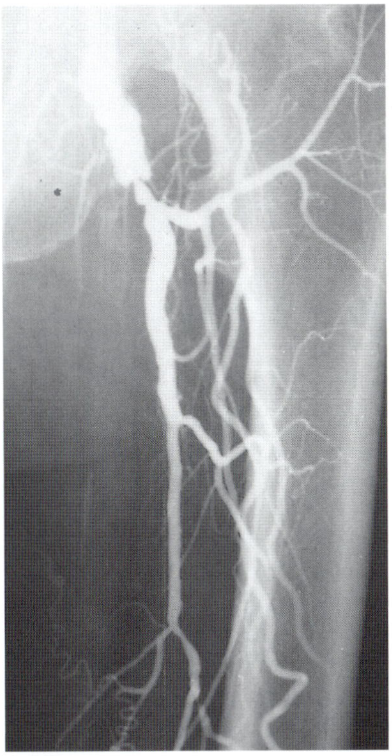

6-59

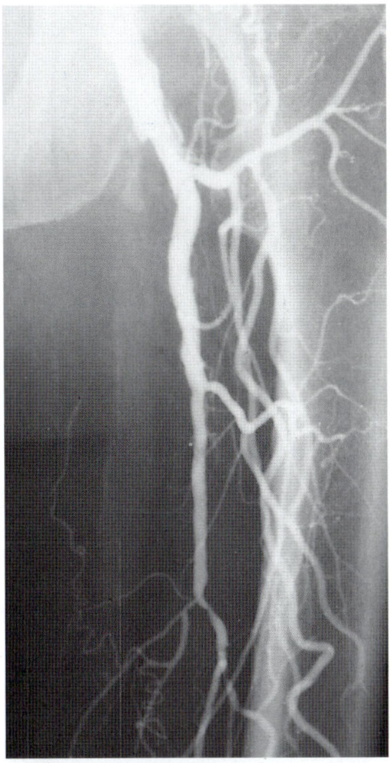

6-60

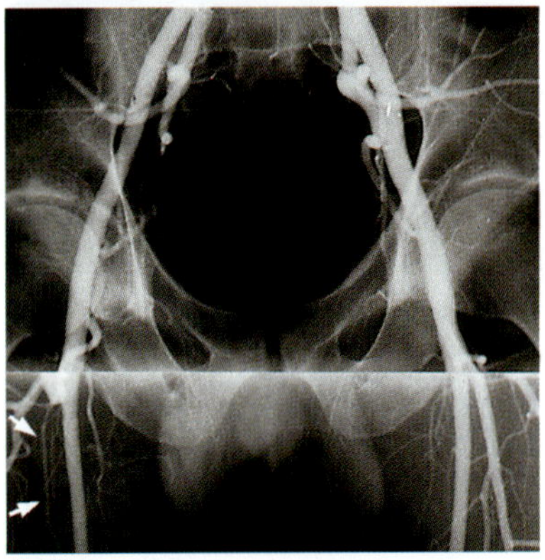

6-61

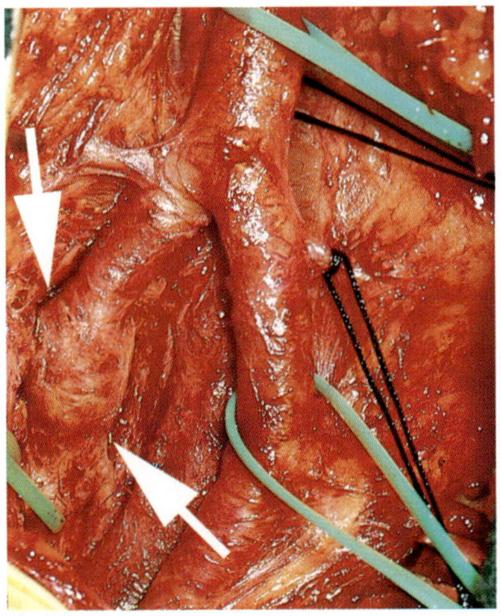

6-62

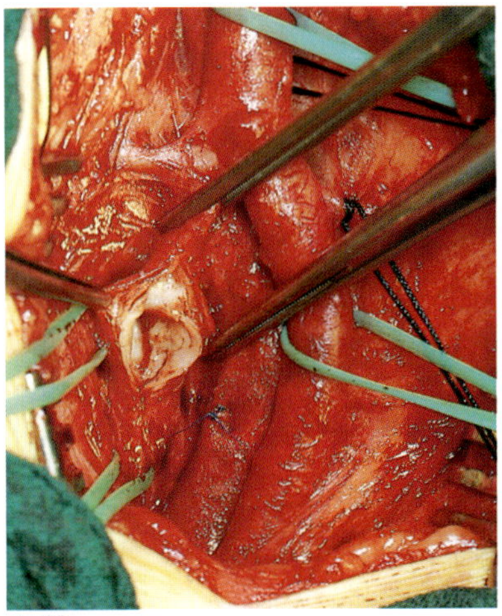

6-63

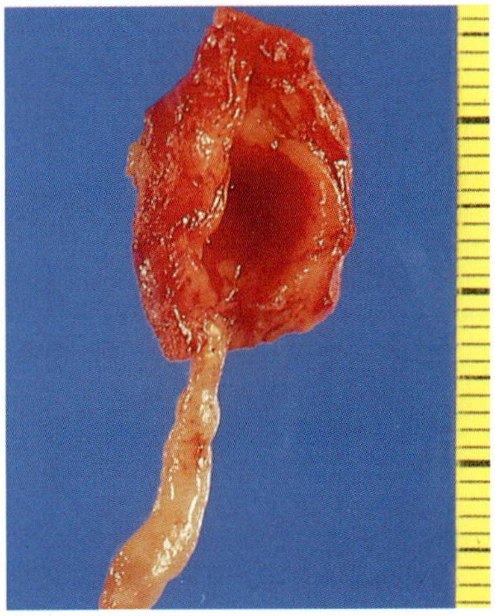

6-64

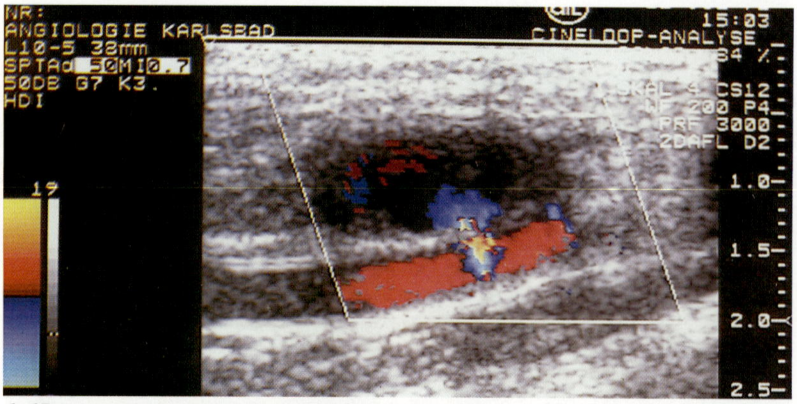

6-65

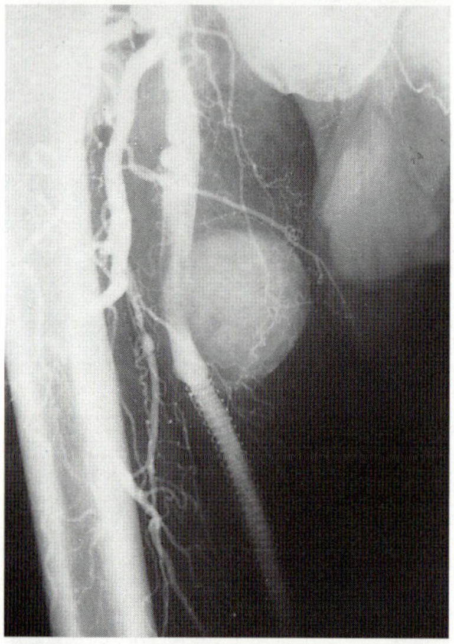

6-66

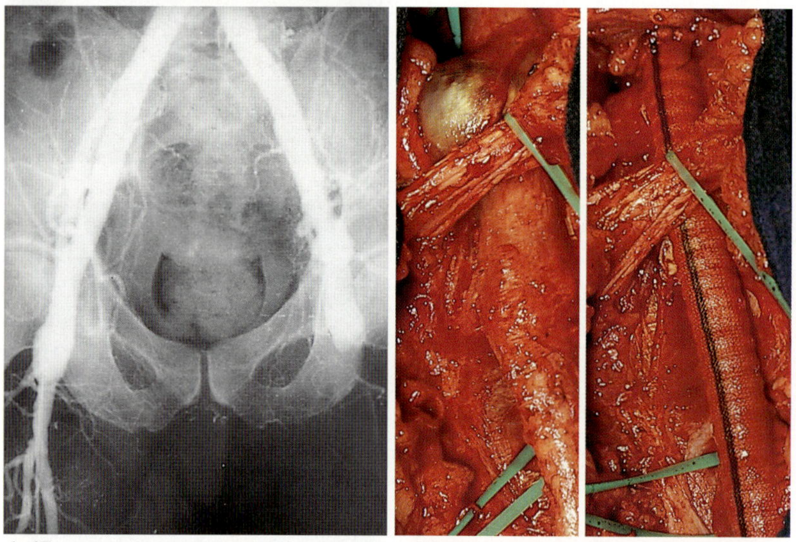

6-67

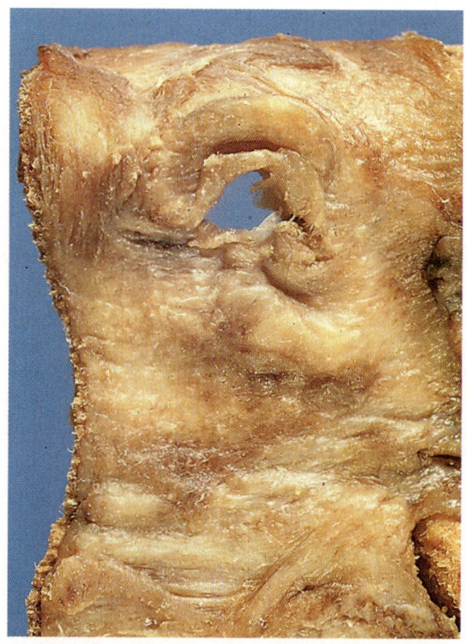

6-68

Fig. 6-65. Color duplex ultrasonography showing a false aneurysm of the femoral artery following angiography

Fig. 6-66. False aneurysm resulting from degenerative changes in a femoro-popliteal, spirally reinforced Dacron graft. The aneurysm arose in a weakened area of the proximal part of the bypass

Fig. 6-67. False aneurysm after rupture of the left limb of an aorto-bifemoral graft below the inguinal ligament. Perhaps because of mechanical irritation the graft ruptured at this site and formed an encapsulated cherry-sized aneurysm. Preoperative angiogram, operative view with aneurysm at inguinal ligament and interposition of a Dacron graft after excising the old anastomosis

Fig. 6-68. Specimen showing the ruptured Dacron graft with the site where the aneurysm developed

Fig. 6-69. Ultrasonographic visualization of an inguinal anastomotic aneurysm following a Dacron aorto-bifemoral bypass (*arrow*)

Fig. 6-70. Operative view after exposing the false aneurysm in the vicinity of the anastomosis. The treatment consists of eliminating the aneurysm by inserting a prosthetic inlay or interposition graft

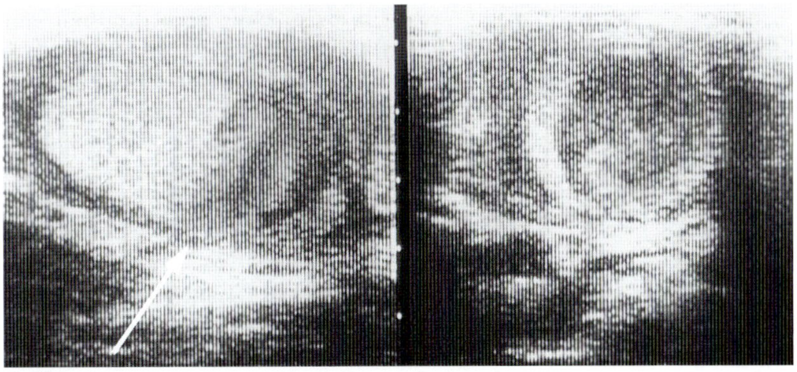

6-69

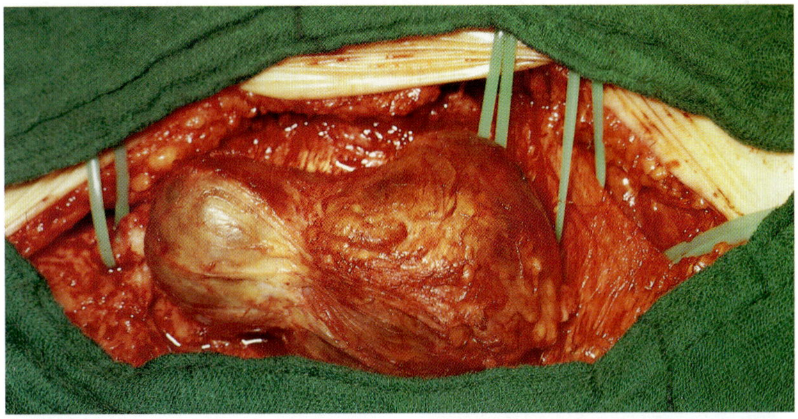

6-70

Figs. 6-71, 6-72. Two examples of a puncture-related A-V fistula following angiography and cardiac catheterization. In the groin there is a typical machinery-like bruit present. Angiography shows rapid passage of contrast material from the arteries into the femoral and iliac veins. The usual location of the fistula is the proximal part of the deep femoral artery (*arrows*), as the deep veins pass in close proximity making fistula development easier. Preoperative localization of the fistula can be difficult, so that it may be necessary to expose the entire femoral bifurcation

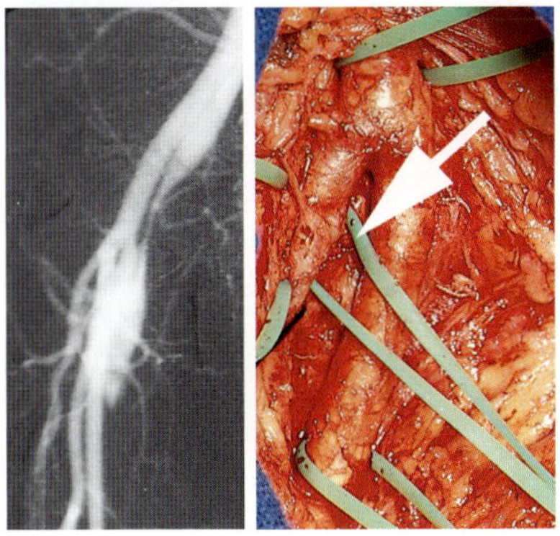

6-71

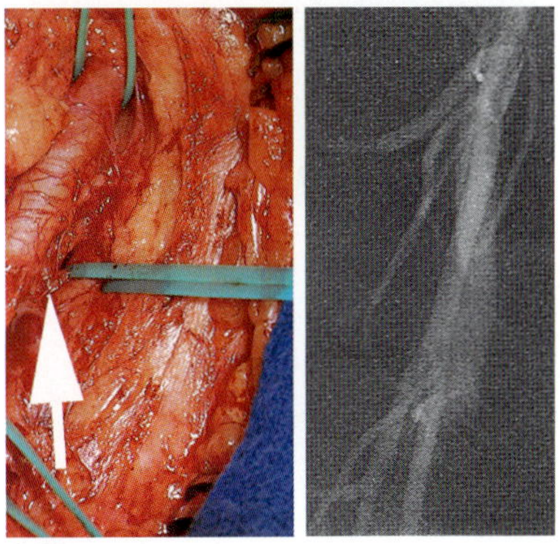

6-72

Fig. 6-73. Destruction of the common femoral artery and part of the deep femoral artery as well as the femur from a bullet wound. Appearance after inserting a vein graft to replace the damaged segment (*arrows*)

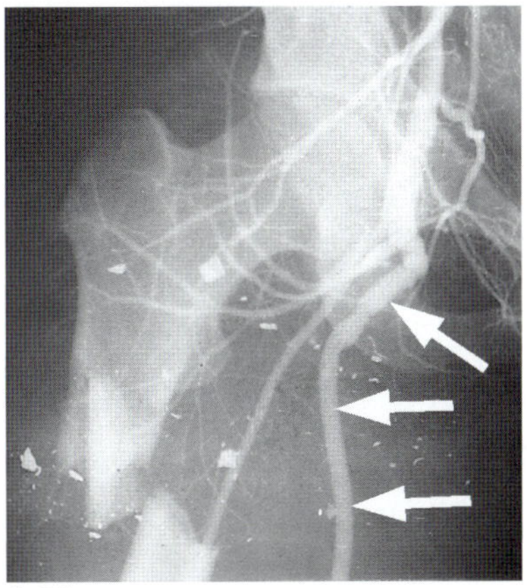

6-73

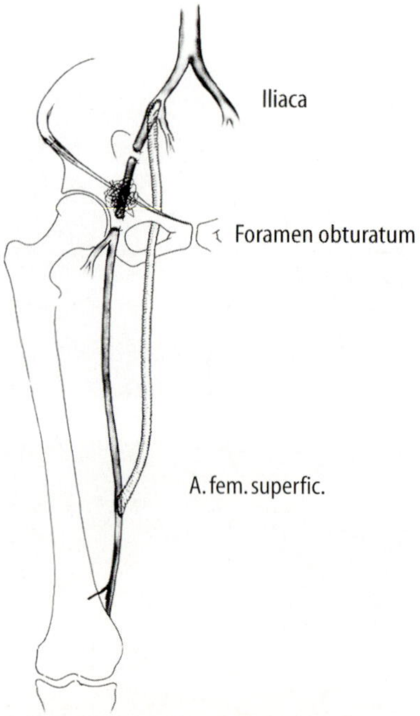

6-74

Fig. 6-74. One can avoid the inguinal canal by using an iliac-to-femoral obturator bypass. The bypass runs from the external or common iliac artery to the superficial femoral artery detouring around the site of infection. After removal of the prosthesis from the infected area, if possible, the native deep and superficial femoral arteries are anastomosed

Fig. 6-75. Primary inguinal infections in the early postoperative period following the insertion of a prosthetic femoro-popliteal bypass

Fig. 6-76. Chronic inguinal infection with exposed PTFE prosthesis

Figs. 6-77, 6-78. Pre- and postoperative angiography showing a left iliac-to-femoral obturator bypass following a prosthetic infection in the groin

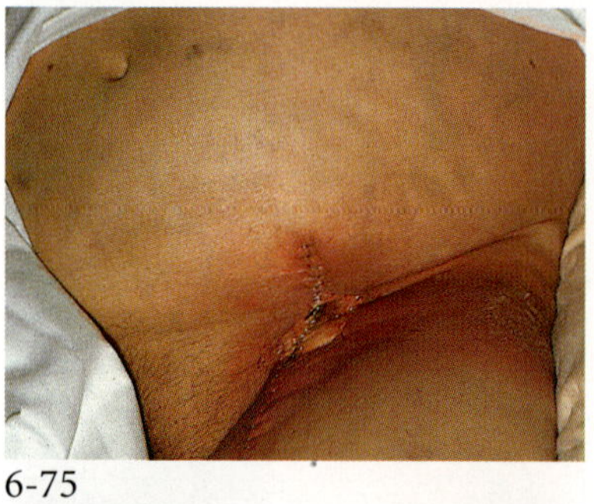

6-75

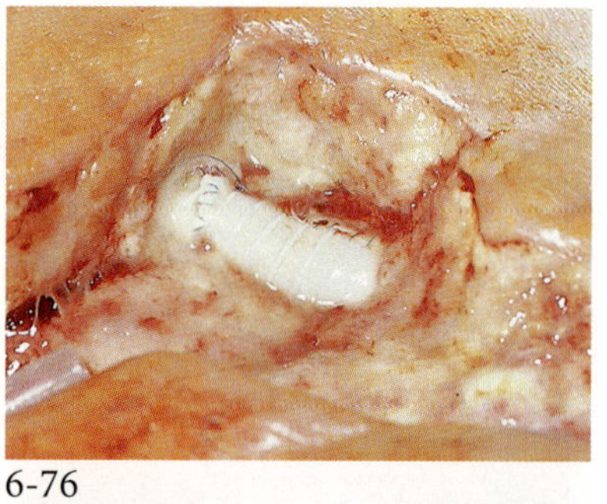

6-76

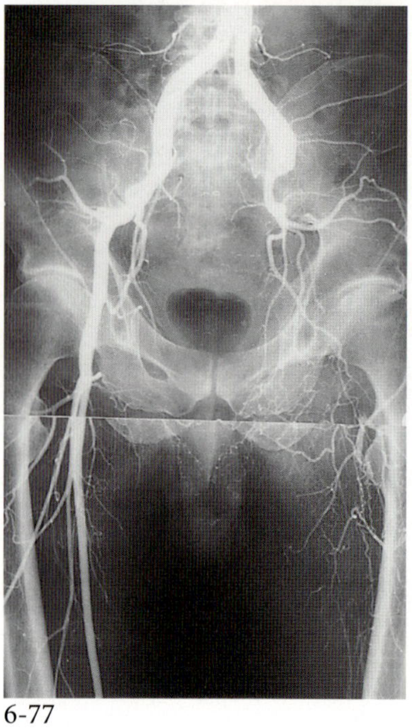

6-77

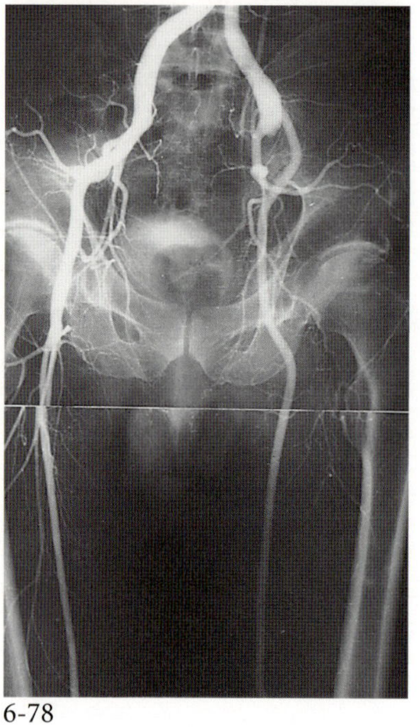

6-78

Fig. 6-79. Perigraft reaction following placing an axillo-femoral Dacron bypass. The graft is surround by a fluid enclosed by a pseudo-membrane, producing a cystic change clinically

Fig. 6-80. Ultrasonography of the inguinal region showing the cystic bulge. A prosthesis within the fluid is shown clearly in both the lateral and cross-sectional views

Fig. 6-81. Perigraft reaction about a Dacron graft in the right inguinal region. In this view, taken 2 months after surgery, the cystic bulges are unmistakable

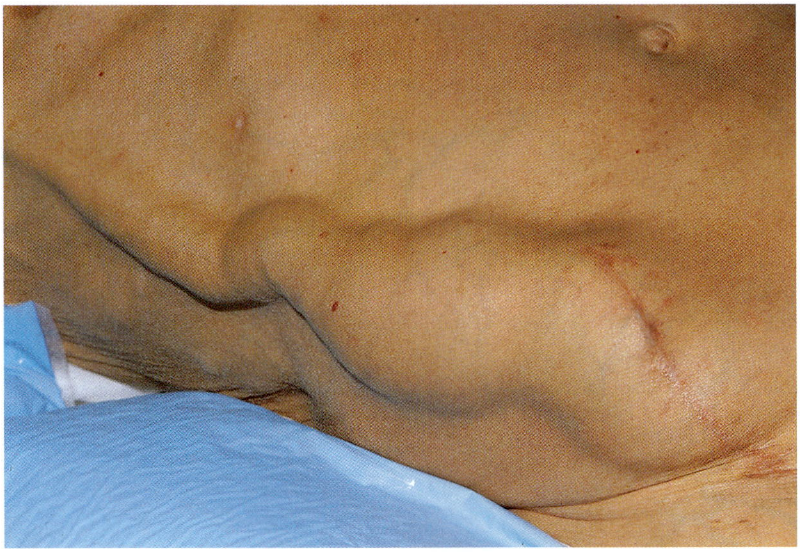

6-79

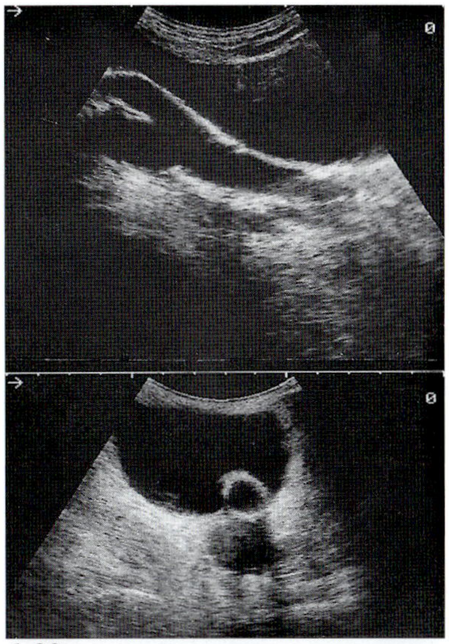

6-80

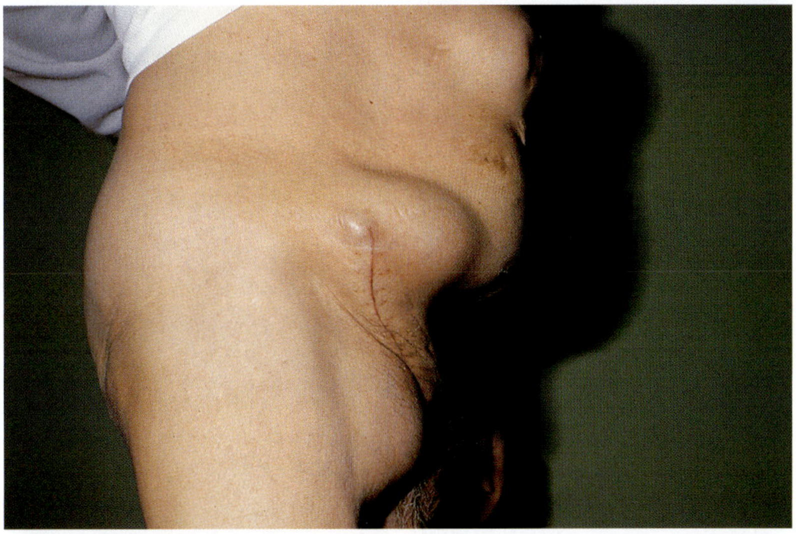

6-81

Fig. 6-82. The wall of the Dacron prosthesis, attached in an end-to-side manner, is easily seen in a sea of fluid

Fig. 6-83. After opening the perigraft space, the pseudocystic membrane is apparent. The repair consists of excising the membrane and changing the prosthesis, using a different material such as PTFE

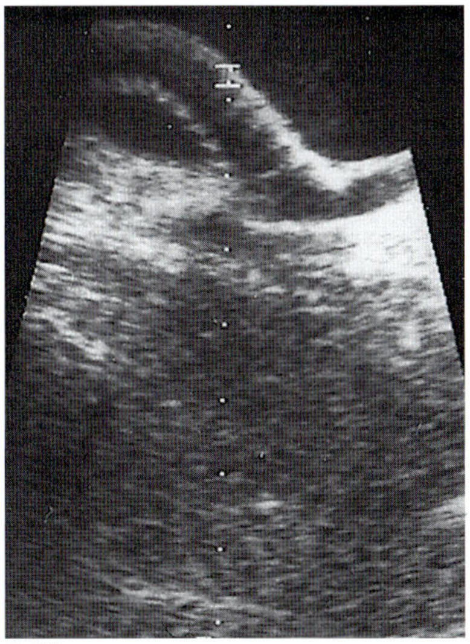

6-82

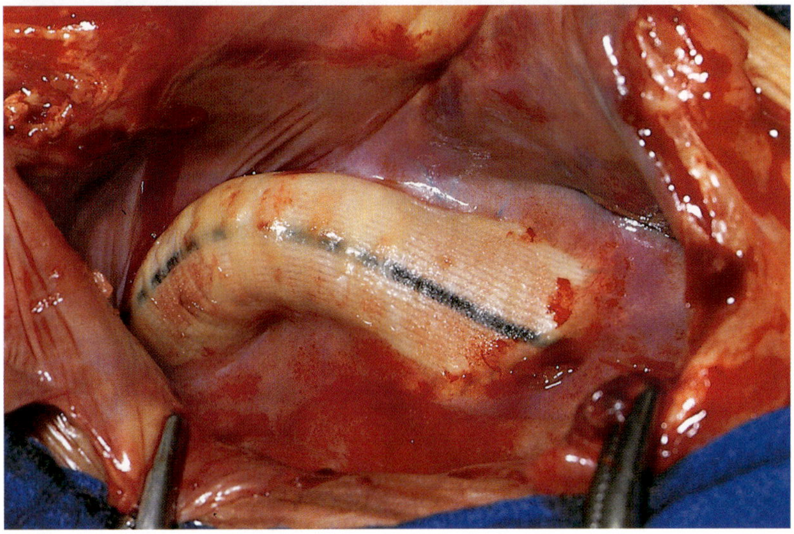

6-83

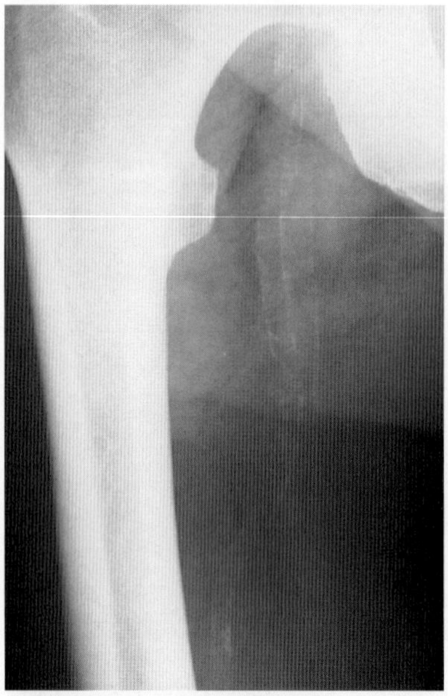

6-84

Fig. 6-84. Routine X-ray picture of the proximal thigh showing the deep and superficial femoral arteries, visible without contrast material because of extensive medial calcification

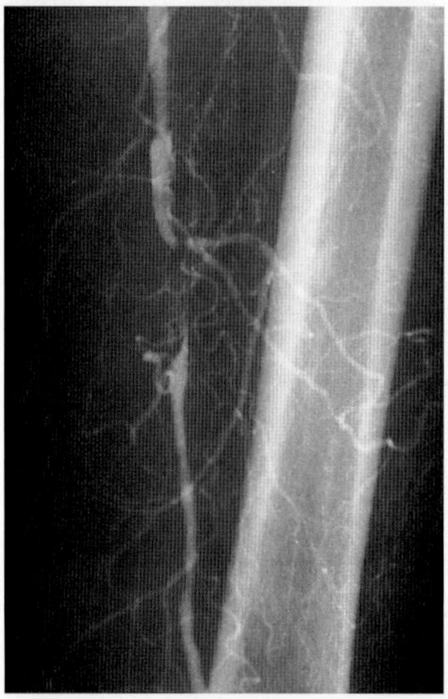

6-85

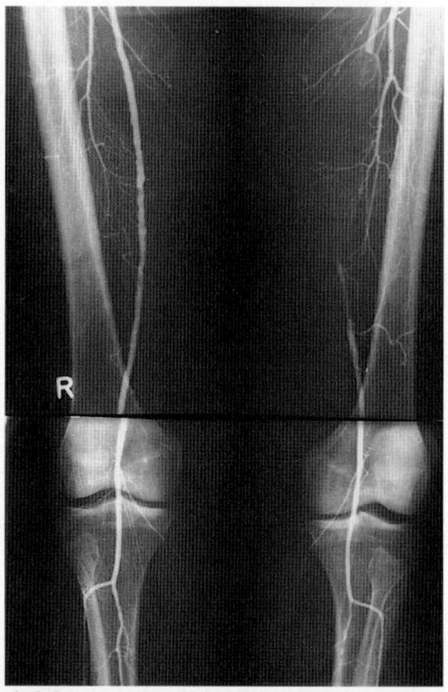

6-86

Fig. 6-85. Short occlusion of the superficial femoral artery in the adductor canal, which is a common site for disease

Fig. 6-86. Longer occlusion of the left superficial femoral artery with filling of the popliteal artery above the knee joint. Early arteriosclerotic changes can be observed on the right side in the same regions, showing the symmetry of arteriosclerotic disease

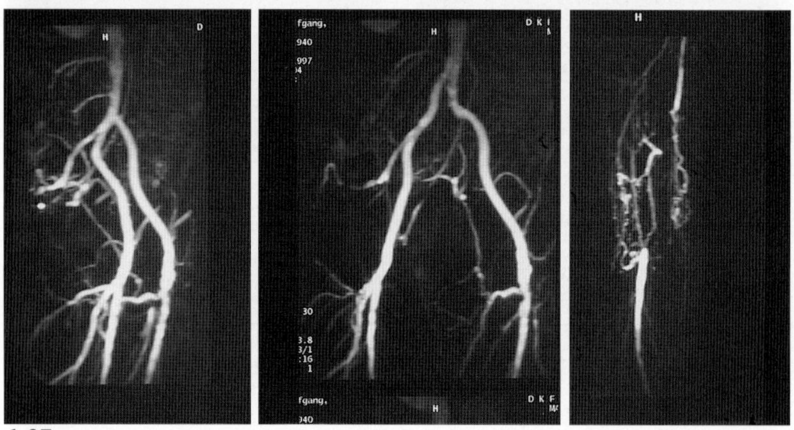

6-87

Fig. 6-87. Magnetic resonance angiography. In this modern imaging technique, occlusion of both the deep and superficial femoral arteries on the left is demonstrated in a patient with severe claudication and a walking distance of only 50 m. As magnetic resonance imaging continues to improve, such angiographic procedures will become well-established

Fig. 6-88. Spontaneous arteriosclerotic aneurysm of the right superficial femoral artery with a typical small aneurysm of the left popliteal artery. The distal vessels are dilated and show embolic occlusion

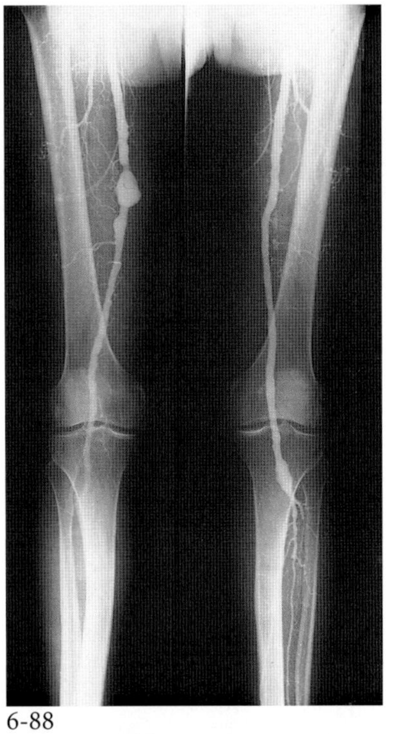

6-88

Fig. 6-89. BUERGER's syndrome with marked vasospasm. The phenomenon of the standing wave is shown in the superficial femoral artery in a 30 year old woman. The same changes can be a normal finding or occur following catheter manipulation

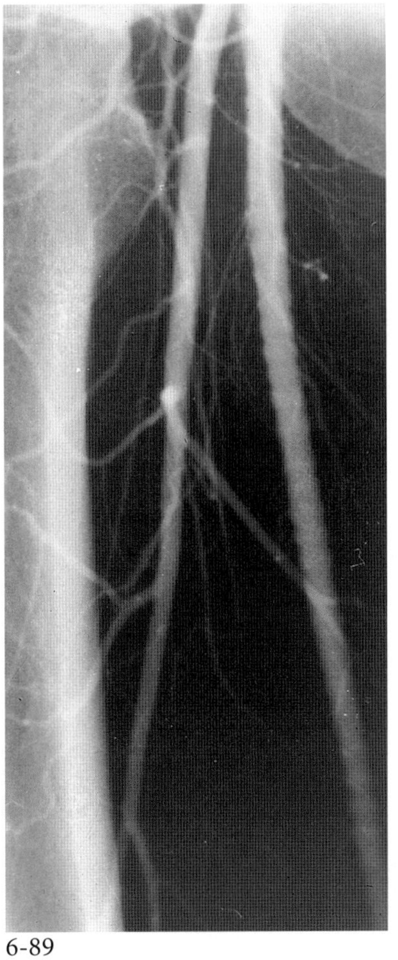

6-89

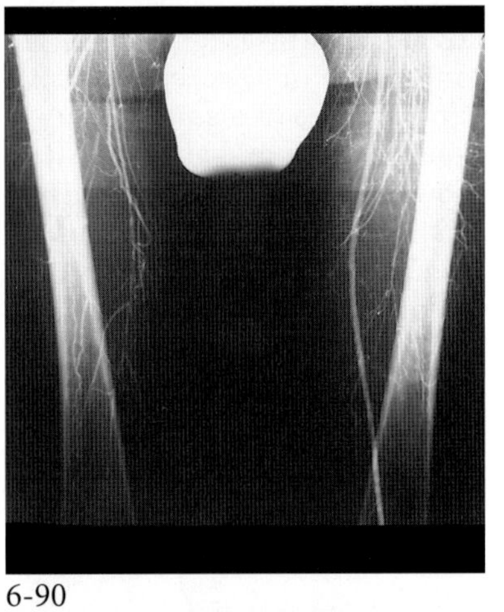

6-90

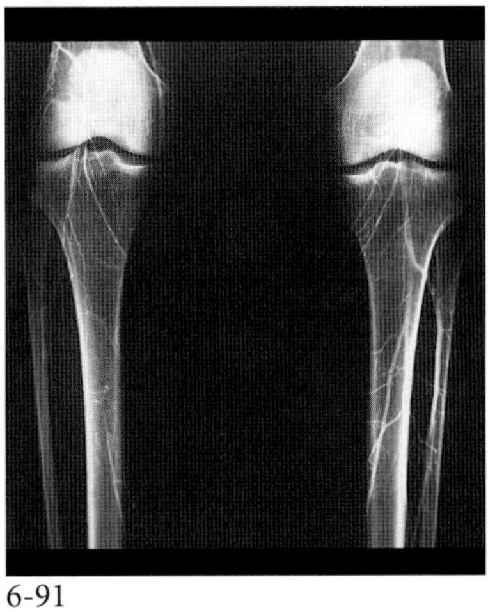

6-91

Figs. 6-90, 6-91. Ergotism. Angiography of both legs in a 48 year old women who had been treated for years with ergot-containing products because of migraine headaches. She had severe circulatory problems in both legs, but once the medication was stopped, the problems completely reversed and her pulses became normal

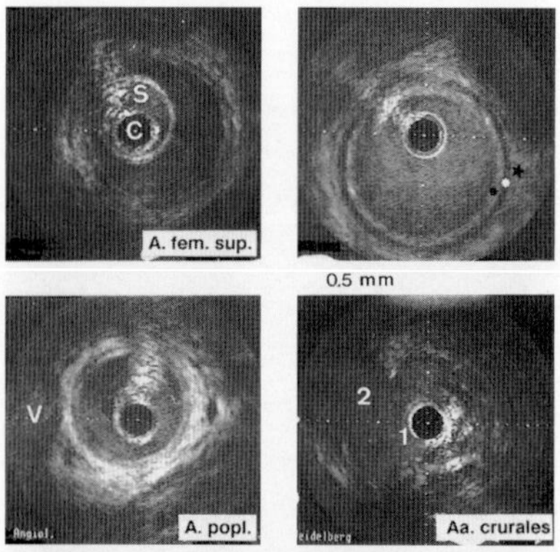

6-92

Fig. 6-92. Intravascular ultrasonography of normal vessels. The femoral and popliteal arteries and the trifurcation of the popliteal artery are shown. A 5-F, 30-MHT catheter (*C*) (Cardiovascular Imaging Systems, Sunnyvale, CA) was used. Typical three-layered wall of a muscular artery. *Black star*, ultrasound intima; *white star*, media; *gray star*, adventitia; *1*, tibio-peroneal trunk; *2*, anterior tibial artery; *V*, accompanying vein; *S*, sheath

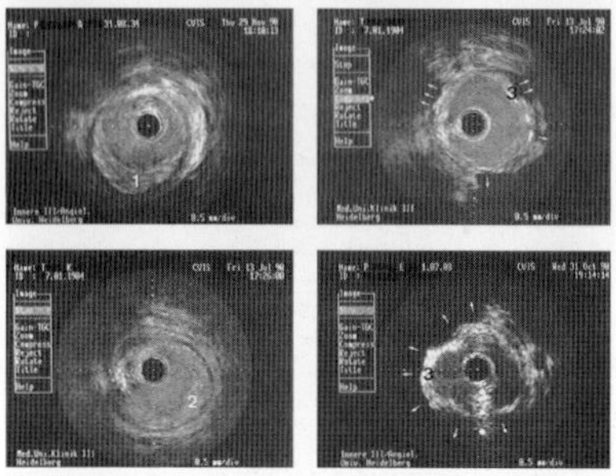

6-93

Fig. 6-93. Intravascular ultrasonography of diseased vessels. Various types of plaques in the superficial femoral artery are shown. *1*, fibrous plaque; *2*, lipid-rich plaque; *3*, calcified plaque, ≠, echo-free shadows; *asterisk*, artifact

Intravascular Ultrasonography

Intravascular ultrasonography creates a detailed two-dimensional cross-sectional image of an artery. It allows an exact quantification of all cross-sectional parameters of a vessel. Intimal plaques can be precisely identified because of the different echogenic properties of fat, connective tissue and calcium. Occlusive thrombi can be identified. This method is much better than contrast angiography or transcutaneous ultrasonography in quantifying and characterizing vessel wall changes. Fine structures such as dissection membranes and intima flaps can be shown even if they cannot be detected by angiography. Another advantage is that this detailed information allows one to choose the most appropriate catheter therapy (conventional PTA, stent, atherectomy or others). Moreover, the success of the therapy can be immediately and accurately documented

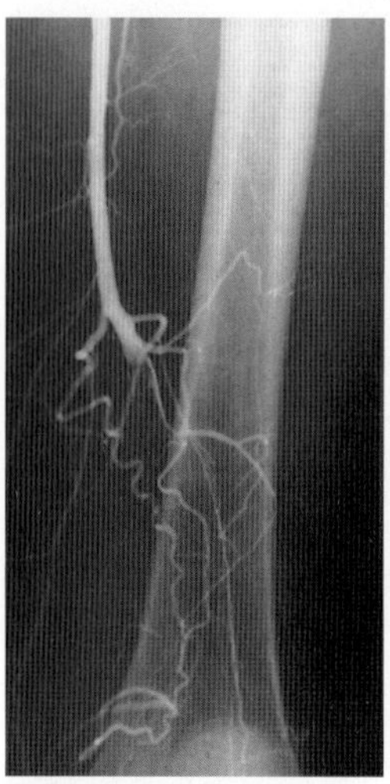

6-94

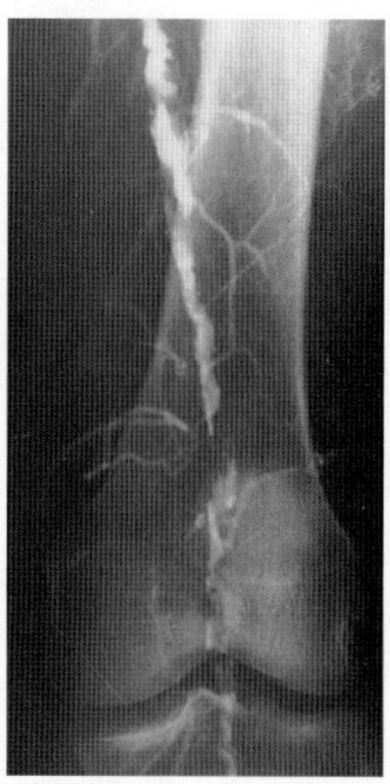

6-95

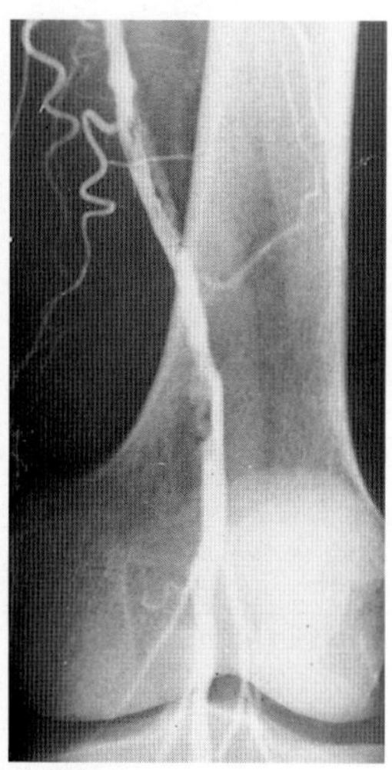

6-96

Figs. 6-94–6-96. Complete occlusion of the superficial femoral artery at the transition to the first part of the popliteal artery in the adductor groove. Local lysis was performed with a catheter using the pulse-spray technique, followed by PTA of the unmasked stenosis. During the PTA a dissection at the level of the adductor canal was created

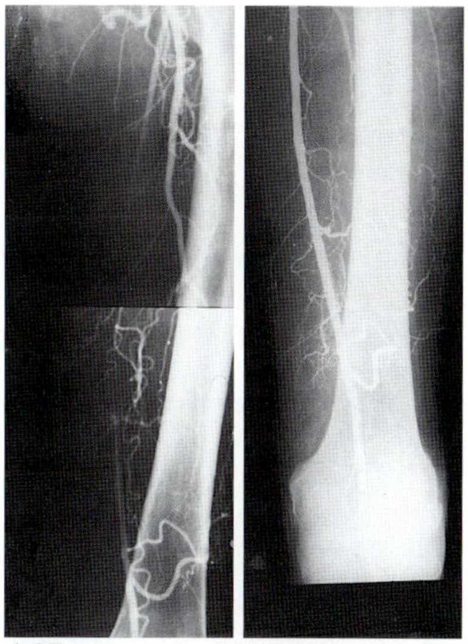

6-97

Fig. 6-97. Long arteriosclerotic occlusion of the superficial femoral artery. At right, follow-up after thromboendarterectomy

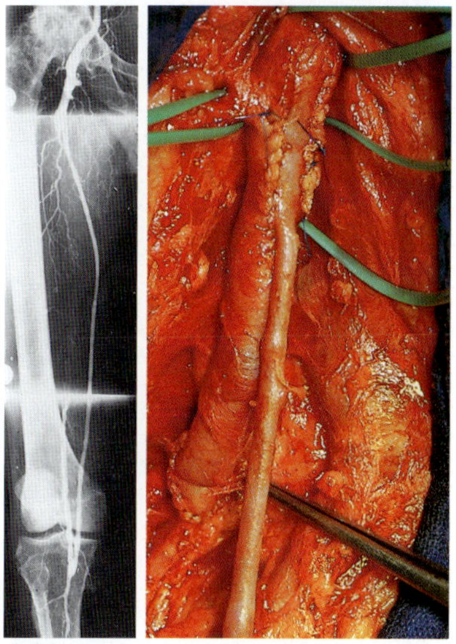

6-98

Fig. 6-98. Lengthy occlusion of the superficial femoral artery. There was a patent popliteal artery with occlusion of all the calf arteries. A femoro-popliteal vein bypass to the isolated segment of the popliteal artery below the knee was performed

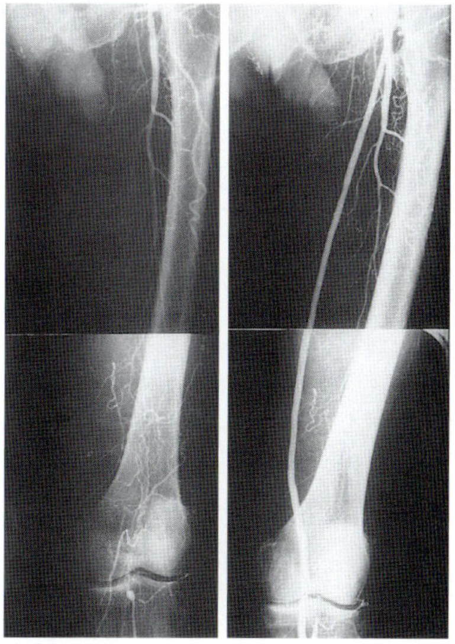

6-99

Fig. 6-99. Extensive occlusion of the superficial femoral artery, as well as the first and second parts of the popliteal artery in a patient with stage III peripheral arteriosclerotic disease. Follow-up angiography after performing a reversed femoro-popliteal vein bypass with a distal end-to-side anastomosis to the third part of the popliteal artery (below the knee)

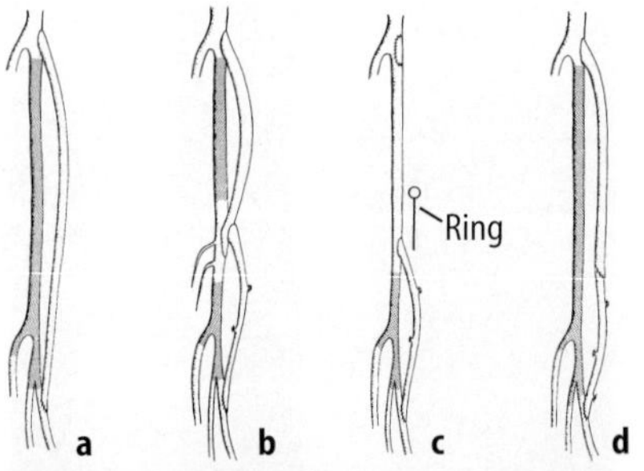

6-100

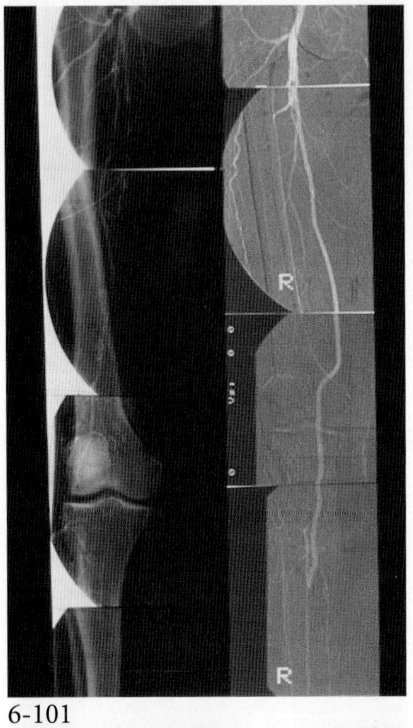
6-101

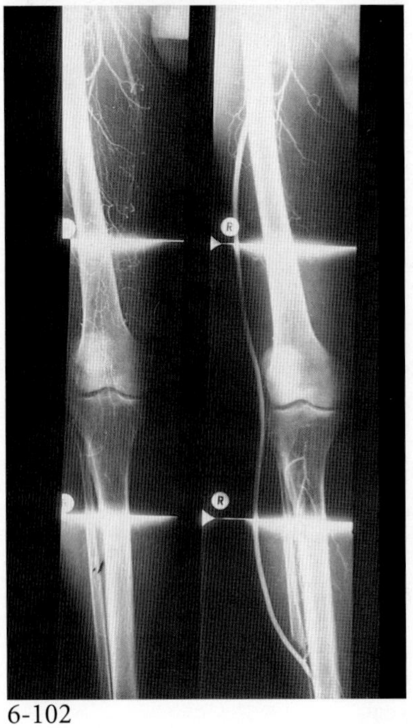
6-102

There are a number of possible bypass procedures which can be performed in patients who are at risk for amputation from advanced peripheral arterial disease

Fig. 6-100.
a Femoro-tibial or femoro-peroneal bypass, using either vein or prosthesis.
b Composite femoro-popliteal bypass. The proximal graft is usually synthetic, but the distal graft spanning the knee joint is usually a vein.
c Retrograde superficial femoral artery disobliteration using vascular ringed endarterectomy instrument, combined with a popliteal-to-tibial graft to span knee joint.
d Femoro-tibial composite graft, with an end-to-end anastomosis of the synthetic and vein grafts to create a long bypass

Fig. 6-101. Lengthy occlusion of the superficial femoral artery, popliteal artery and several of the calf arteries (anterior and posterior tibial arteries). Follow-up angiogram after insertion of a femoro-peroneal vein bypass with partial filling of the anterior tibial artery. (see Fig. 6-100 a)

Fig. 6-102. Widespread occlusion of the superficial femoral artery and the popliteal artery as well as the calf arteries. Retrograde filling of the distal peroneal artery as the only patent target vessel in the lower leg. The patient was at high risk for amputation with stage IV disease. A lateral femoro-peroneal bypass with a synthetic prosthesis was performed to avoid amputation after resection of the distal fibula. (see Fig. 6-100 a)

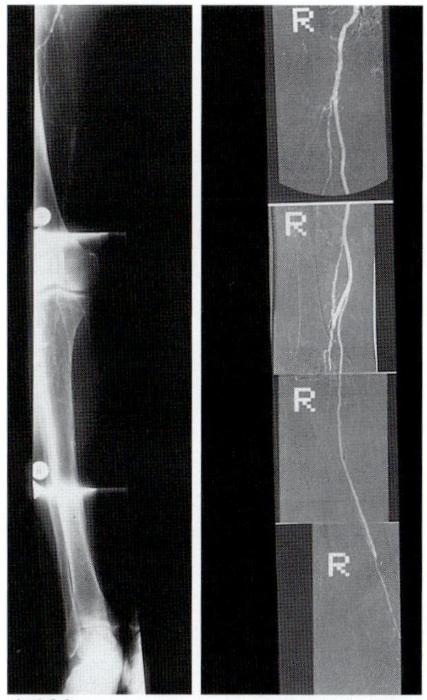

6-103

Fig. 6-103. Severe occlusive disease with arteriosclerotic changes in the thigh, knee and calf regions with an almost avascular preoperative angiogram. A femoro-popliteal-to-tibial jump graft was performed. (see Fig. 6-100b)

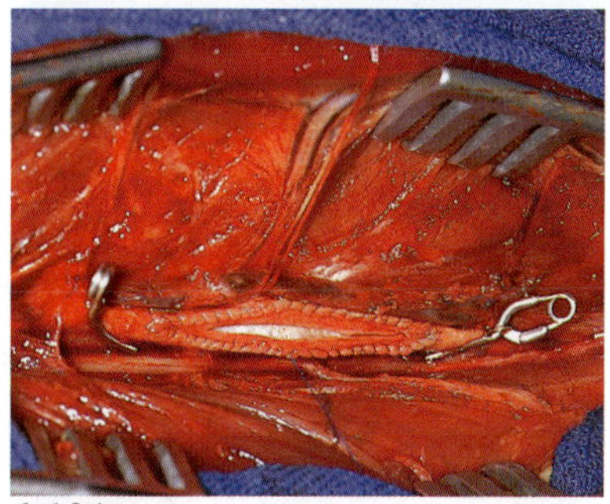

6-104

Fig. 6-104. Operative view showing the placement of a Linton patch anastomosis. A strip of vein has already been used as a patch after being opened in a linear fashion

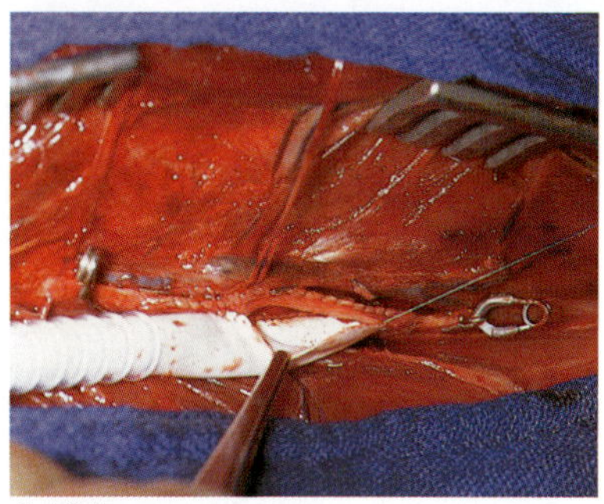

6-105

Fig. 6-105. The synthetic prosthesis is joined end-to-side with the vein patch using a running suture

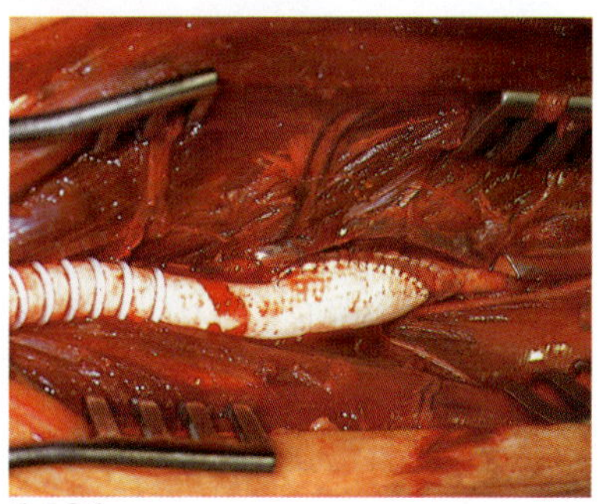

6-106

Fig. 6-106. A wide distal anastomosis is obtained. The segment of vein may decrease the difference in compliance between the prosthesis and the recipient artery

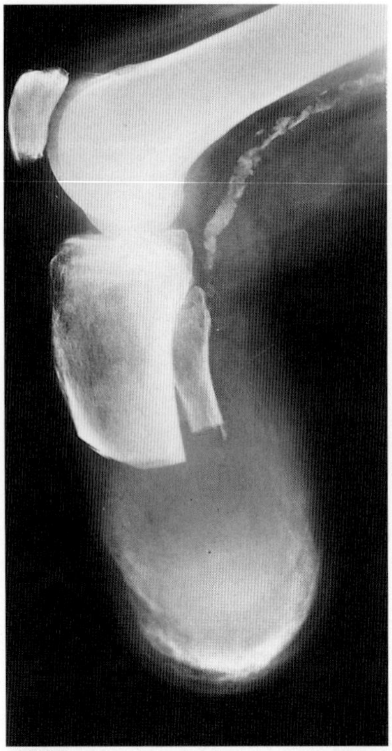

6-107

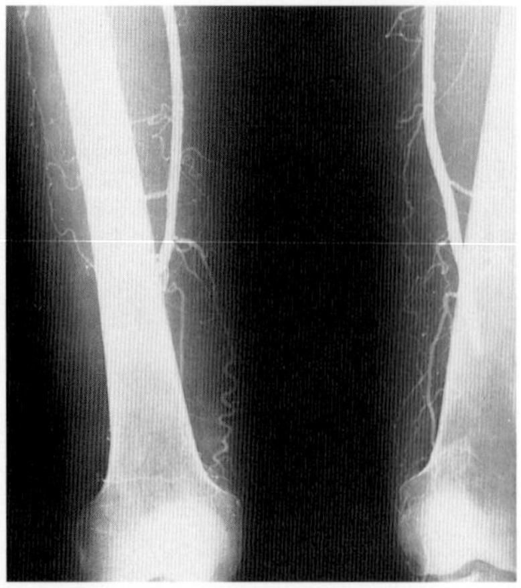

6-108

Fig. 6-107. Patient requiring chronic renal dialysis with severe medial sclerosis in the entire popliteal artery following below-knee amputation

Fig. 6-108. Angiographic view of bilateral popliteal emboli. The proximal vessels appear entirely normal with no sign of arteriosclerosis. On both sides, the vessels are abruptly occluded at the level of the adductor canal by emboli from the heart

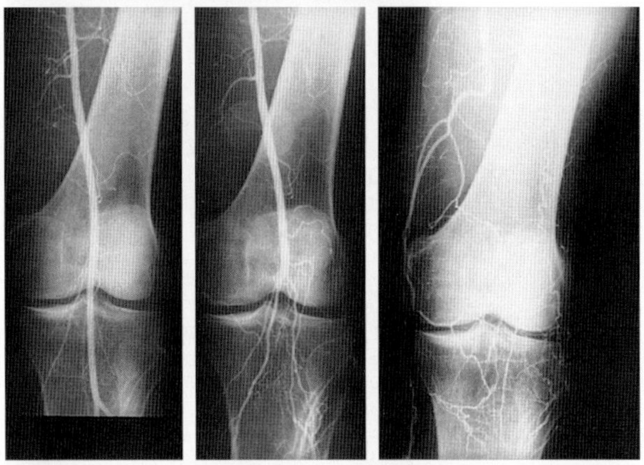

6-109

Fig. 6-109. Course of a lengthy popliteal artery occlusion. The initial angiogram shows a patent popliteal artery and a diagnosis of entrapment syndrome was made. The second image, 6 months later, shows complete occlusion of the distal popliteal artery with early signs of small collaterals. The final view, after another 6 months, shows extensive collateral formation as the result of a thrombosis of the entire popliteal artery

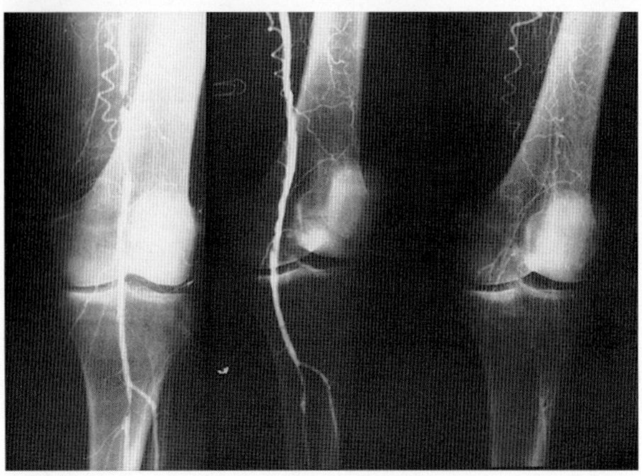

6-110

Fig. 6-110. Short stenosis at the femoro-popliteal transition as well as stenosis of the tibio-peroneal artery causing intermittent claudication. In the second image, the proximal and distal stenoses have been successfully dilated. At *right*, an early occlusion of the tibio-peroneal trunk and multiple distal arteries because of thrombosis. Intraoperative thrombolysis and a femoro-tibial bypass were required

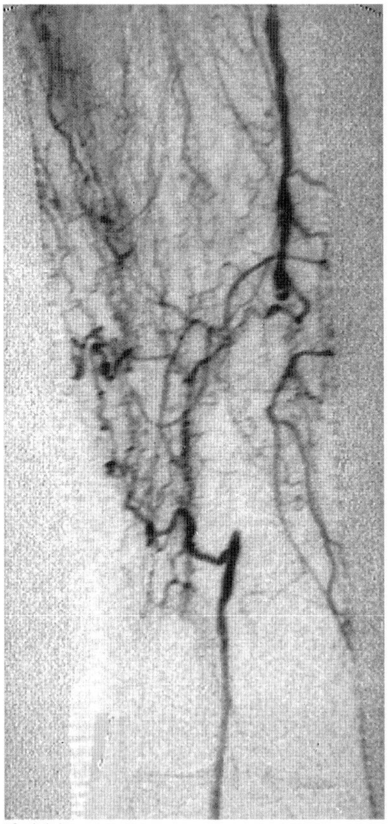

6-111

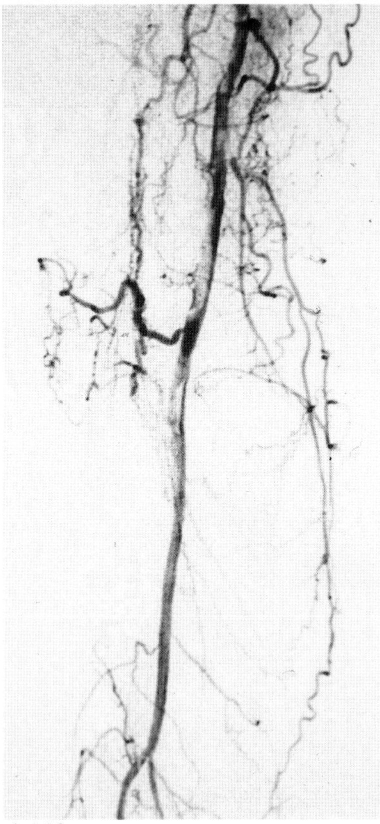

6-112

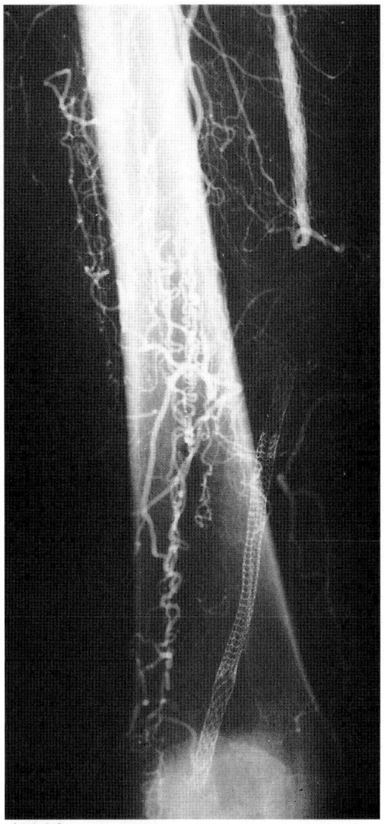

6-113

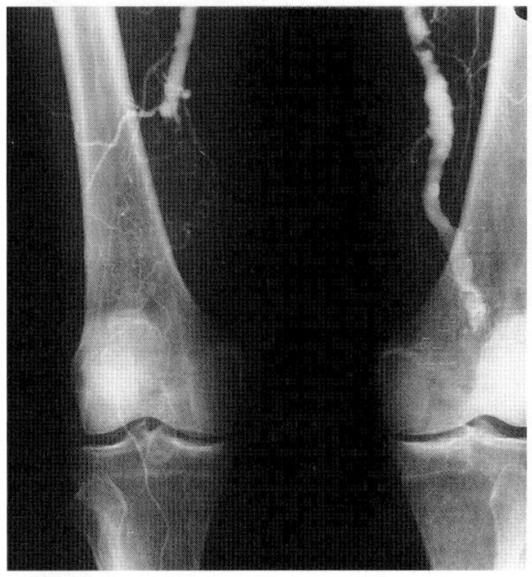

6-114

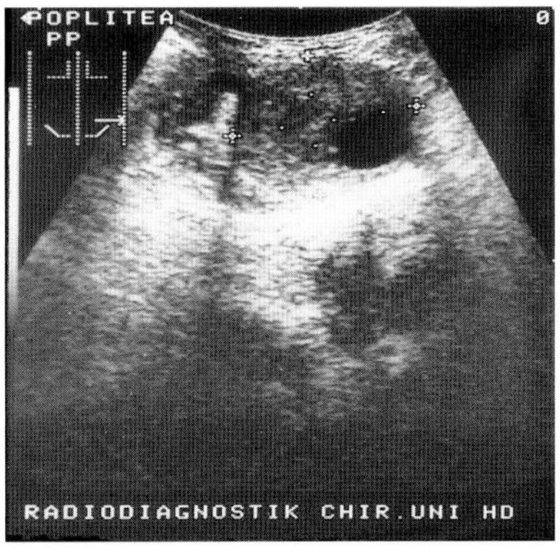

6-115

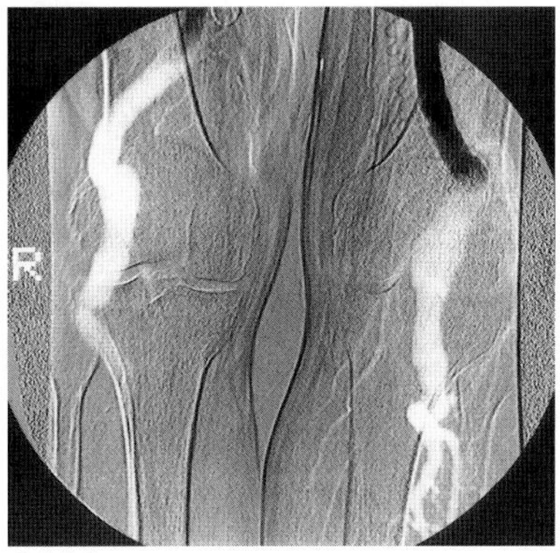

6-116

Fig. 6-111. Femoro-popliteal artery occlusion secondary to arteriosclerosis with good collateral formation

Fig. 6-112. Recanalization by percutaneous transluminal angioplasty (PTA) followed by dissection and partial thrombosis. Multiple stents were inserted reaching as far as the popliteal artery

Fig. 6-113. Recurrent occlusion of the arterial segment treated by stenting. A femoro-popliteal bypass was required

Fig. 6-114. Severe artherosclerosis with marked dilatation and obstruction in the femoral and popliteal arteries with occlusion of multiple distal arteries

Fig. 6-115. Ultrasonography showing a popliteal aneurysm with areas of thrombosis

Fig. 6-116. Angiographic views of the vessel lumina in a case of bilateral popliteal aneurysms. The patient received bilateral Dacron interposition grafts

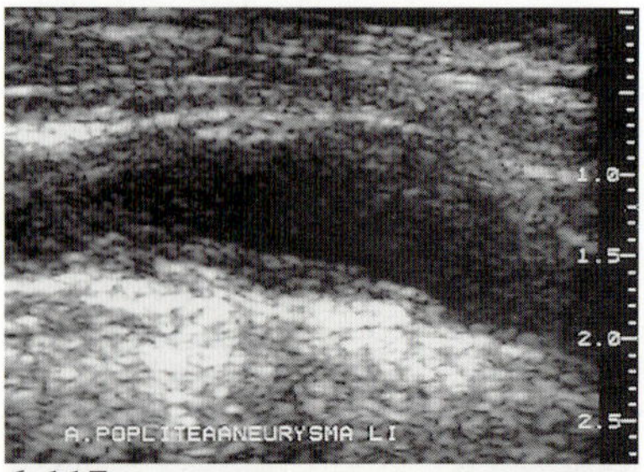

6-117

Fig. 6-117. Popliteal artery aneurysm shown with ultrasonography. Bruits are audible in no more than half the cases. Diagnose is most easily confirmed by B-mode ultrasonography and colour duplex imaging

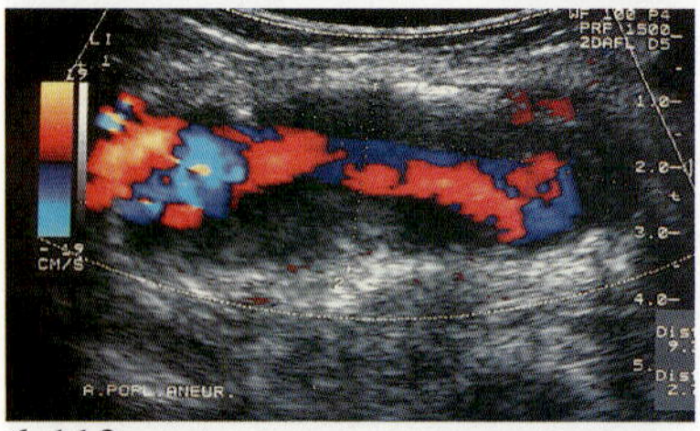

6-118

Fig. 6-118. Color duplex ultrasonography showing a partially thrombosed popliteal artery aneurysm

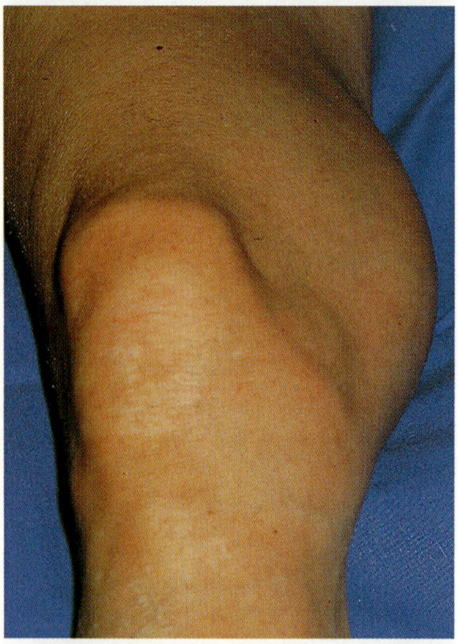

6-119

Fig. 6-119. Expanded aneurysm of the proximal popliteal artery with a visible mass which was non-pulsatile because the vessel was completely thrombosed

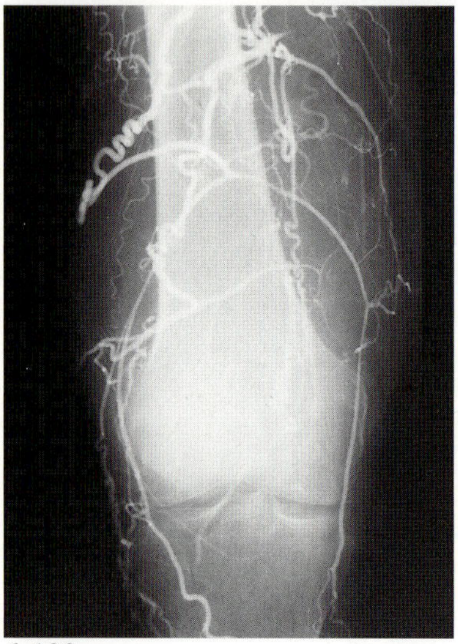

6-120

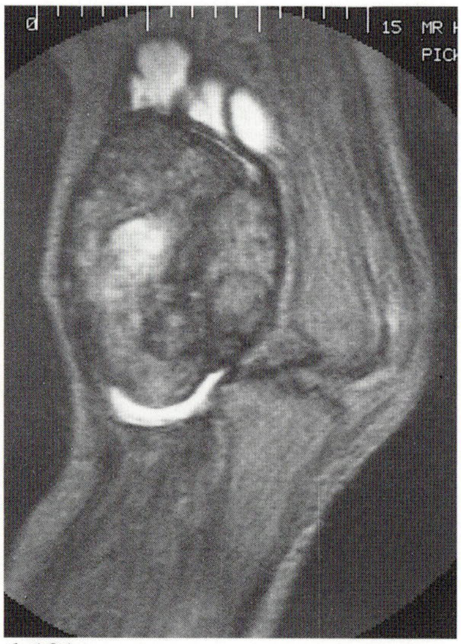

6-121

Fig. 6-120. Angiography of same case showing simultaneous proximal and distal apposition as well as a good superficial collateral system

Fig. 6-121. The accompany magnetic resonance image shows the expanded thrombosed vessel which mimics a malignant tumor

Fig. 6-122. Operative view of popliteal artery aneurysm. The large aneurysm is easily visualized after incising through the skin and subcutaneous tissue

Fig. 6-123. After the aneurysm is opened, several thrombi are seen

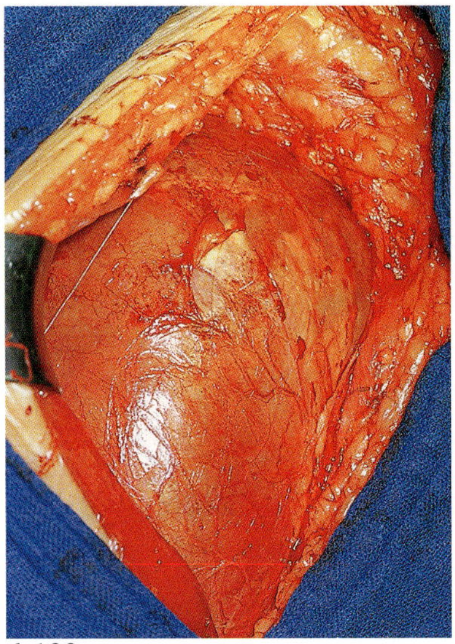

6-122

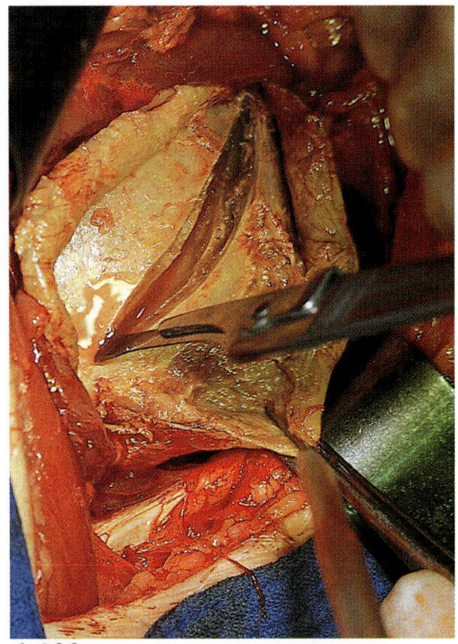

6-123

Fig. 6-124. The layers of the thrombus which are laid down over the years have led to the expression "onion-like aneurysm," referring to the concentric layers of the clot

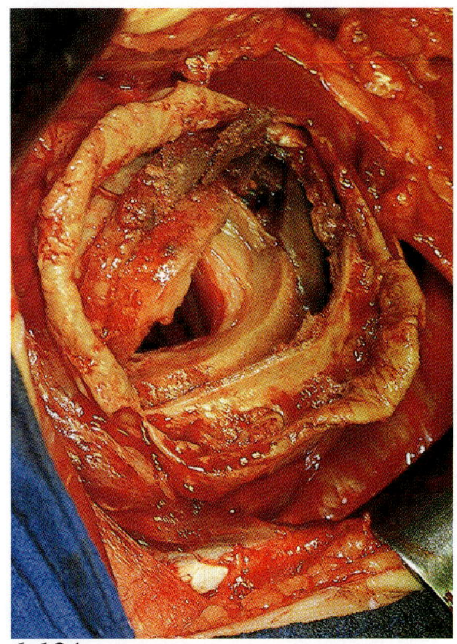

6-124

Fig. 6-125. Small aneurysms can be bypassed. Because this lesion was so large, it was excised and a Dacron prosthesis reinforced with spiral rings was interposed

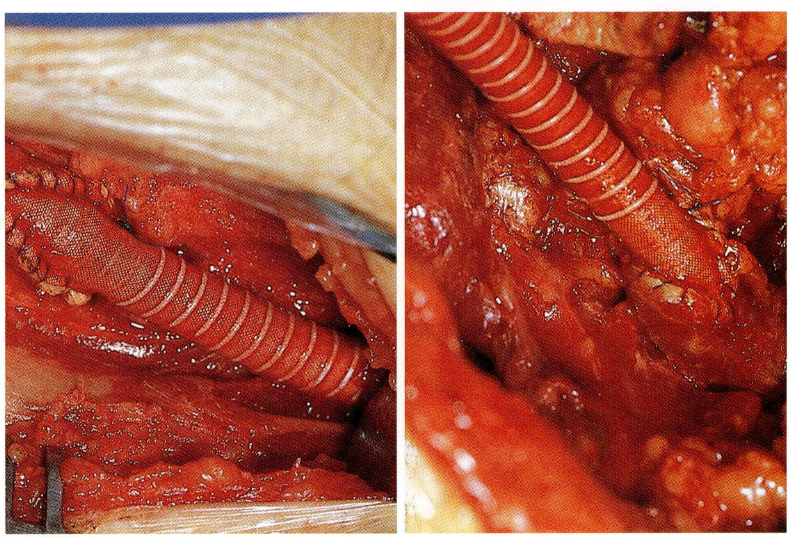

6-125

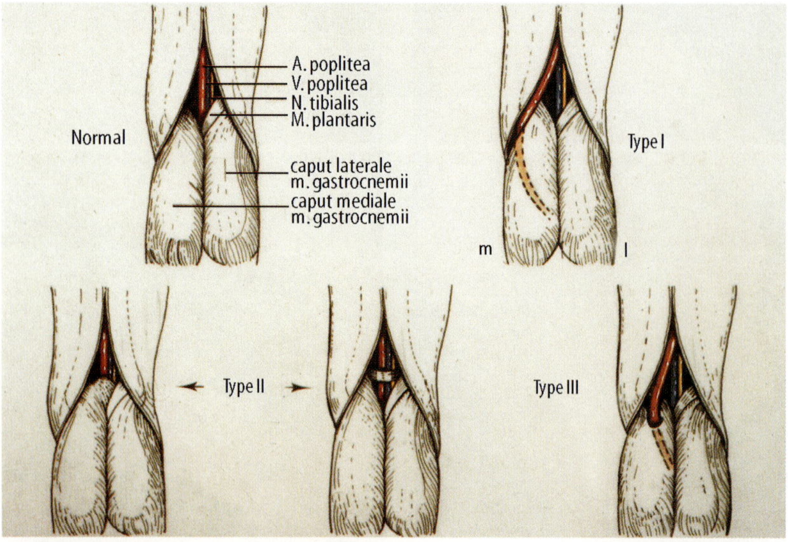

6-126

Fig. 6-126. Classification of the popliteal artery entrapment syndrome. Three different types are identified, based on anatomic variations
Type I: atypical course of the popliteal artery medial to the attachment of the gastrocnemius muscle
Type II: compression of a normally positioned popliteal artery by an abnormal insertion of the gastrocnemius
Type III: a combination of type I and type II

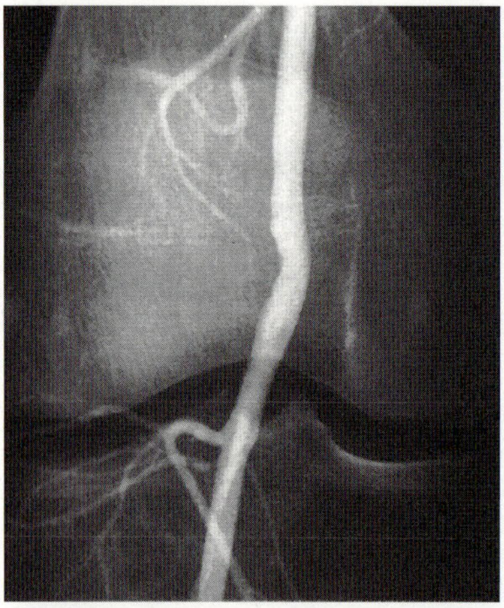

6-127

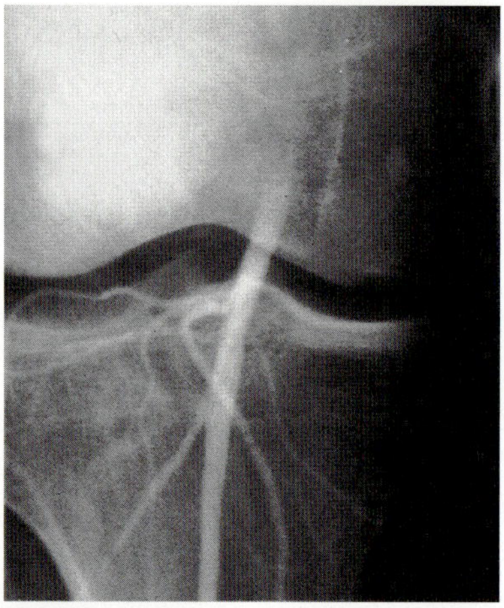

6-128

Figs. 6-127, 6-128. Angiographic presentation of a typical popliteal artery entrapment. When the muscles are relaxed, a slight indentation of the artery is seen. When the foot is dorsally flexed and the gastrocnemius tightened in a provocative test, the popliteal artery is abruptly occluded

Figs. 6-129, 6-130. Angiograms showing bilateral entrapment syndrome, at rest and with the provocative test

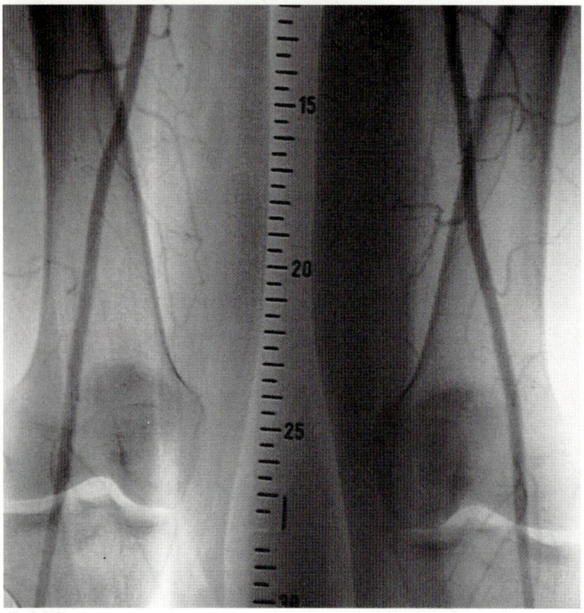

6-129

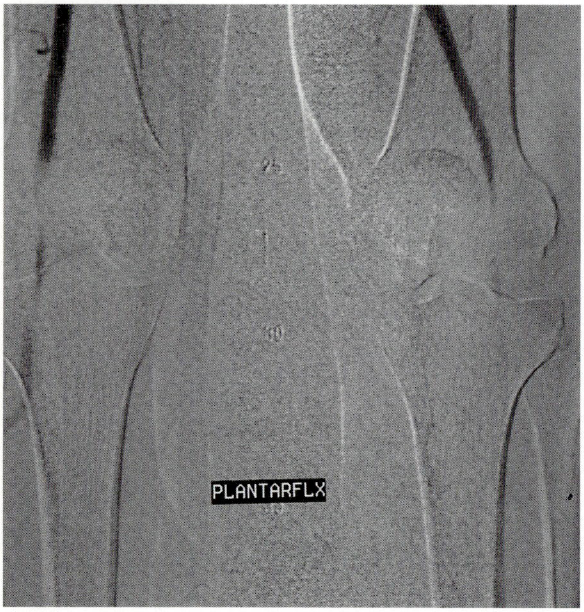

6-130

Fig. 6-131. Operative view showing the popliteal artery from a posterior exposure. The medial head of the gastrocnemius is exposed, revealing the ligaments of the medial head surrounding the artery

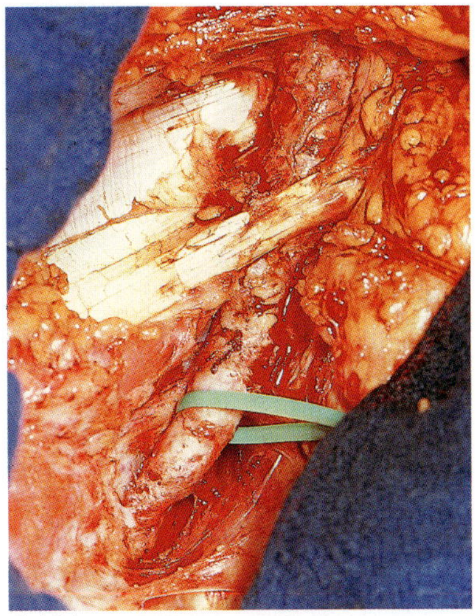

6-131

Fig. 6-132. After the muscle and ligaments have been divided, the entire popliteal artery can be visualized, showing multiple pseudo-aneurysms secondary to compression. The artery will be replaced by a vein graft

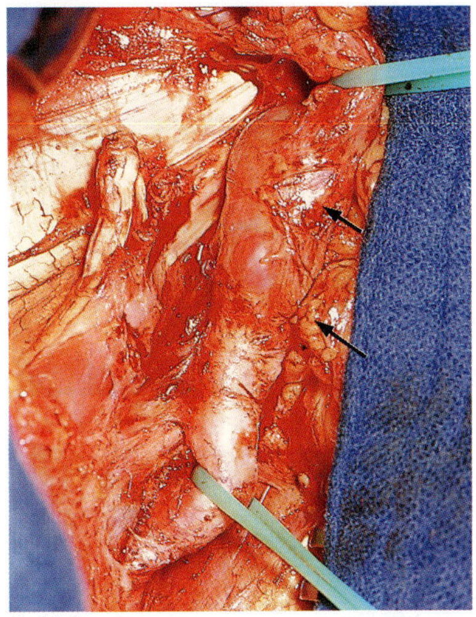

6-132

Fig. 6-133. A 40 year old patient with intermittent claudication but entirely normal pulses. Clinical evaluation revealed complete occlusion of both popliteal arteries with the gastrocnemius provocative test. The angiogram shows the typical indentation and closure two finger breadths above the knee joint. Treatment consisted of dividing the muscular structures and repairing the partially stenotic artery with a vein patch graft

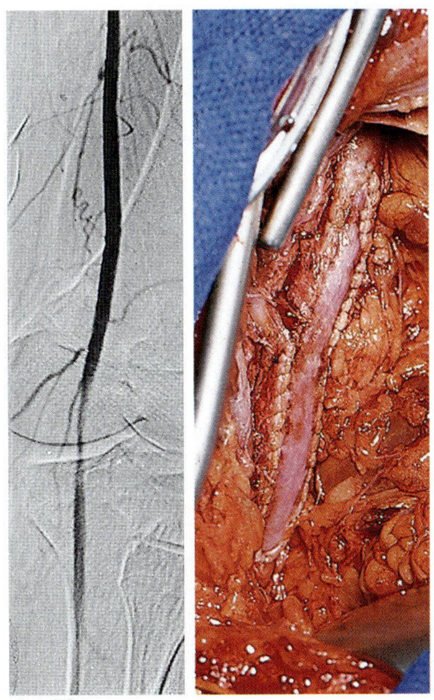

6-133

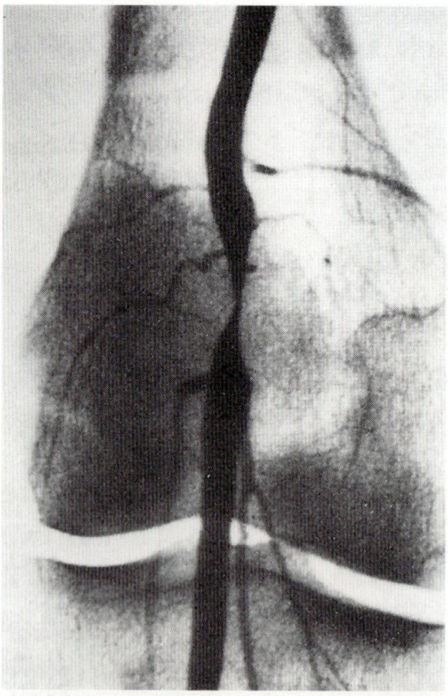

6-134

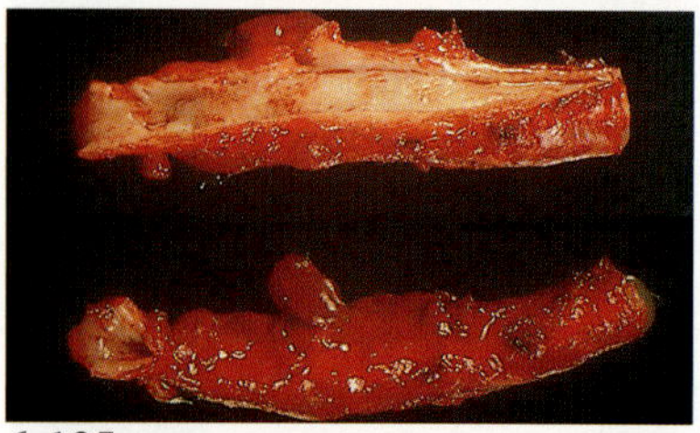

6-135

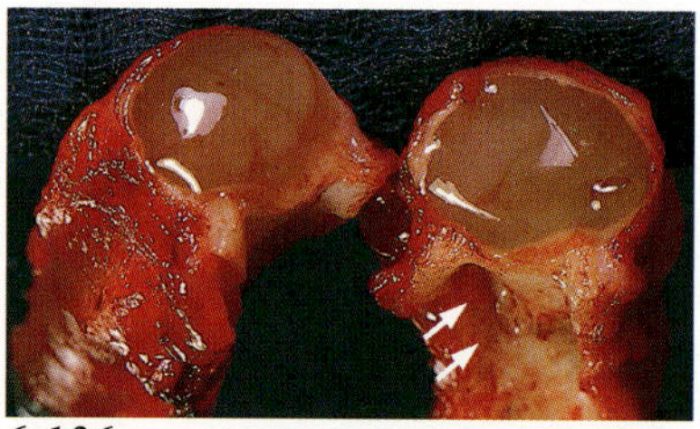

6-136

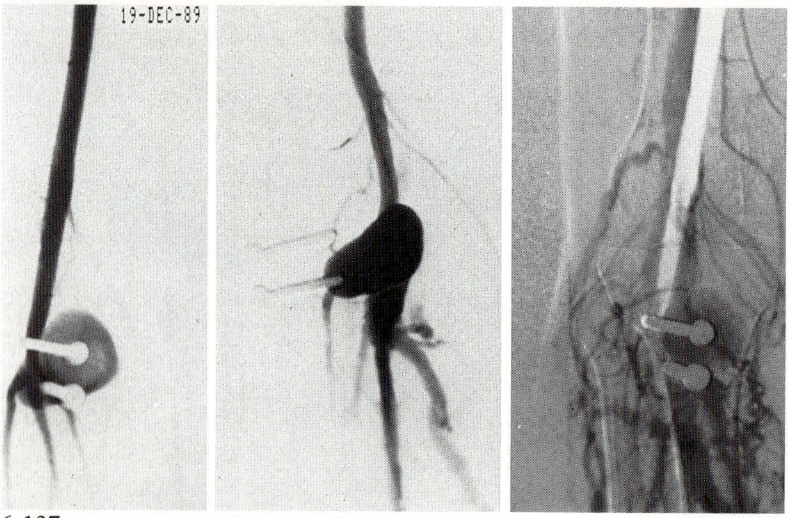

6-137

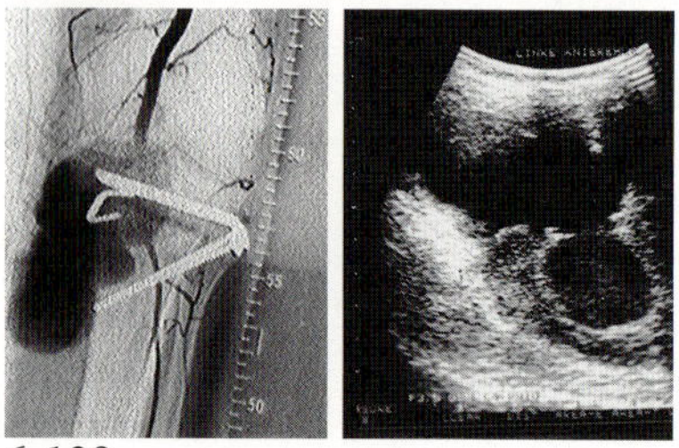

6-138

Fig. 6-134. Angiographic findings in cystic adventitial degeneration. The popliteal artery shows an hourglass deformity at the transition from the first to second part. Another typical finding is a broad-based watch-glass-like indentation in the vessel wall

Fig. 6-135. Surgical specimen of a popliteal artery with cystic adventitial degeneration (*bottom*). The longitudinally opened lumen clearly shows the stenosis induced by the compression (*top*)

Fig. 6-136. In cross-section, one can see cystic changes partially surrounding the media. The lumen of the artery is marked (*arrows*). Gelatinous material oozes out of the cyst. The usual surgical approaches are resection with vein graft or excision of the cystic material while maintaining the vessel integrity

Fig. 6-137. Injury to the right popliteal artery by two orthopedic screws. The false aneurysm was resected and an end-to-end anastomosis performed

Fig. 6-138. Iatrogenic popliteal artery injury. The ultrasonography (*right*) shows a false aneurysm while angiography (*left*) shows leakage at the level of the orthopedic repair

An uncommon cause of arterial occlusion about the knee is the development of bony exostoses

Figs. 6-139, 6-140. Femoral exostosis with complete occlusion of the femoral artery in the above-knee popliteal artery. The exostosis was surgically removed

Figs. 6-141, 6-142. Tibial exostosis completely occluding the third part of the popliteal artery and the trifurcation. After the exostosis was removed, the popliteal artery required reconstruction

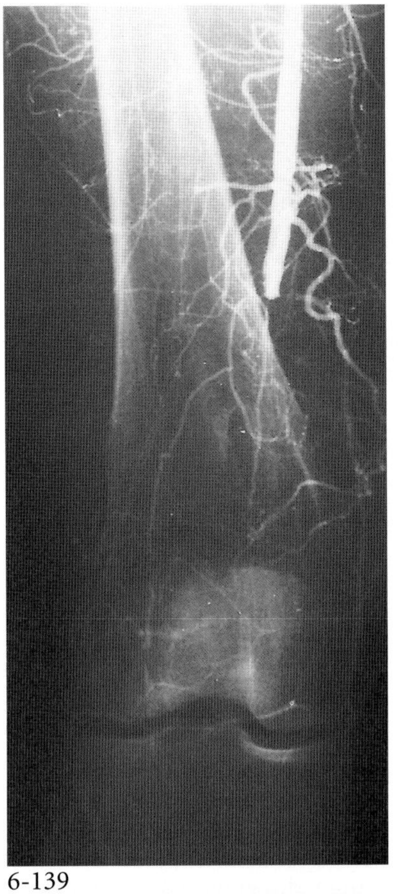

6-139

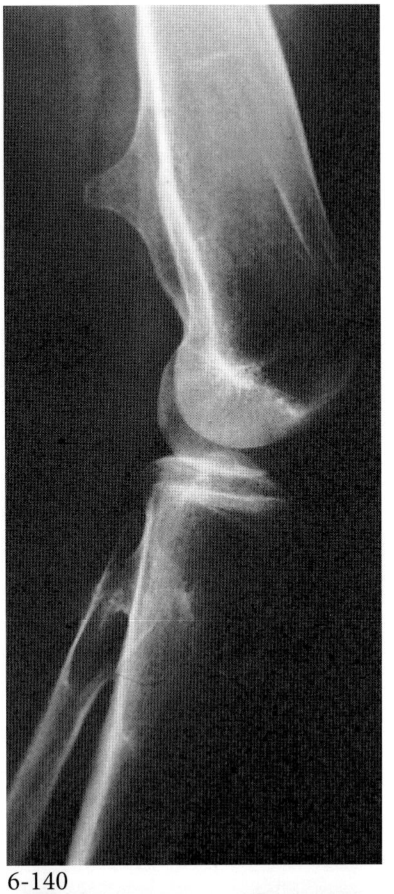

6-140

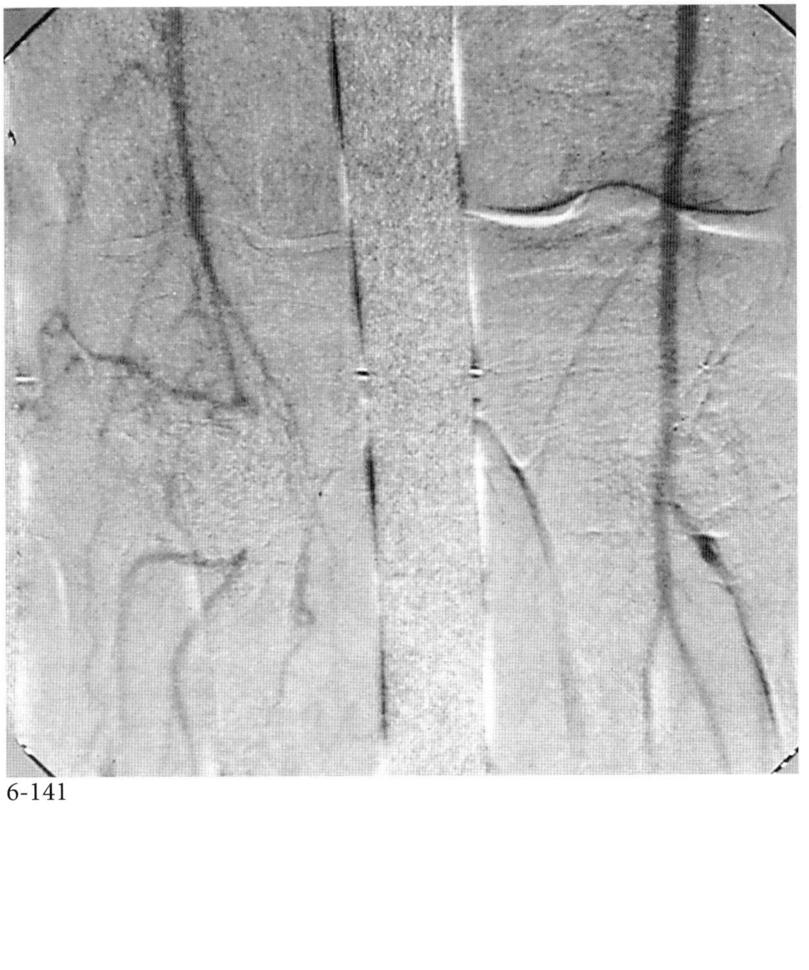

6-141

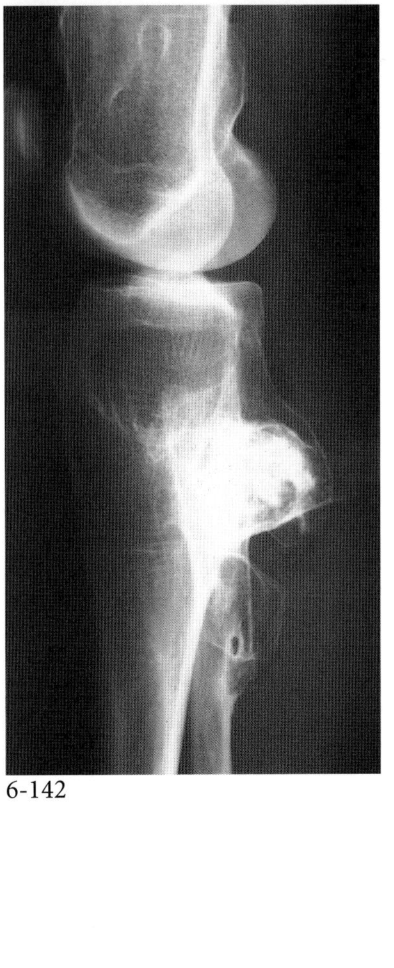

6-142

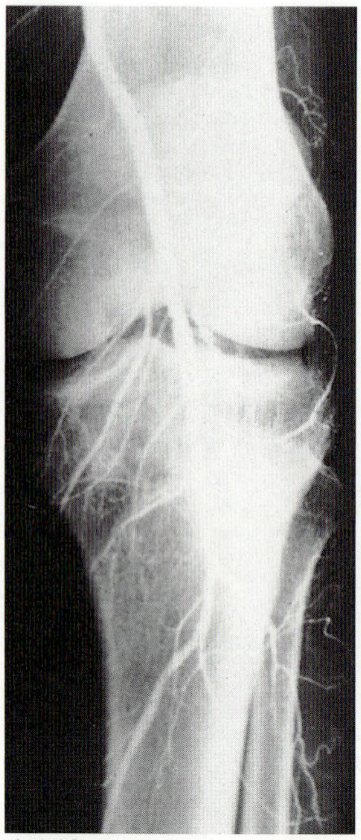
6-143

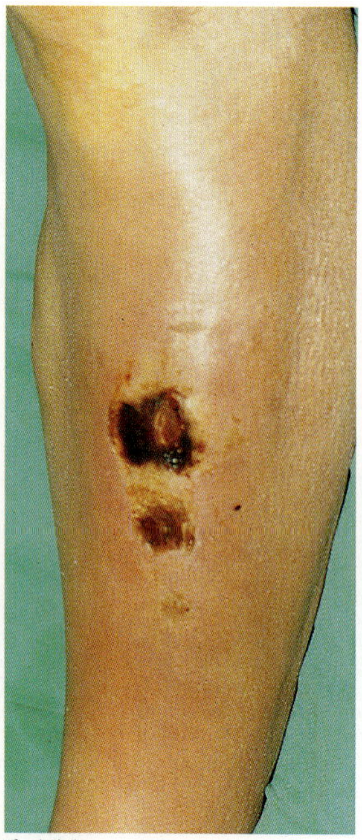
6-144

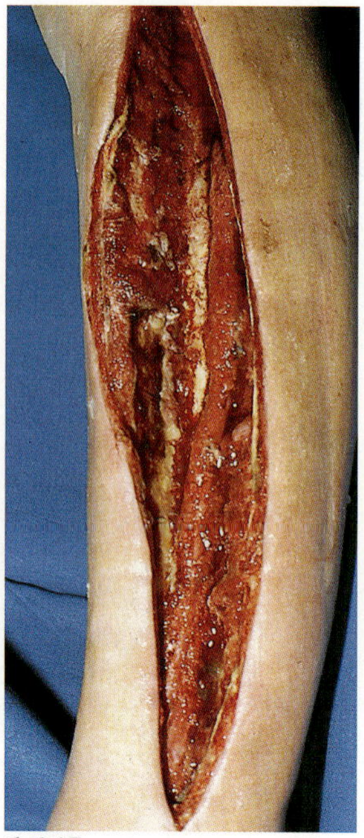
6-145

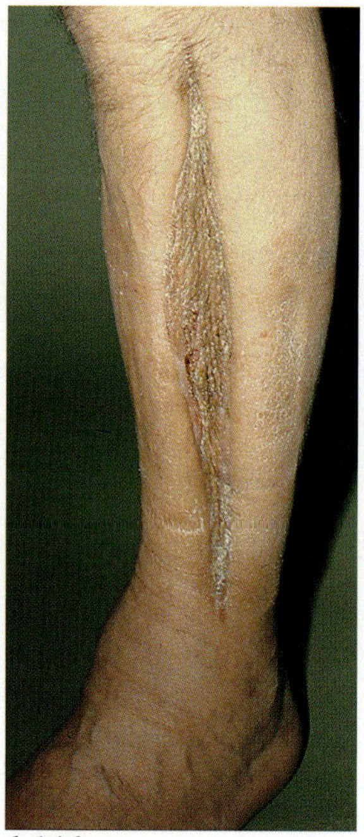
6-146

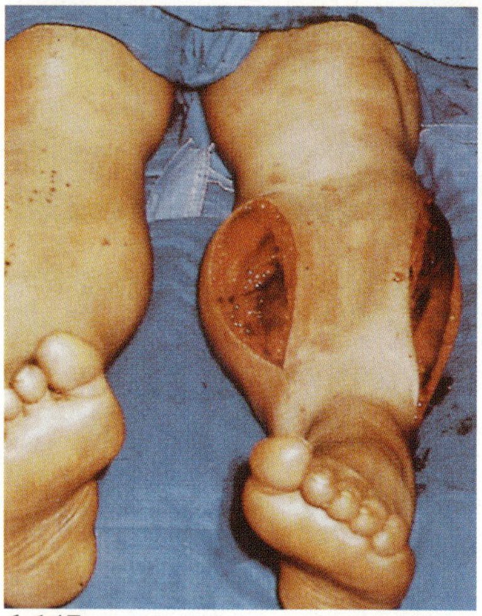
6-147

Fig. 6-143. Angiogram showing occlusion of the anterior tibial artery

Fig. 6-144. Clinical appearance of a patient with compartment syndrome, showing swollen anterior tibial compartment with skin necrosis

Fig. 6-145. Operative view following debridement of necrotic muscle

Fig. 6-146. Healed wound with split-thickness skin graft. The compartment syndrome is defined as the functional impairment of neuro-muscular structures because of increased pressure within a closed fascial compartment. The main causes are revascularization following ischemia, trauma, burns and vascular injuries

Fig. 6-147. Bilateral shin compartment syndrome in a 32 year old patient following marijuana abuse. The patient fell asleep in the tailor position (with legs crossed) and awoke after 8 h with massive swelling of both lower legs. The four compartments of the left lower leg have been opened with medial and lateral fasciotomies. The incision of the fascia to open the muscle compartment is accomplished following proximal exposure with a long scissors. The right side has yet to be treated

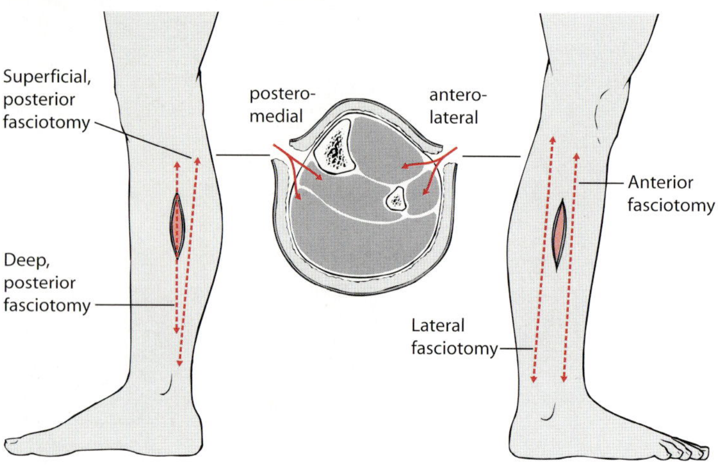

6-148

Fig. 6-148. Schematic representation of posterio-medial and antero-lateral skin incisions and fasciotomies to open the four compartments of the lower leg

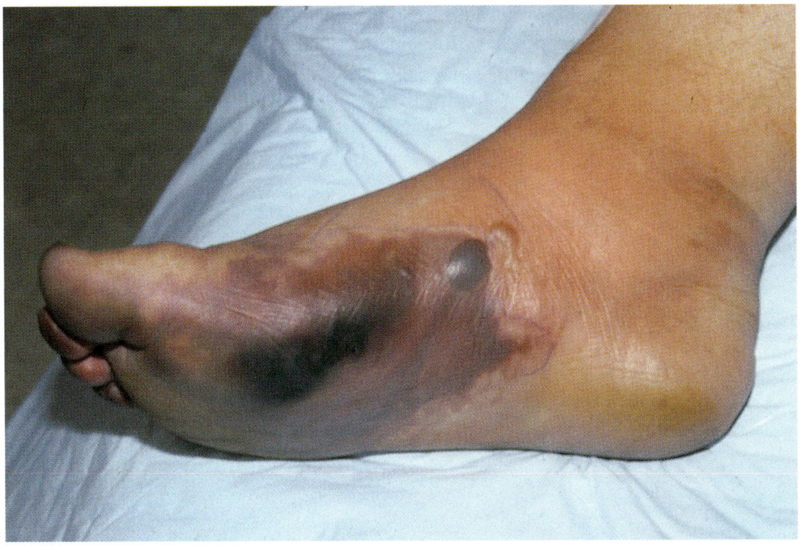

6-149

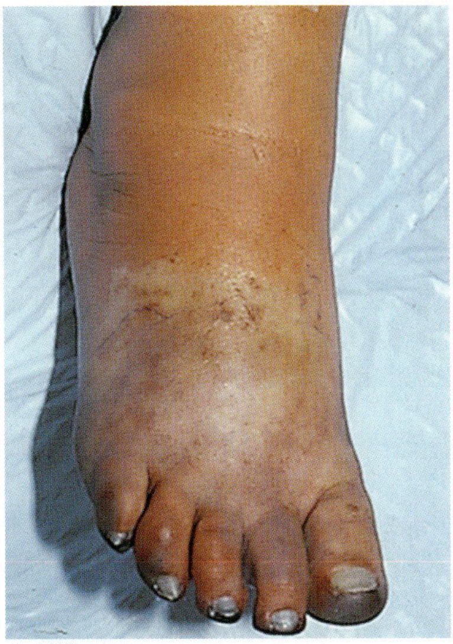

6-150

Figs. 6-149, 6-150. Phlegmasia caerulea dolens is a fulminant form of a deep venous thrombosis. Rarely the swelling can be so severe that the leg arteries are compressed and mottled cyanosis appear, a condition known as phlegmasia caerulea dolens. In this patient there was a complete four stage thrombosis and impaired arterial circulation. Because of the restricted venous drainage, the venous pressure was increased altering the microcirculation and leading to the compartment syndrome. In this patient, a venous thrombectomy was required

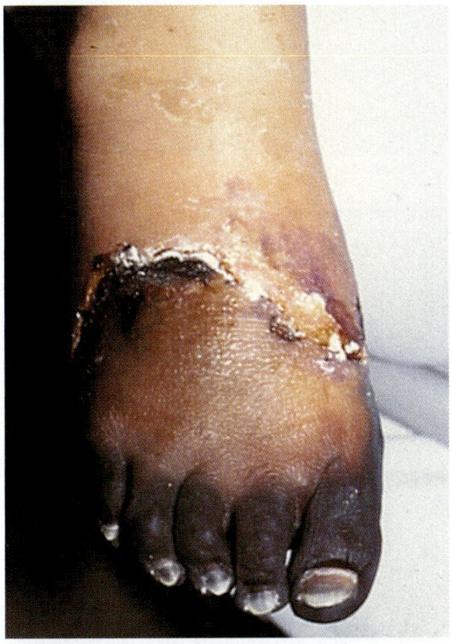

6-151

Fig. 6-151. After 4 weeks, the toes are mummified

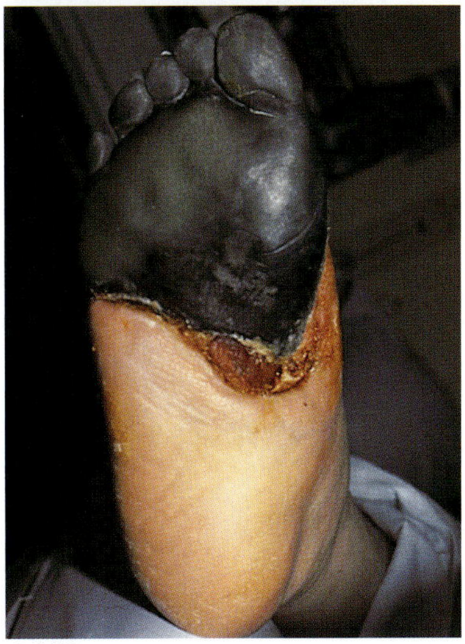

6-152

Fig. 6-152. After 4 months, the mummification was unchanged and an amputation was needed

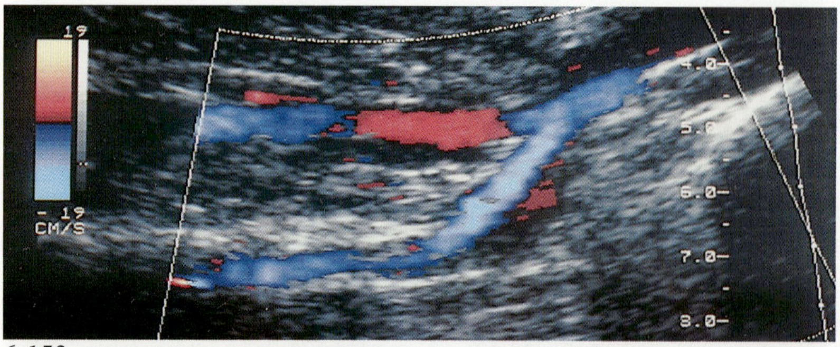

6-153

Fig. 6-153. Color duplex ultrasonography showing the take-off of the anterior tibial artery in the popliteal space

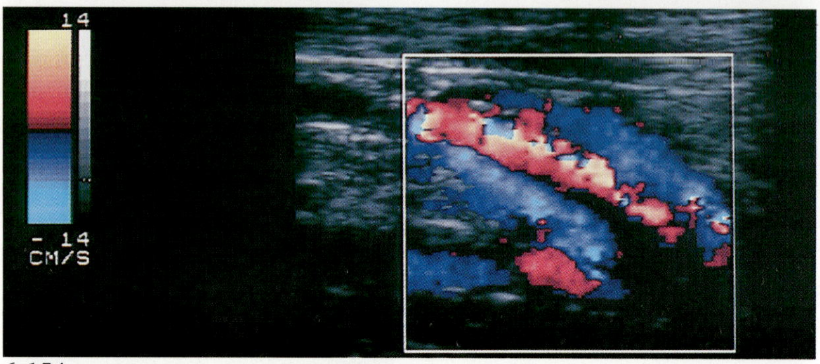

6-154

Fig. 6-154. Color duplex ultrasonography showing the anterior tibial artery with two accompanying veins (anterior tibial veins)

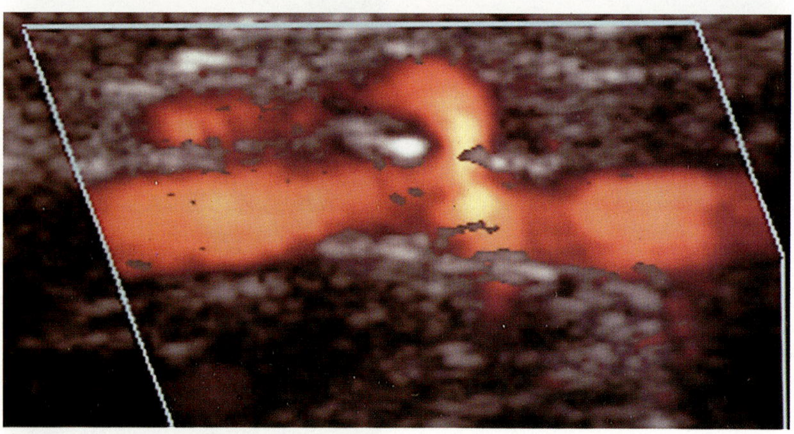

6-155

Fig. 6-155. Stent in the tibioperoneal trunk. The device was implanted 6 months previously. The origin of the anterior tibial artery is patent, without anticoagulation, even though it was very close to the stent

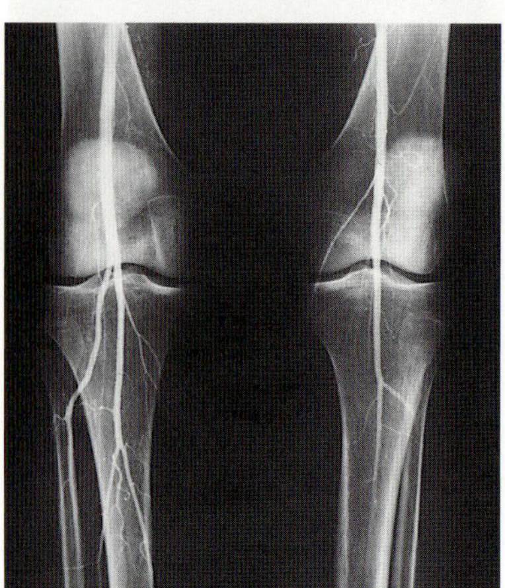

6-156

Fig. 6-156. Conventional angiography of the popliteal artery and vessels of the lower leg. The higher take-off of the anterior tibial artery on the right popliteal artery is unusual

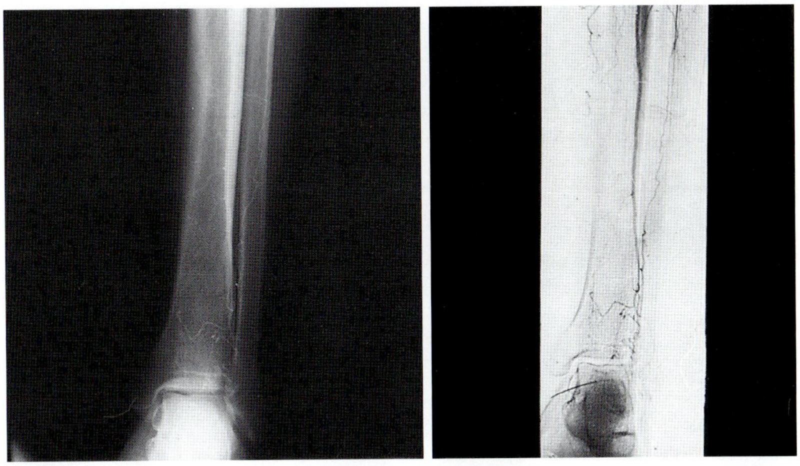

6-157

Fig. 6-157. Conventional angiography in a patient with occlusion of the vessels of the lower leg. An „empty" angiogram is shown on the *left*, while at the *right* subtraction angiography allows the vessels to be visualized. These views were obtained 20 years ago

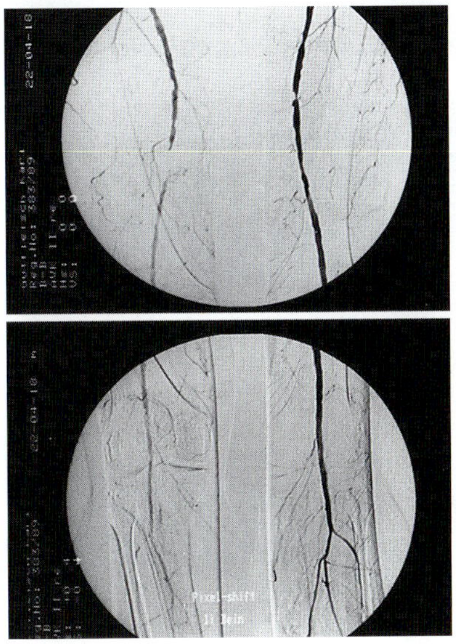

6-158

Fig. 6-158. Digital subtraction angiography. When the background, the bone and the soft tissues are subtracted, the contrast of the vessels is enhanced. Multiple stenoses and partial occlusions are seen at several levels, including the arteries of the thigh, the popliteal artery and the arteries of the lower leg

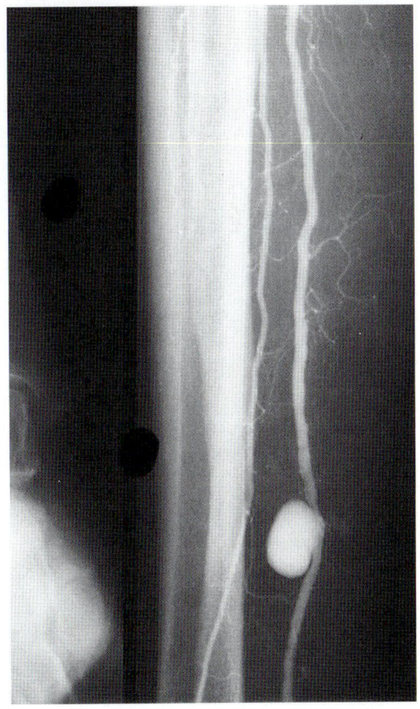

6-160

Fig. 6-160. Angiographic view of a false aneurysm following thrombectomy. Thrombosis of the arteries of the lower leg with acute ischemia. Condition following Fogarty thrombectomy with perforation of the posterior tibial artery and formation of a false aneurysm

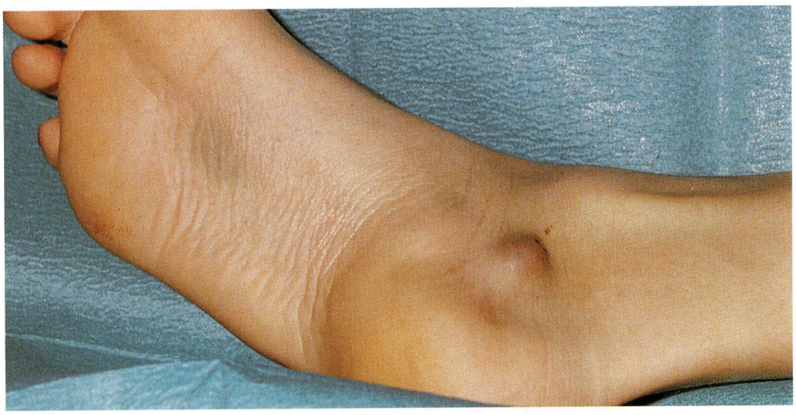

6-159

Fig. 6-159. A small mycotic aneurysm of the posterior tibial artery near the ankle

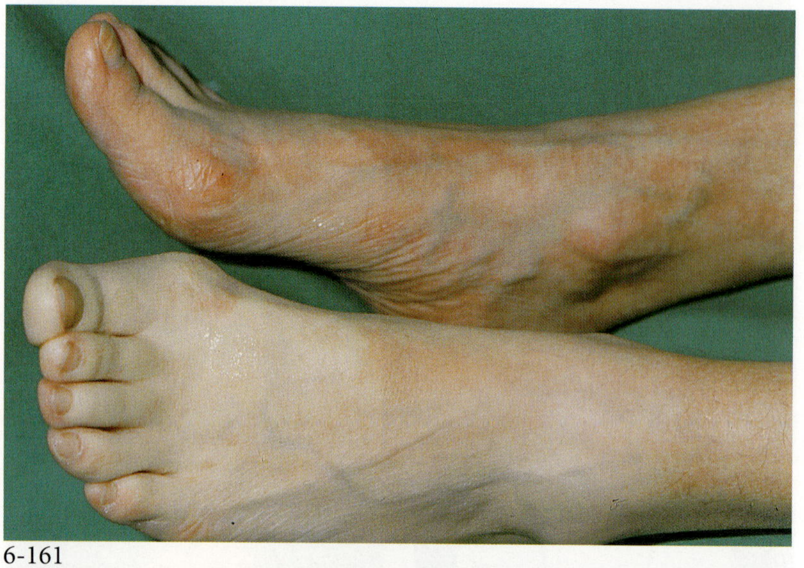

6-161

Fig. 6-161. Pale white ischemia of the left foot following an embolic occlusion. In addition, venous filling is absent

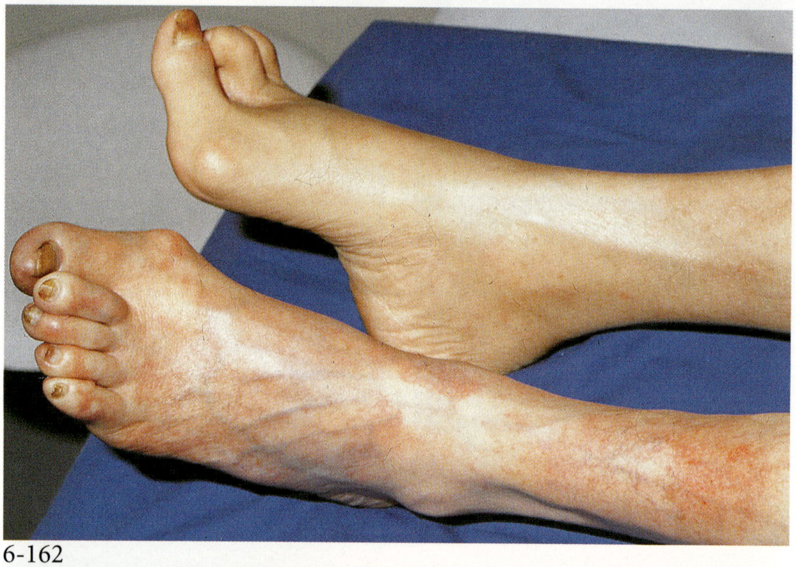

6-162

Fig. 6-162. In contrast to the above picture, here a more chronic stage of acute ischemia is shown with patchy erythema speckling, a generally pale and cool left lower extremity

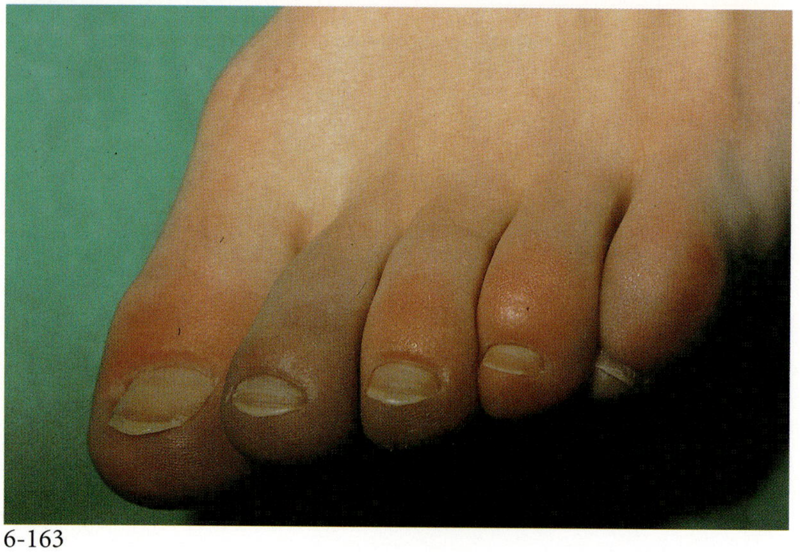

6-163

Fig. 6-163. Pernio of the toes. Chronic exposure to cold and moisture is the cause of pernio, manifest here as erythema of the toes. The post-ischemic edema coupled with thrombotic occlusion of small and mid-sized veins and arteries can lead to permanent tissue damage

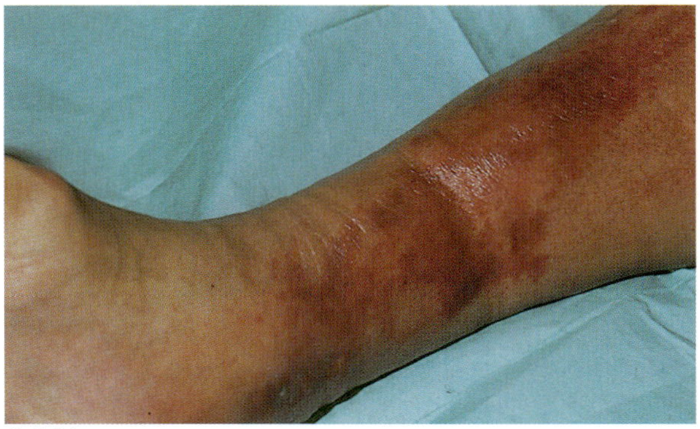

6-164

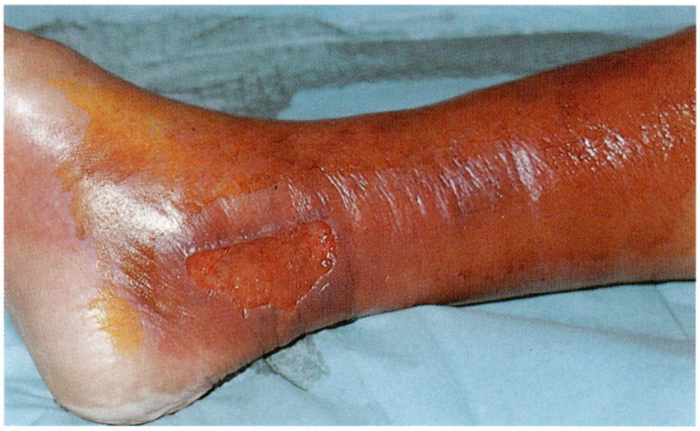

6-165

Figs. 6-164, 6-165. Freezing of the skin following a knee joint injury. The patient applied ice packs to the knee and lower leg for 48 h following an injury. Initially there were painful erythematous patches, but eventually necrosis developed

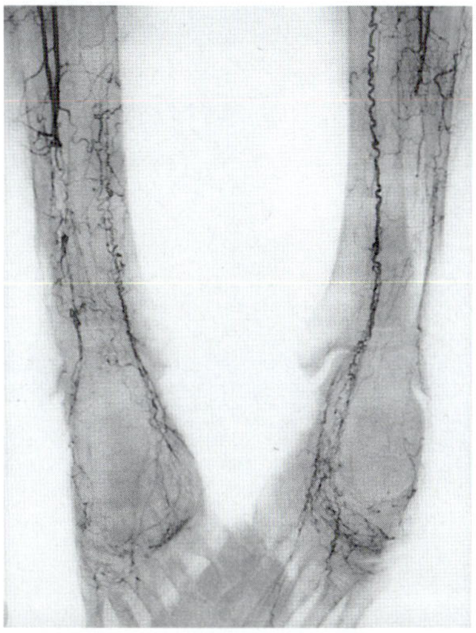

6-166

Fig. 6-166. Angiography of the vessels of the lower leg and foot following freezing. The main arteries are not seen. The original adventitial arteries have developed into cork screw-shaped collaterals

Fig. 6-167. Grade IV frostbite with gangrene of the foot. A 21 year old student under the influence of alcohol fell asleep in the woods in winter and was only found 24 h later. An amputation was unavoidable

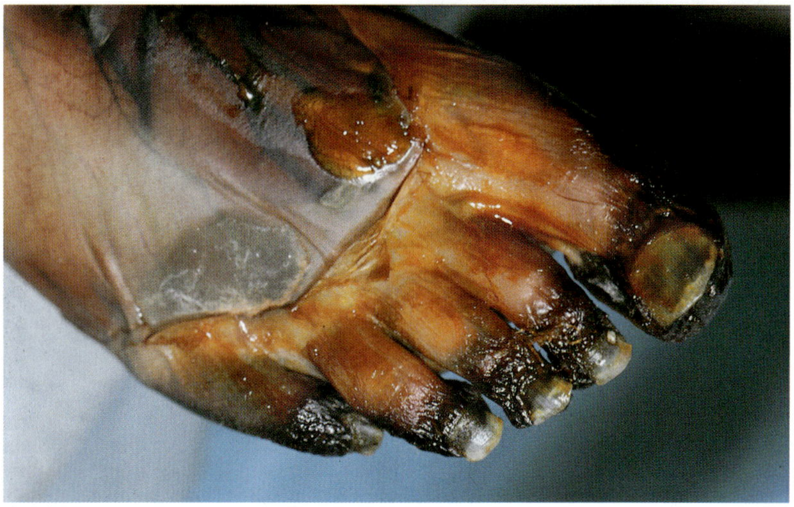

6-167

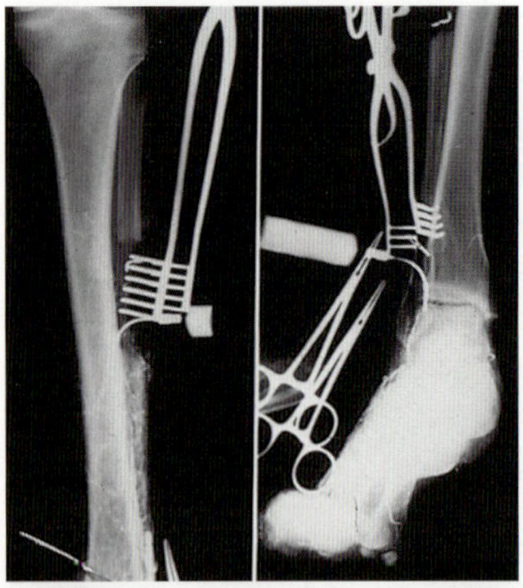

6-168

Fig. 6-168. If the arterial occlusion extends quite peripherally, the angiogram may show no arteries. In such cases, it is wise to expose a vessel and perform intraoperative angiography. In this case, the peroneal artery was identified and the angiogram revealed the dorsal pedis artery, suggesting the possibility of a popliteal-to-pedal bypass

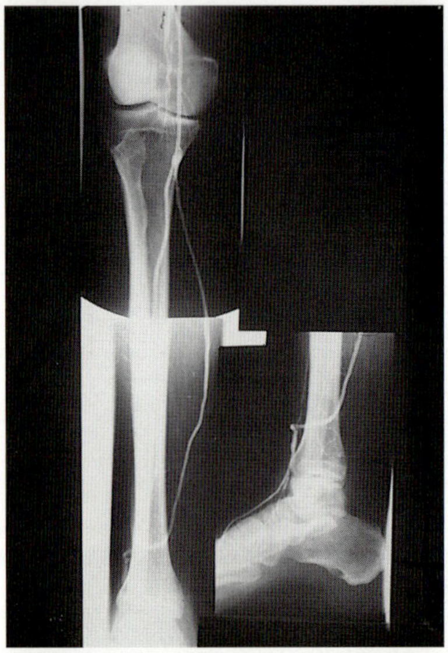

6-169

Fig. 6-169. Follow-up angiography after performing the popliteal-to-pedal bypass

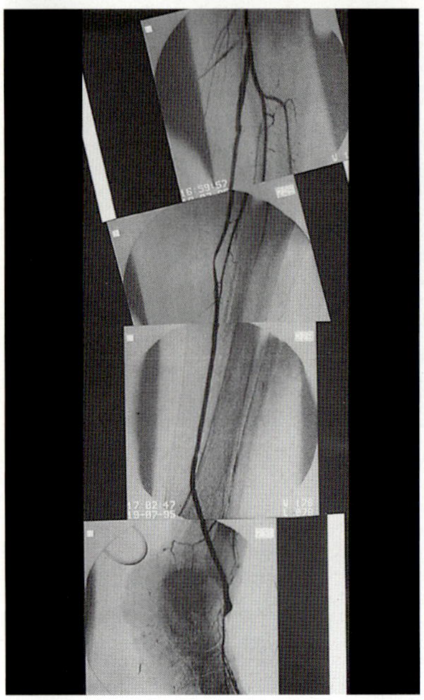

6-170

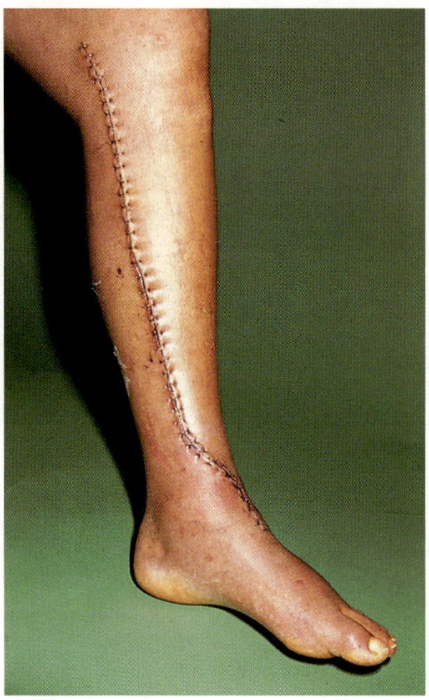

6-171

Fig. 6-170. Postoperative appearance of a bypass from the below-knee popliteal artery (end-to-side) to the dorsalis pedis artery (end-to-end)

Fig. 6-171. Skin incision required for a popliteal-to-pedal bypass

Fig. 6-172. Angiography showing placement of a femoro-plantar vein bypass with follow-up appearance after 2 years

Fig. 6-173. Operative view showing attachment of a vein bypass to the medial plantar artery

Fig. 6-174. Acute ischemia of the left lower leg with occlusion following a complex fracture after the patient was in a car accident. External fixation was employed and a femoro-posterior tibial PTFE bypass was placed

Fig. 6-175. Following the bypass, the sole showed patchy erythema as a sign of successful restoration of circulation following 8 h of ischemia. The entire limb was saved without amputation

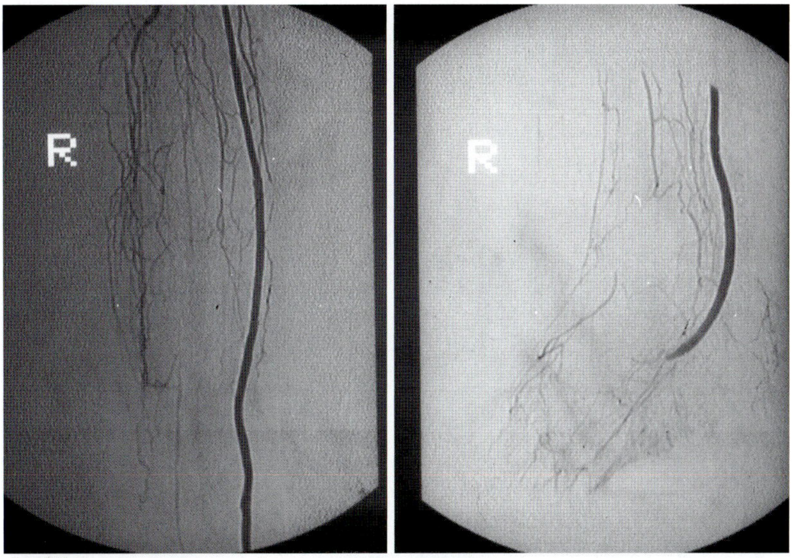

6-172

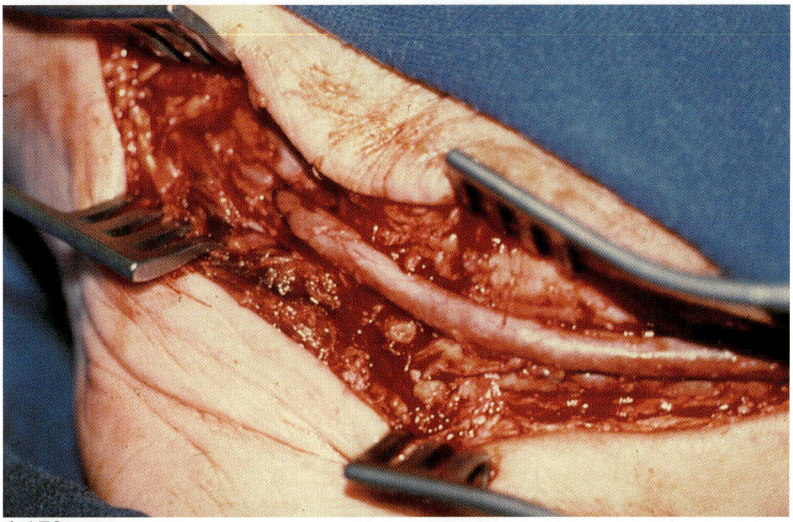

6-173

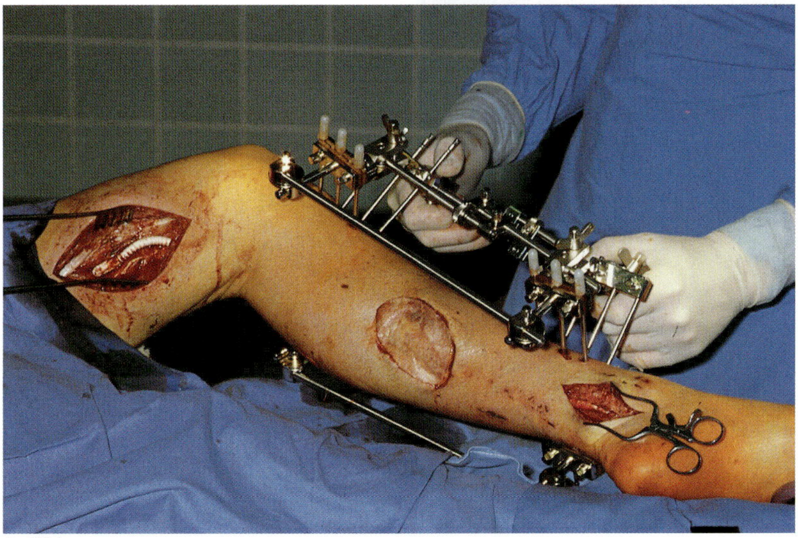

6-174

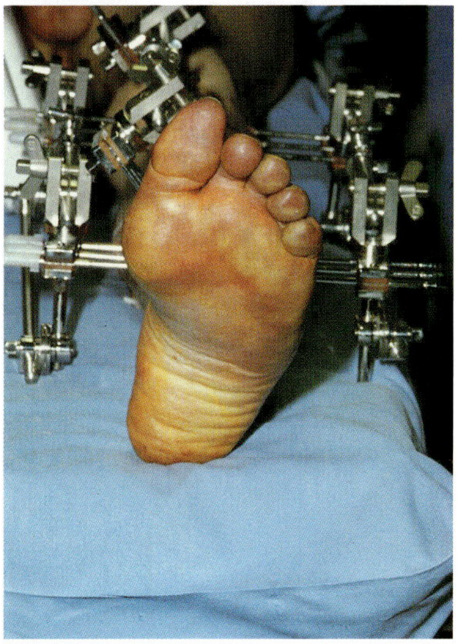

6-175

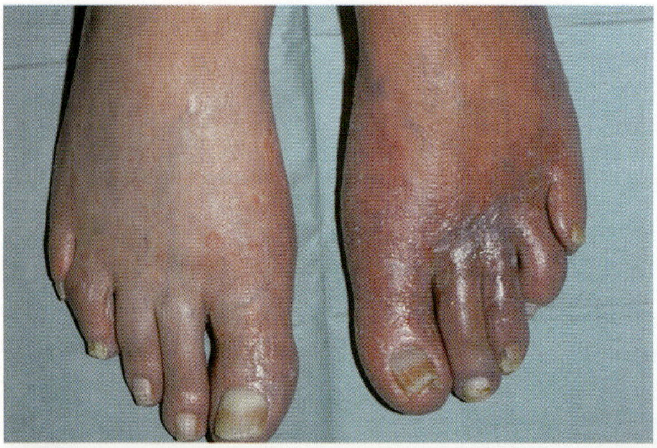

6-176

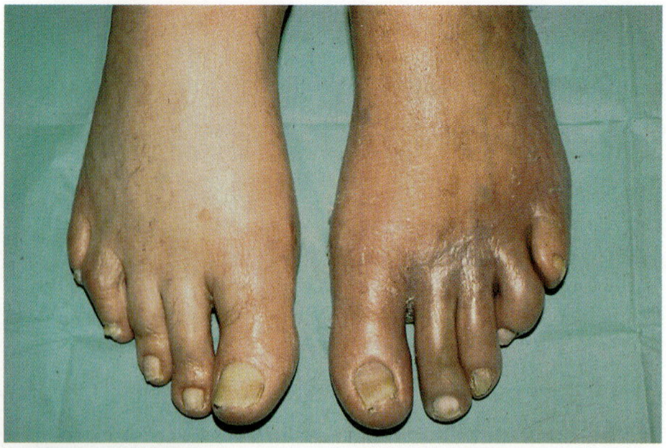

6-177

Figs. 6-176, 6-177. Patients with impaired peripheral circulation are susceptible to dermatophytic infections of the feet. In most cases, topical antimycotic treatment is effective

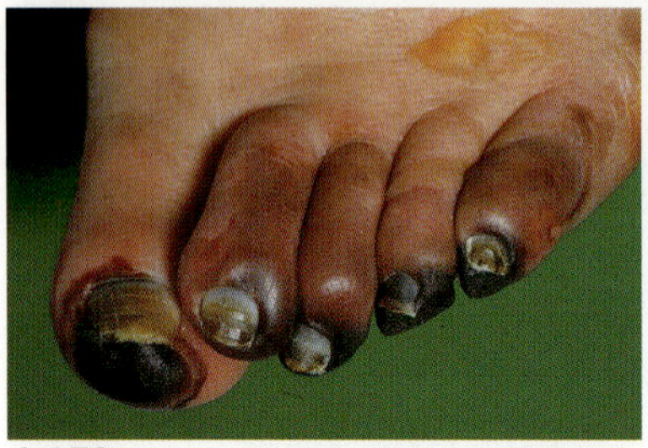

6-178

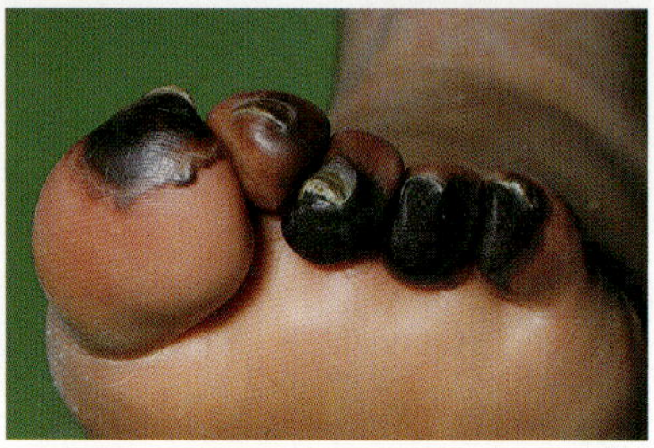

6-179

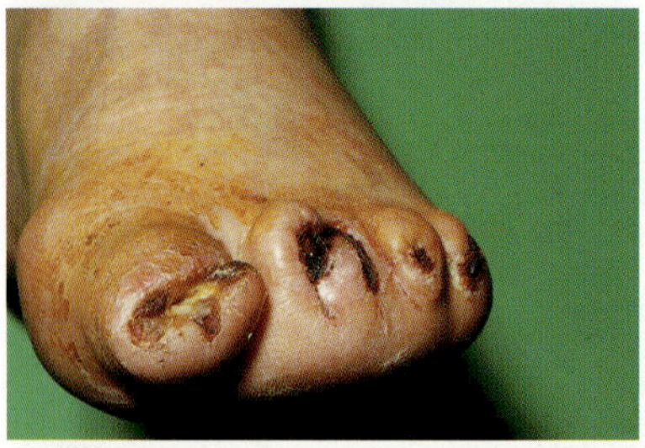

6-180

Figs. 6-178–6-180. Sharply demarcated dark digital necrosis 8 days after insertion of a femoro-tibial bypass. A minimal amputation was performed at the border between the damaged and healthy tissue

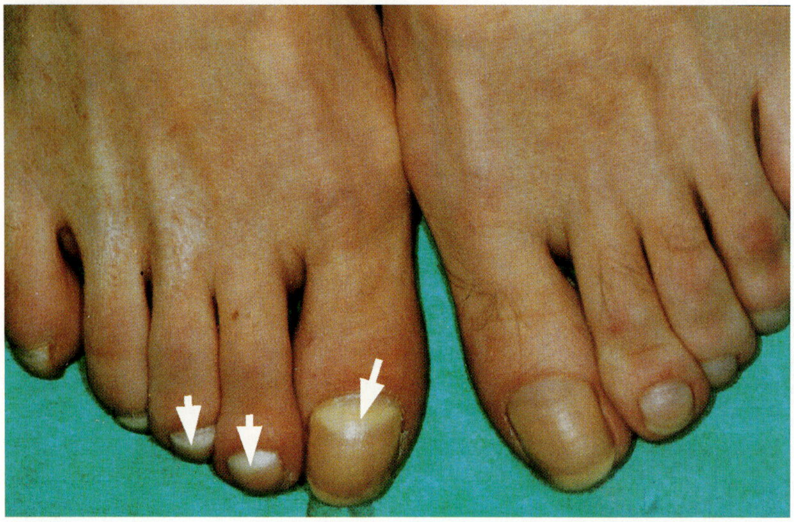

6-181

Fig. 6-181. A patient with bilateral peripheral arterial disease and severe ischemia of the legs. On the right, PTA of the tibio-peroneal artery was successfully performed. The improved blood supply led to an increase in the rate of growth of the toenails (*arrows*)

Fig. 6-182. Lumbar sympathectomy guided by computerized tomography. After all conservative measures have been tried, a sympathectomy can be performed to improve peripheral circulation. The sympathectomy leads to dilatation of the smallest arteries, reduced peripheral resistance and improved skin circulation. Possible indications include:

- Peripheral circulatory disturbances of the skin
- Thrombangitis obliterans
- Peripheral nerve injuries that produce causalgia
- Hyperhidrosis

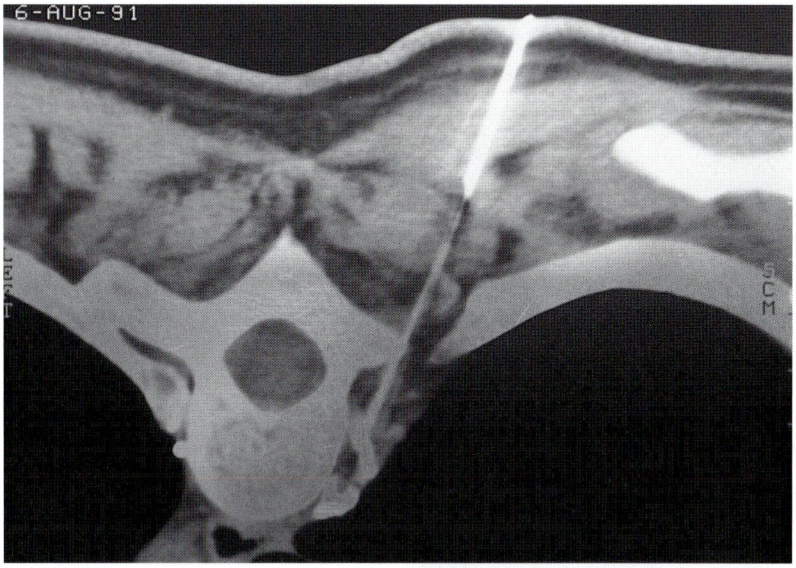

6-182

Fig. 6-183. Epidural spinal cord stimulation. SHEALY and MORTIMER, in 1967, introduced epidural spinal cord stimulation to treat therapy-resistant pain of varying etiologies. In 1976, COOK and colleagues described its effectiveness in treating patients with peripheral arterial disease and pain at rest. Diagram showing placement of a spinal cord stimulation system (Medtronic).The quadrupolar electrode is introduced percutaneously with a special needle under local anesthesia with imaging control and passed into the epidural space. In order to determine the correct location of the electrode, intraoperative paresthesias should be produced in the involved areas. The electrode can be left in place for a stimulation period lasting many days, in order to test the effectiveness of the procedure

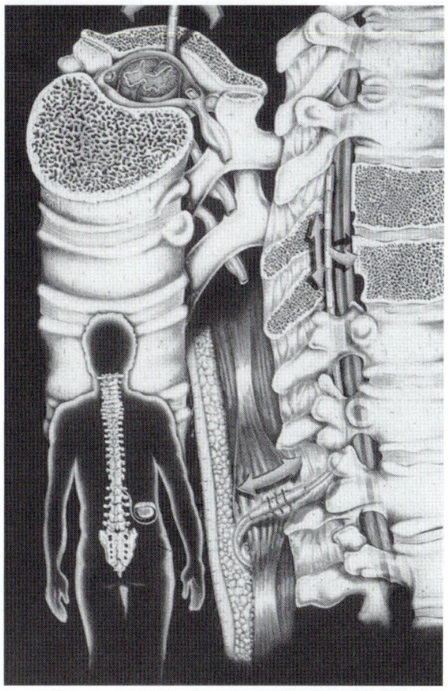

6-183

Fig. 6-184. If the external stimulation is successful, a permanent impulse generator is implanted

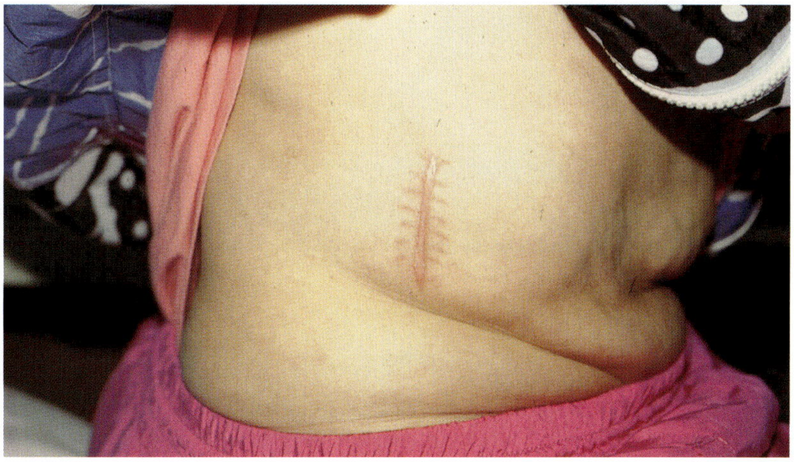

6-184

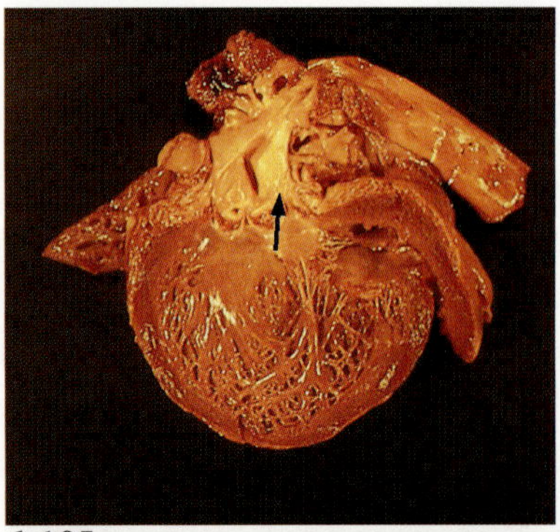

6-185

Fig. 6-185. Appearance of a chronic aortic and mitral valve endocarditis (*arrow*). Cardiac emboli play an important role in acute peripheral arterial occlusion, Patients with vegetative valve lesions are at highest risk

Source of cardioembolism

Cause	Frequency
Pneumatic heart disease	10
Prosthetic cardiac valves	10
Nonvalvular atrial fibrillation	45
Left ventricular aneurysm	10
Acute myocardial infarction	15
Other	10

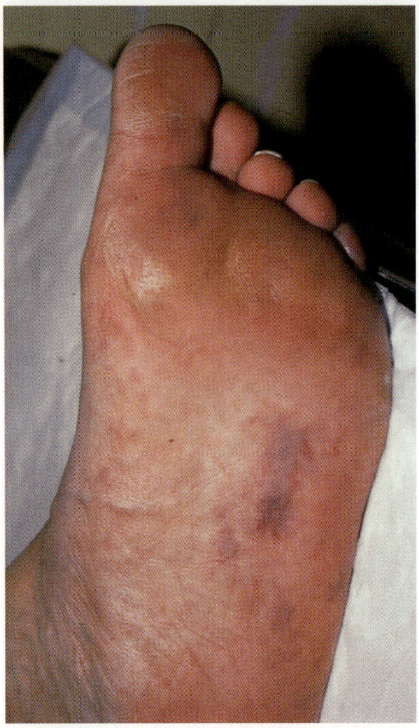

6-186

Fig. 6-186. Distal circulatory impairment following emboli from a popliteal artery aneurysm

Figs. 6-187, 6-188. Blue toe phenomenon as a paraneoplastic sign in a 60 year old patient with a bronchial carcinoma. The deep cyanosis of the distal digits is striking. The differential diagnostic considerations in blue toe phenomenon include:

- Emboli (cardiac, arterial, cholesterol)
- Peripheral arterial occlusive disease
- Paraneoplastic sign (usually from hyperviscosity)
- Drug reaction, such as from cyclosporine A

Fig. 6-190. Marked cholesterol emboli arising from a thoraco-abdominal aneurysm in a 65 year old man. Even though the foot pulses were intact, acute necrosis of the toes and feet developed. At the same time, emboli caused occlusion in the renal arteries, gastrointestinal arteries and other skin sites. The patient died as a result of multi-organ failure from the many areas of occlusion

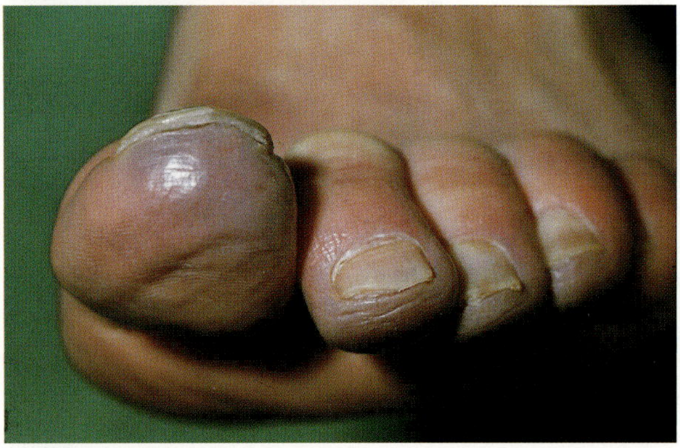

6-187

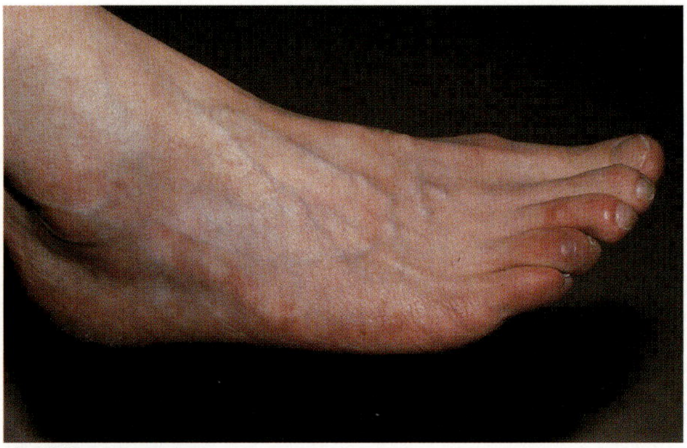

6-188

Microembolism of atherosclerotic debris consisting of lipid and thrombotic material may originate from the aorta or more distal arteries and lead the occlusion of small distal limb arteries

Fig. 6-189. Light microscopic view of cholesterol crystals with tears in the intima and media in a patient with an aneurysm of the abdominal aorta. Tiny fragments of such cholesterol-rich deposits can break away causing emboli and occlusion in small peripheral or visceral vessels

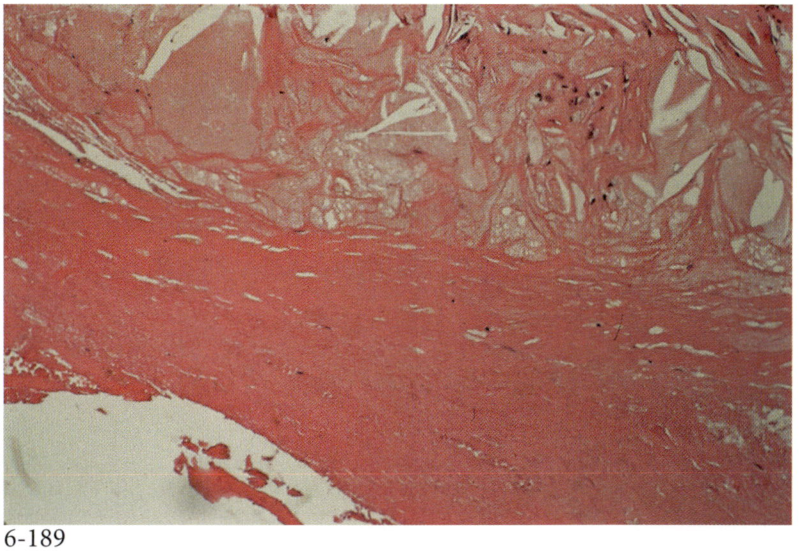

6-189

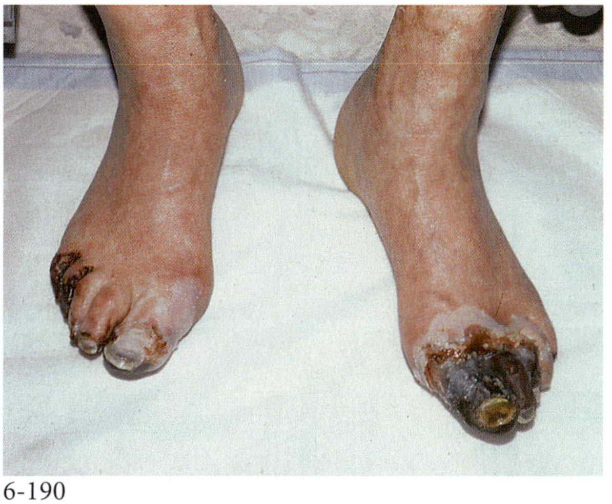

6-190

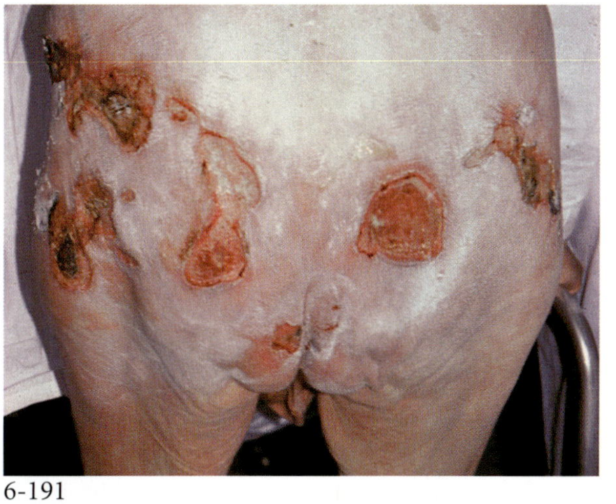

6-191

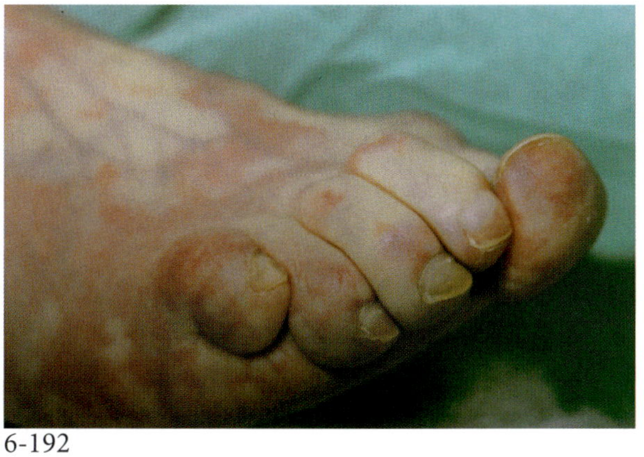

6-192

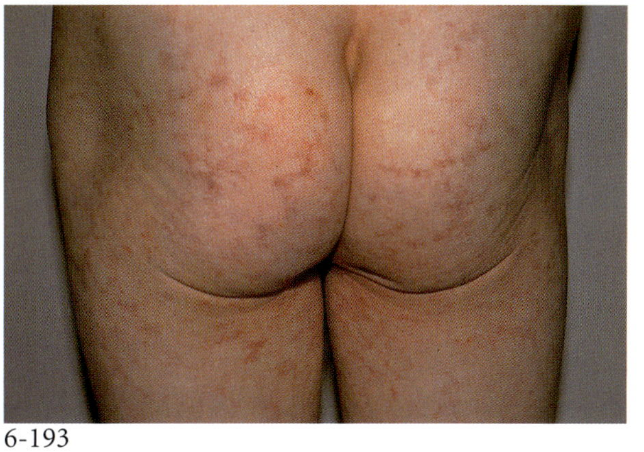

6-193

Fig. 6-191. Prominent ulcerations and necrotic areas on buttocks of same patient

Fig. 6-192. Necrosis from cholesterol crystals in a 70 year old woman following cardiac catheterization

Fig. 6-193. Cholesterol emboli in a 55 year old man following aortography with the use of a pigtail catheter which dislodged the cholesterol-rich fragments

Chapter 7: Diabetic Foot Syndrome

Contents

A: Introduction

Diabetic Foot Syndrome

Synonyms. Diabetic foot, diabetic angiopathy

Definition

The term diabetic foot syndrome refers to the combination of organ system disorders which together produce a variety of clinical problems in the feet of patients with diabetes mellitus. They include:

- Vascular system with angiopathy
- Peripheral nervous system with polyneuropathy
- Skeletal system with osteoarthropathy
- Skin and soft tissue with trophic changes

Diabetic neuropathy alone is responsible for 45%–60% of diabetic foot problems, angiopathy for 7%–13%, and a combination of these two for 25%–45%.

As far back as 1843, A. Faber, a pathologist in Heidelberg, wrote that "*Vascular wall disease is the cause of the tendency of patients with diabetes mellitus to develop infections and gangrene.*"

Epidemiology

- Some 3%–7% of patients have diabetes mellitus.
- Diabetic patients have about a 30-fold increased risk of having a major leg amputation when compared to non-diabetics.
- Yearly, 50,000 – 100,000 leg amputations are performed in the United States; of this group, more than one-third involve diabetics.
- In the 2 years following their amputation, over 25% of the patients experience severe enough problems in the other leg to make a second amputation likely. More than 50% of foot amputations in diabetics can be avoided if the patients are better informed about foot care and receive professional help as needed (St. Vincent Declaration, 1989)

Etiology and Pathogenesis

The macroangiopathy of diabetes mellitus is indistinguishable pathologically from atherosclerosis in a non-diabetic patient. The changes develop earlier in diabetics and lead more often to complications. Women with diabetes mellitus have about the same risk of macroangiopathy as men.

Diabetic microangiopathy is a combined term used to describe the functional and degenerative changes in the small vessels (capillaries, veins, arteries). Diabetic microangiopathy is a generalized process that leaves no capillary bed spared. The most severe changes involve the retina, heart, kidneys and feet. Changes can also be found in the muscle capillaries, the vasa vasorum et nervorum and the nail fold capillaries.

Actually, vessel destruction is not seen; the changes are functional. It would be more appropriate to speak of a disturbed microcirculation, but the term microangiopathy has become firmly established.

In addition, changes in the rheological or flow properties of blood play a major role. The erythrocytes are more rigid and less easily deformed in diabetics. The plasma viscosity is higher and the erythrocytes tend to aggregate. Platelet function is increased, while platelet life span is shortened.

Both increased glycosylation of myelin sheath proteins and metabolic changes in the structural lipids may contribute to the neuropathy. The osteoarthropathy describes all the bone and soft tissues changes which typically involve the metatarso-phalangeal joints and tarsal bones. They can range from subluxation to destruction of the joints with osteolysis.

Most diabetic feet have atrophic skin changes. The most common lesion is a solitary, usually painless, punched-out ulcer on the plantar surface over the metatarsal heads, known as a mal perforans ulcer.

Diagnosis

- History
- Clinical vascular evaluation (inspection, palpation, auscultation, oscillography, Doppler ultrasonography, angiography)
  Caution: Doppler pressure readings are often incorrect because of medial sclerosis.
- Neurological evaluation
- Orthopedic evaluation
- Laboratory investigations
- Bacteriological smears and cultures
- Radiological evaluation (bone lesions, vessel calcification)

Table 7-1. Differential diagnosis of foot lesions in diabetes mellitus

Feature	Neuropathic, infected foot	Ischemic, gangrenous foot
Skin	Pink and warm	Blue and cool
Pulses	Intact	Diminished/absent
Pain	Painless	Painful (sometimes painless)
Location	Often over metatarsal head	Often involve tips of toes, heel
Deep sensation (Tuning fork test)	Reduced	Intact, no other risk factors for arteriosclerosis
Transcutaneous pO_2	Normal to raised	Markedly reduced
Arteriography	Not indicated	Indicated early in course

Table 7-2. Special features of peripheral vascular disease in diabetes

- Earlier onset
- More common
- Diffuse atheroma
- Distal vessel disease

Therapy

Preventive Measures

- Careful education and training of patient
- No walking barefoot
- Avoiding trauma (pressure, burns, minor injuries)
- Appropriate shoes, often custom-made
- Daily inspection of shoes for rough spots, foreign objects
- Skilled foot care, keeping nails trimmed and calluses pared while avoiding injury. Some patients can achieve this themselves; others will require podiatric care.
- Appropriate foot hygiene including daily lukewarm baths followed by clean socks, most often wool or cotton
- Daily inspection of feet, using a hand mirror, searching for minor injuries, dermatophyte infections, changes in color
- No heating pads or hot water bottles; caution about avoiding sunburn.

Treatment of Diabetic Gangrene

- Local therapy is usually required for diabetic ulcers and gangrene unless a tendon or bone is exposed, provided the circulation is adequate.
- In many instances surgical debridement is required. Pockets of pus should be drained and sequestered bones removed. In the case of mal perforans ulcers, it may be necessary to remove the underlying metatarsal head.
- Elimination of weight bearing is usually required.
- Systemic antibiotics should be used following culture and sensitivity studies if there is evidence of soft tissue infection, ascending lymphangitis, osteomyelitis or sepsis.
- If a lesion does not heal and diminished pedal pulses are present, full lower extremity angiography should be performed.
- Surgical revascularization: The lesions with a neurological basis usually heal with avoidance of pressure and local care. In contrast, if ischemia is present, healing may be indolent and revascularization procedures may be needed.
- Percutaneous transluminal angioplasty

No amputation should be performed prior to evaluation by a well-qualified vascular surgeon!

Table 7-3. Information given to diabetics (taken from British Diabetic Association leaflet on foot-care

Do:
- Inspect feet daily
- Wash feet regularly in warm water
- Dry feet carefully, especially between the foer
- Check bath water temperature before stepping in
- Avoid dry skin (use lotion after washing)
- Cut toenails straight across
- Have feet measured professionally before buying shoes
- Inspect the inside of shoes daily for foreign bodies
- Ensure feet are examined at each clinic visit
- Seen early advice from your doctor or chiropodist about any foot problems

Do not:
- Walk barefoot
- Wear new shoes for long periods
- Use razors, knifes or corn remedies on feet
- Smoke

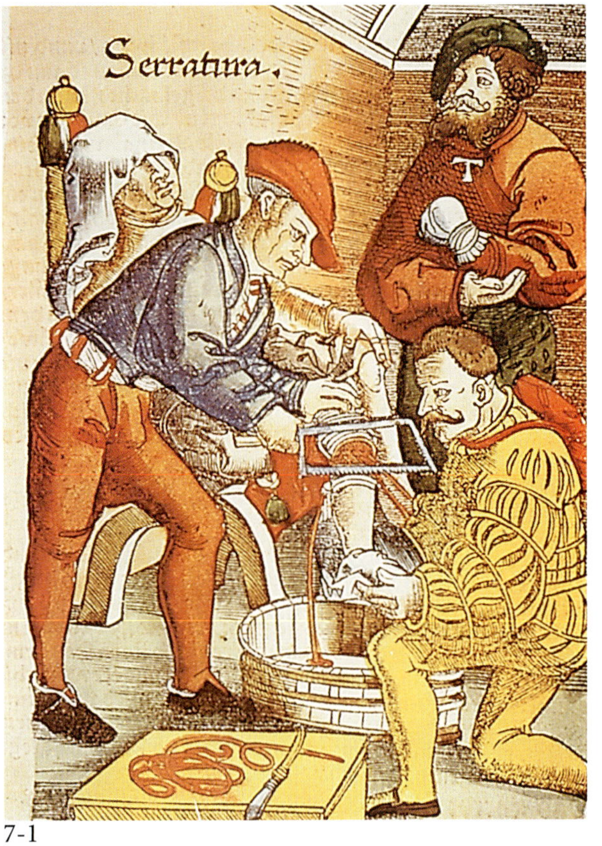

7-1

Fig. 7-1. The leg amputation. This woodcut, by J. WETCHLIEN, was prepared for the *Feldbuch der Wundarztney (Field Book for Military Doctors)*, by GERSDORFF, published in Strasbourg in 1540 (Philadelphia Museum of Arts, USA). This is the first known illustration of a leg amputation. The injured patient, whose face is covered with a veil, appears to be under the influence of some type of narcotic or sedative, perhaps derived from a plant. GERSDORFF himself developed the technique shown here

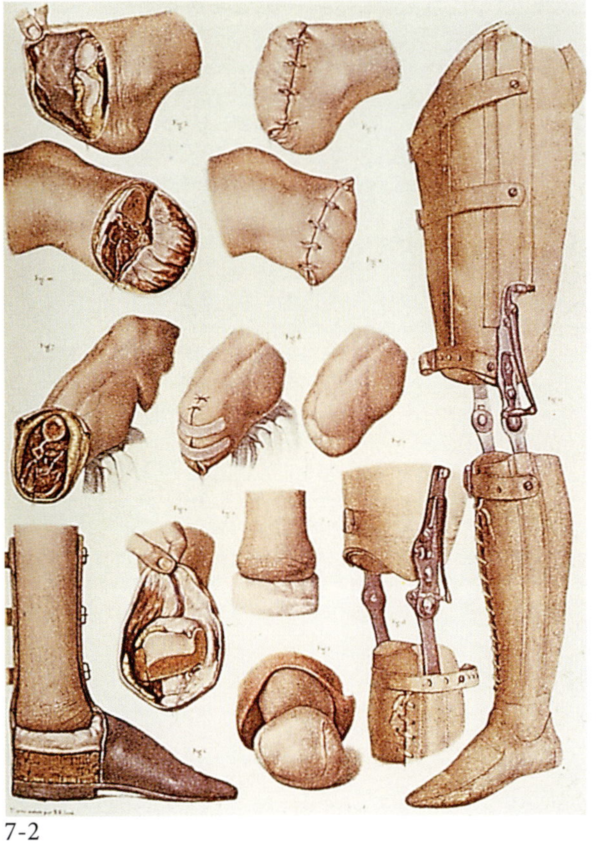

7-2

Fig. 7-2. Different methods of amputation and a surprisingly modern leg prosthesis. (From J. B. M. BOURGERY and C. BERNARD, *Traité complet de l'anatomie de l'homme*, Paris, 1866/1867)

B: Supplementary Figures and Legends

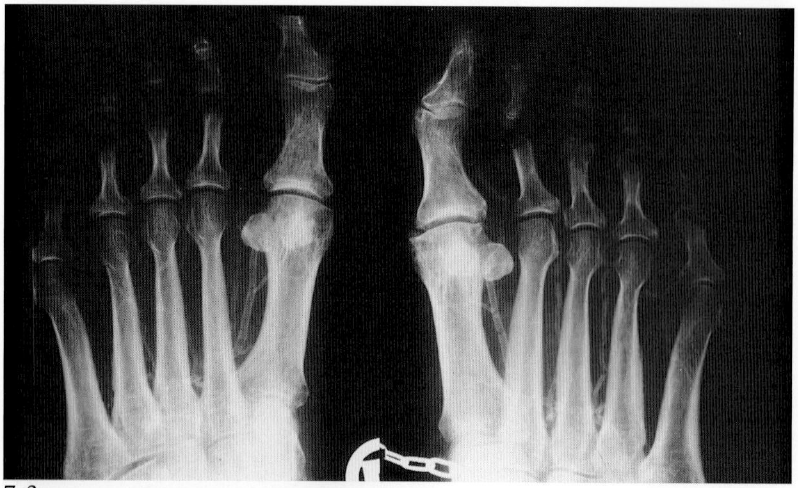

7-3

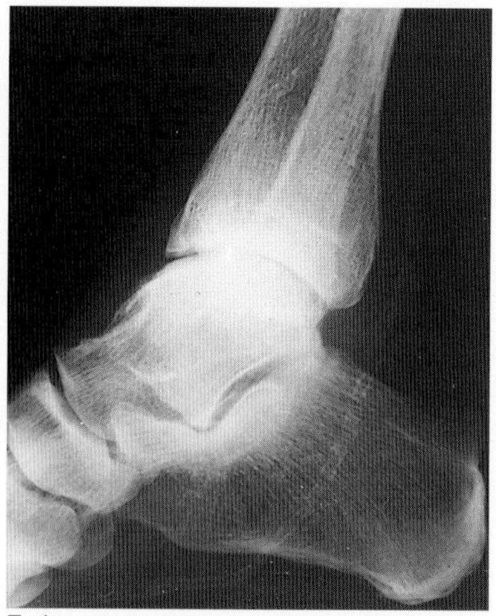

7-4

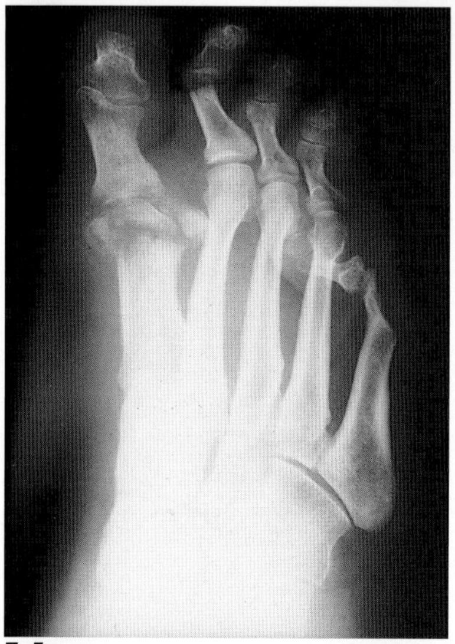

7-5

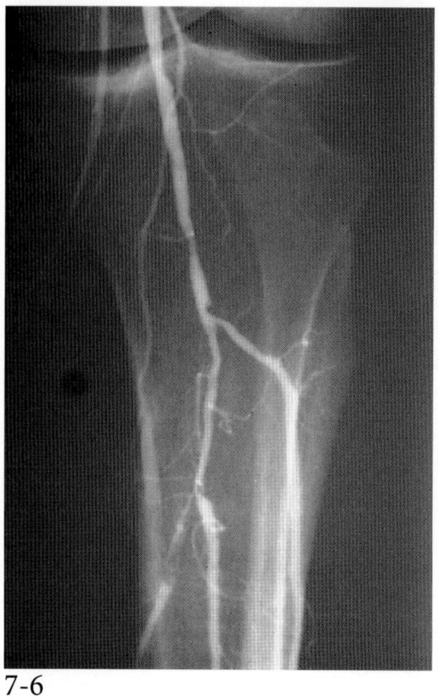

7-6

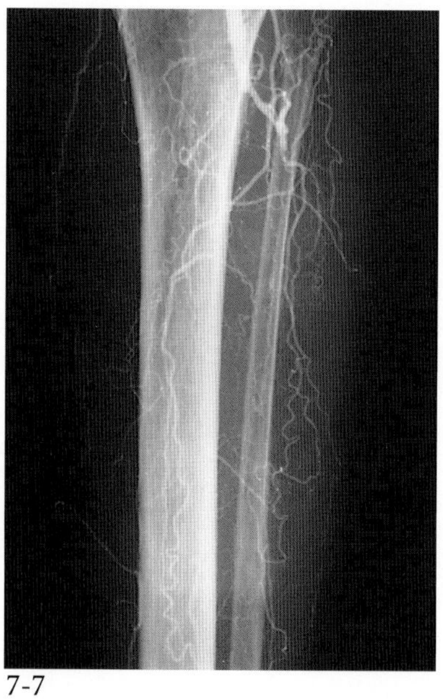

7-7

Fig. 7-3. Marked medial sclerosis of the foot arteries in a patient with diabetes mellitus

Fig. 7-4. Marked medial sclerosis (Mönckeberg medial sclerosis) in a patient with long-standing diabetes mellitus. These changes were discovered on a routine orthopedic X-ray; the patient had no clinical signs of peripheral vascular disease

Fig. 7-5. Diabetic osteopathy with damage to the interphalangeal joints

Figs. 7-6, 7-7. Two angiograms showing peripheral vascular disease with occlusions in the lower leg. The localization of the stenoses and occlusions are typical for chronic diabetes mellitus

Arteriography demonstrates three common patterns of vessel involvement in diabetics

1. Isolated superficial femoral artery disease
2. Combined superficial femoral and popliteal trifurcation disease
3. Tibial and peroneal disease

Fig. 7-8. Superficial burns with blisters. This diabetic with neuropathy burned his foot on a copper hot water bottle. There was no associated pain

Fig. 7-9. Severe burn of the toes and anterior part of foot. This patient wanted to take a warm foot bath, but failed to check the water temperature with either a thermometer or his elbow

Fig. 7-10. Mal perforans ulcer and secondary hyperkeratosis in a patient with diabetic foot syndrome. The chronic pressure causes both the ulcer and the extensive thickening of the skin

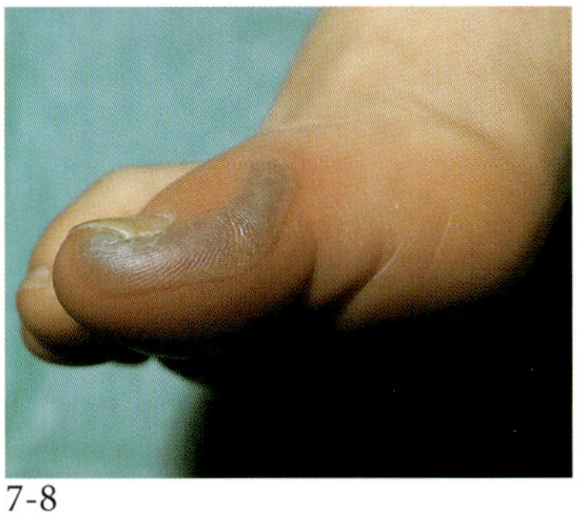

7-8

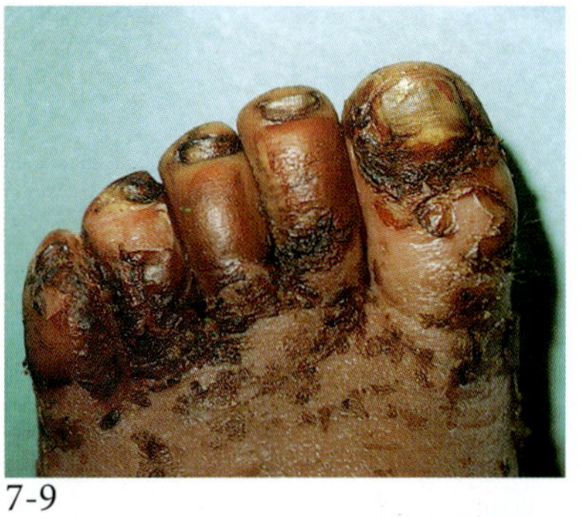

7-9

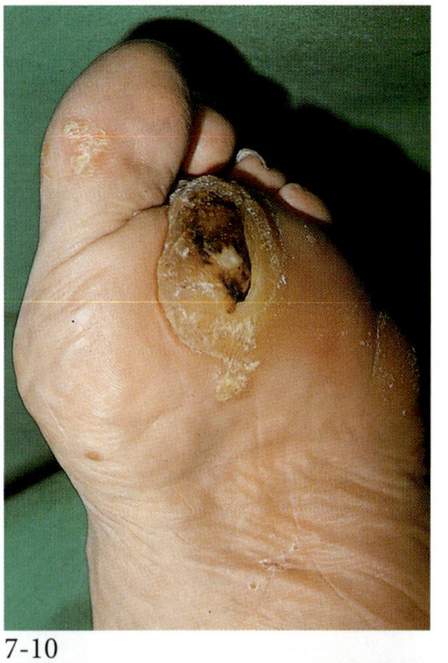

7-10

Figs. 7-11, 7-12. Full-blown Charcot syndrome (J. M. Charcot, 1825–1893, French neurologist). The foot is swollen and distorted from deformed joints, so that the risk of pressure points and ulcerations is great. It is important to diagnosis Charcot syndrome early before extensive damage has occurred. Treatment consists of minimizing the demands upon the foot and making available special shoes

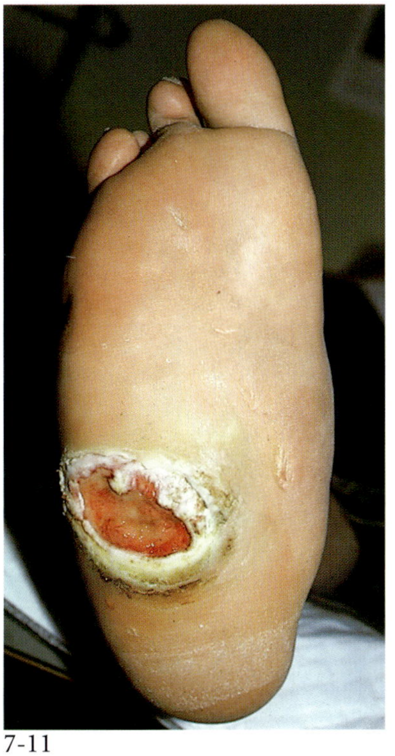

7-11

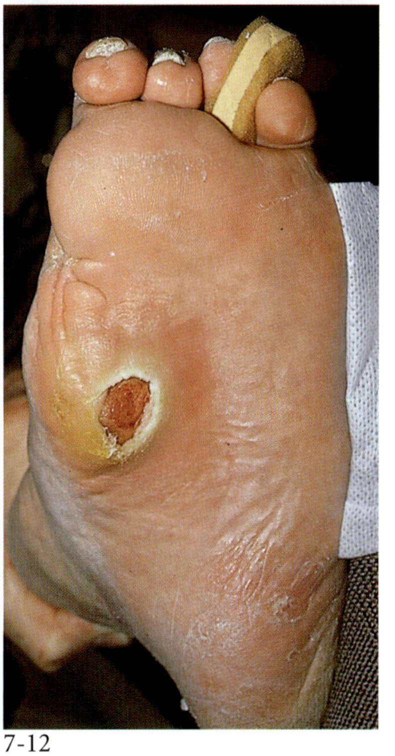

7-12

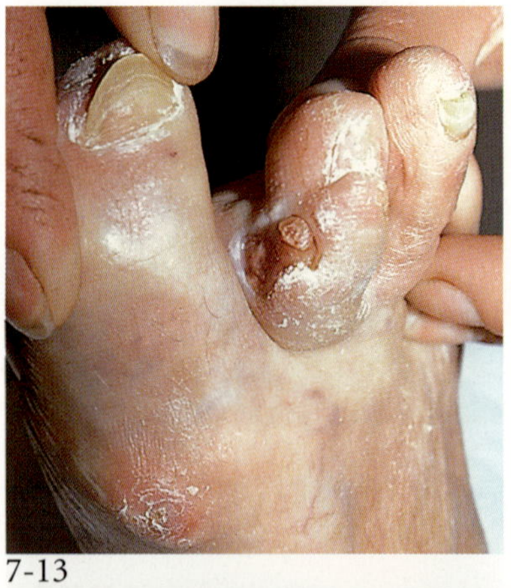
7-13

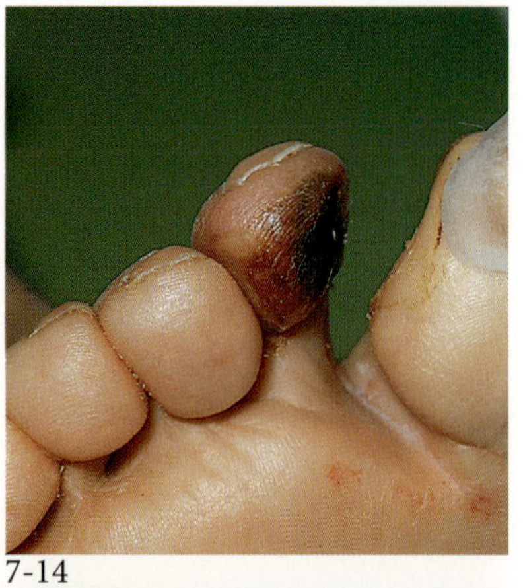
7-14

Figs. 7-13, 7-14. Pressure-induced necrosis of the toes and interdigital spaces in a patient with diabetic neuropathy

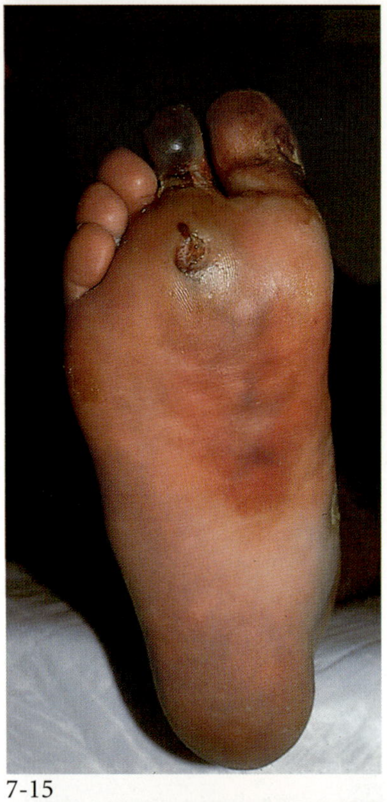
7-15

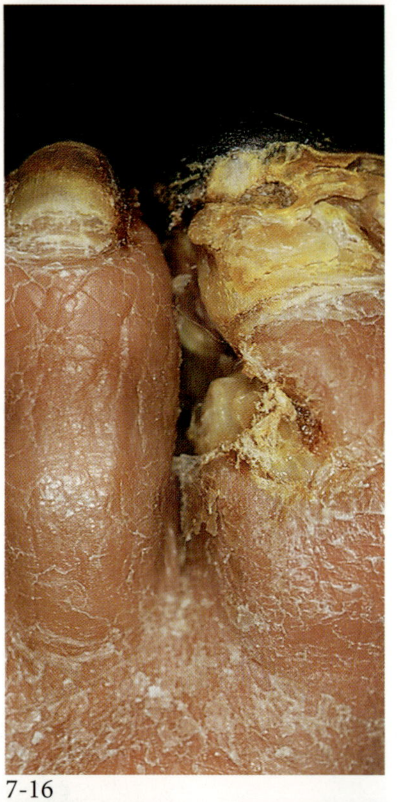
7-16

Fig. 7-15. Gangrene of the toes with deep cellulitis extending into the mid-part of the foot. Mal perforans ulcer over the second metatarsal head

Fig. 7-16. Onychomycosis and severe interdigital tinea pedis in a patient with diabetes mellitus

Fig. 7-17. Typical gangrene of the big toe in diabetes mellitus

Fig. 7-18. A differential diagnostic consideration is podagra or gout, shown here in its most typical site – the first metatarsal-phalangeal joint. In podagra, ulcerations do not occur

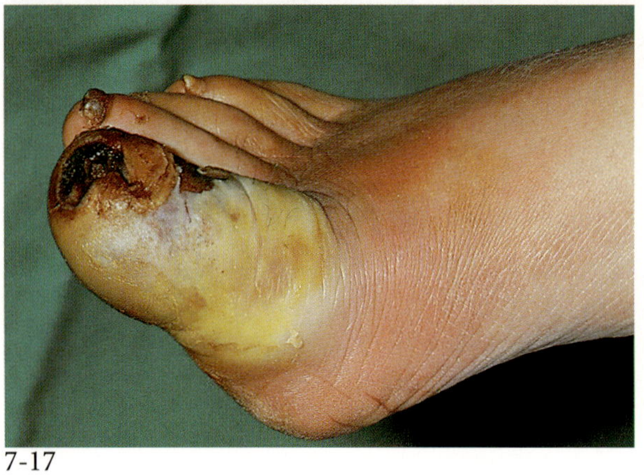
7-17

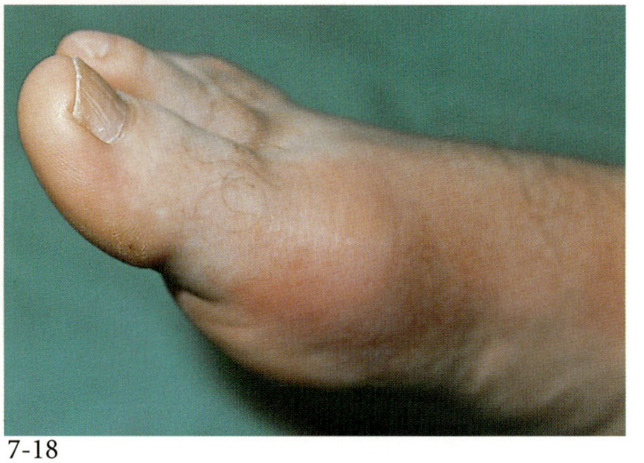
7-18

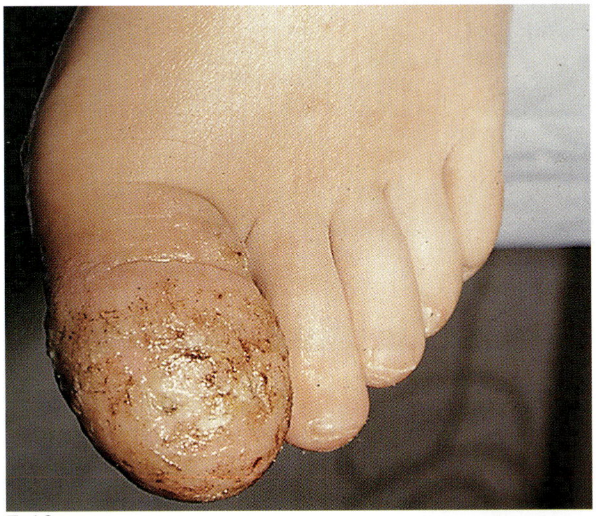
7-19

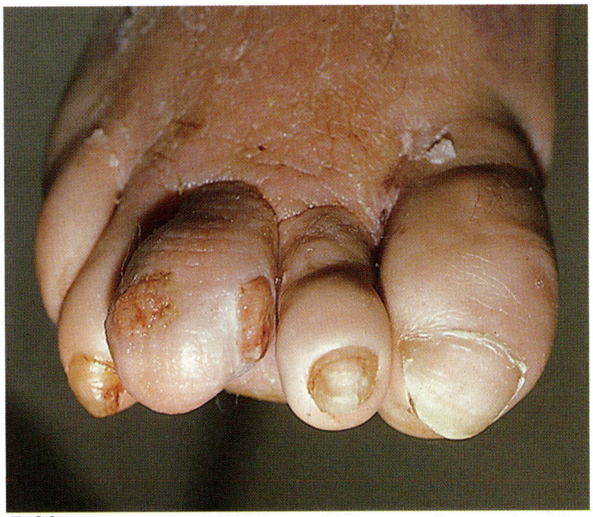
7-20

Figs. 7-19, 7-20. Lymphedema of the toes in diabetes mellitus

Additional Acral Circulatory Problems in Non-diabetic Neuropathy

Acro-osteolysis

Synonyms. Familial acro-osteolysis, disappearing bone disease

This disorder may be sporadic or familial. The distal phalanges of the fingers and toes show loss of bone (distal osteolysis) usually with rarefaction of the bones. In blacks there may be spontaneous amputation of the little toes with bone necrosis and presumably small vessel disease; this is known as ainhum.

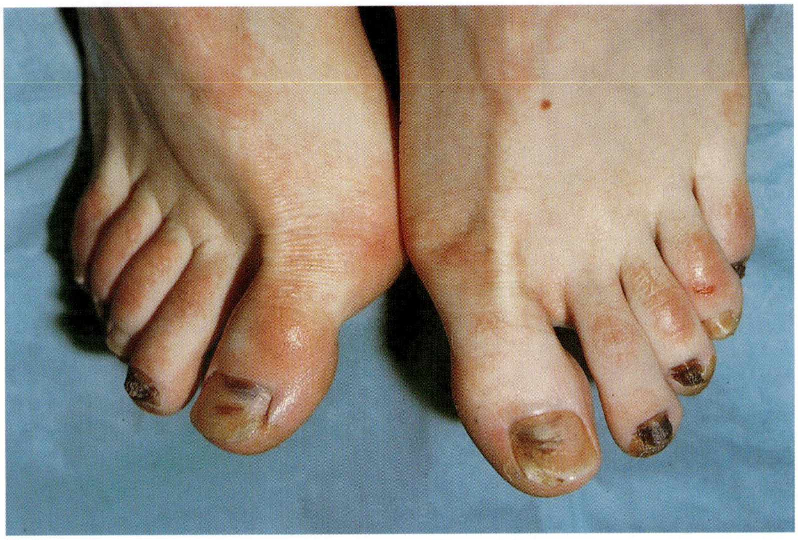
7-21

Fig. 7-21. The toes and foot of a 23 year old patient with acro-osteolysis. The patient had experienced multiple painless necrotic lesions at pressure points associated with subungual hematomas. Wearing new shoes or engaging in sports seemed to be likely triggers. The neurological examination revealed markedly diminished deep sensation and a distal polyneuropathy

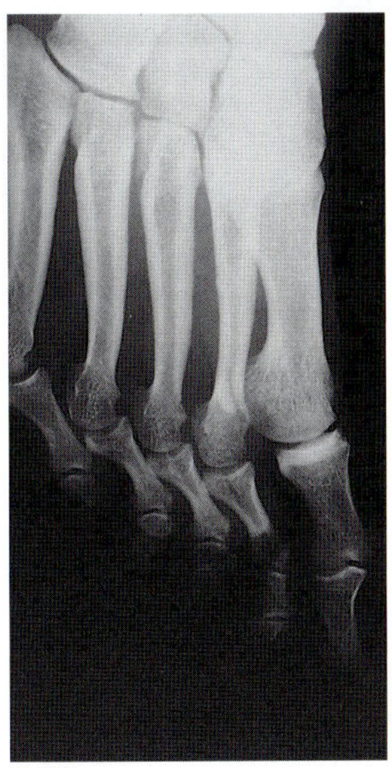
7-22

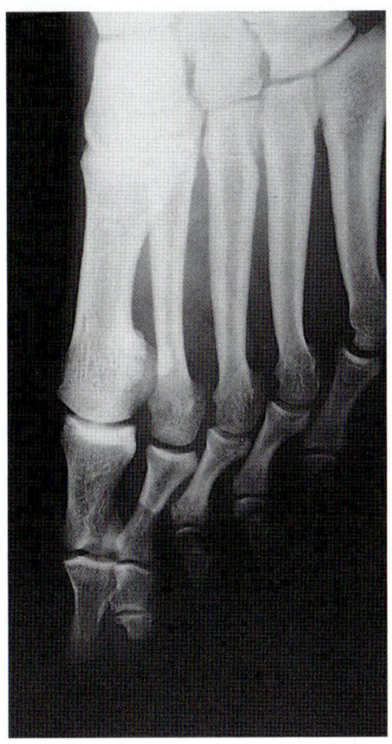
7-23

Figs. 7-22, 7-23. X-rays from the same patient. The angled view shows a clear shortening of the distal phalanges on both sides

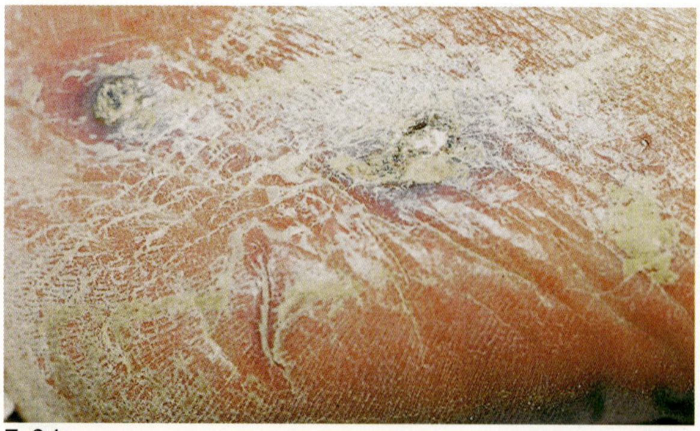
7-24

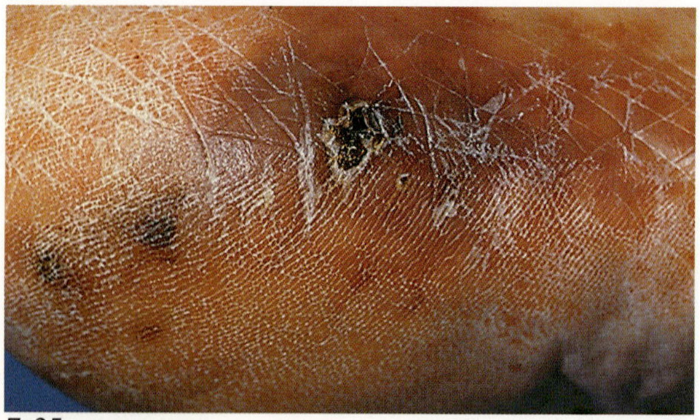
7-25

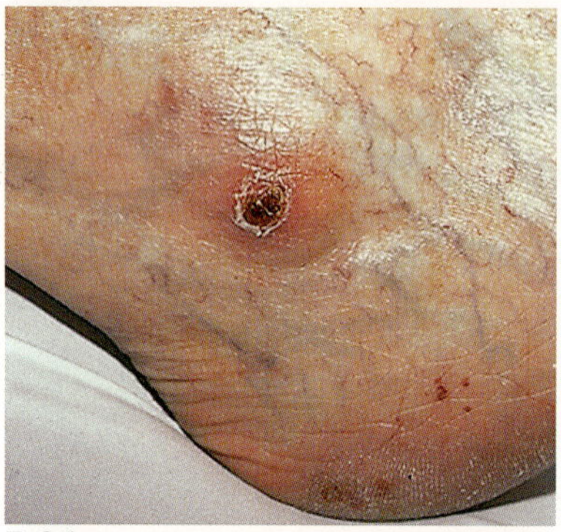
7-26

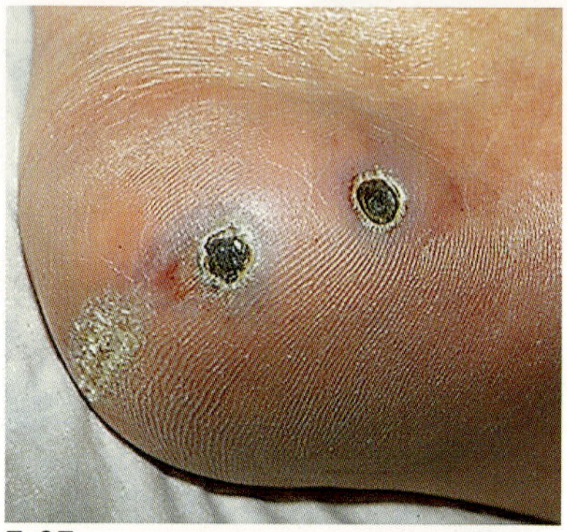
7-27

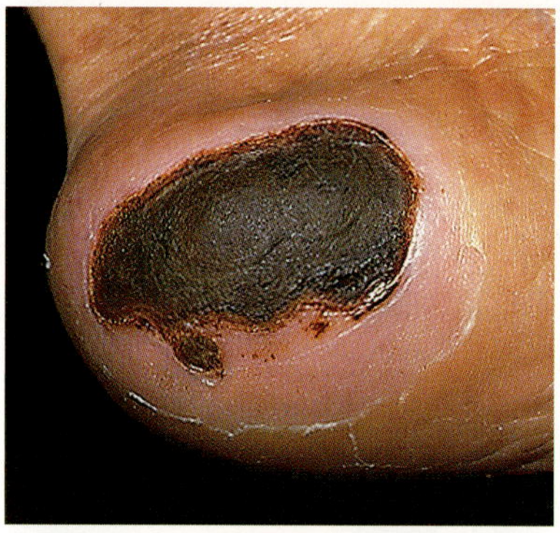
7-28

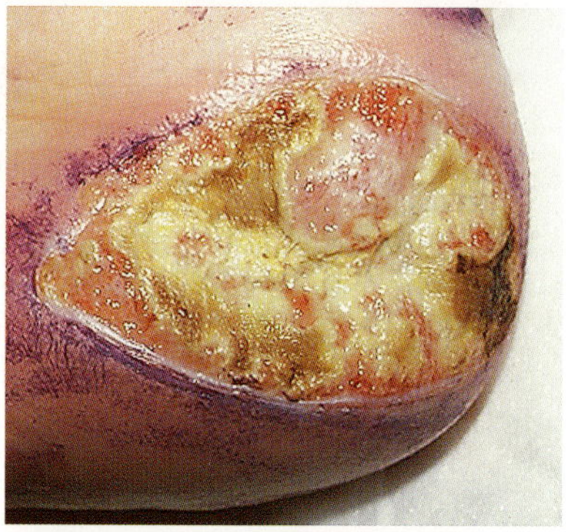
7-29

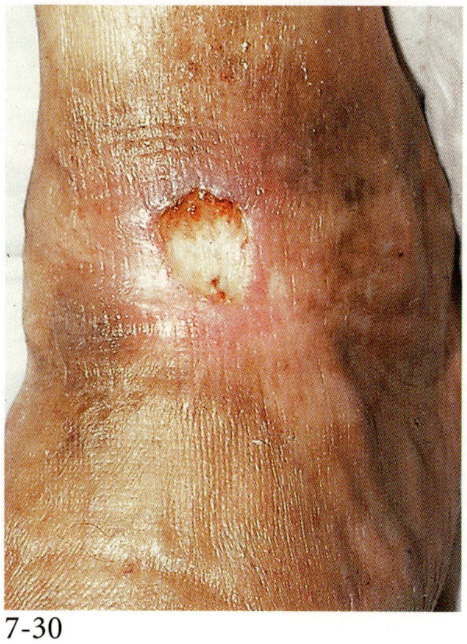
7-30

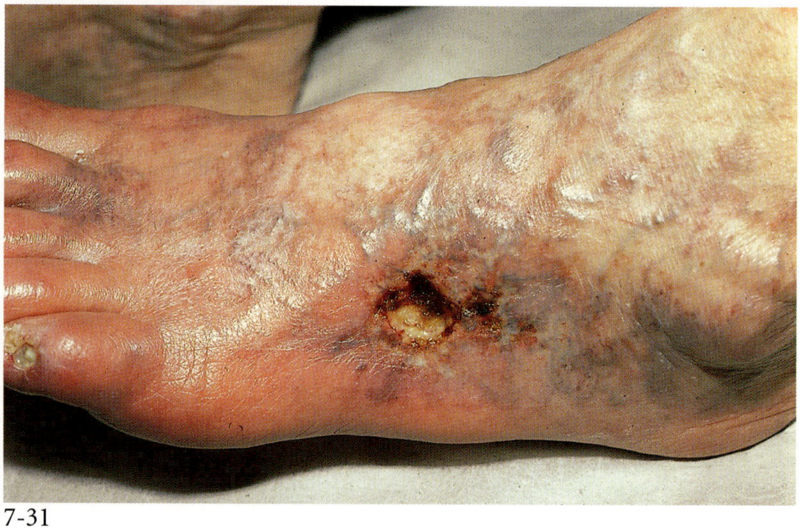
7-31

Figs. 7-24, 7-25. Fissures or gangrenous patches on the heel in a patient with diabetes mellitus. The reduced sympathetic innervation leads to a hypohidrosis, or drying of the skin, which facilitates fissuring

Figs. 7-26 – 7-29. Typical necrotic lesions about the ankle and heel, showing varying degrees of severity. The main causes are mechanical pressure, neurological disease, vascular impairment, altered blood viscosity and metabolic problems, usually in combination

Figs. 7-30, 7-31. Diabetic ischemic ulcer in an unusual location on the dorsal surface of the foot

Figs. 7-32–7-37. A 57 year old women with insulin-dependent diabetes mellitus. In addition to the usual complications (angiopathy, retinopathy, neuropathy, renal disease), she had marked mutilating osteopathy. Her feet and toes are deformed both from the bone destruction and from previous operations. The matching X-ray pictures show marked osteolysis and bone destruction (Charcot arthropathy). Charcot arthropathy (diabetic osteopathy) leeds to severe foot deformity. The exact pathogenesis of this problem is unknown

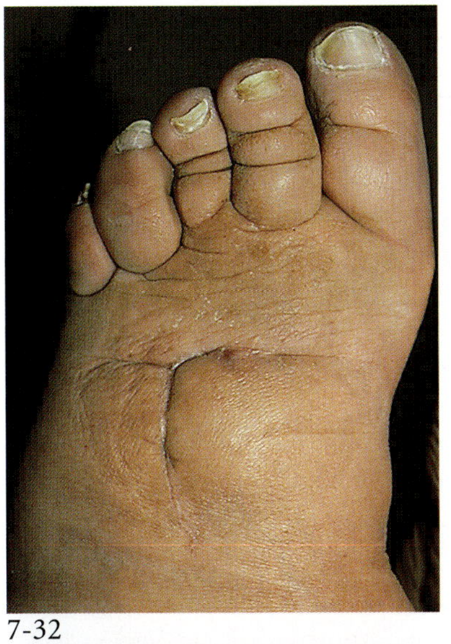

7-32

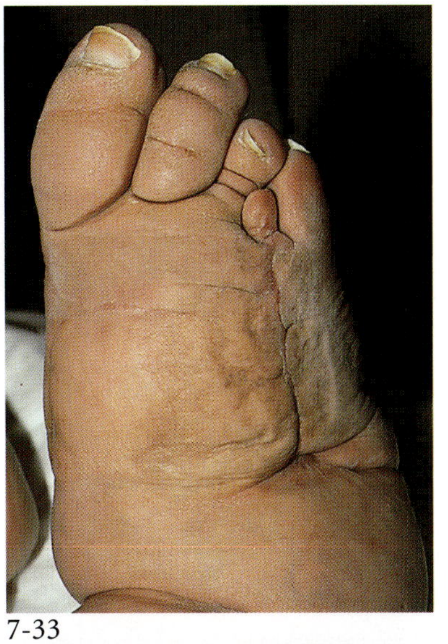

7-33

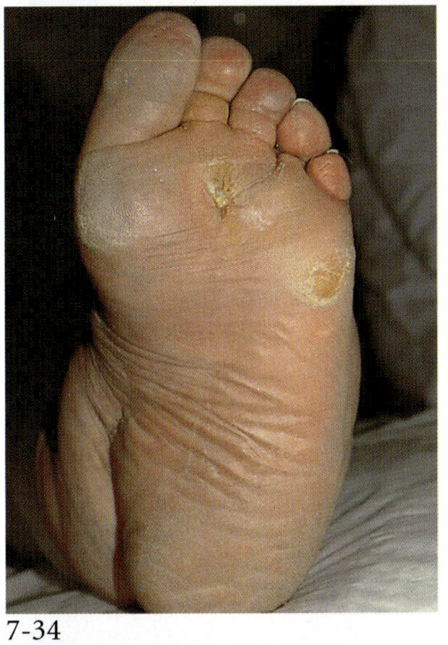

7-34

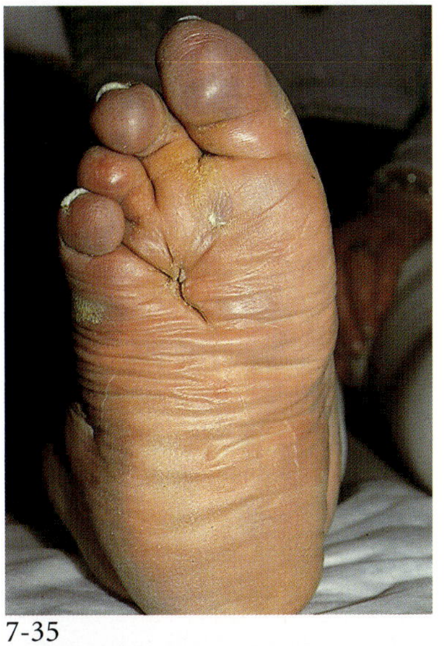

7-35

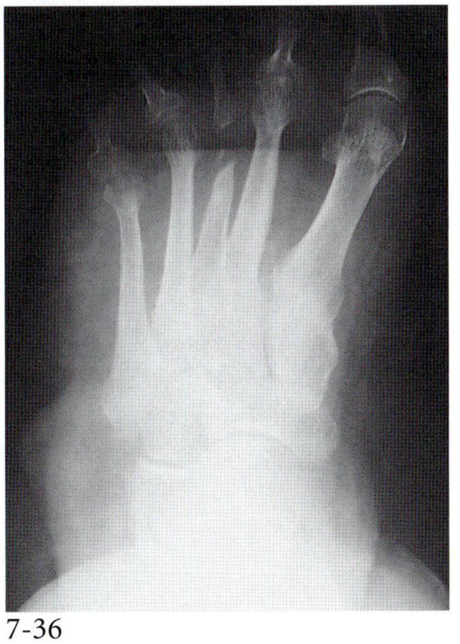

7-36

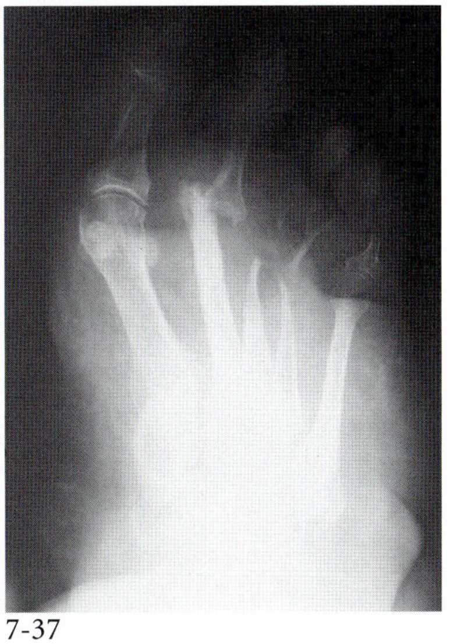

7-37

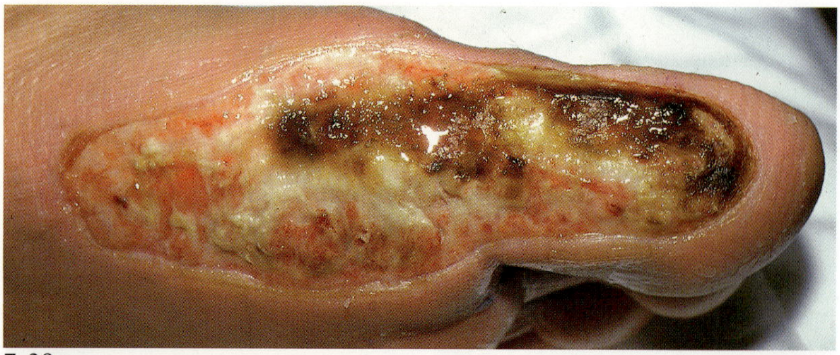
7-38

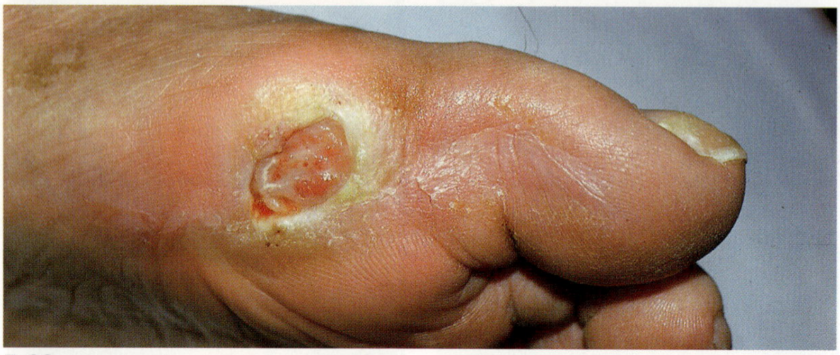
7-39

Figs. 7-38, 7-39. Extensive diabetic ulcer treated conservatively. The healing process took over 1 year

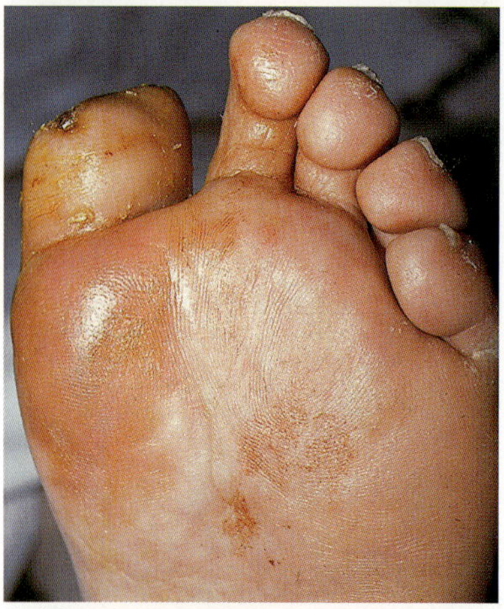
7-40

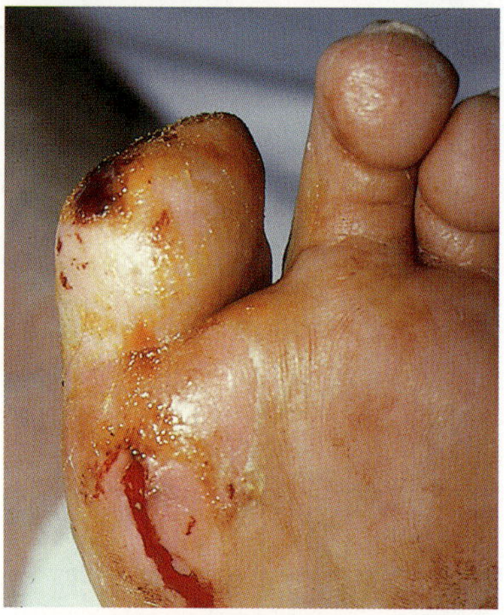
7-41

Figs. 7-40, 7-41. Acute infection in a 57 year old diabetic women. When an abscess forms, it is often helpful to make a deep incision opening it

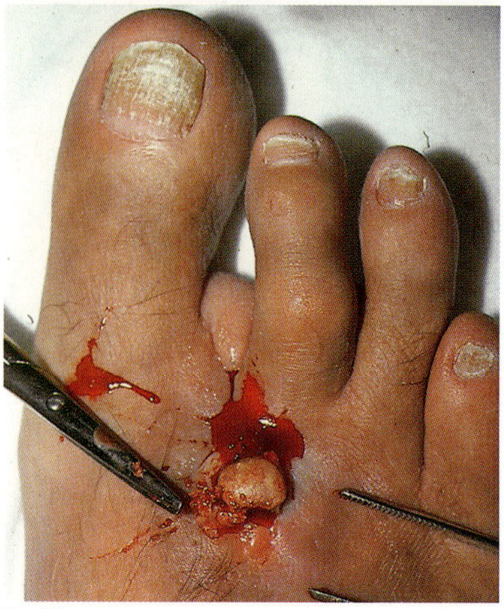
7-42

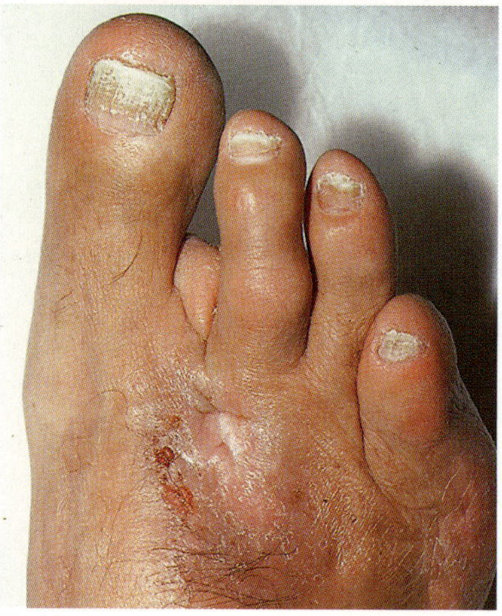
7-43

Figs. 7-42, 7-43. Removal of a sequestered bone. This patient had a toe amputation with a persistent draining sinus. After the loose metatarsal head was removed, the area healed well

Figs. 7-44, 7-45. A 23 year old patient with insulin-dependent diabetes mellitus and cellulitis. Insertion of a drain through the foot facilitated healing

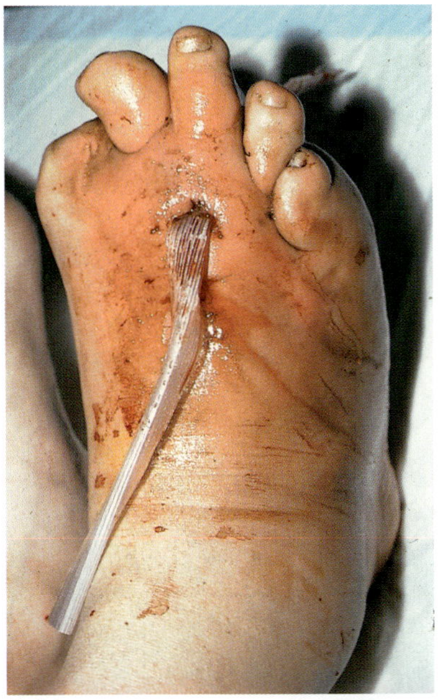

7-44

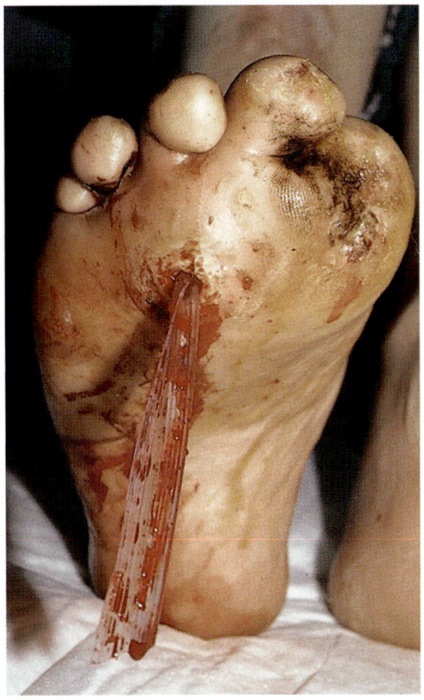

7-45

Figs. 7-46, 7-47. A 58 year old patient with diabetes mellitus. Angiography showed multiple occlusions of the arteries of the lower leg. He developed therapy-resistant painful necrosis of the big toe and an anaerobic infection of the sole. Appropriate antibiotics and percutaneous transluminal dilatation of a stenosis in the peroneal artery restored function to the foot, allowing him to walk again. Three toes were amputated

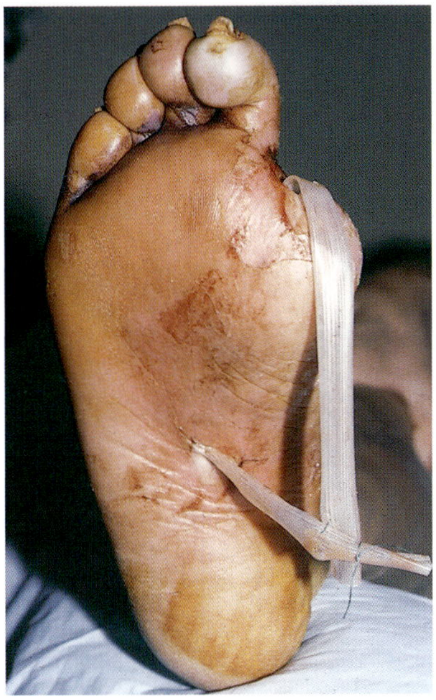

7-46

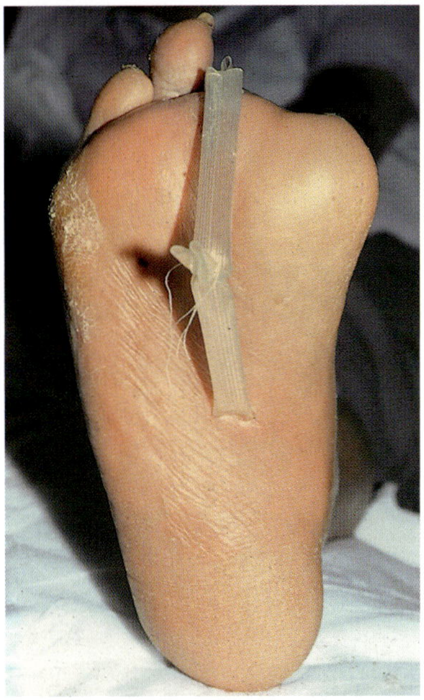

7-47

Figs. 7-48, 7-49. Necrosis of the toes in a 70 year old women with diabetes mellitus. Angiography showed femoral artery stenosis and multiple occlusions of the arteries of the lower leg. After percutaneous transluminal angioplasty of the femoral artery, a limited amputation of the toes was performed

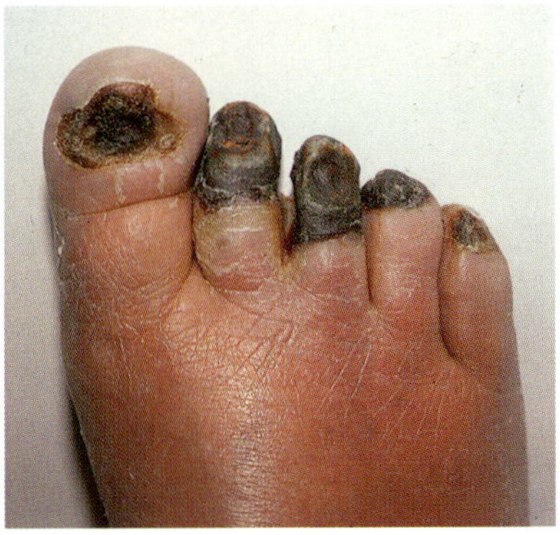

7-48

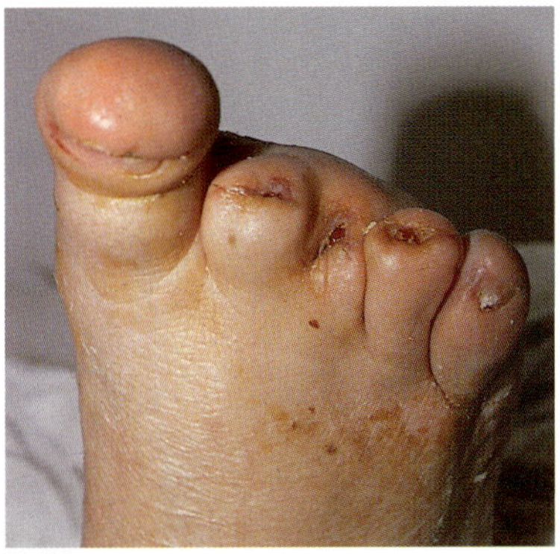

7-49

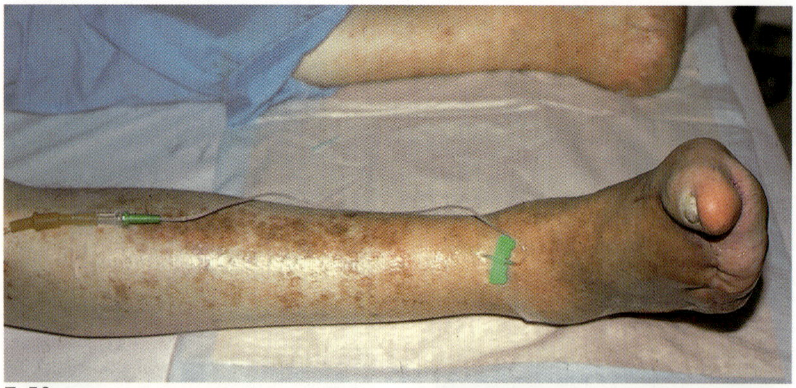

7-50

Figs. 7-50–7-52. Bony fragment removal with retrograde venous perfusion. An 80 year old diabetic patient with a therapy-resistant mal perforans ulcer. After the sequestered bone was removed, the healing process was accelerated

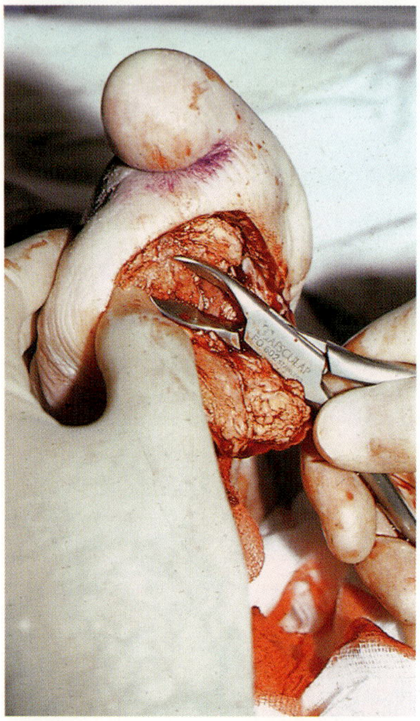

7-51

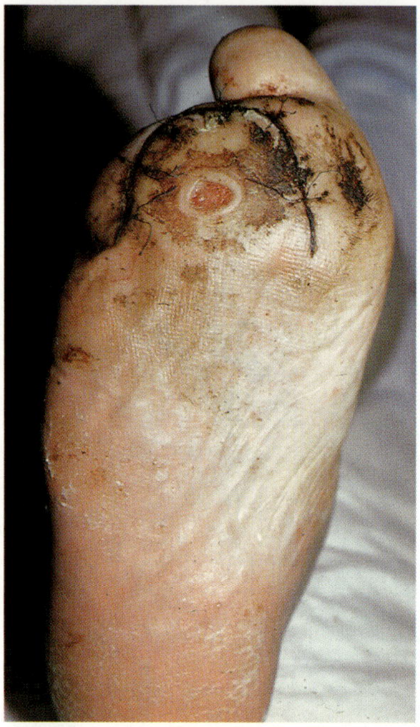

7-52

Figs. 7-53, 7-54. Retrograde intravenous perfusion was first employed by August Bier in 1908 to anesthetize limbs. A variety of Bier tourniquets are used and many different medications (fibrinolytic agents, prostaglandins, antibiotics) can be infused. In experienced hands this method is helpful in treating limbs in jeopardy of amputation

Procedure: A blood pressure tourniquet is inflated around the thigh to 80–90 mm Hg. This stops the venous return. A butterfly needle is inserted into a vein on the dorsal surface of the foot. To reduce the blood volume, the leg is elevated to 60°–80° for 2 min. Then the arterial flow is stopped with a pressure of 300 mm Hg. The medication is administered through the butterfly needle with a pressure pump

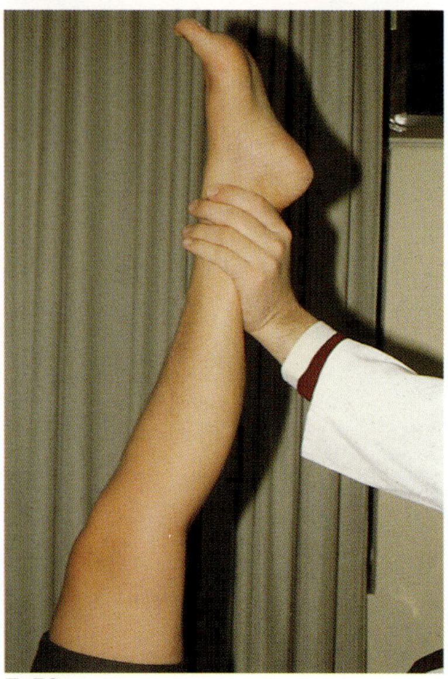

7-53

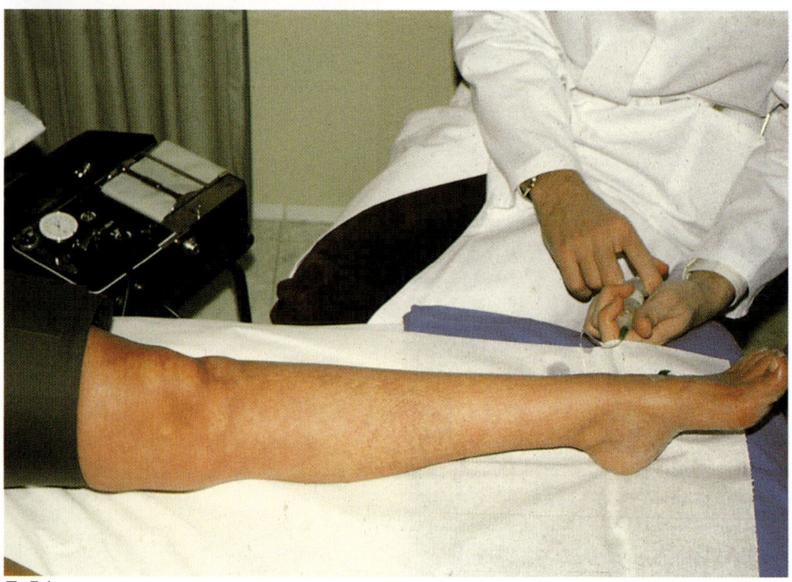

7-54

Figs. 7-55–7-58. A 55 year old women with diabetic angiopathy and polyneuropathy had multiple necrotic areas and a deep cellulitis. After the infected area was surgically opened, both antibiotics and prostaglandin E_1 were infused. After 4 months the foot was once again able to bear weight

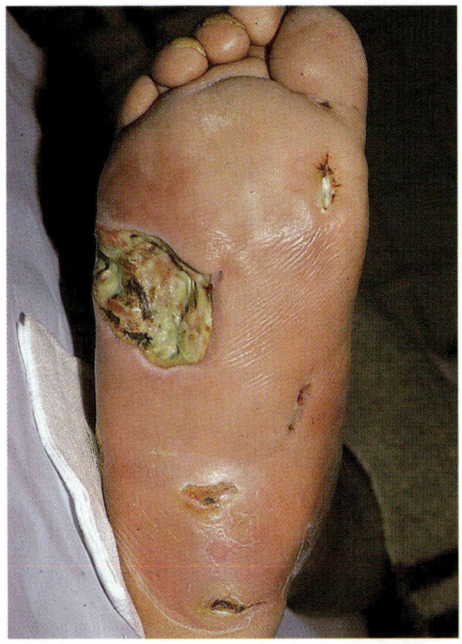

7-55

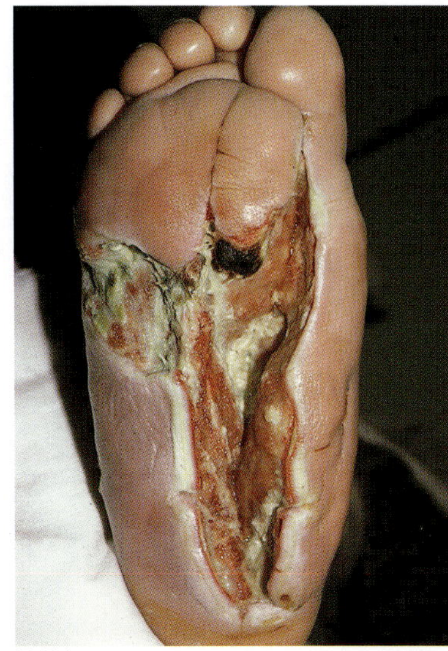

7-56

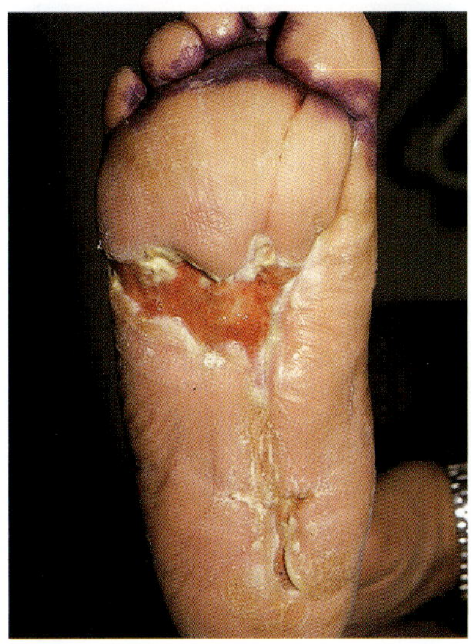

7-57

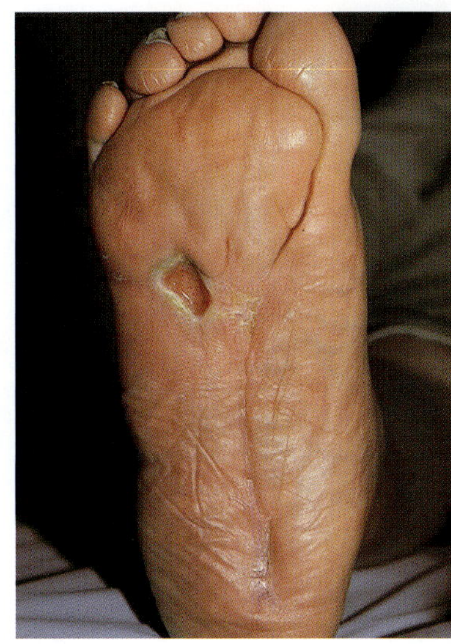

7-58

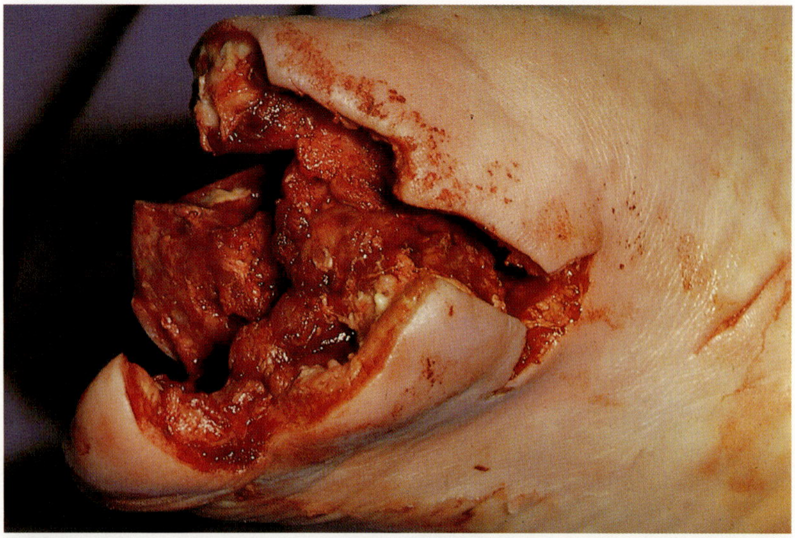

7-59

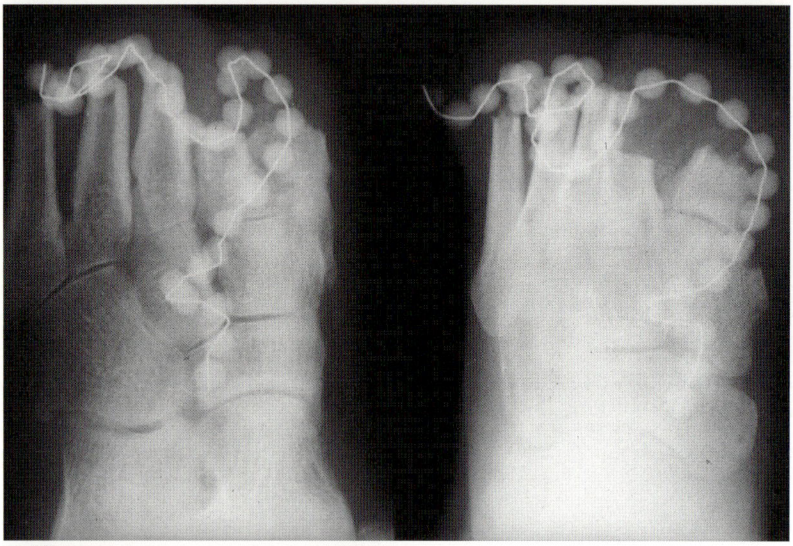

7-60

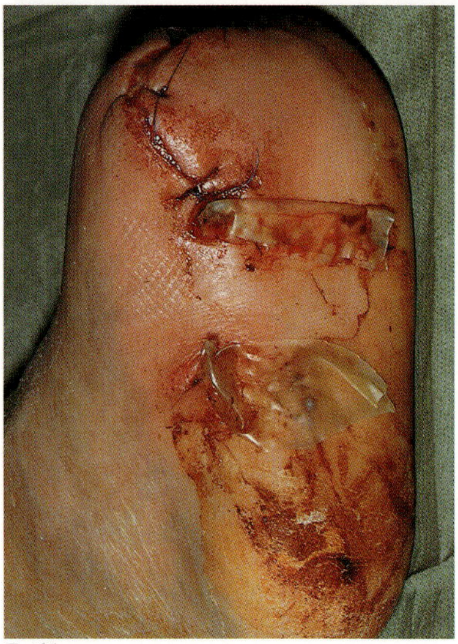

7-61

Figs. 7-7-59 – 7-61. Surgical approach in a 53 year old patient with severe diabetic gangrene of the forefoot. The figures show, from *top* to *bottom*:

- Forefoot amputation with radical debridement
- Implantation of a chain containing gentamicin
- Treating the stump with dilatation sutures and rubber drains

Complete healing occurred after months

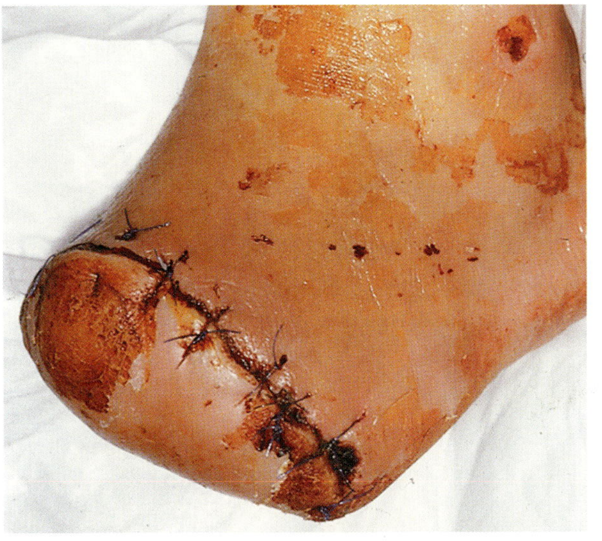

7-62

Fig. 7-62. Transmetatarsal amputation

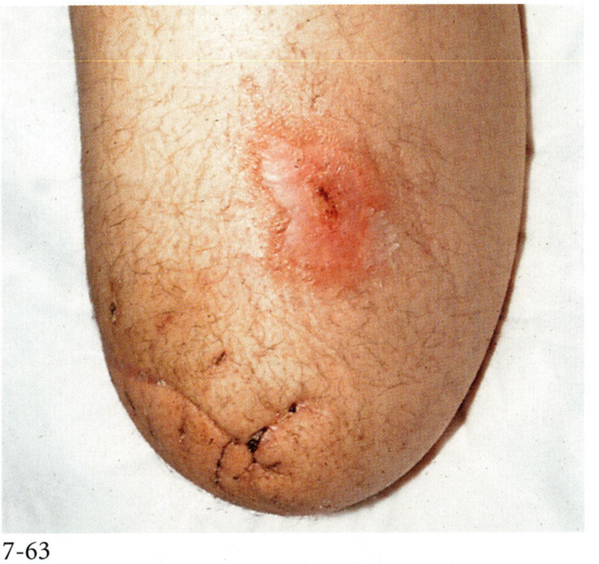

7-63

Fig. 7-63. Appearance after below-the-knee amputation in a 58 year old patient with a pressure ulcer from his prosthesis

Figs. 7-64, 7-65. Knee-joint disarticulation (through knee amputation) in a 44 year old women with diabetes mellitus

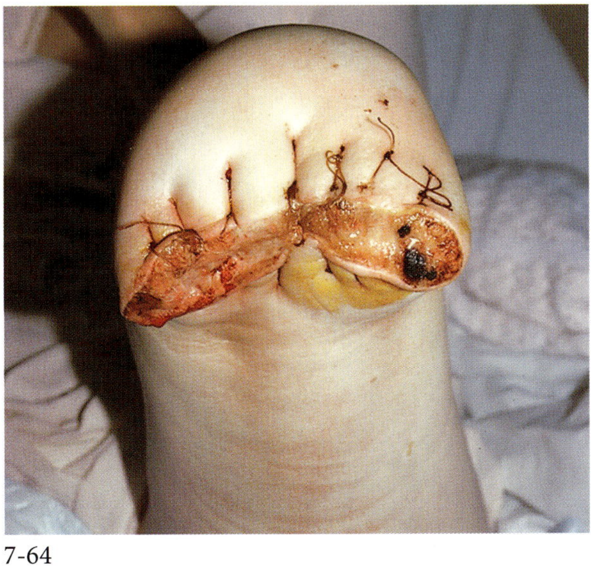

7-64

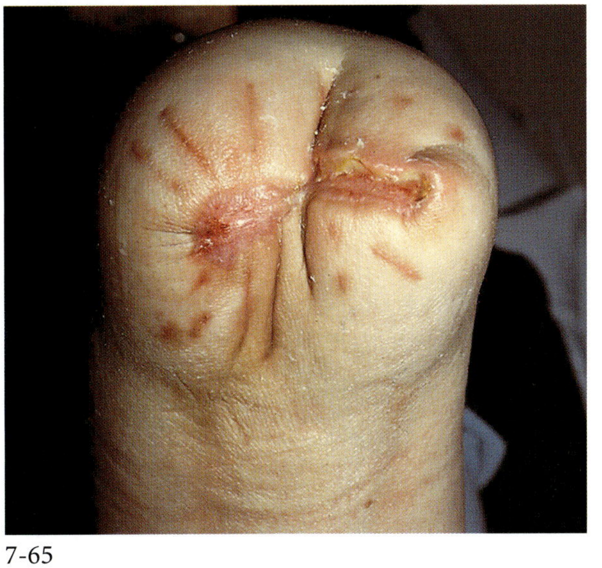

7-65

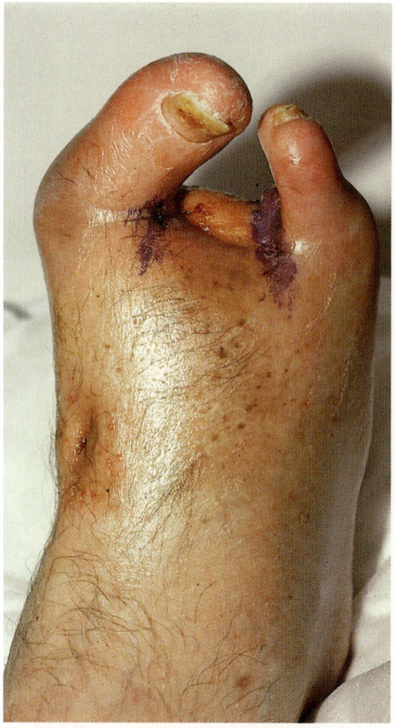
7-66

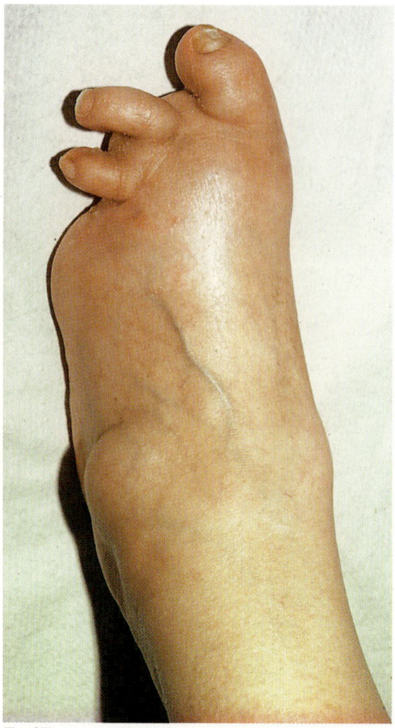
7-67

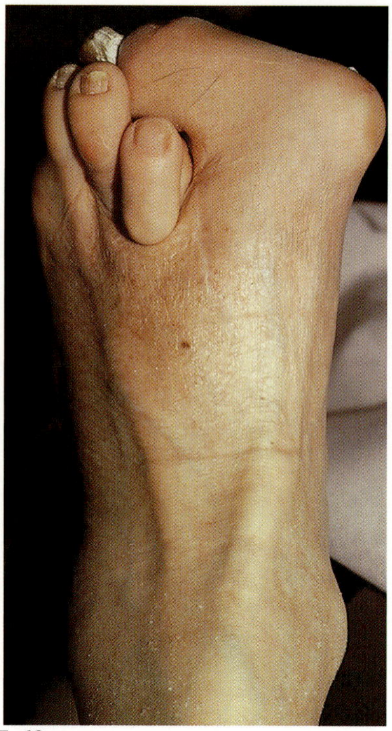
7-68

Figs. 7-66 – 7-68. Foot deformities in patients with diabetes mellitus

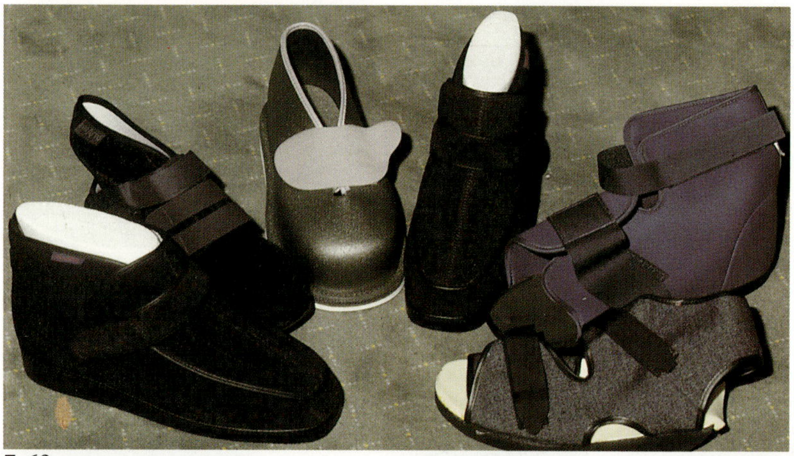
7-69

Figs. 7-69–7-71. Various orthopedic shoes to reduce pressure in patients with diabetic foot syndrome. Once a necrotic area has healed, special shoes of some type are essential to re-distribute the pressure and avoid new lesions

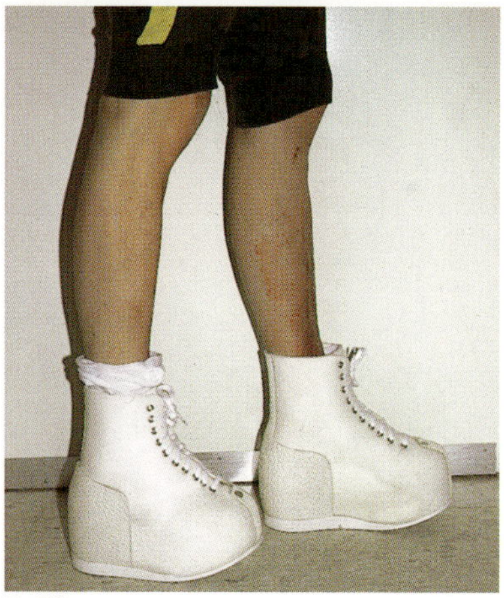
7-70

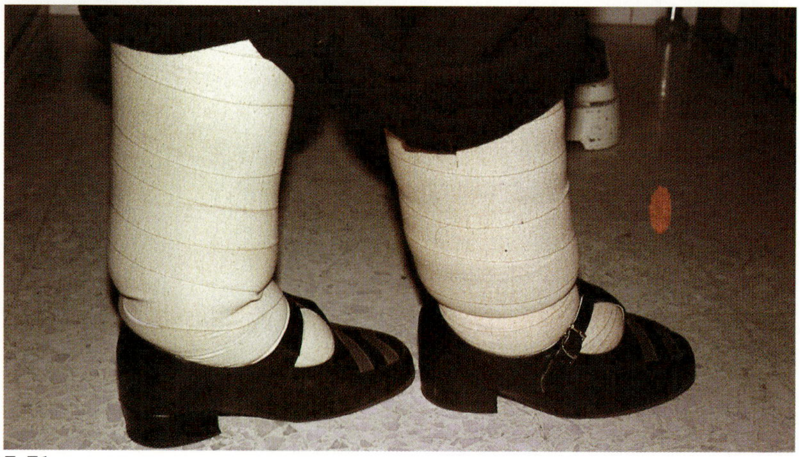
7-71

Fig. 7-72. Prostheses: After below-knee amputation, the course of the patient is determined primarily by the type of procedure, their age and associated diseases. The role of physical therapy is essential. The patient must learn to walk again, almost from the start, once he has a prosthesis. He must also be taught how to most effectively use crutches or a cane.
In addition, the good leg must be preserved. The indications for an artificial limb should be carefully followed, since not every patient can use one

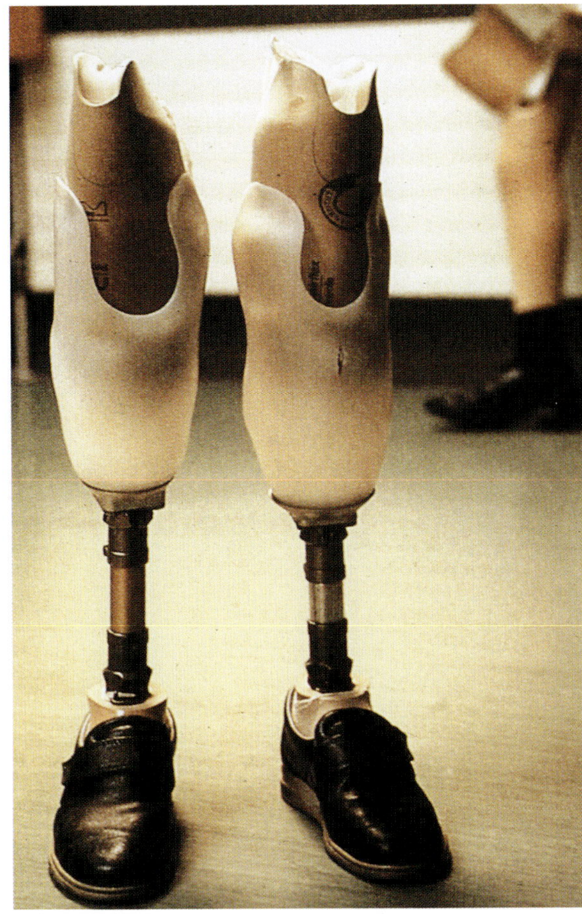

7-72

Chapter 8:
Buerger's Disease

CONTENTS

A: Introduction

Buerger's Disease

Synonyms. Thromboangiitis obliterans (TAO), endangiitis obliterans

Definition

Non-arteriosclerotic multifocal segmental progressive inflammation of the small and medium vessels of the limbs, which often leads to secondary thrombosis. TAO is in the same general category of generalized, necrotic inflammation, along with polyarteritis nodosa, giant cell arteritis and necrotizing angiitis.

History

The Viennese pathologist Felix von Winiwarter, in 1879, described an "unusual form of endarteritis and endophlebitis with gangrene of the foot." In 1908, Leo Buerger, a surgeon at Mount Sinai Hospital in New York City, published a paper in the American Journal of Medical Science with the title "Thromboangiitis obliterans: A study of the vascular lesions leading to presenile spontaneous gangrene." In this paper, Buerger for the first time delineated this disorder as a distinct entity.

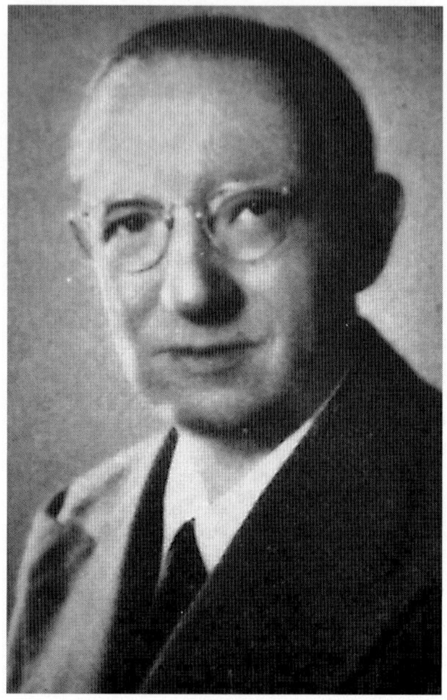

Fig. 8-1. Portrait of Leo Buerger (1879–1943)

Epidemiology

The share of patients with TAO in the general collection of peripheral arterial diseases is 1%–2% in Western Europe, 4% in Eastern Europe, 6% in Israel, but 16% in Japan.

- Men are much more often involved than women; the ratio is about 3.5–5 : 1.
- Recent surveys in the USA have indicated many more involved women, up to 30% of the group.
- Patients with TAO have the same life expectancy as age-matched controls. In contrast, the incidence of amputation in the first 5 years after diagnosis is about 25%.

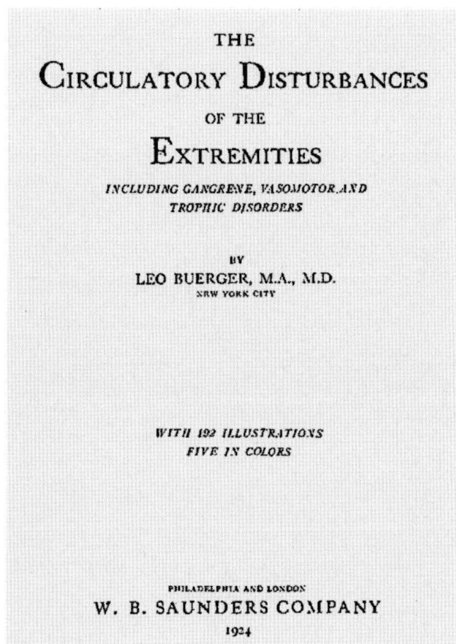

THE

CIRCULATORY DISTURBANCES

OF THE

EXTREMITIES

INCLUDING GANGRENE, VASOMOTOR AND TROPHIC DISORDERS

BY

LEO BUERGER, M.A., M.D.

NEW YORK CITY

WITH 192 ILLUSTRATIONS FIVE IN COLORS

PHILADELPHIA AND LONDON

W. B. SAUNDERS COMPANY

1924

Fig. 8-2. Title page of Buerger's book "*Circulatory Diseases of the Extremities*," published in 1924

Etiology and Pathogenesis

The exact cause of TAO is unknown. Among the hypotheses are autoimmune, immunogenetic, and infectious factors as well as abnormalities of clotting and clot lysis. Probably a combination of these is the answer. The most reliable trigger is cigarette smoke; almost all patients are smokers and many do this to great excess. Thus the theory that some component of smoke induces an immune-mediated or toxic vessel wall damage appears attractive. Almost all patients improve when they stop smoking. Passive smoking also appears to play a role.

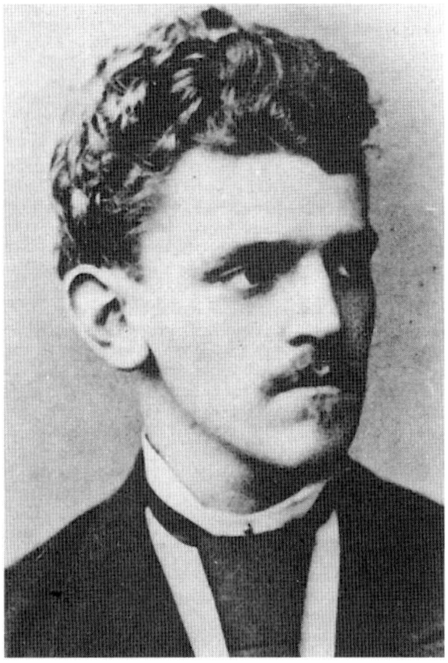

Fig. 8-3. Portrait of Felix von Winiwarter (1852–1931)

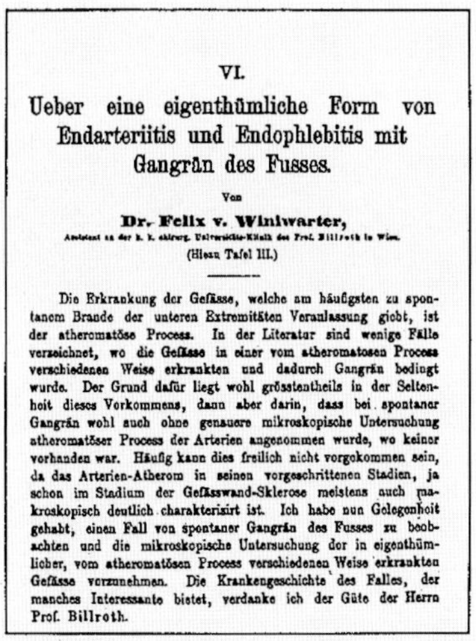

VI.

Ueber eine eigenthümliche Form von Endarteriitis und Endophlebitis mit Gangrän des Fusses.

Von

Dr. Felix v. Winiwarter,

Assistent an der k. k. chirurg. Universitäts-Klinik des Prof. Billroth in Wien.

(Hiezu Tafel III.)

Die Erkrankung der Gefässe, welche am häufigsten zu spontanem Brande der unteren Extremitäten Veranlassung giebt, ist der atheromatöse Process. In der Literatur sind wenige Fälle verzeichnet, wo die Gefässe in einer vom atheromatosen Process verschiedenen Weise erkrankten und dadurch Gangrän bedingt wurde. Der Grund dafür liegt wohl grösstentheils in der Seltenheit dieses Vorkommens, dann aber darin, dass bei spontaner Gangrän wohl auch ohne genauere mikroskopische Untersuchung atheromatöser Process der Arterien angenommen wurde, wo keiner vorhanden war. Häufig kann dies freilich nicht vorgekommen sein, da das Arterien-Atherom in seinen vorgeschrittenen Stadien, ja schon im Stadium der Gefässwand-Sklerose meistens auch makroskopisch deutlich charakterisirt ist. Ich habe nun Gelegenheit gehabt, einen Fall von spontaner Gangrän des Fusses zu beobachten und die mikroskopische Untersuchung der in eigenthümlicher, vom atheromatösen Process verschiedenen Weise erkrankten Gefässe vorzunehmen. Die Krankengeschichte des Falles, der manches Interessante bietet, verdanke ich der Güte der Herrn Prof. Billroth.

Fig. 8-4. Title page of Winiwarter's original description in *Archiv für Klinische Chirurgie* 23: 202 (1879)

Clinical Features

- TAO is a clinical diagnosis.
- Most patients are smokers under the age of 40 years.
- Typically the patients complain of Raynaud's phenomenon, paresthesias and more persistent painful cold pale digits. Often they present with digital, usually pulp bed, ulcerations. The necrosis spreads rapidly to involve bones and tendons. The pain is intense, deep and considerably more severe than that associated with arteriosclerosis.
- The Fontaine classification does not help when studying TAO.
- Only 10%–15% have claudication and it usually involves the instep.
- Superficial thrombophlebitis may be the first sign, appearing months before other problems.
- The acral skin tends to be cyanotic, while with arteriosclerotic disease, it tends to be pale.
- The disease runs in spurts; acute flare-ups may be followed by long periods with few problems. The disease tends to burn out over the years and may merge into a secondary arteriosclerosis.
- The only clear trigger is smoking. Psychosomatic factors have also been suggested, such as aggressive behavior.

Diagnosis

There are no specific laboratory tests which are helpful. There appears to be an increased prevalence of HLA-A9 and -B5 antigens (Antielastan Antikollagen AK).
The main diagnostic criteria are:

- Age <40 years
- Smoker
- Peripheral vascular occlusion, distal to knees and elbows
- Raynaud's phenomenon

And two of the following three factors:

- History or presence of superficial thrombophlebitis
- Involvement of the arm
- Characteristic angiographic findings

Angiographic Findings in TAO

- Absence of arteriosclerotic lesions
- Segmental occlusion in peripheral vessels
- Smooth-walled contours to the uninvolved vessels
- Sharp cut-off character to the proximal occlusions
- Pointed or drawn out closure of the distal arteries
- Standing wave phenomenon
- Vasospasm

Unique Collateral Patterns

- Martorell sign: direct or corkscrew collaterals
- Collaterals resembling "trees roots", "spiders' feet" or "grapes on a vine"
- Rippling of the vessels
- Slow collateral flow
- Early vein filling as a result of shunting

Table 8-1. Diagnostic differences between TAO and arteriosclerotic occlusion

Factor	*TAO*	*Atherosclerosis*
Cause	???	Arteriosclerosis
Immunopathological findings	Occasionally positive	Negative
Distribution	Localized, segmental	Generalized
Coronary artery involvement	Rare	Common
Risk factors		
Endogenous	Unknown	Multiple
Exogenous	Smoking	Diet, smoking, diabetes
Onset	20–40 years	>40 years
Claudication	+/–	+++
Course	Waxes and wanes, life-long	Progressive, life expectancy reduced ~10 years

Therapy

- Conservative
  - With pain at rest or necrosis, the patient should be admitted.
  - Often very difficult, may be useful to use nicotine patches or nicotine gum during withdrawal.
  - Pain therapy, perhaps including peridural anesthesia or neurostimulatory techniques.
  - The agent of choice is intravenous prostaglandin E_1 (alprostadil).
  - Systemic corticosteroids can be helpful in a acute flare.
  - Aspirin 100–300 mg daily as platelet inhibitor.
  - Calcium channel antagonists such as nifedipine 5 mg b.i.d. to 10 mg t.i.d.
  - Vasoactive agents such as pentoxifylline (Trental) and naftidrofuryl (Dusodril) are often employed although proof of their efficacy is not available.
  - Systemic and local thrombolysis is usually ineffective.
- Surgical
  - In selected cases, thoracic and lumbar sympathectomy can be considered.
  - Percutaneous transluminal angioplasty and bypass surgery have little value. In acute flare-ups, there is a high rate of re-occlusion.
  - Compression-distraction osteosynthesis of Ilisarow may or may not be effective.

B: Supplementary Figures and Legends

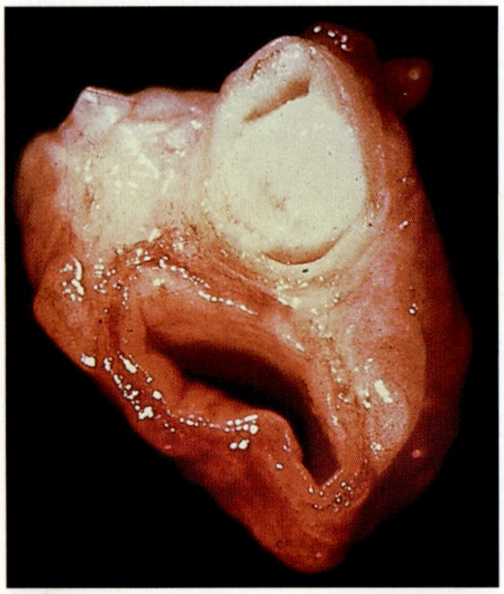

8-5

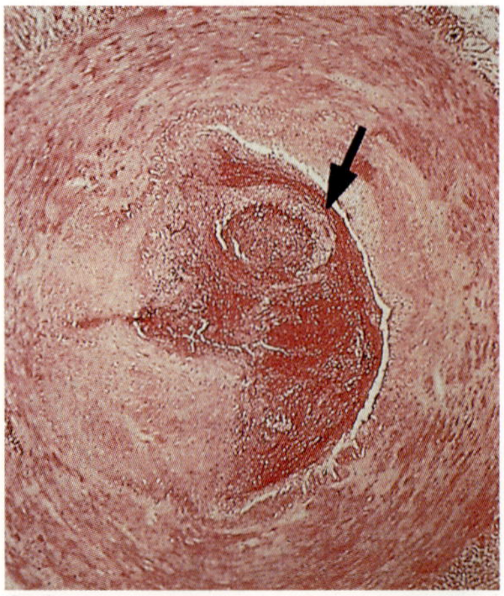

8-6

Figs. 8-5, 8-6. Gross specimen and microscopic section of TAO. The early stage of TAO is characterized by intimal edema with fibrinoid necrosis, fibroblast proliferation and infiltration of the vessel wall with lymphocytes, plasma cells and neutrophils. Cell-rich thrombi with giant cells usually lead to rapid occlusion. In contrast to arteriosclerotic lesions, neither cholesterol clefts nor calcification is seen. The microscopic section on the *right* shows an acute thrombus with an intra-luminal microabscess (*arrow*).

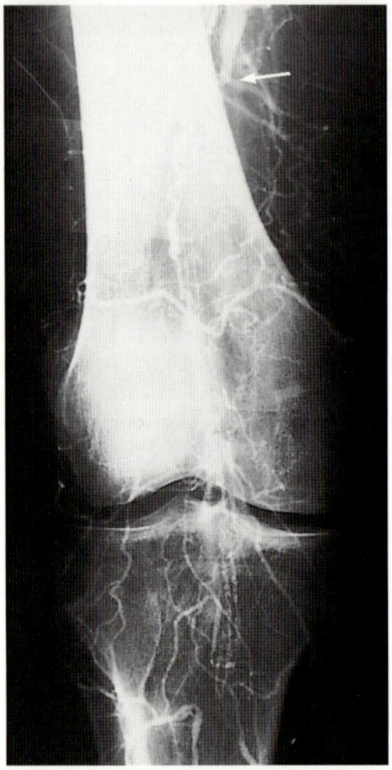

8-7

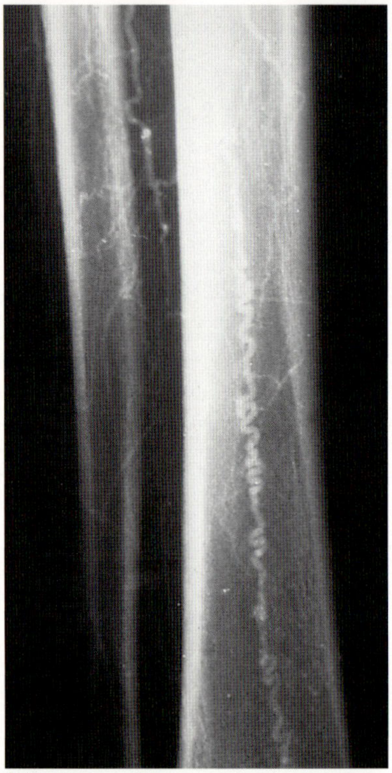

8-8

Fig. 8-7. Typical angiographic picture of occlusion of a thigh artery by TAO with a sharp, pointed cut-off (*arrow*) and grapevine-like collaterals

Fig. 8-8. Corkscrew collaterals (MARTORELL sign). All three calf arteries are occluded; the calf and foot are served by the smallest of collaterals. The corkscrew collaterals probably evolve out of the vasa vasorum of the original arteries

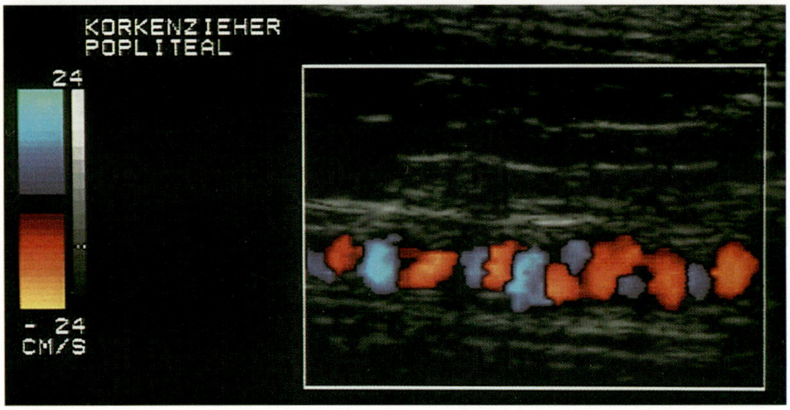

8-9

Fig. 8-9. Corkscrew collaterals in duplex color ultrasonography

Figs. 8-10, 8-11. Fluorescent angiogram and clinical picture in a 24 year old TAO patient who had occlusion of arteries in both calves. The angiogram shows marked restriction of flow in the right foot. After a lumbar sympathectomy, the right great toe was amputated

Fig. 8-12. Acute flare-up in a 32 year old patient with TAO. His symptoms began at age 17. As he continued to smoke, the disease advanced on both his hands and feet

Fig. 8-13. Condition of same patient 1 year later, just prior to below knee amputation

Fig. 8-14. Severe ischemia of the foot during an acute attack of TAO. A blister as a result of the edema can be seen on the dorsal aspect of the foot. In this case, a below knee amputation was also needed

Fig. 8-15. Extreme damage to the toes in TAO. The great toe has already been amputated; the second toe is necrotic and the bones are exposed, necessitating another amputation. In TAO, there is little direction connection with occlusion of major arteries, as seen with arteriosclerotic occlusion. Disturbances in microcirculation, often not identified with angiography, seem to play a key role in TAO and often lead to sequential amputations

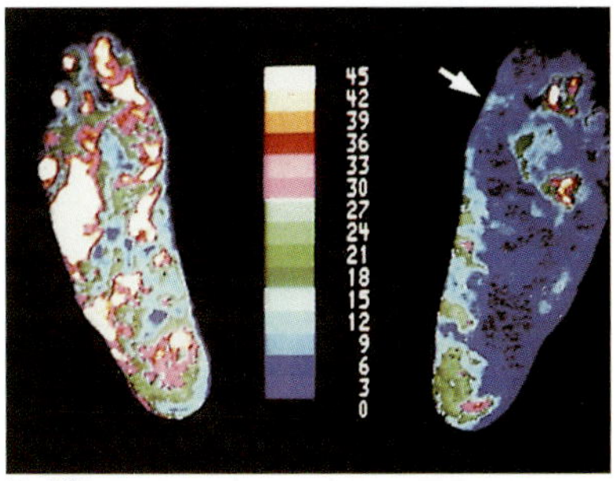

8-10

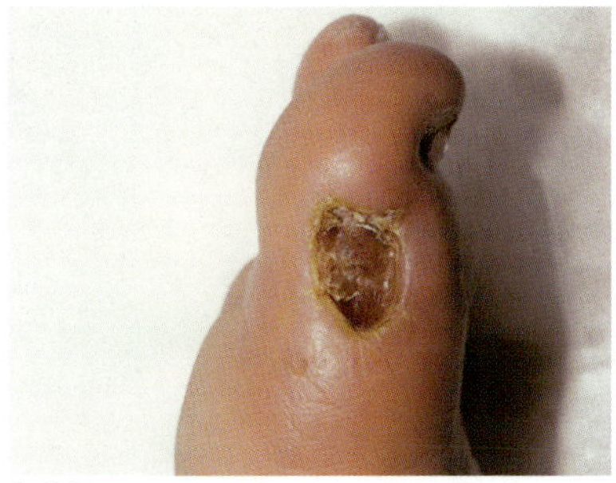

8-11

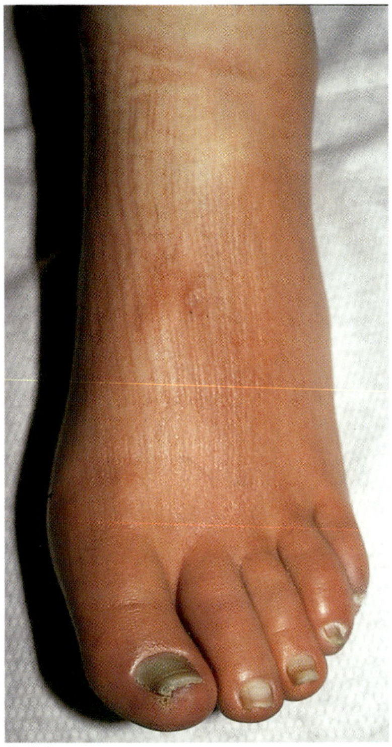

8-12

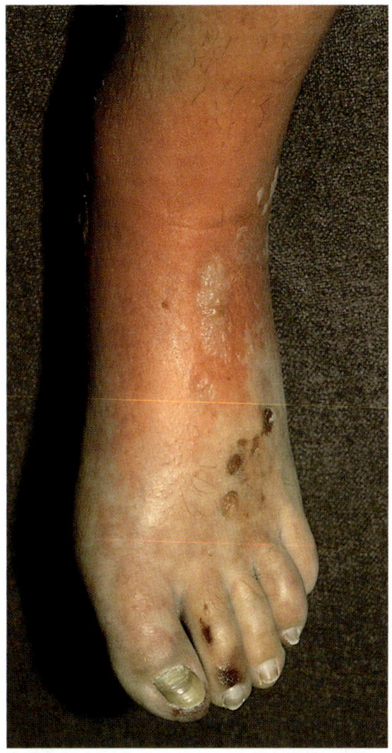

8-13

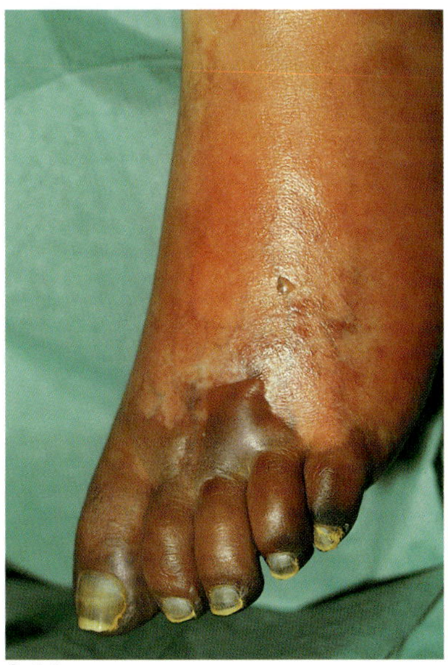

8-14

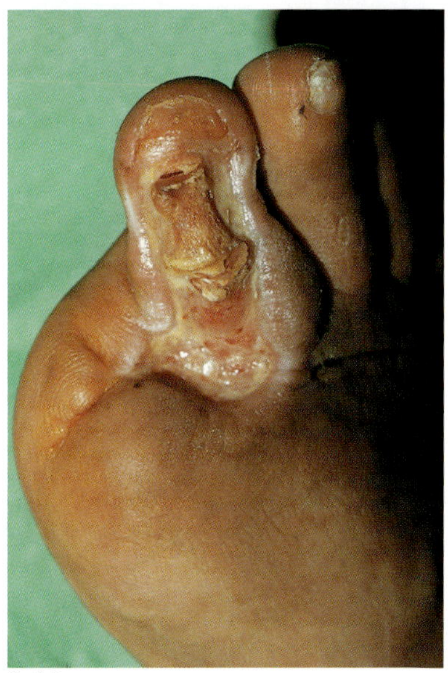

8-15

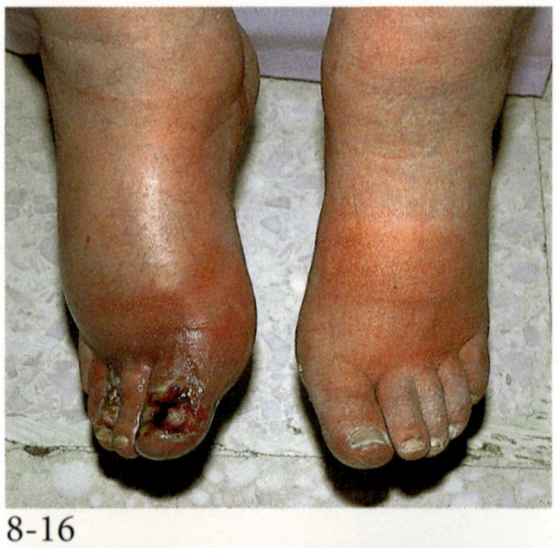
8-16

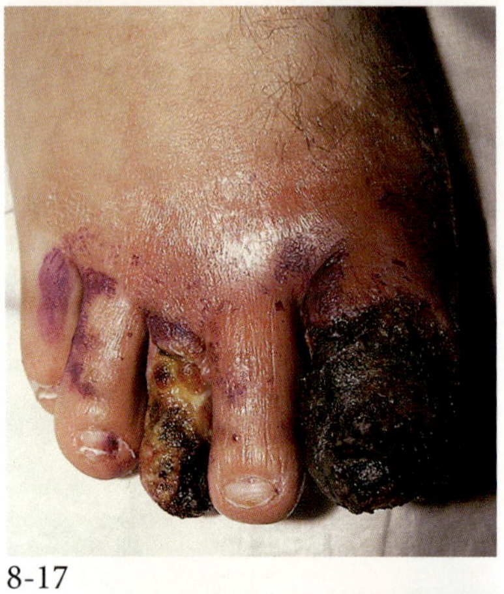
8-17

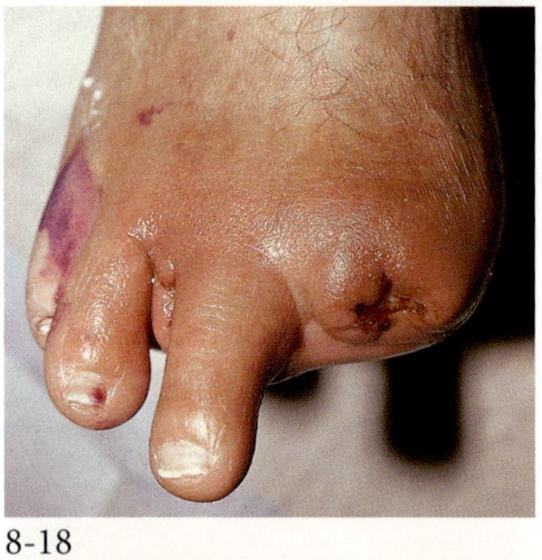
8-18

Figs. 8-16 – 8-18. Typical course of TAO in a 38 year old man with calf artery occlusion

Fig. 8-16. Marked edema of the feet, worsened because the patient always kept his legs down to ameliorate the pain

Fig. 8-17. Reduction of edema following peridural anesthesia and infusion of alprostadil. The extensive necrosis of the great and third toes is clear

Fig. 8-18. Appearance after partial amputation of the most severely involved digits

Fig. 8-19. Extensive necrosis of the toes and distal aspect of the foot in a 23 year old student with occlusion of all three calf arteries

Fig. 8-20. Appearance after conservative treatment and limited amputation. The only arterial supply to the foot was through corkscrew collaterals but healing was still satisfactory

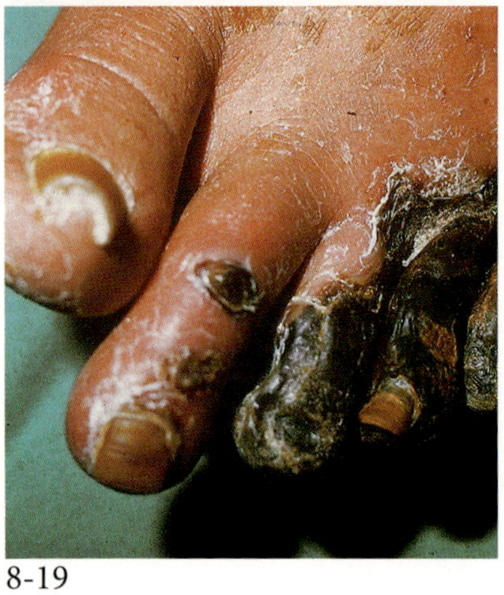
8-19

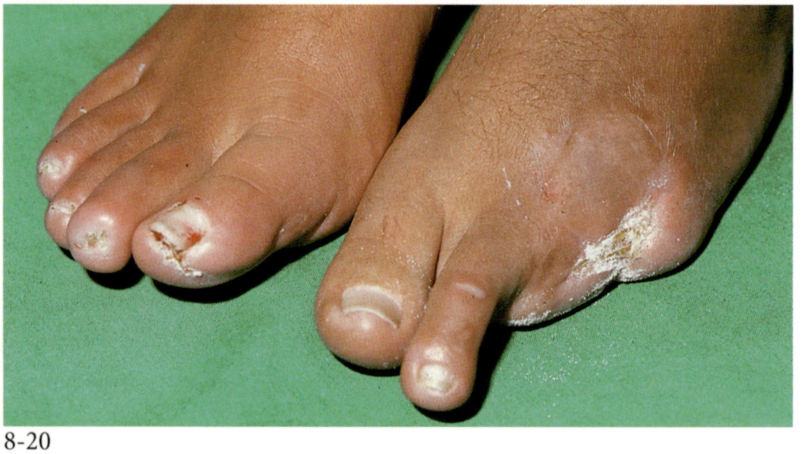
8-20

Figs. 8-21, 8-22. Appearance after a forefoot amputation in a 40 year women with TAO. Often after multiple amputations, a stable condition is first reached when the patient stops smoking

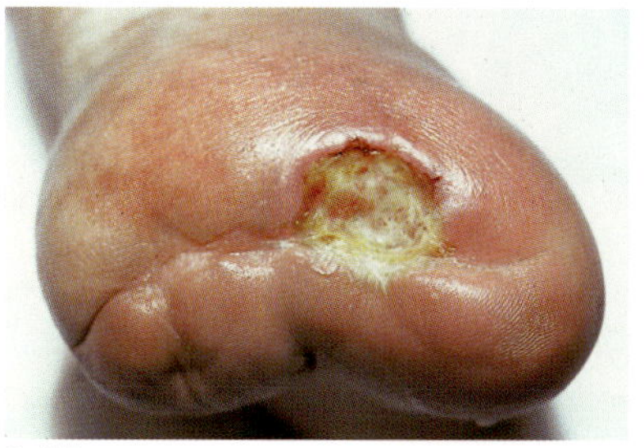

8-21

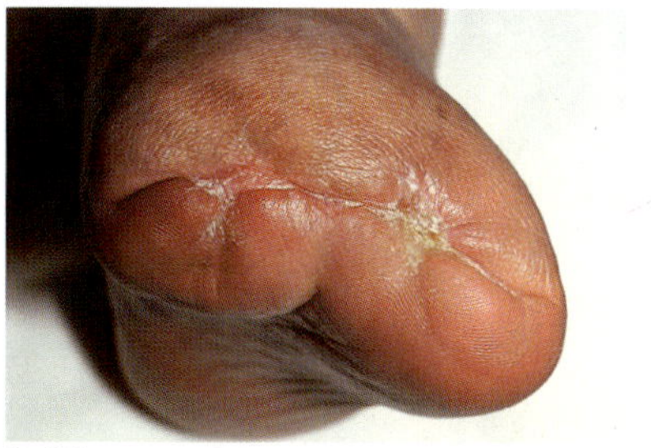

8-22

Figs. 8-23, 8-24. Extensive amputation of toes and distal part of foot in a 41 year old man. After about 6 months, the wound had healed well

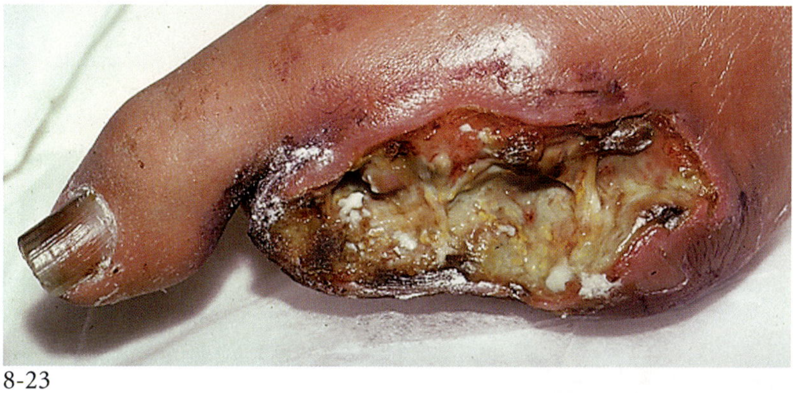

8-23

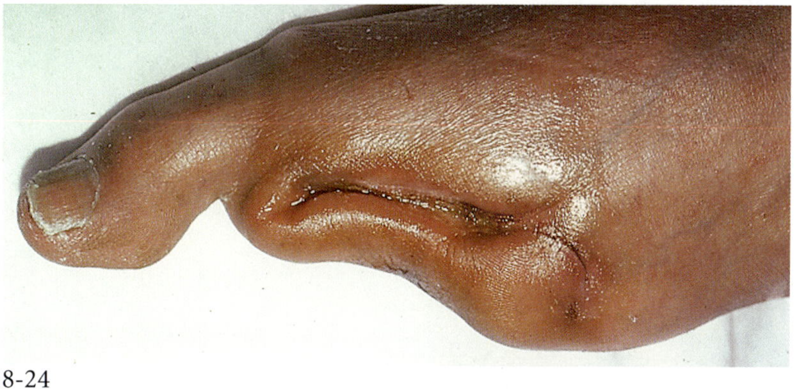

8-24

Fig. 8-25. Extreme necrosis of the foot in a 34 year patient with TAO. He had multiple bilateral segmental occlusions of his calf arteries. The patient had been treated by a faith healer with dirt and honey. He was septic when this picture was taken and required a below knee amputation

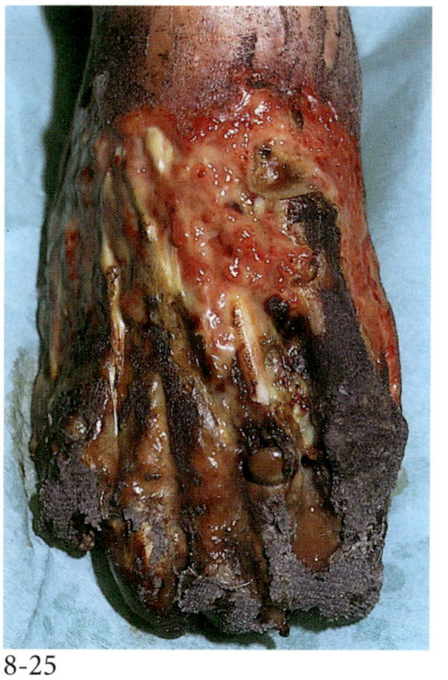

8-25

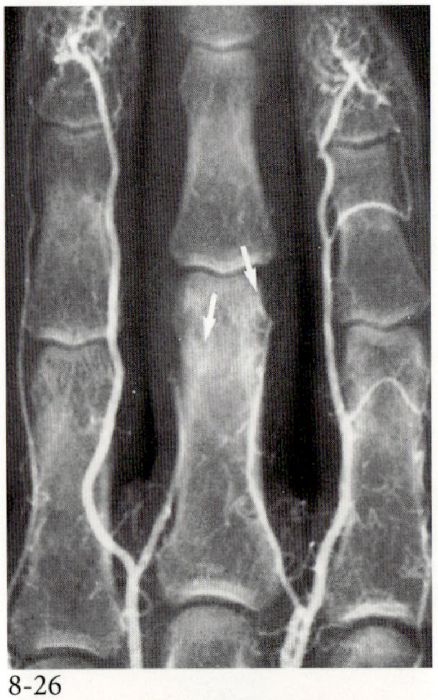

8-26

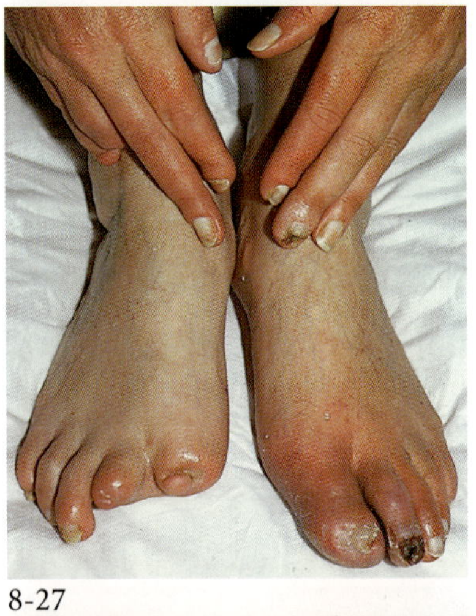

8-27

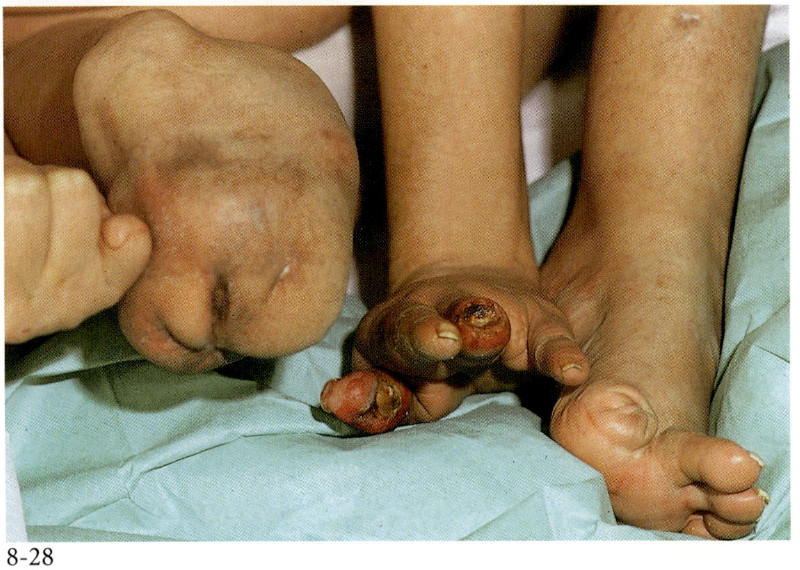

8-28

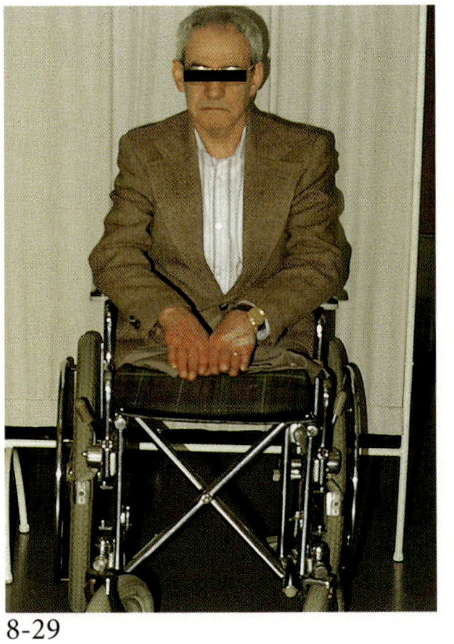

8-29

Fig. 8-26. Typical digital artery occlusion (*arrow*) in a 32 year old patient with TAO

Fig. 8-27. A 42 year old women with multiple digital amputations and some residual necrosis

Fig. 8-28. Flare of TAO on the fingers in a patient with multiple previous amputations

Fig. 8-29. A 52 year old man with a typical end-stage of a TAO "career" prolonged by continued smoking. A series of leg amputations were carried out bilaterally in an ascending fashion. Many of the his finger tips were also excised

Fig. 8-30. Post-operative appearance of a 30 year patient following amputation of the distal part of the foot and ILISAROW procedure

Figs. 8-31, 8-32, Radiological image and sketch of ILISAROW procedure. The traction wires extend from the tibia through the fragment of bone lifted from the tibia through the skin surface where they are attached to the fixation apparatus. The *arrows* show the direction of traction

Comments: This method was suggested by ILISAROW in 1983 and further developed by FOKIN and colleagues. It extends the repertoire of surgical procedures to indirectly improve the peripheral circulation when the arteries of the calf are occluded and the arteries of the dorsal arch are absent or inadequate. The principle is that when a piece of bone is separated and then stabilized with external fixation, the arterial circulation is stimulated. The goal is to develop collaterals out of the small muscular, fascial and bone vessels

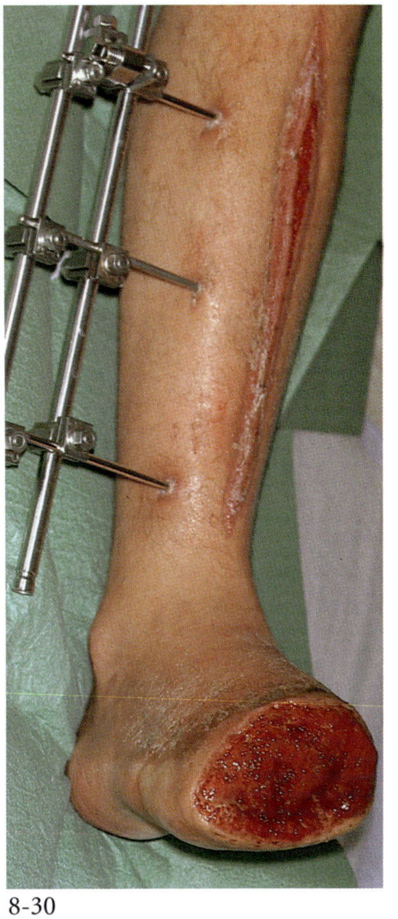

8-30

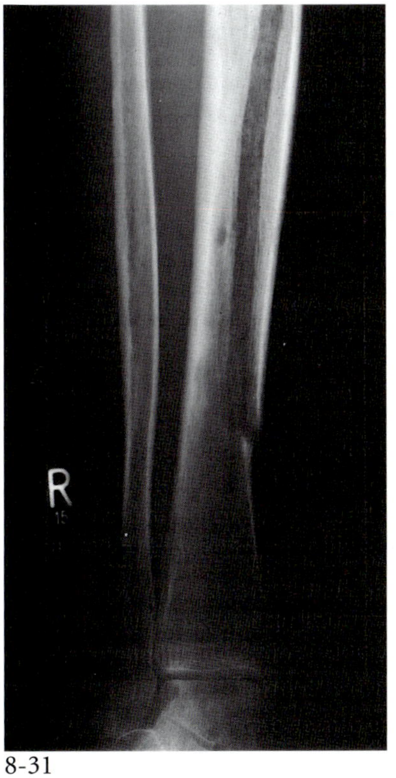

8-31

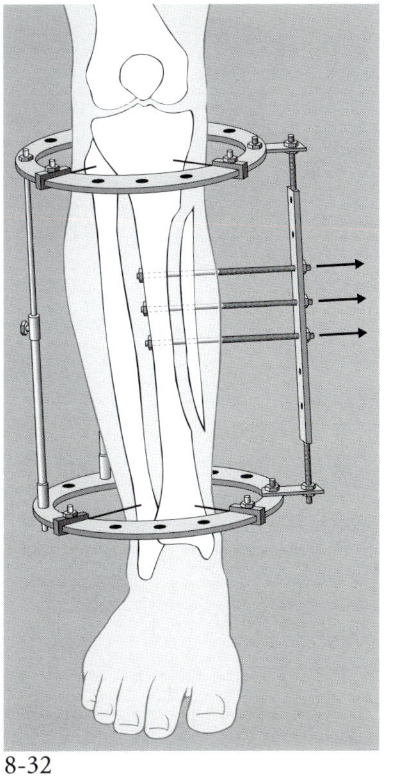

8-32

Chapter 9: Functional Circulatory Disorders and Vasculitides

Contents

A: Introduction

1. Raynaud's Syndrome

Synonyms. RAYNAUD's disease, RAYNAUD's phenomenon, vasomotor acroasphyxia, dead finger syndrome, vibration white finger syndrome

Definition

Vasospasm of the acral or distal vessels, often triggered by cold or stress and relieved by warmth or pharmacological agents. One distinguishes between primary RAYNAUD's disease as an idiopathic vasospastic symptom complex of unknown etiology with no associated diseases and secondary RAYNAUD's syndrome with organic vascular damage associated with systemic disorders such as collagen vascular diseases. Occasionally RAYNAUD's phenomenon is the first sign of a connective tissue disease such as systemic sclerosis (scleroderma), so that the initial diagnosis of primary RAYNAUD's disease later has to be adjusted to secondary RAYNAUD's syndrome.

Epidemiology

Women are twice as likely to be affected as men. Most cases begin in young adult life. The prevalence in the Western Hemisphere is about 5 % in women, and 2 % – 3 % in men. Patients with systemic sclerosis, thromboangiitis obliterans and Sjögren's syndrome are especially likely to be affected. The symptom complex is also common in workers who are exposed to vibration, such as those working with jack hammers, tampers, motor saws, drills and other power tools.

Etiology and Pathogenesis

There are many causes of RAYNAUD's syndrome as shown in Table 9-1.

Clinical Features

Symmetrical intermittent ischemia of the digits. Occasionally the toes, nose and ears are affected. Most commonly the thumbs are spared. The attacks are painful and have a typical tricolor change of the digits.

- White blanching as the arterioles and venules constrict
- Blue cyanosis
- Red reactive hyperemia

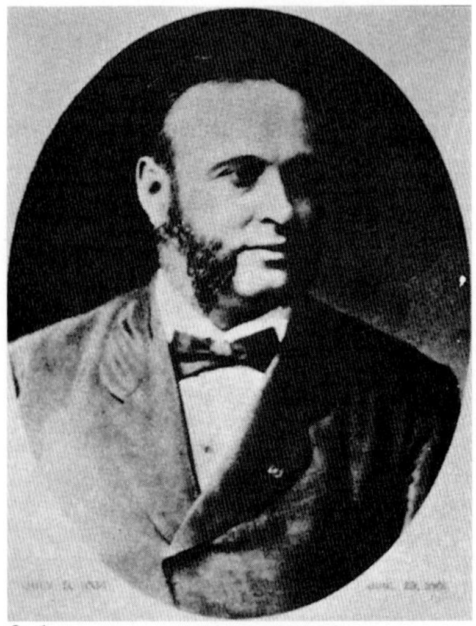

9-1

"I attempt to prove that a variety of dry gangrenes affect the extremities and cannot be explained by vascular obliteration – these forms of gangrene show a remarkable tendency to symmetry in that the same parts of the body are always affected, the hands or feet or in some cases both, as well as in other cases the nose and ears.

I hope to demonstrate that this type of gangrene is caused by an abnormal innervation of the capillary vessels whose nature I will explain."

Maurice Raynaud, 1862

9-2

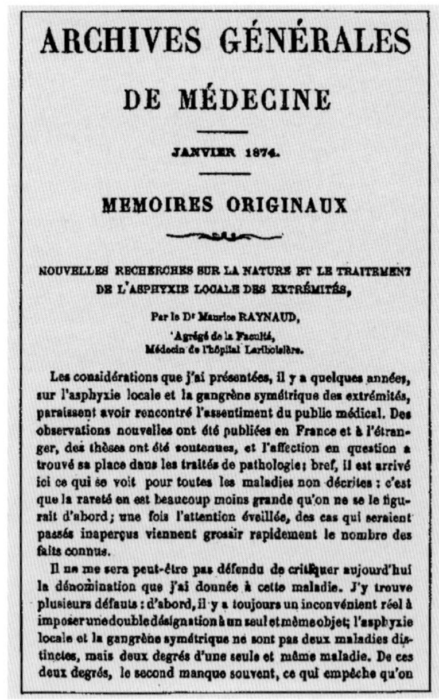

ARCHIVES GÉNÉRALES

DE MÉDECINE

JANVIER 1874.

MEMOIRES ORIGINAUX

NOUVELLES RECHERCHES SUR LA NATURE ET LE TRAITEMENT DE L'ASPHYXIE LOCALE DES EXTRÉMITÉS,

Par le Dr Maurice RAYNAUD,
Agrégé de la Faculté,
Médecin de l'hôpital Lariboisière.

Les considérations que j'ai présentées, il y a quelques années, sur l'asphyxie locale et la gangrène symétrique des extrémités, paraissent avoir rencontré l'assentiment du public médical. Des observations nouvelles ont été publiées en France et à l'étranger, des thèses ont été soutenues, et l'affection en question a trouvé sa place dans les traités de pathologie; bref, il est arrivé ici ce qui se voit pour toutes les maladies non décrites : c'est que la rareté en est beaucoup moins grande qu'on ne se le figurait d'abord; une fois l'attention éveillée, des cas qui seraient passés inaperçus viennent grossir rapidement le nombre des faits connus.

Il ne me sera peut-être pas défendu de critiquer aujourd'hui la dénomination que j'ai donnée à cette maladie. J'y trouve plusieurs défauts : d'abord, il y a toujours un inconvénient réel à imposer une double désignation à un seul et même objet; l'asphyxie locale et la gangrène symétrique ne sont pas deux maladies distinctes, mais deux degrés d'une seule et même maladie. De ces deux degrés, le second manque souvent, ce qui empêche qu'on

9-3

Fig. 9-1. MAURICE RAYNAUD, 1834 – 1881, French physician

Fig. 9-2. Translation of the first case description of RAYNAUD's phenomenon

Fig. 9-3. The title page of RAYNAUD's first paper on asphyxia of the extremities

Table 9-1. Causes of RAYNAUD's syndrome

Causes of RAYNAUD's syndrome
Digital artery occlusion Arterial microemboli
Proximal stenosis and occlusion of subclavian artery
Costoclavicular compression syndrome (e.g. cervical rib)
Vibration syndrome (vibration white finger disease)
Hypothenar hammer syndrome
Cold injury
Arterial occlusion or compression (secondary to a cervical rib or anomalous first thoracic rub)
Inflammatory vascular disease
Collagen-vascular disease, especially systemic sclerosis (scleroderma), systemic lupus erythematosus and SJÖGREN's syndrome
WEGENER's granulomatosis
Rheumatoid arthritis
Thromboangiitis obliterans
Hypersensitivity vasculitis
Hematological diseases
Cold agglutinins
Cryoglobulinemia
Polycythemia vera
Essential thrombocythemia
Paraproteinemia
Toxic substances and medications
Ergot-containing compounds and other migraine therapies
β-blockers
Oral contraceptives
Chemotherapy agents especially bleomycin, vinca alkaloids
Neoplastic
Noradrenaline
Polyvinyl chloride
Bromocriptine
Cyclosporine A
Functional vasospasm
Acrocyanosis
Digitus mortuus (dead or white finger)
Paroxysmal finger hematoma
Pernio
Degenerative spinal column changes
Other causes
A-V fistulas
Hepatitis B
Malignancy
Uraemia
Reflex lympathetic dystrophy

Diagnosis

The diagnosis is clinical. Primary RAYNAUD's disease is likely when:

- The vasospasm appears in attacks, often triggered by cold or emotions.
- The fingers are symmetrically involved and the thumbs spared.
- There are no underlying disorders and no trophic changes.
- RAYNAUD's phenomenon has been present for at least 2 years.

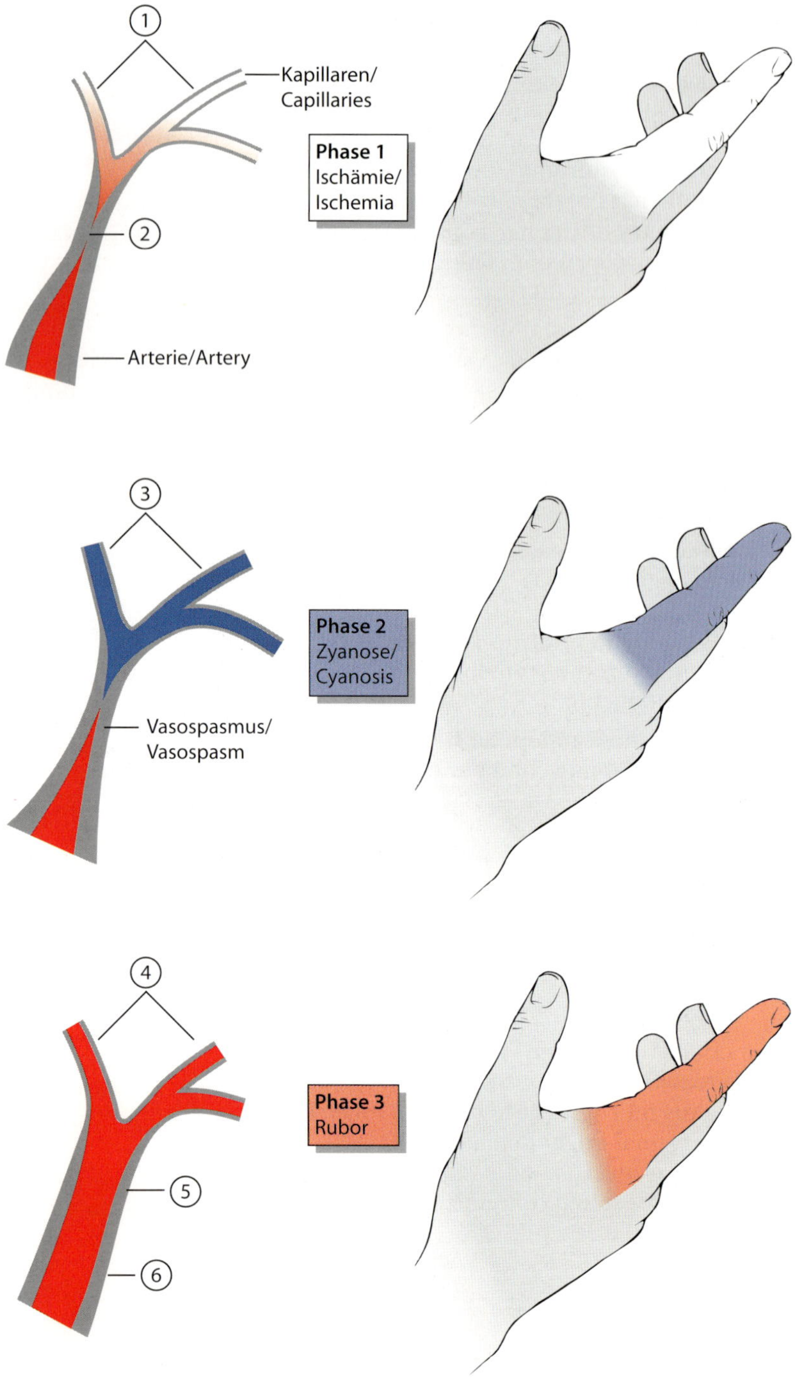

Fig. 9-4. Symmetrical intermittent ischemia of the extremities

① Blood flow through the capillaries is reduced, resulting in digital ischemia
② Arterial vasospasm produces vascular occlusion
③ Ischemia leads to dilation of the capillaries and venules; they fill with deoxygenated blood
④ The capillaries are still dilated, but oxygenated blood now flows through them
⑤ Markedly increased blood flow
⑥ Relaxation of vasospasm

The acral circulation can also be studied with oscillometry, Doppler pressure measurements and finger plethysmography with and without cold provocation.

Doppler Pressure Measurement/Measurement of the Digital Blood Pressure

A finger tourniquet is applied and the pressure in the digital arteries measured. Cold provocation by immersing the fingers in ice water for 2–3 min helps separate organic and functional digital artery occlusion.

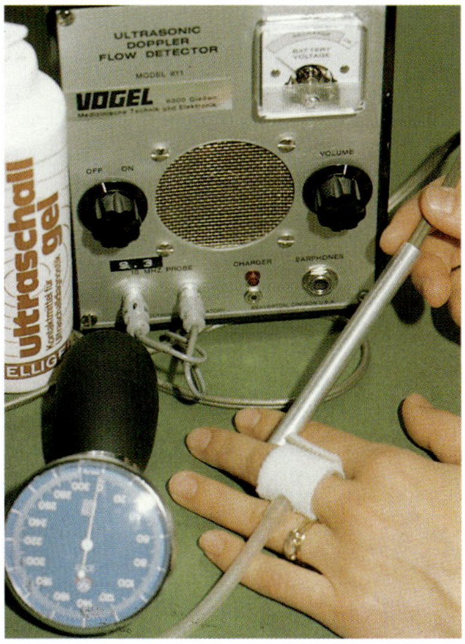

Fig. 9-5. Systolic Doppler pressure measurement of a finger

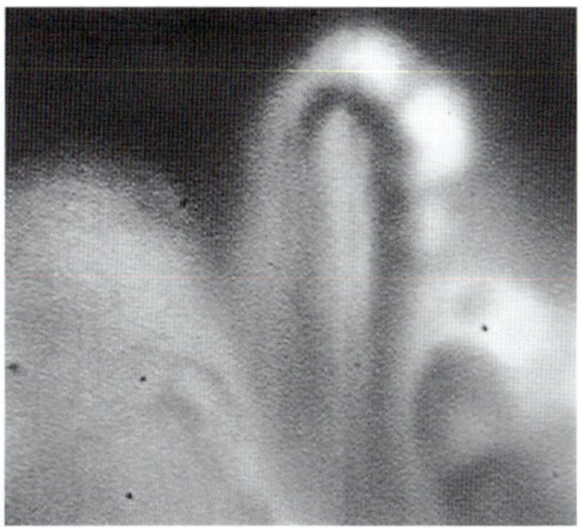

Fig. 9-6. Typical giant capillaries on capillary microscopy

- Normal findings: After cold provocation, the digital pressure swings by a maximum of 20% – 30% of the normal value.
- Vasospasm: The digital artery pressure drops to less than 50% of the normal value.

Capillary Microscopy

The evaluation of the nail fold capillaries is important in RAYNAUD's phenomenon. Key criteria are giant capillaries, avascular areas and hemorrhage.

Laboratory Evaluation

- CBC, differential white blood cell count, hematocrit, platelet count
- Erythrocyte sedimentation rate
- C-reactive protein
- Cryoglobulins, cryofibrinogen and cold agglutinins
- Platelet function
- Plasma viscosity
- Immunoelectrophoresis
- Autoimmune screening: anti-nuclear antibodies, anti-DNA antibodies, SSA, SSB, Scl 70, anti-centromere antibodies

Table 9.2 shows the main features used to separate primary RAYNAUD's disease from secondary RAYNAUD's syndrome.

Table 9-2. Separating primary and secondary RAYNAUD's phenomenon

Criterion	*Primary*	*Secondary*
Age at onset	10 – 45 years	Follows underlying disease, often > 50 years
Involvement of fingers	Symmetrical, thumb spared	Asymmetrical, often only 1 – 2 fingers involved
Systemic involvement	None	Follows underlying disease
Acral necrosis	Never	Common
Serological changes	None	Follows underlying disease
Acral light plethysmography following topical nitroglycerin	Normal	Often abnormal
Capillary microscopy	Normal	Often abnormal
Arteriography of the hand	Vasospasm, no permanent changes	Both vasospasm and organic changes

After CREUTZIG 1933.

Therapy

Prophylactic measures include:

- Wearing mittens or heated gloves
- Protection from cold and moisture
- Avoiding vibrating tools (power saws, jack hammers, and the like)
- Often changing duties at work is required.
- Many patients benefit from regularly making repeated fists or wind milling their arms.
- Psychosomatic therapy is often helpful, including autogenous training, yoga and biofeedback.
- Medications which could be triggers, such as β-blockers, ergot-containing substances and oral contraceptives should be avoided.

Active therapy is indicated in patients with frequent and severe attacks or signs of ulceration or scarring (Table 9-3) The best prophylactic measures are topical nitroglycerin ointment or oral calcium channel blockers such as nifedipine. The calcium channel blockers inhibit the calcium-driven contraction of vascular smooth muscle in a dose-related fashion. The use of nitroglycerin tablets is limited by the frequent occurrence of headaches. Among the ointments, nitroglycerin appears better absorbed through the skin than isosorbide dinitrate, perhaps because of its lower molecular weight and higher lipid solubility.

Course and Prognosis

The prognosis for RAYNAUD's disease is good. In secondary RAYNAUD's syndrome, the outlook depends on the underlying disorder. Digital amputations are often necessary.

Table 9.3. Medical management of RAYNAUD's phenomenon

Goal of therapy	Possible agents
Reducing vascular tone	Calcium channel blockers, nitroglycerin
Peripheral vasodilatation	α-adrenergic antagonists (prazosin, phenoxybenzamine), angiotensin-converting enzyme inhibitors (captopril, lisinopril)
Blocking mediators of platelet adhesion and vasoconstriction	Prostaglandins, thromboxane synthetase inhibitors, serotonin inhibitors
Reducing blood viscosity	Plasmapheresis, hemodilution, removal of fibrinogen

2. Other Functional Circulatory Disorders

A. Digitus Mortuus

Digitus mortuus is also known in German as "Leichenfinger" which could be translated as corpse finger or dead finger. A single finger suddenly becomes pale and cold as the result of digital artery vasospasm. The cause of this disease is unknown. Some view it as RAYNAUD's syndrome limited to one finger; others argue it is slightly different because the three color phases are often not seen. The main differential diagnostic point is an infarct of a digit, known as digitus moriens (Table 9-4).

Table 9-4. Differences between digitus mortuus (functional vasospasm) and digitus moriens (actual occlusion)

Digitus mortuus	Digitus moriens
Very pale	Pale-cyanotic and often mottled
Episodic	Permanent
Little pain	Very painful

B. Acrocyanosis

Synonym. Acroasphyxia

Definition

Idiopathic acrocyanosis clinically features cool, livid hands and feet. There is a uniform, painless cyanosis of all four extremities, usually with hyperhidrosis and cooling. Just as with RAYNAUD's disease, young women are most often affected, but the disease is not paroxysmal.

History

Acrocyanosis was described by CROCQ (1896) and then more extensively studied by CASSIRER (1901).

Etiology and Pathogenesis

In acrocyanosis, there is constriction of the arterioles and pre-capillary sphincters associated with venous dilatation. The microcirculation is slowed and discordant between the adjacent capillary loops, leading to increased removal of oxygen from hemoglobin. The reasons for this dysregulation are unclear.

Clinical Features

The hands are most often involved, although the feet, nose and ears may also be affected. The skin is permanently cold and blue. Almost all patients are young women, often with low blood pressure. Often other family members are affected. The lesions are generally painless, but may be symptomatic in cold weather. Hyperhidrosis is frequently found. There are no episodic attacks, and ulcerations or other trophic changes almost never occur.

Therapy

- Reassuring the patient, reminding them of the good prognosis
- Protection against cold
- Active medical therapy is not usually needed.

C. Erythrocyanosis

Definition

This variant of acrocyanosis also has idiopathic autonomic dysregulation of vascular tone. Often there are associated follicular keratoses. Based on localization, three different names are attached:

- Erythrocyanosis faciei
- Perniosis retiformis mammae
- Erythrocyanosis cruris puellarum

Clinical Features

There is a diffuse, patchy, blue-gray-purple discoloration of the skin, usually on the face, breasts, thighs and upper aspects of the arms. Keratosis pilaris-like follicular plugging may be seen, especially on the arms.

Therapy

Usually none is needed, just as with acrocyanosis. Lotions or creams containing urea may help the keratoses.

D. Erythromelalgia (EM)

Synonyms. Erythermalgia, erythralgia, WEIR-MITCHELL syndrome

The first reported case was diagnosed by GRAVES (1834) and the syndrome itself was described by MITCHELL (1874).

Definition

Episodic attacks of erythema, warmth and pain usually involving the hands. Cold usually brings relief. For the physician and the patient erythromelagia is a distressing, debilitating disaster.

Etiology and Pathogenesis

The cause of idiopathic or primary erythromelalgia is unknown. The distal vascular channels react inappropriately to warmth. Sometimes physical activity or simply letting the limbs hang in a dependent position may be a sufficient trigger.
Erythromelalgia may be secondary to a variety of disorders:

- Arterial occlusive disease
- Diabetic and alcoholic polyneuropathy
- Hyperviscosity, such as in polycythemia vera or leukemia (especially chronic myeloid leukemia)
- Hypertension
- Heavy metal poisoning
- Systemic diseases such as rheumatoid arthritis or systemic lupus erythematosus
- Hyperviscosity (leukaemias particularly chronic myeloid leukaemia)
- Thrombocytosis (Thrombocythaemia, Polycythaemia)

Diagnosis

- History and clinical examination
- Laboratory tests: CBC, differential white blood cell count, plasma viscosity, glucose, relevant immunologic tests
- Vascular laboratory evaluation: Doppler, thermography, percutaneous pO_2 measurement, laser Doppler percutaneous flow measurements

Therapy

Physical therapy with hydrotherapy, iontophoresis, electrostimulation or cold can reduce the complaints. Transcutaneous nerve stimulation (TENS) may be helpful. The limbs should be elevated at night. Low-dose aspirin is often beneficial. β-blockers help some of the patients, while sedatives may allow the patient to better tolerate the pain at night. Patients should be advised to avoid extremes of temperatures, e.g. direct heat and cooling below 15 °C.

E. Ergotism

Synonyms. Ergot poisoning, ergotismus, St. Anthony's fire

Definition

Acute or chronic vasospasm of muscular arteries caused by ergot-containing compounds.

Etiology and Pathogenesis

The most common cause of ergotism is medications containing ergot, usually used for migraine. Women are more often affected and usually they have exceeded the recommended dose or duration of therapy. Occasionally dihydroergotamine is used for thrombosis prophylaxis and can cause similar problems. On rare occasions grains from ecological farmers can become contaminated with organisms producing ergot, so a dietary history should be obtained. Mushroom poisoning (*Claviceps purpura)* is another cause originally described in the Middle Ages.

Clinical Features

The limbs may be cold, pale and progress to gangrene. Patients have a variety of symptoms including nausea, vomiting, diarrhea, confusion, headache, chills, paresthesias and visual disturbances. There may also be spasms of visceral arteries, leading to renal damage as well as mesenteric and myocardial infarctions (Table 9-5).

Table 9-5. Symptoms of ergotism

CNS	Extremities	Endocrine
Nausea	Paleness	Menstrual disturbances
Vomiting	Coolness	
Confusion	Paresthesias	
Headache	Claudication	
Visual disturbances		
(double vision, seeing stars)	Gangrene	

Therapy

- If the ergot intake is stopped soon enough, reversal is spontaneous and complete.
- In more advanced cases, vasodilatation with nitrates (also sodium nitroprusside), calcium-channel blockers and prostaglandin E_1 infusions (intravenous or intra-arterial) may be necessary.

F. Reflex Sympathetic Dystrophy

Synonyms. SUDECK's dystrophy, SUDECK's syndrome, algodystrophy

Definition

Post-traumatic vasomotor disturbance associated with patchy osteoporosis and pain in the involved extremity.

Clinical Features

The skin is usually smooth; it may be cool or excessively warm, moist, and sometimes cyanotic or edematous. Occasionally there is an associated RAYNAUD's syndrome. In later stages, disuse osteoporosis may develop.

Therapy

- Adequate pain therapy following limb injuries
- Early and consistent physical therapy with effective mobilization of injured limbs
- Measures to stimulate circulation, such as intravenous prostaglandin E_1
- Calcitonin

G. Pernio/Cold Injury

Synonym. Chilblains

The first thermal insults to military personal we reported as far back as XENOPHON's experience in Persia about 400 BC.

Definition

Peripheral occlusive disease developing after cold exposure without freezing.

Etiology and Pathogenesis

Cold exposure may lead to contraction and occlusion of peripheral arteries and arterioles with resultant ischemic tissue damage.

Clinical Features

Pernio is primarily a disease of women in the fall and early winter. The individual lesions are livid, round and swollen; they may advance to blisters and ulcerations. The most common sites as the anteriolateral aspects of the shins, as well as the dorsal sides of the hands, feet and toes. Associated symptoms may include acrocyanosis, chills, hypesthesias, paresthesias and hyperhidrosis. Recurrent lesions may produce atrophy and scarring.

Differential Diagnosis

Erythema nodosum, erythema induratum of Bazin and various forms of vasculitis

Therapy

Avoidance of cold is the most important step. With acute lesions, careful re-warming is useful. Early local or systemic fibrolytic therapy can resolve fresh thrombi in small vessels. A trial of nifedipine 5–20 mg t.i.d. is warranted as this may help relieve pain.

H. Cold-Induced Injuries

Synonyms. Frostbite, non-freezing and freezing injuries

Definition

Combination of vascular occlusion and direct tissue damage producing localized injury. Systemic cold injury is hypothermia.

Etiology and Pathogenesis

Exposure to freezing temperatures causes profound constriction of the peripheral arteries and arterioles, leading to ischemic damage to skin, muscles and the autonomic nervous system. In addition, there is crystal formation in tissues; the freeze-thaw cycle causes direct damage.

Clinical Features

Four grades of cold injuries are identified:

1. Erythema and edema of the skin, often lasting for weeks
2. Blister formation
3. Irreversible skin damage with superficial necrosis and pain
4. Deep necrosis and gangrene

Therapy

- Frozen tissues should be slowly warmed in 40 °C (38 – 42 C) water.
- Higher temperatures, as with a heating pad or other sources of dry heat, are contraindicated.
- Analgesics are usually required.
- Massaging the tissue brings no benefit and may cause harm.
- Pale homogenous serous blisters suggest a good outlook. Blood-filled blisters as well as dark areas of skin suggest deeper, more permanent damage.
- The involved extremities should be actively moved.

  Recommended medications include:
- Intravenous prostaglandin E_1 or Iloprost
- Broad spectrum antibiotics
- Tetanus prophylaxis
- Platelet aggregation inhibitors
- Topical *Aloe vera* is occasionally recommended because of its bactericidal effect and possible inhibition of thromboxane synthesis.

Other Types of Cold Injury

The combination of moisture and cold, but not freezing, temperatures can cause vasospasm and tissue damage similar to frostbite. In severe cases gangrene may develop. Chronic cases often include increased cold sensitivity and hyperhidrosis. Several different terms have been employed, but all are similar.

Trench foot was described in soldiers, such as those in World War I, standing for long periods of time in cold, wet boots in the trenches. Outdoor activities with exposure to melting snow and ice can produce the same effect.

Immersion foot refers to the situation where the feet are actually immersed in cold water, as following a ship disaster.

Shelter foot was first coined to describe extremity damage in Londoners forced to spend many evenings in cold, damp air raid shelters during World War.

3. Inflammatory Vascular Disease: The Vasculitides

Definition

Vasculitis includes the inflammatory reactions that begin in and primarily involve the walls of vessels. Vasculitides are uncommon disorders with heterogeneous clinical patterns. Recent classification schemes (Tables 9-6, 9-7, Fig. 9-7) attempt to simplify the complex nature of this family of disorders. Primary and secondary vasculitides are separated from difficult-to-classify special variants. The new classifications consider etiologic, clinical, pathological and laboratory aspects. Many areas of overlap are present.

Etiology and Pathogenesis

The usual trigger for the primary vasculitides is circulating immune complexes which cause localized or generalized vascular damage via histamine, anaphylotoxins and other mediators. Typical laboratory findings include signs of humoral immune reactions, such as hypergammaglobulinemia, cryoglobulinemia, rheumatoid factor, anti-nuclear antibodies, hypo- or hypercomplementemia and circulating immune

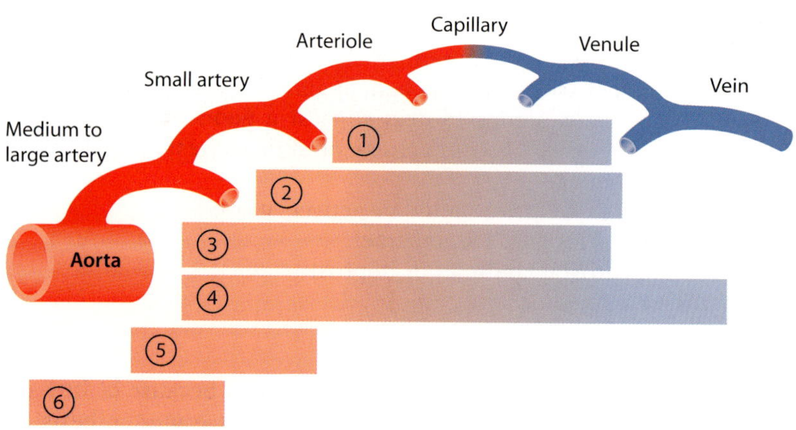

Fig. 9-7. Typical sites of involvement for various vasculitides

① Leukocytoclastic cutaneous angiitis
② Henoch-Schönlein purpura and essential cryoglobulinemia
③ Microscopic polyangiitis
④ Wegener's granulomatosis and Churg-Strauss syndrome
⑤ Polyarteritis nodosa and Kawasaki syndrome
⑥ Giant cell (temporal) arteritis and Takayasu's arteritis

complexes. The stimulus for and the target of the inflammation is the blood vessels themselves. The severity of the vessel damage is often determined by the extent of the repair mechanisms called into play.

Secondary vasculitides are more common than primary. The blood vessels are one showplace for an inflammatory reaction that arises elsewhere. A typical example is systemic lupus erythematosus, in which vasculitic lesions almost always involve serosal surfaces. Secondary vasculitides are seen in other connective tissue disorders. Cerebral, pulmonary, cardiac or renal vasculitis may be seen.

Tumors can also cause the clinical picture of vasculitis. For example, an atrial myxoma may produce not only fever, weight loss, arthritis, renal and hepatic symptoms, but also painful acral nodules with tiny ulcerations. In the following sections we have concentrated on those vasculitides that are of practical importance for vascular surgeons and physicians.

Table 9-6. Types of vasculitis: definitions based on Chapel Hill Consensus Conference

Large-vessel vasculitis[a]	
Giant cell (temporal) arteritis	Granulomatous arteritis of the aorta and its major branches with a predilection for the extracranial branches of the carotid artery; often involves the temporal artery; usually occurs in patients more than 50 years old and is often associated with polymyalgia rheumatica
TAKAYASU's arteritis	Granulomatous inflammation of the aorta and its major branches; usually occurs in patients less than 40 years old
Medium-sized-vessel vasculitis[a]	
Polyarteritis nodosa	Necrotizing inflammation of medium-sized or small arteries without glomerulonephritis or vasculitis in arterioles, capillaries or venules
KAWASAKI disease	Arteritis involving large, medium-sized and small arteries and associated with mucocutaneous lymph node syndrome; coronary arteries often affected; aorta and veins may be involved; usually occurs in children
Small-vessel vasculitis[a]	
WEGENER's granulomatosis[b]	Granulomatous inflammation involving the respiratory tract and necrotizing vasculitis of the small to medium-sized vessels (e.g., capillaries, venules, arterioles and arteries); necrotizing glomerulonephritis is common

Churg-Strauss syndrome[b]	Eosinophil-rich, granulomatous inflammation involving the respiratory tract and necrotizing vasculitis affecting small to medium-sized vessels and associated with asthma and eosinophilia
Microscopic polyangiitis[b]	Necrotizing vasculitis with few or no immune deposits affecting small vessels (capillaries, venules or arterioles). Necrotizing arteritis involving small and medium-sized arteries may be present. Necrotizing glomerulonephritis is very common. Pulmonary capillaritis often occurs.
Henoch-Schönlein purpura	Vasculitis with IgA-dominant immune deposits affecting small vessels (capillaries, venules or arterioles). Typically affects the skin, gut and glomeruli and is associated with arthralgias or arthritis.
Essential cryoglobulinemic vasculitis	Vasculitis with cryoglobulin immune deposits affecting small vessels (capillaries, venules or arterioles) and associated with cryoglobulins in serum. Skin and glomeruli are often involved.
Cutaneous leukocytoclastic angiitis	Isolated cutaneous leukocytoclastic angiitis with systemic vasculitis or glomerulonephritis.

[a] Large vessel refers to aorta and its major branches, such as those serving the head or limbs. Medium-sized vessels are the major visceral arteries, including the coronary, renal and mesenteric arteries. Small vessels include small arteries as well as capillaries, arterioles and venules.
[b] ANCA -positive.

Table 9-7. Classification of inflammatory vessel diseases

- Primary vasculitides
  1. Polyarteritis nodosa
     (a) Generalized polyarteritis nodosa
     (b) Cutaneous polyarteritis nodosa
  2. Hypersensitivity angiitis
     (a) Generalized form (Henoch-Schönlein purpura)
     (b) Localized forms
     - Necrotizing venulitis
     - Urticarial vasculitis
     - Erythema elevatum diutinum (Radcliff-Crocker)

3. Granulomatous vasculitis
   (a) Systemic forms
   - WEGENER's granulomatosis
   - CHURG-STRAUSS syndrome (allergic granulomatosis)
   - BEHÇET's disease
   - Polyangiitis overlap syndrome (Fauci)
   (b) Localized forms
   - Nasopharynx/trachea : Midline granulomatosis (angiocentric lymphoma)
   - Lungs: Lymphomatoid granulomatosis (angiocentric lymphoma)
   - CNS: Isolated granulomatous CNS vasculitis (angiocentric lymphoma)
   - Skin: Cutaneous CHURG-STRAUSS granulomatosis
4. Giant cell arteritides
   (a) Medium-sized and small arteries
   - Temporal (cranial) arteritis
   - Polymyalgia rheumatica
   (b) Aortic arch
   - TAKAYASU's arteritis

- Secondary vasculitides
  1. Autoimmune disease
     - Rheumatoid arthritis
     - Systemic lupus erythematosus
     - Systemic sclerosis
     - Dermatopolymyositis
     - Chronic active hepatitis
     - Primary biliary cirrhosis
     - Sarcoidosis
     - CROHN's disease
  2. Infections
     - Streptococci (rheumatic fever)
     - Spirochetes (syphilis, borreliosis)
     - Viruses (hepatitis, herpes, Coxsackie)
     - Parasites
  3. Tumors
     - Solid tumors
     - Atrial myxomas
     - Leukemia
     - Lymphoma
  4. Toxins
     - Ergotism
     - Snake toxins
     - Nicotine
  5. Medications
     - Non-steroidal anti-inflammatory drugs
     - Antibiotics
     - D-penicillamine
     - Gold salts
     - Cytostatic agents
- Special types of vasculitis
  - Thromboangiitis obliterans (BUERGER's syndrome)
  - Purpura fulminans (WATERHOUSE-FRIEDRICHSEN syndrome)
  - Thrombotic thrombocytopenic purpura (MOSCHKOWITZ)
  - Embolic vasculitis (OSLER)

A. Polyarteritis Nodosa (PAN)

Synonyms. Panarteritis nodosa, periarteritis nodosa, Kussmaul-Maier syndrome

KUSSMAUL and MAIER first described PAN in 1866 as a necrotising vasculitis affecting small and muscular arteries in multiple systems throughout the body.

Definition

Necrotizing inflammation of medium-sized or small arteries without glomerulonephritis or vasculitis in arterioles, capillaries or venules.

Epidemiology

The incidence of polyarteritis nodosa is about 4.6 per million. The male:female ratio is 2.5 : 1. The disease typically starts in the fourth to sixth decade of life; the mean age of onset is 48 years.

Etiology and Pathogenesis

The etiology of polyarteritis nodosa is unknown. In some cases, it appears to be associated with infections.

The disease is characterized by involvement of many organs. The necrotizing inflammation affects medium-sized and small arteries, as well as neighboring veins and occasionally arterioles and venules. The vessel damage is segmental but widely distributed. The coronary, mesenteric, renal and muscular arteries can be affected, as well as the vasa vasorum. Capillaries are not involved.

Clinical Features

General symptoms include:

- Malaise
- Arthralgias and myalgias
- Anorexia and weight loss
- Headache
- Fever

Typical organ involvement produces or includes:

- Abdominal pain and other symptoms (60% – 70% of cases).
- In over 50% of cases there is renal disease including aneurysms at the bifurcations of the arteries, infarcts and parenchymal hematomas following vessel rupture.
- When the arteries of the extremities are involved, small nodules can be palpated along the vessel course as aneurysms are formed.
- Polyneuropathies with motor and sensory components may develop. A mononeuritis multiplex or an isolated brachial plexus neuritis can also be seen, depending on which vessels are affected.
- Testicular pain and swelling may occur.
- Skin changes include mottled lividity (livedo reticularis) and small nodules, as well as rare infarcts.
- Mesenteric vasculitis can lead to gastrointestinal bleeding, small bowel infarcts or perforation. The liver and gall bladder can also be affected.

Diagnosis

There is no specific laboratory test for polyarteritis nodosa. Signs of inflammation (erythrocyte sedimentation rate, C-reactive protein) and organ damage are seen. ANCA, ANA and rheumatoid factor are negative. The diagnosis is based on the histological demonstration of necrotizing inflammation of the appropriate vessels, often seen in skin, subcutaneous or muscle biopsies. Angiographic demonstration of aneurysms of the renal or mesenteric arteries supports the diagnosis but is not specific. Table 9-8 lists diagnostic criteria for polyarteritis nodosa.

Table 9-8. Diagnostic criteria for polyarteritis nodosa (based on American College of Rheumatology suggestions)

1. Weight loss >4 kg, malaise, other general symptoms
2. Livedo reticularis
3. Testicular pain and swelling
4. Myalgias, weakness and tenderness of the leg muscles
5. Mono- or polyneuropathy, CNS symptoms
6. Hypertension (diastolic pressure >90 mg Hg)
7. Serum creatinine >1.5 mg/dl
8. Hepatitis B virus carrier status
9. Arteriographic findings: aneurysms and occlusions
10. Typical histological picture of necrotizing vasculitis of small and medium-sized vessels.

At least three of the ten criteria should be present to make the diagnosis. The sensitivity is 82.2%; the specificity, 86.6%.

Course and Prognosis

Poor prognostic signs are hypertension, cardiac failure and renal damage. Without therapy, two-thirds of patients die within 1 year. The course is unpredictable; some patients go rapidly downhill, in others the disease smolders over years. Remissions are rare.

Therapy

Systemic corticosteroids (prednisone 100 mg daily with gradual tapering) usually produce prompt improvement. In the usual Fauci regimen, systemic corticosteroids are combined with cyclophosphamide. Other immunosuppressive agents such as azathioprine may also be effective.

B. Giant Cell Arteritis (GCA)

Synonyms. Temporal arteritis, cranial arteritis, senile arteritis, HORTON's syndrome (BAYARD TAYLOR HORTON, 1895–1980, American clinician), HORTON-MAGATH-BROWN syndrome

Definition

Granulomatous arteritis of the aorta and its major branches with a predilection for the extra-cranial branches of the carotid artery, especially the temporal artery. There is often an association with polymyalgia rheumatica.

Table 9-9. History of giant cell arteritis

Year	Author	Findings	Terminology
1889	Hutchinson	Thrombotic arteritis in older patients, with gangrene	
1930	Schmidt	Intracranial aneurysms	
1932–34	Horton, Magath, Brown	Temporal arteritis, with clinico-pathological description	Temporal arteritis
1938	Jennings	Temporal arteritis	
1941	Gilmour	Chronic giant cell arteritis	Giant cell arteritis

History

Table 9.9 shows the history of giant cell arteritis.

Epidemiology

The incidence in the USA and Europe is around 7/100,000. In individuals older than 50 years, it is 16–19/100,000. The incidence has increased in recent years in several countries, such as Sweden. The male: female ratio is 2:1. Onset is typically between ages 65–75; appearance before age 50 is rare except in HIV positive patients.

Etiology and Pathogenesis

The etiology is unknown. Giant cell arteritis can involve the larger aortic branches but most typically affects the temporal arteries. Polymyalgia rheumatica is a fibromyalgia which most often involves the muscles of the shoulder girdle. The two disorders show frequent clinical overlaps, cannot be separated with certainty, and probably represent variants of the same disease process.

The inflammatory changes damage the large and medium-sized arteries in a segmental fashion. The arterioles and capillaries are not affected. Histologically there is an infiltrate of histiocytes, epithelioid cells, multi-nucleated giant cells, lymphocytes and plasma cells which damages the inner layers of the vessel wall, destroying the elastic fibers.

Clinical Features

The main features are shown in Table 9-10. Initially the complaints are typically vague, including fatigue, loss of appetite, loss of weight, night sweats, fleeting muscle and joint pain and low-grade fever.

After days to weeks, uni- or bilateral headache develops, typically in the temporal region. Sometimes the skin of the scalp is painful. About 50% of patients have visual changes. Inflammation and occlusion of the ophthalmic or central retinal arteries can lead to blindness. Without

Table 9-10. Main features of temporal arteritis

Pain in the temple or nape regions, or in the cheeks or tongue when chewing.

Thickening, hardening, tenderness and even loss of pulse in the temporal artery.

Uni- or bilateral visual disturbances.

Pain in the shoulder or back muscles.

Marked elevation of erythrocyte sedimentation rate.

Table 9-11. Comparison of the most common symptoms in temporal arteritis and polymyalgia rheumatica

Symptom	Temporal arteritis	Polymyalgia rheumatica
Poor general condition	(+)	+
Weight loss	(+)	+
Loss of appetite	+	+
Fatigue	+	+
Depression	(+)	(+)
Headache	+	(+)
Neck pain	(+)	+
Shoulder pain	(+)	+
Back pain	(+)	+
Fever	+	(+)
Intermittent claudication	(+)	(+)
Visual disturbances	+	(+)
Joint swelling	(+)	(+)
Muscle weakness	(+)	(+)

prompt treatment, irreversible often bilateral loss of vision can rapidly evolve. In about 20% of cases, other organs are affected. Involvement of the coronary, mesenteric or limb arteries can produce ischemia and infarcts of the respective tissues with accompanying clinical signs and symptoms.

In the case of polymyalgia rheumatica, stiffness and pain in the neck, shoulder girdle, upper parts of the arms, back and occasionally pelvic tissues are most common. Morning stiffness is common and marked. Fever, loss of appetite and weight loss show the relationship to temporal arteritis. The symptoms of both diseases are compared in Table 9-11.

Diagnosis

The laboratory pattern is dominated by signs of inflammation:

- Marked elevation in erythrocyte sedimentation rate which is usually greater than 50 mm/hour. A normal value is most uncommon.
- Elevated C-reactive protein
- Elevated levels of $_2$-globulins and fibrinogen
- Mild leukocytosis with left shift
- Normo- to hypochromic anemia
- Reactive thrombocytosis

The diagnosis is confirmed by a biopsy of the temporal artery. Because the involvement is segmental with skip-areas, it is wise to take a 3 cm segment of artery which can be serially sectioned. Even if both temporal arteries are clinically unremarkable, if the diagnosis is suspected bilateral biopsies should be carried out. The yield is close to 80%. An ophthalmologic examination is also mandatory. Table 9-12 shows the diagnostic criteria for temporal arteritis.

Table 9-12. Diagnostic criteria for temporal arteritis (based on American College of Rheumatology suggestions)

Age at onset of disease >50 years
Headache of recent origin
Changes in the temporal arteries
Erythrocyte sedimentation rate >50 mm in first hour
Typical histological findings on biopsy
Three of the five criteria should be present.

Differential Diagnosis

- Migraine headache
- Cluster headaches (Bing-Horton syndrome)
- Trigeminal neuralgia
- Cervical spine disease
- Maxillary or frontal sinusitis
- Polymyositis
- Sepsis
- Paraneoplastic syndrome

Course and Prognosis

While temporal arteritis can remit spontaneously, more typically it has a long course with remissions and relapses.

Therapy

If there is clinical suspicion of temporal arteritis, systemic corticosteroid therapy should be instituted. One should start with 100 mg prednisone daily, tapered over 3–4 weeks. The general symptoms disappear rapidly with this dosage and eye complications are avoided. In those patients who already have visual disturbances, more than 50% improve. As soon as the clinical symptoms are better and the laboratory values start to return towards normal, one can taper the maintenance dose to around 7.5–10 mg daily. This dose should be continued for at least 6–12 months. Sometimes treatment for years is needed.

Excision of the temporal arteries for diagnostic purposes often relieves the headache but of course does not otherwise influence the disease process.

If the symptoms of polymyalgia rheumatica dominate, then nonsteroidal anti-inflammatory drugs, such as salicylates or indomethacin, may be helpful. Most often systemic corticosteroids are also needed for these patients. Here one must balance the risk of a recurrence against the side effects of the corticosteroids.

C. Wegener's Granulomatosis (WG)

Synonyms. WEGENER's disease (FRIEDRICH WEGENER, 1907–1990, German pathologist), KLINGER-WEGENER-CHURCH syndrome, lethal granulomatosis

Definition

Granulomatous inflammation involving the respiratory tract and necrotizing vasculitis of the small to medium-sized vessels (e.g., capillaries, venules, arterioles and arteries). Necrotizing glomerulonephritis is common. WEGENER's granulomatosis is one of the ANCA-associated vasculitides (ANCA, anti-neutrophil cytoplasmic antibody).

Epidemiology

The disease affects both sexes equally and can appear in every age group. The peak incidence falls between 30 and 50 years of age.

Etiology and Pathogenesis

The etiology of Wegener's granulomatosis is unknown.

Clinical Features

- General symptoms (weight loss, night sweats, fever)
- Granulomatous inflammation of the respiratory tract, involving the nose, mouth, trachea and bronchi. Symptoms include cough, dyspnea, hemoptysis, rhinorrhea and sinusitis.
- Granulomatous changes in the lungs which lead to liquefaction and hemorrhage
- Eye involvement with scleritis, episcleritis and retinal vasculitis
- Chronic or rapidly progressive glomerulonephritis with renal failure; often dialysis is needed.
- Arthralgias and arthritis
- Cutaneous leukocytoclastic vasculitis

Diagnosis

The diagnostic criteria are shown in Table 9-13.

Table 9-13. Diagnostic criteria for WEGENER's granulomatosis (based on suggestions of the American College of Rheumatology)

Inflammation in nose and mouth (ulcers, hemorrhages, purulent discharge). Infiltration of the lungs as seen on chest X-ray (round lesions, cavitation, fixed infiltrates). Nephritic urinary sediment: >5 erythrocytes/high power field or with erythrocyte casts or cylinders Histological demonstration of granulomatous inflammation in the vessel wall (peri- and extravascular)
If two of the four criteria are present, the disease can be diagnosed as Wegener's granulomatosis. Clinical signs of vasculitis are not part of the criteria but are often present.

Course and Prognosis

Untreated, the outlook is dismal. Typically the disease smolders at first for months or years but can also take a fulminant course with severe renal and pulmonary disease. In untreated patients the most frequent cause of death is renal and/or pulmonary failure, with a mortality rate of 90% at 2 years.

Therapy

Initially one can try trimethoprim-sulfamethoxazole (160–800 mg [double strength]) b.i.d. If this fails, then cyclophosphamide and prednisone, or perhaps low-dose methotrexate, should be employed.

D. Behćet's Disease

Synonyms. BEHÇET's syndrome, ADAMANTIADES-BEHÇET syndrome, Gilbert syndrome, trisymptom complex, generalized aphthosis, cutaneous-mucosal-uveal syndrome.

Definition

Behçet's disease is a systemic disorder that features oral and genital ulcerations as well as eye involvement, probably on a vasculitic basis.

Epidemiology

The disease is most common in Turkey, Iran, Japan and Korea. The prevalence in the West is about 5/100,000, while in the Near East and Asia it is much higher. The peak age of onset is in young adult life.

Etiology and Pathogenesis

The etiology is unknown. The histological sign of early lesions is a vasculitis involving small vessels with a lymphocytic infiltrate, intimal proliferation and thrombosis.

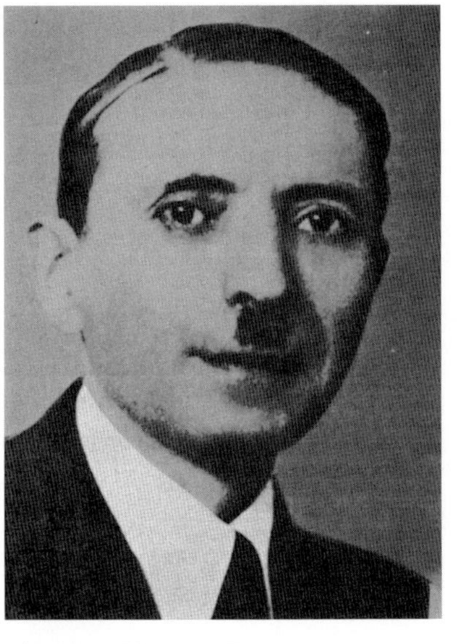

Fig. 9-8. HULUSI BEHÇET, 1889–1948, Turkish dermatologist, Istanbul

Diagnosis

The diagnostic criteria of the Japanese BEHÇET's Syndrome Research Committee as shown in Table 9-14 are most generally used.

Therapy

There is no specific therapy leading to cure. Treatment is symptom- and organ system-directed.

- In severe forms with vasculitis and eye findings, immunosuppressive drugs are required. Cyclosporine A may be most effective for acute ocular inflammation; other choices include azathioprine, chlorambucil, methotrexate and cyclophosphamide. In Japan, colchicine is often employed for acute flare-ups.
- Systemic corticosteroids can be used alone or combined with the immunosuppressive agents. They appear especially important in patients with neurological disease. The dosage should be adjusted to the inflammatory activity.

Table 9-14. Diagnostic criteria for BEHÇET's disease

Obligate symptom: Recurrent oral aphthae at least twice yearly, plus two of the following: • Genital ulcerations • Uveitis/ iritis with hypopyon, retinitis • Skin changes (erythema nodosum, folliculitis, sterile pustules) • Thrombophlebitis (also migratory forms) and phlebothrombosis • Positive pathergy test. When the skin is traumatized with a simple needle stick (such as from drawing blood) or the test injection of physiologic NaCl solution, pathergy is diagnosed when a pustule develops at the site of minor trauma after 24–48 h. Additional symptoms: • Skin: extragenital ulcerations, erythema multiforme • Eyes: keratitis, retinal exudates and hemorrhage (can lead to blindness) • Joints: recurrent or chronic oligo- or polyarthritis • CNS: cerebellar syndrome, pyramidal signs, meningoencephalitis and others • Gastrointestinal tract: duodenal ulcer, esophageal ulcerations, bleeding, enteritis and recto-colitis • Miscellaneous: epididymitis, inguinal lymphadenopathy, glomerulonephritis, pneumonia, pleurisy, pericarditis and myositis The individual symptoms often appear in isolated fashion with considerable time intervals separating them. Thus a detailed history is needed and a plausible historical description of a symptom is sufficient to include it.

- The arthritis often responds to non-steroidal anti-inflammatory drugs, sometimes in combination with systemic or intra-articular corticosteroids. Cold packs may help relieve acute pain. In some instances a synovectomy may be required.

E. Henoch-Schönlein Purpura (HSP)

JOHANN LUKAS SCHÖNLEIN, 1793–1864, German internist and pathologist, Berlin; EDUARD HEINRICH HENOCH, 1820–1908, German pediatrician, Berlin

Definition

Vasculitis with IgA-dominant immune deposits affecting small vessels (capillaries, venules or arterioles) which typically involves the skin, gut and glomeruli and is associated with arthralgias or arthritis.

Epidemiology

HENOCH-SCHÖNLEIN purpura is a relatively common disorder, seen primarily in children and adolescents.

Clinical Features

Typically there is a respiratory tract infection followed by malaise, fever, acral purpura, arthralgias, myalgias and abdominal colic.

Diagnosis

The diagnostic features are shown in Table 9-15.

Table 9-15. Diagnostic criteria for HENOCH-SCHÖNLEIN purpura (based on American College of Rheumatology suggestions)

Palpable purpura
Age < 21 years
Abdominal pain
Histological evidence for leukocytoclastic angiitis

Therapy

Usually only symptomatic therapy is required, as spontaneous improvement is the rule. Non-steroidal anti-inflammatory drugs can be used if the arthritic pain is severe. Systemic corticosteroids may be occasionally be used for edema and severe abdominal pain, once other surgical causes of pain are ruled out. The overall prognosis for paediatic HSP is good.

F. Autoimmune Diseases

F-1. Systemic Sclerosis

Synonyms. Scleroderma, progressive systemic sclerosis

Definition

Systemic connective tissue disease with increased collagen accumulation and fibrosis of the skin and internal organs. Obliterative acral angiopathy (intimal proliferation) leads to skin and internal infarcts.

Epidemiology

The incidence is about 1/100,000. Women between 30 and 50 years of age are most often affected.

Clinical Features

Clinically one usually distinguishes between systemic sclerosis with limited skin involvement (face and distal to knees and elbows) such as in CREST syndrome and systemic sclerosis without skin involvement. The main features are:

- Thickening and hardening of the skin (especially fingers and toes)
- RAYNAUD's phenomenon
- Acral ulcerations
- Exertional dyspnea
- Difficulty swallowing

Diagnosis

- Dermatosclerosis of the fingers, toes, hands and feet
  - The skin is tight and firm often producing painless contractures
  - Ulcerations and necrosis of the finger tips (rat bite necrosis)
  - Fixed facial expression, inability to open mouth widely, radial folds at corner of mouth (tobacco pouch mouth), sclerosis of frenulum
- Pulmonary function tests to document lung fibrosis
- Esophageal studies (manometry, barium swallow examination)
- EKG and echocardiography
- Acral circulatory disturbances: ice water test, Doppler ultrasonography, light plethysmography

Nail Fold Capillary Microscopy

Careful examination of the nail folds can demonstrate capillary damage.

- Slow pattern: dilated giant capillaries, rarefaction
- Active pattern: increased number of avascular areas

Laboratory Tests

- Search for typical antibodies (anti-DNA topoisomerase I, Scl-70, anti-centromere)

Differential Diagnosis

- Morphea does not damage hands
- Mixed connective tissue disease (SHARP syndrome) represents an overlap between systemic sclerosis, systemic lupus erythematosus, polymyositis and rheumatoid arthritis. Usually patient have high ANA titers, directed against nuclear ribonucleoprotein (RNP).
- Pseudoscleroderma caused by chemical exposure (vinyl chloride, silica dioxide)
- Eosinophilic fasciitis (SHULMAN syndrome) features swelling of the proximal extremities without involvement of the hands and feet, with eosinophils in the blood and the fascia, best diagnosed by fascial biopsy.

Therapy

Treatment is symptomatic. Protection against cold is essential. RAYNAUD's phenomenon can be treated with nifedipine. If acral necroses are present. intravenous prostaglandins or even sympathectomy may be tried. In the early edematous phase, systemic corticosteroids may be helpful. With more advanced cutaneous fibrosis, D-penicillamine or methotrexate may bring benefits.

F-2. Systemic Lupus Erythematosus

Definition

Systemic lupus erythematosus (SLE) is a chronic inflammatory autoimmune disease which involves the skin and the vascular connective tissue. Many organs are affected by vasculitis/perivasculitis of the small arteries and arterioles, associated with deposition of immune complexes containing DNA, anti-DNA, complement and fibrin.

Epidemiology

Some 80%–90% of patients are women, usually in young adult life.

Etiology and Pathogenesis

The etiology is unknown in most cases. Some cases may be caused by medications; the best established agents are hydralazine, procainamide, isoniazid, methyldopa, phenytoin, penicillamine, carbamazepine, primidone and thiouracils.

Clinical Features

- General symptoms (fever, weakness, weight loss)
- Musculo-skeletal complaints
- Skin changes (butterfly facial rash, chronic discoid lesions [often hypopigmented, scarring] alopecia
- Photosensitivity
- Oral ulcerations
- Cardio-pulmonary diseases (pleurisy, pericarditis, LIBMAN-SACKS endocarditis, myocarditis)
- Renal disease (glomerulonephritis, nephrotic syndrome, renal failure) plays a major role in determining prognosis.
- Neurological disease (psychosis, seizures, cranial nerve paralysis, extrapyramidal changes)

Diagnosis

- Non-specific signs of inflammation such as erythrocyte sedimentation rate, C-reactive protein, α_2- and γ-globulin levels
- Specific immunological findings
  - Antinuclear antibodies (ANA) high titer in 95%
  - Anti-dsDNA in 50%, more often in severe cases
  - Anti-Sm in 25%
  - Reduced levels of C3, C4
  - Circulating immune complexes
  - LE cell test (30%)
  - False-positive test for syphilis

A skin biopsy with direct immunofluorescent examination may show a band of immunoglobulins (IgG, IgM, C3) along the basement membrane zone (lupus band test).

The diagnostic criteria of the American Rheumatism Association are shown in Table 9-16.

Course and Prognosis

While the course is highly variable, today the 10 year survival is 80%–85%. The main causes of death are renal failure, cardiac failure, neurological complications and sepsis.

Therapy

The wide variety of therapeutic measures are responsible for the improved outlook. If the systemic lupus erythematosus appears drug-induced, stopping the suspected agent leads to rapid improvement.

Table 9-16. Diagnostic criteria for systemic lupus erythematosus (based on American Rheumatism Association suggestions)

Butterfly facial erythema
Discoid lupus erythematosus
Photosensitivity
Oral ulcerations
Non-deforming polyarthritis
Serositis (pleurisy, pericarditis)
Renal disease (proteinuria >0.5 g/dl or casts
CNS disease (psychosis or seizures)
Hematological findings (Coombs-positive hemolytic anemia, thrombocytopenia, leukopenia, lymphopenia)
Immunological findings (anti-dsDNA antibodies, anti-Sm antibodies, LE cell preparation, false-positive syphilis serology)
Antinuclear antibodies, as determined by immunofluorescent test
If four of these 11 criteria are present, the diagnosis of systemic lupus erythematosus is likely.

- Cutaneous disease: sunscreens, topical corticosteroids
- Systemic disease: if mild, non-steroidal anti-inflammatory drugs and anti-malarial drugs (hydroxychloroquine) usually suffice. Regular ophthalmologic examinations are required if anti-malarial drugs are used. Systemic corticosteroids may be useful to control flare-ups.

If the disease is more severe, immunosuppressive agents are usually effective. Plasmapheresis and cyclophosphamide pulse therapy seems the best option for glomerulonephritis. Kidney transplantation may be required for renal failure.

F-3. Rheumatoid Arthritis with Vasculitis

Definition

Chronic, usually progressive disease with immunologic pathogenesis which primarily involves the joints but can affect visceral organs and cause vasculitis.

Etiology and Pathogenesis

A number of types of vasculitis are possible. In rheumatoid nodule, there appears to be an initial involvement of small arteries producing edema and fibrinoid necrosis. Later there is proliferation of fibroblasts and revascularization. Larger arteries can also be involved primarily in the hands and lower aspects of the arms. In addition, leukocytoclastic angiitis may be seen.

Clinical Features

The rheumatoid nodules can be present almost anywhere, but are typically symmetrical and often found on the extensor surfaces of the extremities. The arteritis can lead to:

- Raynaud's phenomenon
- Nail fold and finger pulp infarcts
- Ulcerations (especially on the shins and ankles)

The leukocytoclastic angiitis may cause palpable purpura and ulcerations on the skin, as well as mononeuritis multiplex.

Diagnosis

Typically the hand, knee, metatarsal, elbow and shoulder joints are involved. Muscle atrophy is common. Rheumatoid nodules are present in 20%; sicca syndrome in 10%.

Arteriography reveals irregular vessel lumina with stenoses and occlusions, but usually good collaterals.

Laboratory

- Erythrocyte sedimentation rate and C-reactive protein moderately to markedly elevated
- Anemia in 25% of chronic cases
- Rheumatoid factor present initially in about 40% of cases, later in 80%
- Anti-nuclear antibodies positive in 25%–30% of patients

Therapy

The goal is to reduce pain and swelling, minimizing loss of function. Non-steroidal anti-inflammatory drugs, methotrexate, gold salts, salazosulfapyridine and sulfasalazine are often used. Accompanying physical therapy is very important.

B: Supplementary Figures and Legends

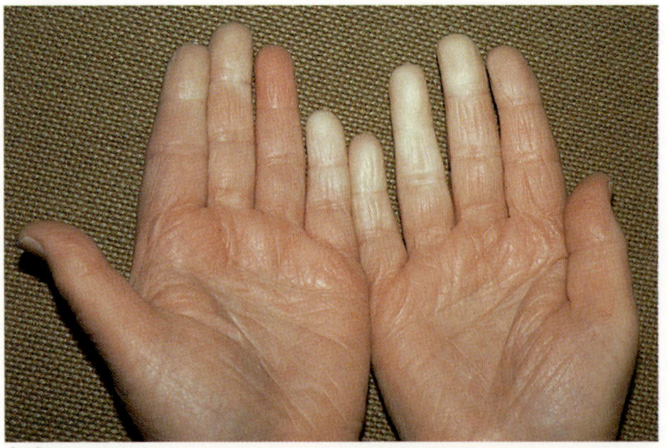
9-9

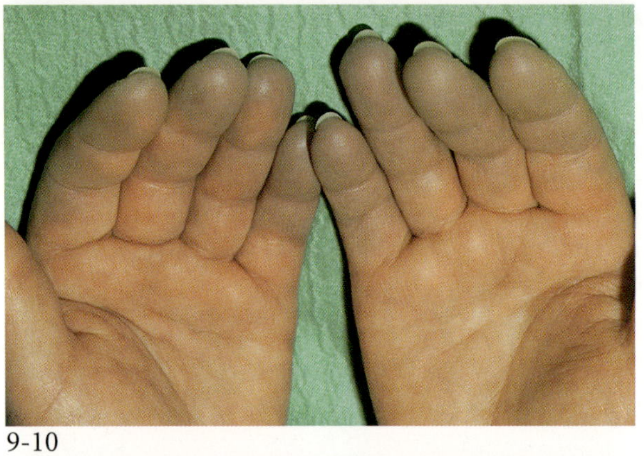
9-10

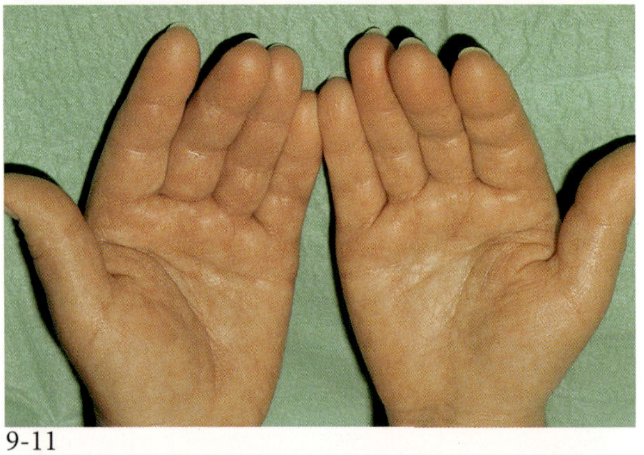
9-11

Figs. 9-9 – 9-11. Primary, vasospastic RAYNAUD's phenomenon. Typically the thumbs are not affected. There is spasm of the digital arteries usually triggered by cold or emotional stress. Most often there are three phases with different colors:

1. White (arterial vasospasm with empty capillary beds)
2. Blue-cyanotic (dilated capillaries and venules)
3. Red (reactive hyperemia as arteries dilate)

Figs. 9-12, 9-13. Severe acral circulatory problem in patient with systemic sclerosis. There is secondary RAYNAUD's syndrome and the fingers are quite edematous and swollen (sausage fingers)

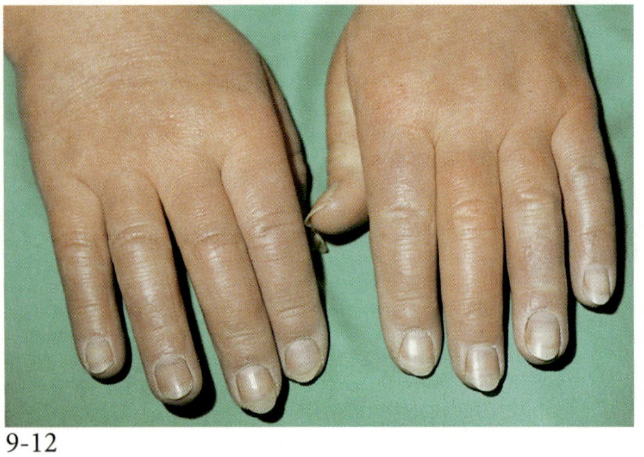
9-12

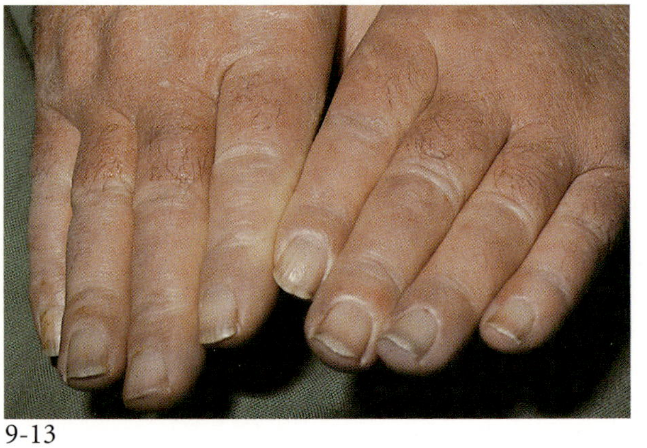
9-13

Fig. 9-14. Acrocyanosis. A 22 year old woman with marked acrocyanosis. Persistent livid discoloration of the hands and feet; the ears and nose can also be affected. There is often a triad of cyanosis, cool skin temperature and hyperhidrosis. Occasionally there is local swelling. The cause is persistent vasospasm of the arterioles and pre-capillary sphincters which is usually caused by cold exposure. Almost all patients are young women, usually with low blood pressure. Often there is a positive family history. Paroxysmal attacks of pain and ulcerations do not develop. The course is benign. There is most often improvement with time. No medical therapy is needed

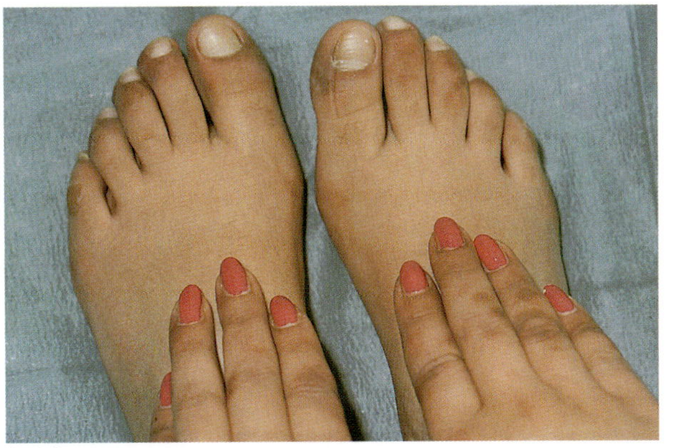

9-14

Fig. 9-15. Erythromelalgia. Hands of a woman with this uncommon idiopathic acral circulatory disorder. There is the paroxysmal appearance of increased acral circulation with erythema, warmth and burning pains. The etiology is unknown, but almost all patients are women. The symptoms can be elicited or worsened by application of heat (warm bath, bed rest)

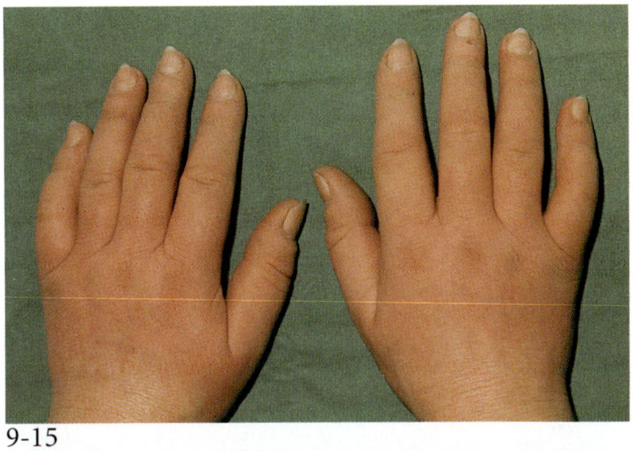

9-15

Fig. 9-16. Pernio in a 38 year old woman. Pernio usually appears in women in the late fall or early winter months. The lesions are oval doughy pruritic areas of swelling which can advance to blisters and ulcerations. Typical locations are on the hands, feet and especially the toes. There appears to be a inadequate adaptability of the terminal vessels. Microscopically one sees inflammatory infiltrates with edema and widened skin capillaries which have thickened walls and later may contain thrombi

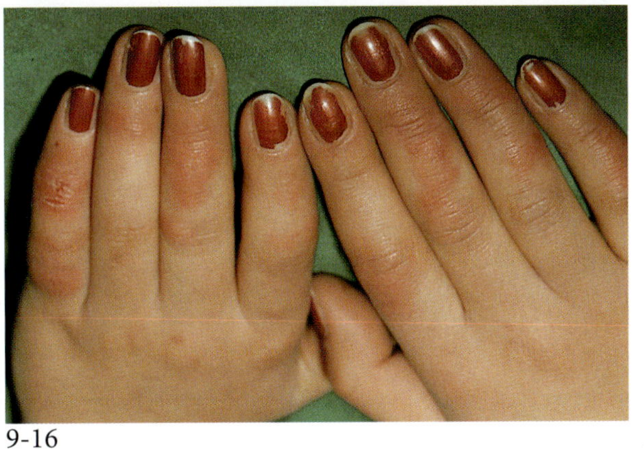

9-16

Fig. 9-17. Palmar erythema in a 48 year old man. One must consider systemic lupus erythematosus, liver cirrhosis, hepatitis, chronic pulmonary disease, subacute bacterial endocarditis, rheumatoid arthritis and dermatomyositis

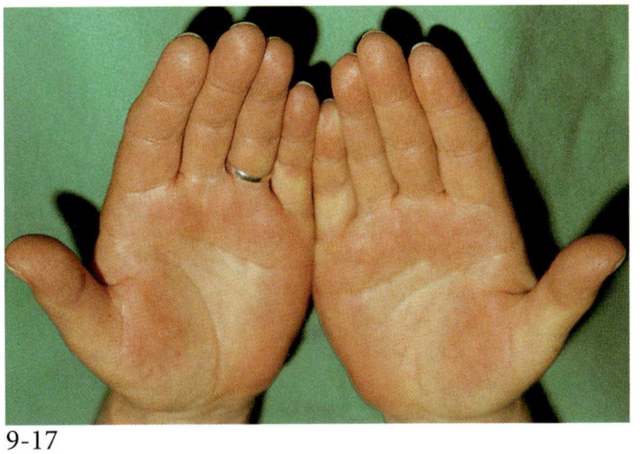

9-17

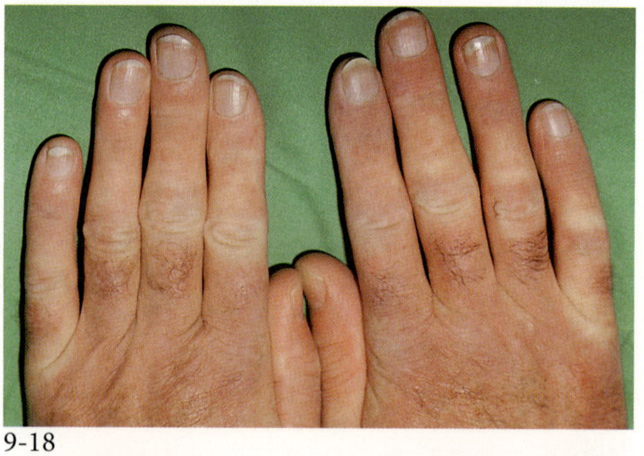
9-18

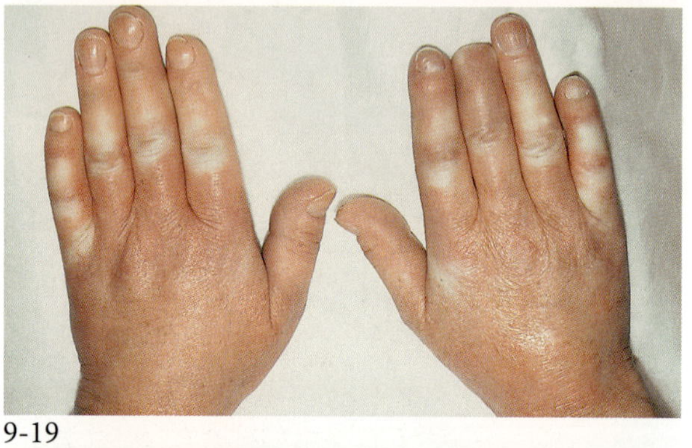
9-19

Figs. 9-18, 9-19. Secondary RAYNAUD's syndrome in a patient with scleroderma. The skin is taut over the indurated deeper tissues. Around the joints, the pressure of motion or flexion typically produces a white color by emptying the capillaries

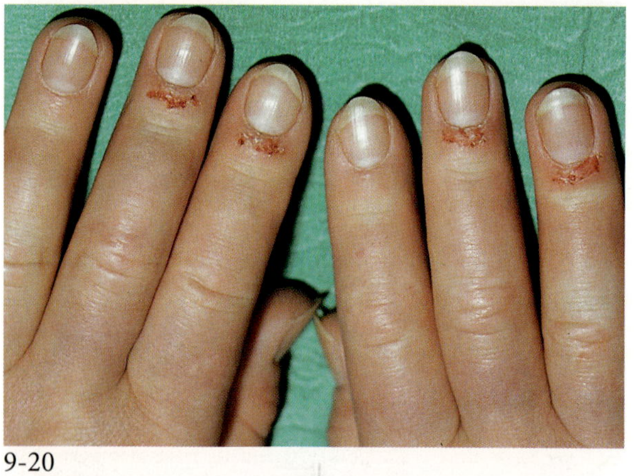
9-20

Fig. 9-20. Nail fold necrosis in a 40 year old woman with systemic sclerosis

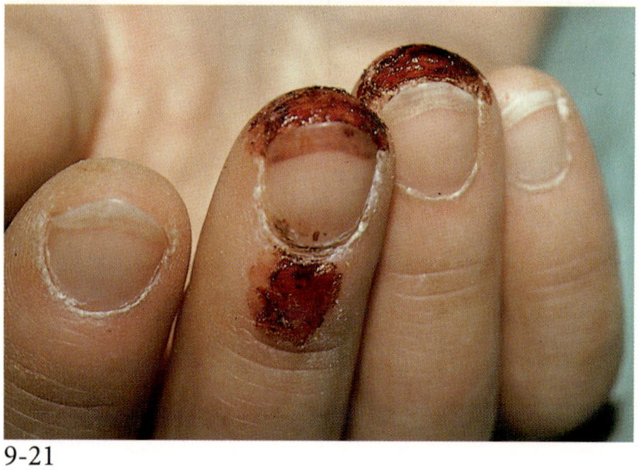
9-21

Fig. 9-21. Finger tip necrosis (rat bite necrosis) in a 55 year old woman with long-standing systemic sclerosis and secondary RAYNAUD's syndrome. Multiple digital artery occlusions could be shown on angiography. A thoracic sympathectomy had already been performed

Figs. 9-22, 9-23. Thibierge-Weissenbach syndrome refers to systemic sclerosis with focal calcification in the skin, subcutaneous tissue, along tendons and about joints. The calcified deposits are usually found on the flexural surfaces, especially of the palms, as well as over the elbows. This patient had severe Raynaud's syndrome. Many consider Thibierge-Weissenbach syndrome as a variant of CREST syndrome

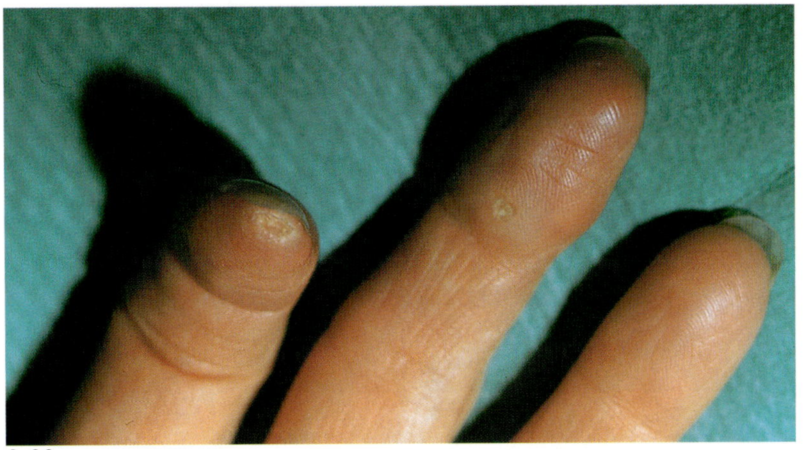

9-22

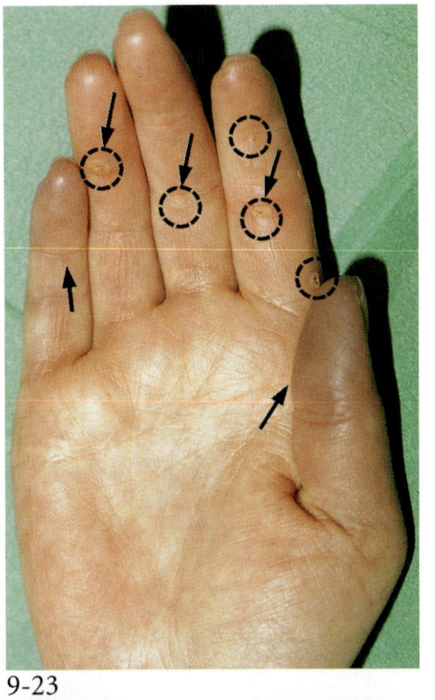

9-23

Figs. 9-24, 9-25. Radiological examples of Thibierge-Weissenbach syndrome with widely scattered subcutaneous calcification

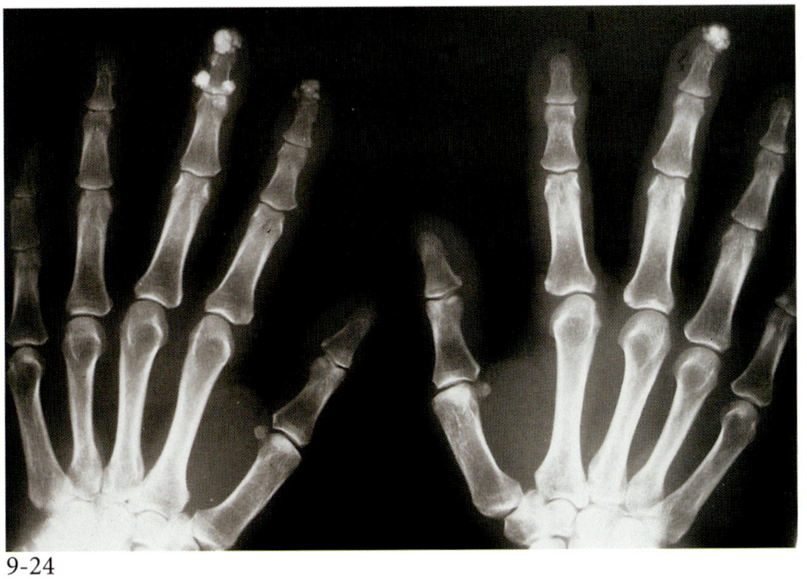

9-24

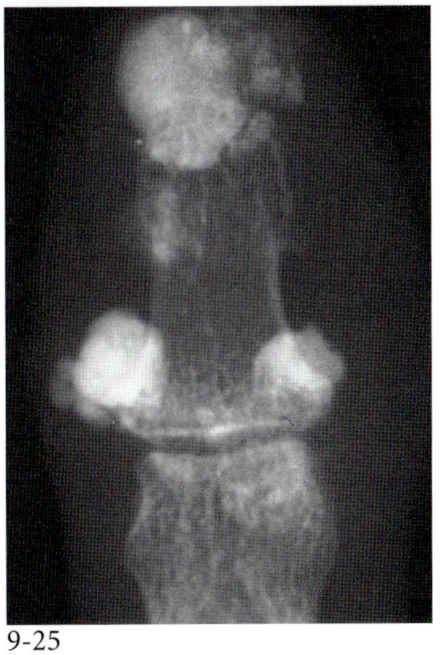

9-25

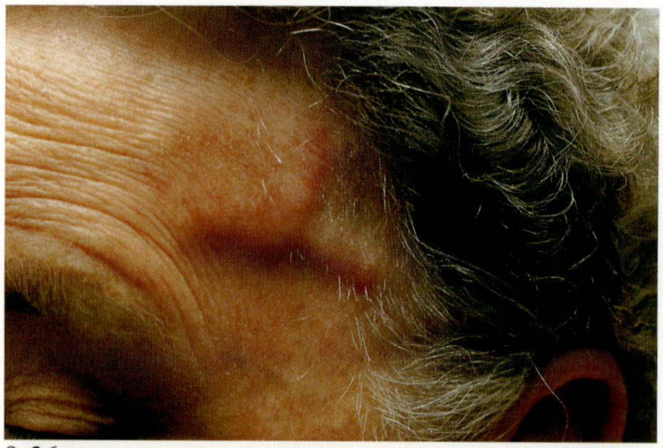

9-26

Fig. 9-26. Temporal arteritis in a 70 year woman. The temporal artery is inflamed, thickened and firm. There is a granulomatous, necrotizing arteritis which can damage any large or medium-sized artery, but favors the temporal arteries. Men and women are equally affected. The disease is almost exclusively limited to individuals greater over 50 years of age. The etiology is unknown. Systemic corticosteroids are the therapy of choice and should be started without delay

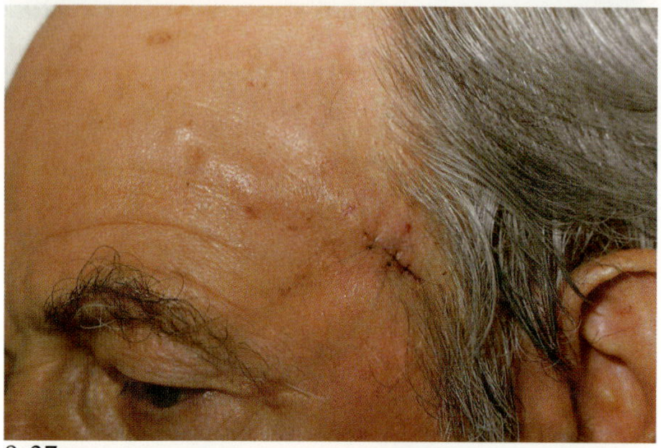

9-27

Fig. 9-27. A 66 year old patient with temporal arteritis following biopsy. The temporal arteries were very swollen and painful to touch. Doppler- and duplex ultrasonography failed to identify any flow. A biopsy is always indicated when there is suspicion of temporal arteritis. Because of the risc of blindness, therapy should be instituted promptly and need not to be delayed whiest awaiting temporal artery biopsy

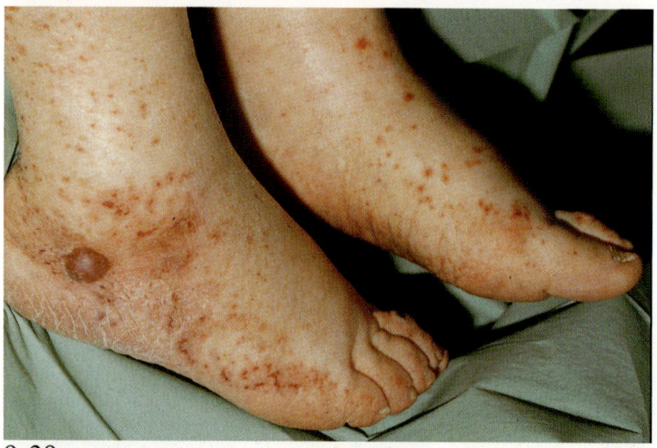

9-28

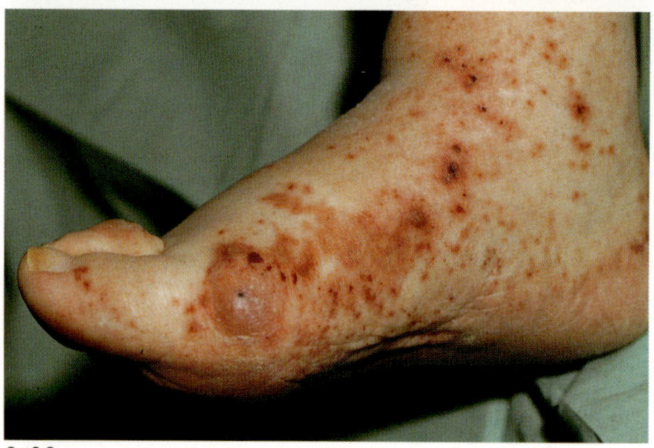

9-29

Figs. 9-28, 9-29. A 21 year old patient who suddenly developed cutaneous necrotizing vasculitis. HENOCH-SCHÖNLEIN purpura is an IgA-related form of hypersensitivity vasculitis with purpura, joint pain, abdominal complaints and glomerulonephritis. The platelet count is normal. Boys are more often affected than girls. Acute phase reactants are elevated and IgA levels can be high. In the biopsy, direct immunofluorescent examination shows deposits of IgA around the dermal and often renal vessels. The outlook is good and systemic corticosteroids are rarely required

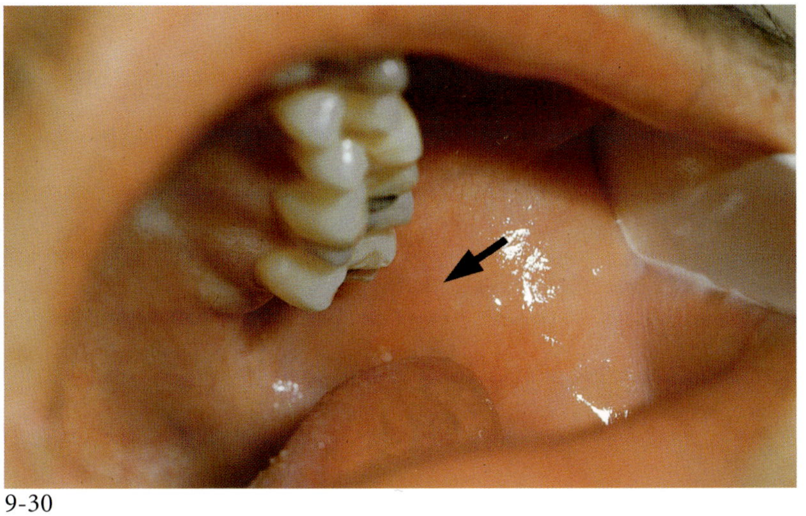

9-30

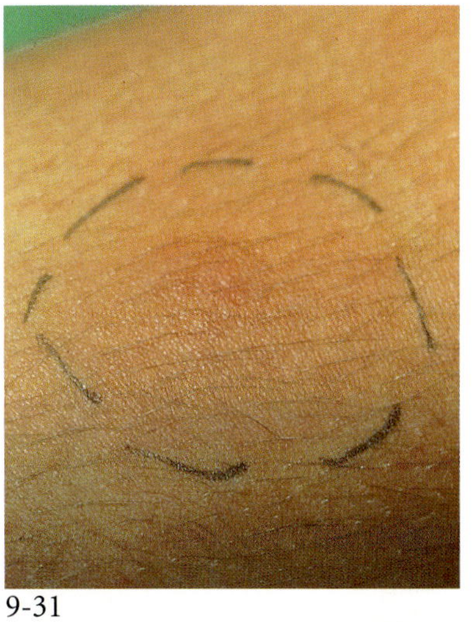

9-31

Figs. 9-30 – 9-32. Typical oral aphthae (*arrow*) in a 22 year old man with BEHÇET syndrome. In addition there were lesions on the penis (*arrow*) and a thrombophlebitis. BEHÇET syndrome is a chronic-recurrent variant of vasculitis characterized by the triad of:

- Oral aphthae
- Genital aphthae
- Ocular lesions (hypopyon and iritis)
- Other lesions include thrombophlebitis, erythema nodosum and pathergy

Men are twice as often affected as women. The disease is most common in Turkey, Iran, Japan and Korea. There is no curative therapy, but symptomatic measures are usually helpful

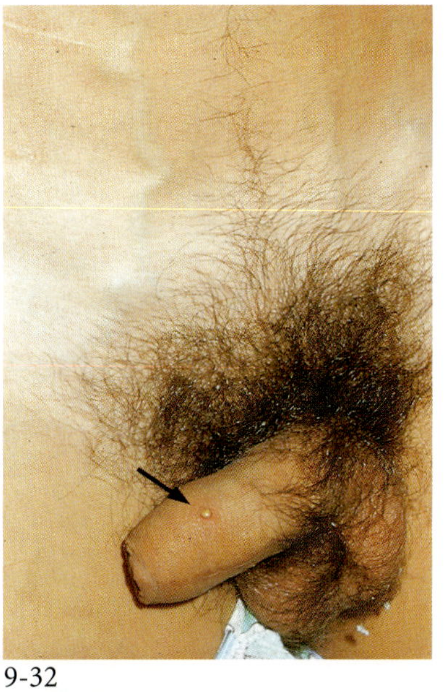

9-32

Figs. 9-33, 9-34. A 45 year old man with acrodermatitis chronica atrophicans (PICK-HERXHEIMER) as a late sequelae of infection with *Borrelia burgdorferi.* There is inflammation of the skin and subcutaneous tissue with eventual atrophy, most typically about distal joints. Histologically there are perivascular infiltrates of lymphocytes, histiocytes and plasma cells. Rarely intimal proliferation and occlusion of small arteries and veins can be seen. (KARL HERXHEIMER, 1861 – 1944, German dermatologist)

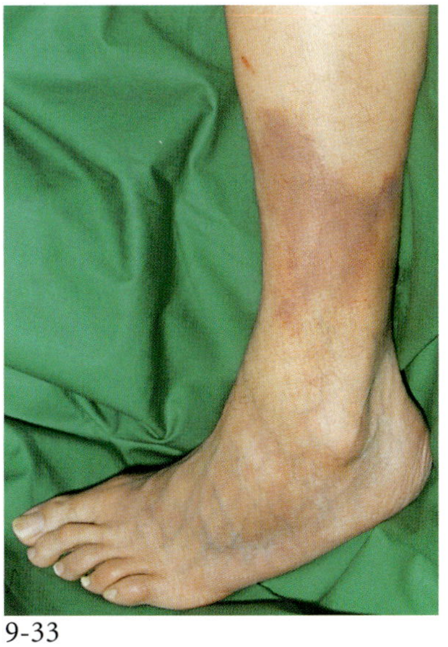

9-33

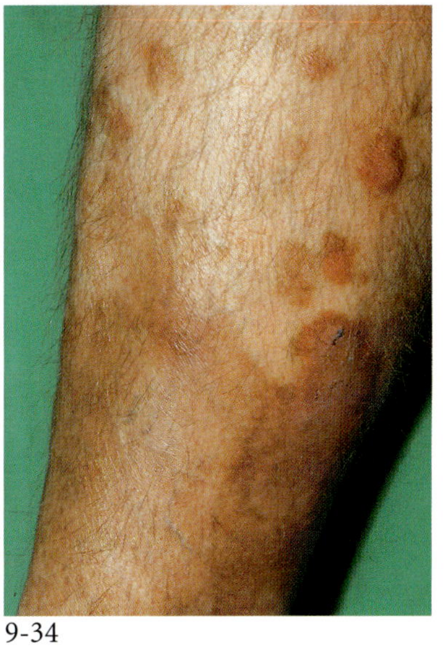

9-34

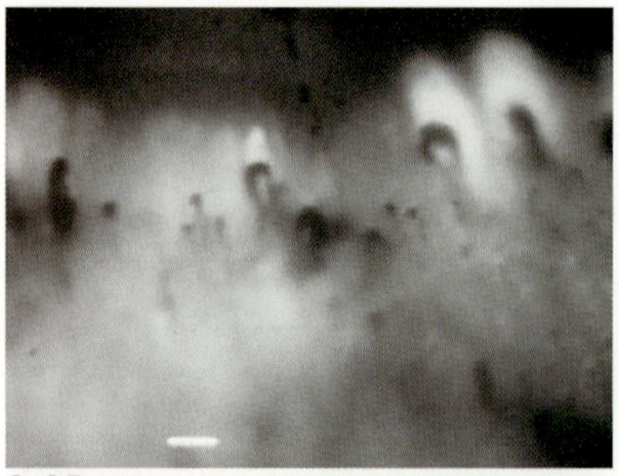

9-35

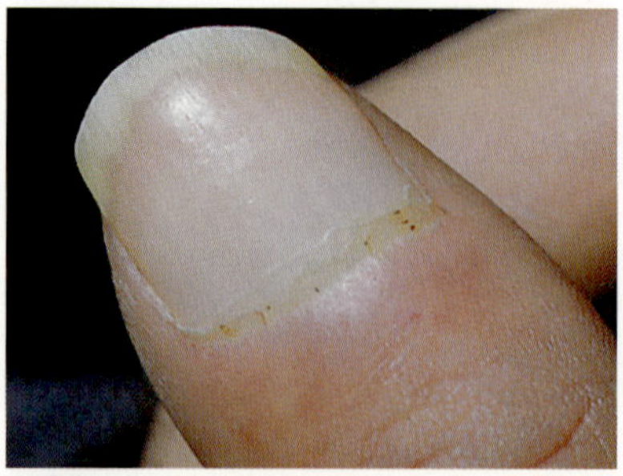

9-36

Figs. 9-35, 9-36. Nail fold microscopy in systemic sclerosis shows avascular zones which probably represent microinfarcts. Rarefaction of the loops is usually seen. Giant capillaries are found in the nail fold; often they are so large that they can be seen with the naked eye. The widened capillaries may have a diameter of 80 μm (normal 8 – 15 μm)

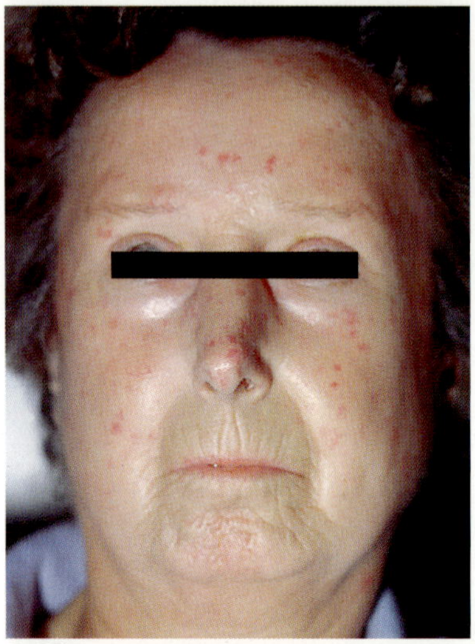

9-37

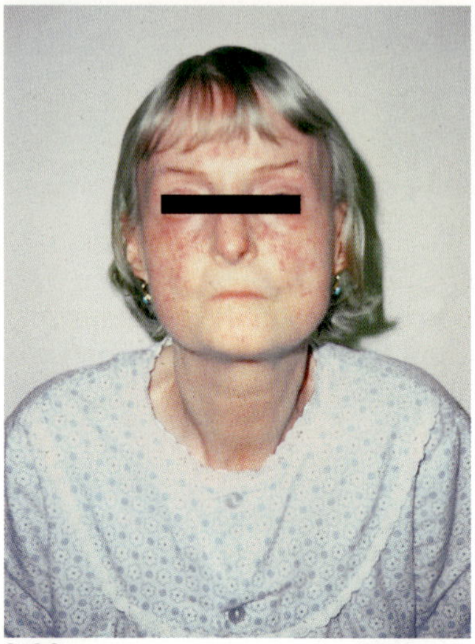

9-38

Figs. 9-37, 9-38. Typical face in scleroderma. The face is mask-like with tight thin lips, narrowed mouth opening and radial folds about the mouth. The retraction of the skin makes the nose appear tight and beaked

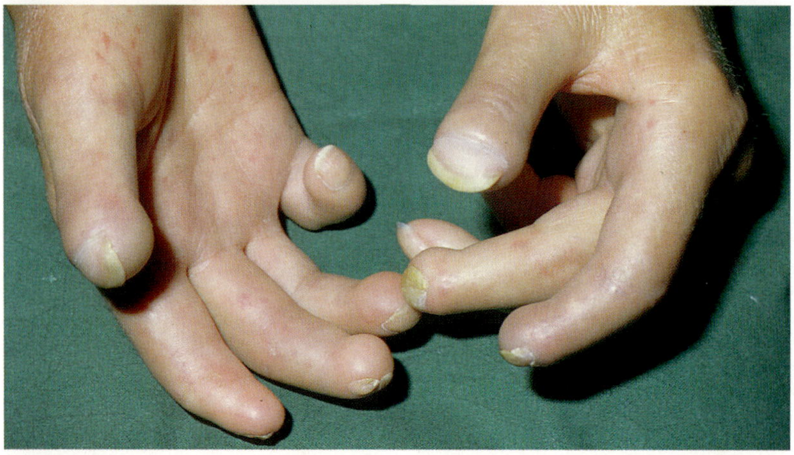

9-39

Fig. 9-39. A 51 year old women with systemic lupus erythematosus and acral problems. Here one sees thickened skin, clubbing and flexed fingers because of the induration. Such fingers have been called "Madonna fingers"

Fig. 9-40. Typical tightened frenulum in 46 year old women with systemic sclerosis

Fig. 9-41. Esophageal swallowing studies in same patient. The patient clinically had trouble with swallowing. Her esophagus is dilated and physiologic contractions are absent

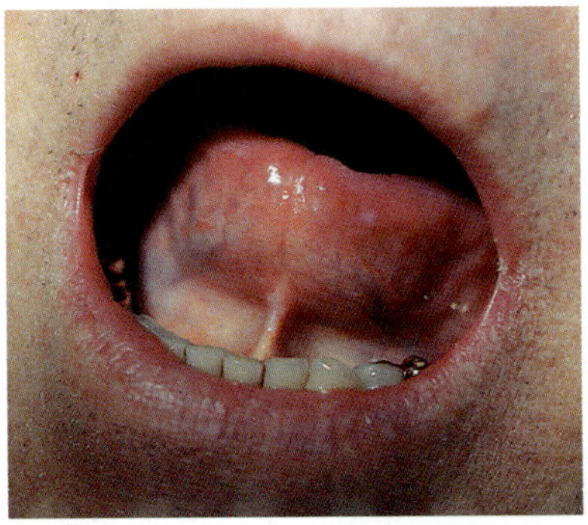

9-40

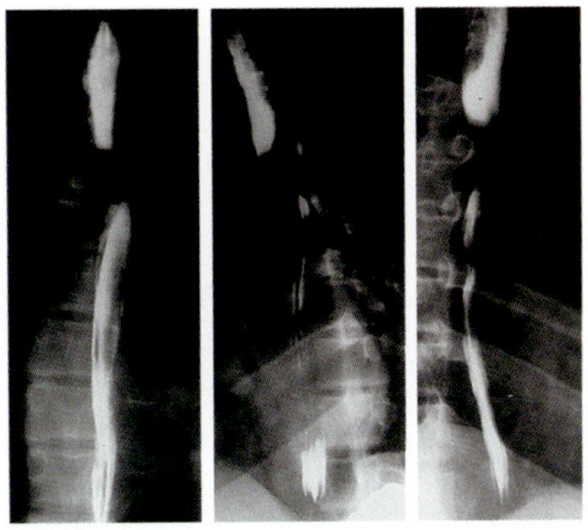

9-41

Fig. 9-42. Severe acral circulatory problems in a 37 year old woman with systemic lupus erythematosus. There is an autoimmune vasculitis, often involving the terminal arteries. Sometimes there are antiphospholipid antibodies which lead to hypercoagulability

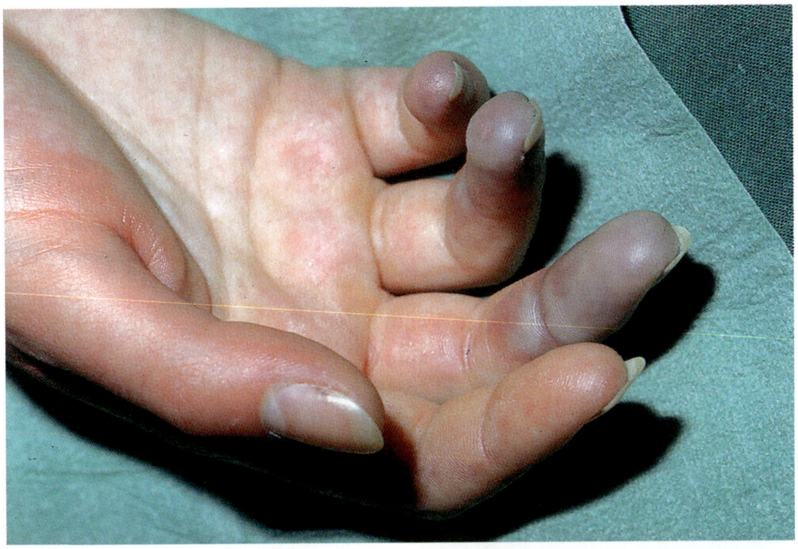

9-42

Figs. 9-43, 9-44. Typical butterfly rash in two young women with systemic lupus erythematosus. The skin findings can be so obvious that they allow a "quick glance" diagnosis. Usually they include erythema, telangiectases, atrophy and mild hyperkeratosis

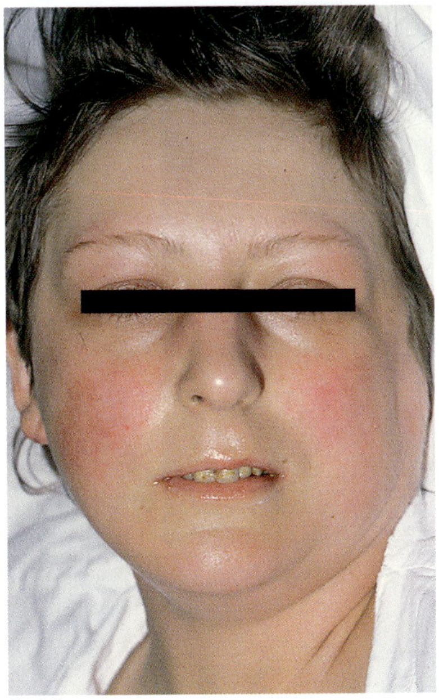

9-43

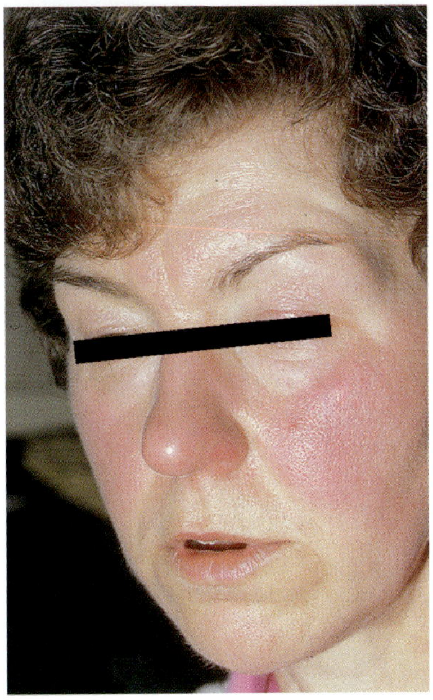

9-44

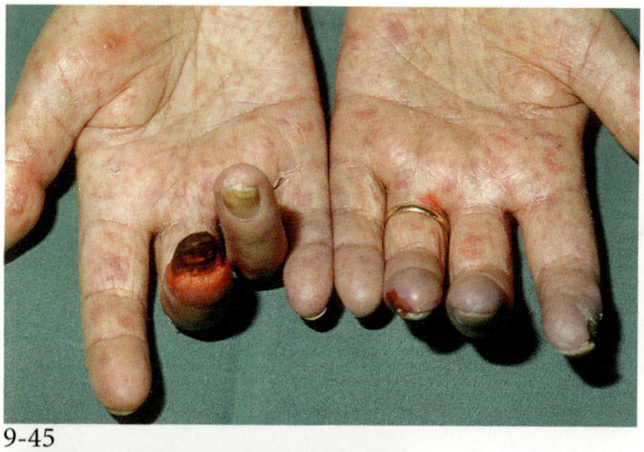
9-45

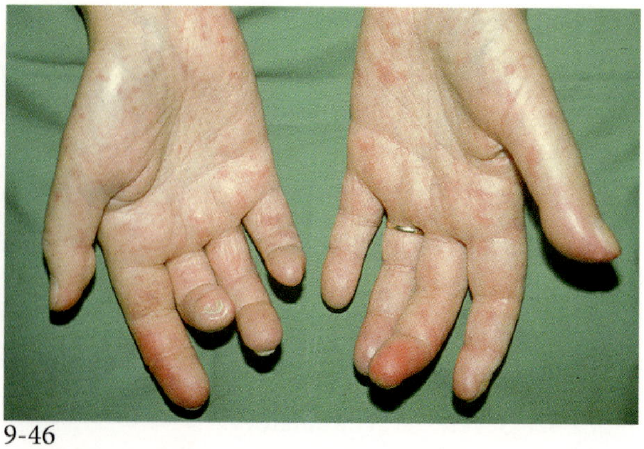
9-46

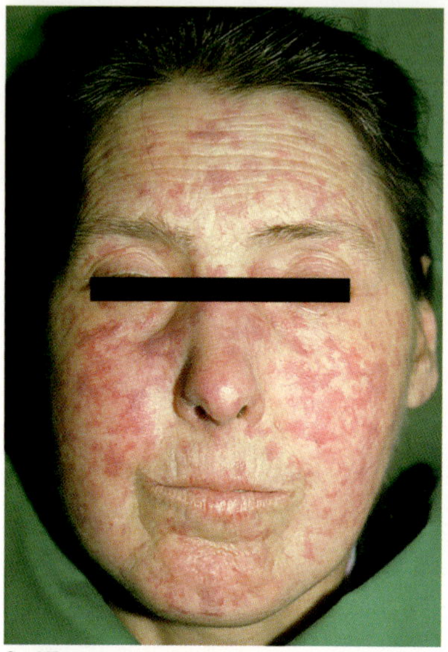
9-47

Figs. 9-45–9-47. CREST is an acronym for calcinosis, RAYNAUD's phenomenon, esophageal motility disturbances, sclerodactyly and telangiectases. It is a limited form of scleroderma with acral cutaneous involvement and anti-centromere antibodies. This patient lost a finger tip because of necrosis. In contrast, in diffuse systemic sclerosis, the internal involvement is more severe and, when skin disease is present, it usually affects the trunk. In about 70% of cases, Scl-70 antibodies are present

Figs. 9-48–9-51. This patient with mixed connective tissue disease died of progressive renal failure. Her skin showed poikiloderma – atrophy, telangiectases and pigmentary changes

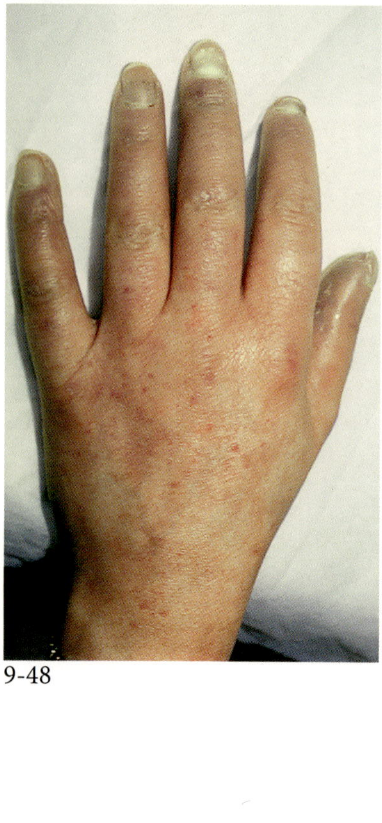
9-48

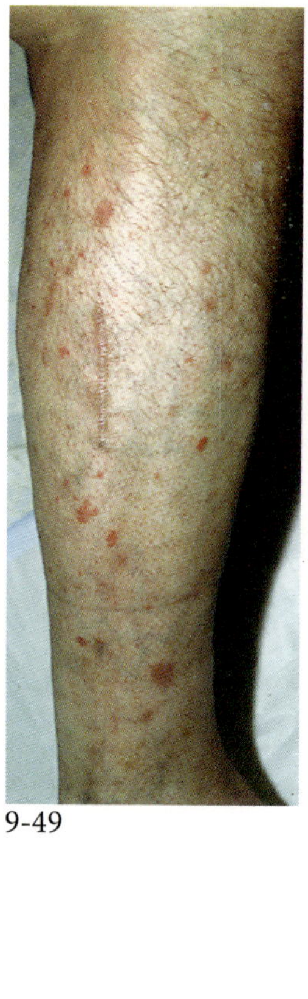
9-49

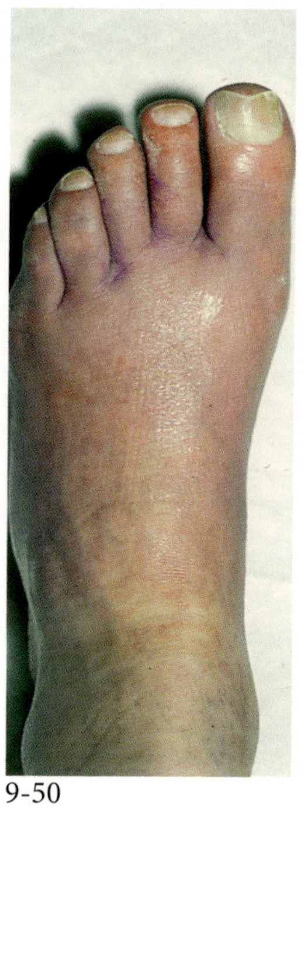
9-50

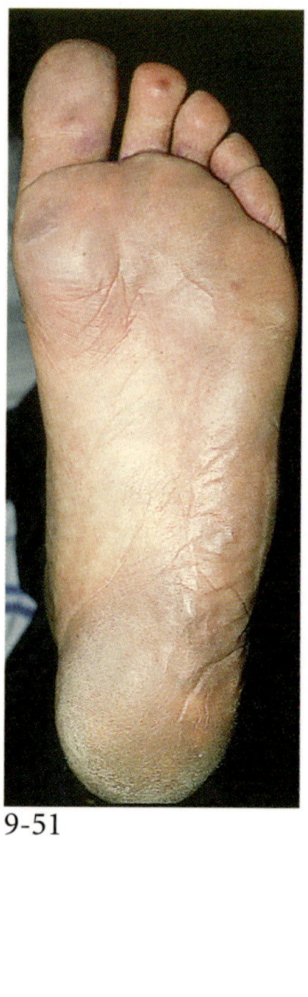
9-51

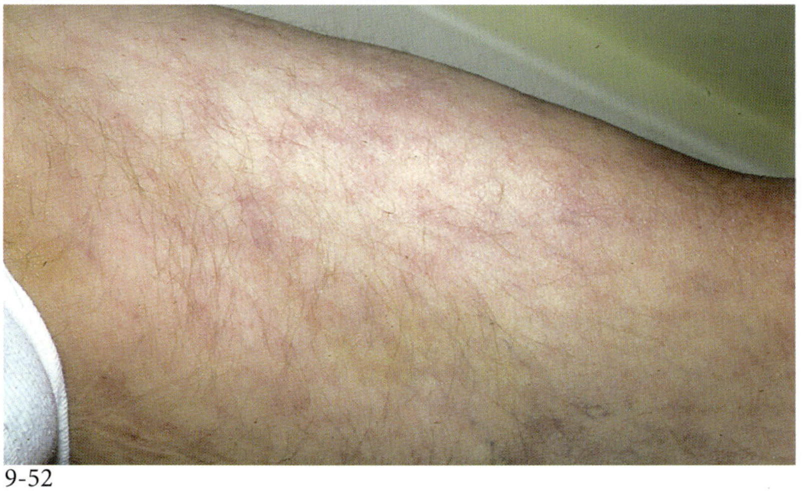

9-52

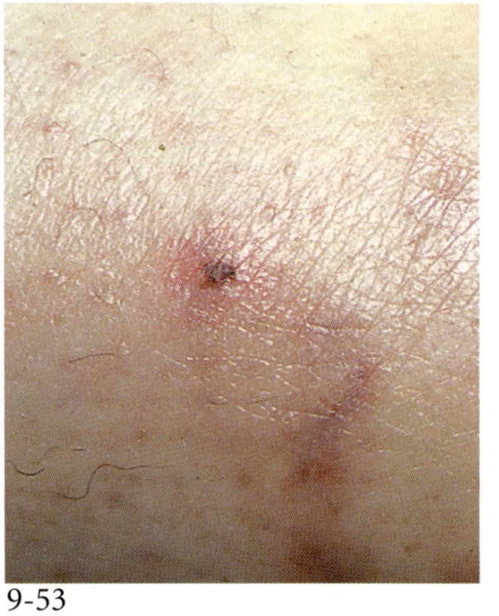

9-53

Figs. 9-52 – 9-55. Vasculitis in a 47 year old patient with long-standing rheumatoid arthritis. There were occlusions of the digital and foot arteries. Clinical changes included:

- Livedo reticularis on the thigh
- Early skin lesion
- Severe vasculitic ulcerations on both shins; the lower figure shows the same ulcer after 6 weeks of conservative therapy

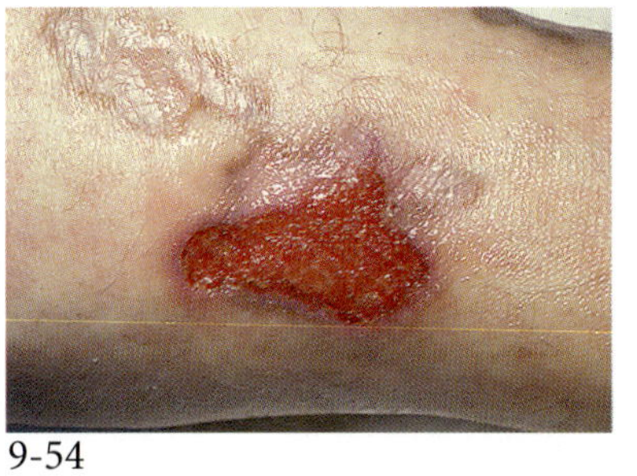

9-54

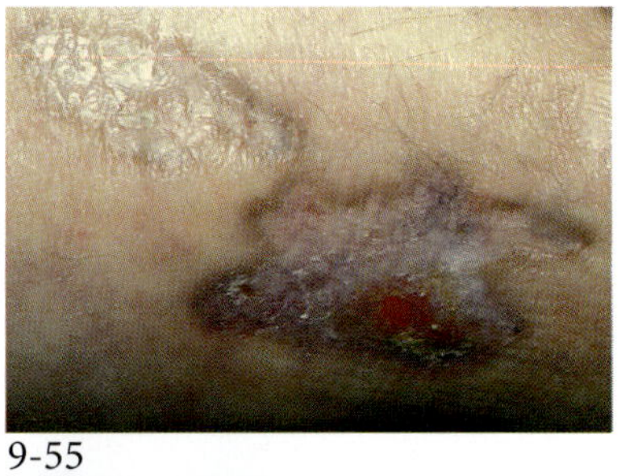

9-55

Figs. 9-56, 9-57. Livedo reticularis on the extensor surface of the forearm (also on the legs), as well as multiple painful vasculitic ulcers on the shin and about the ankle

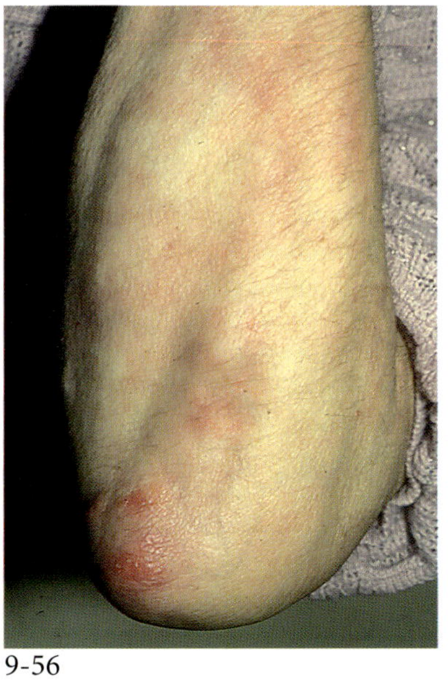

9-56

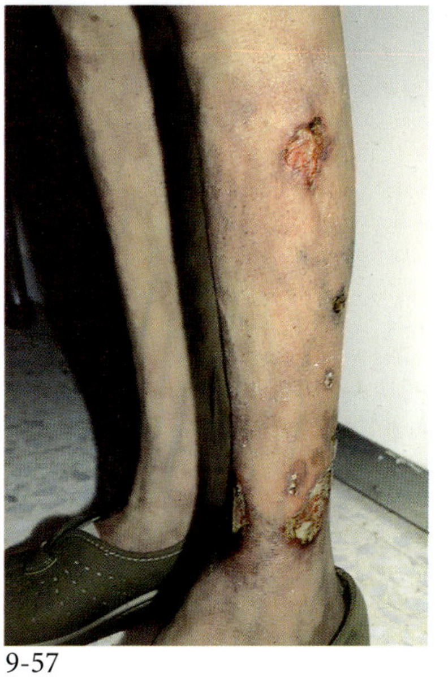

9-57

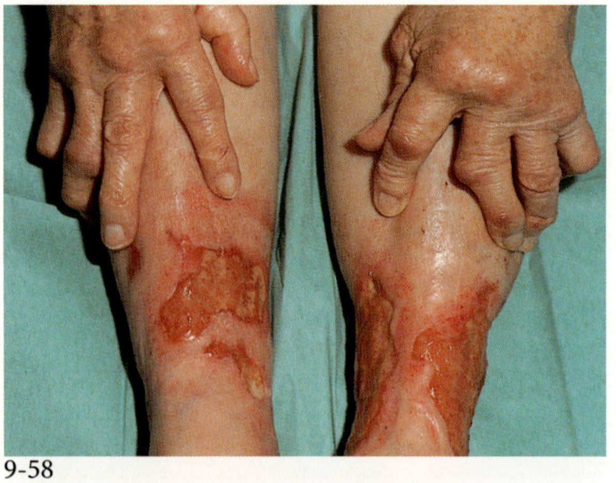

9-58

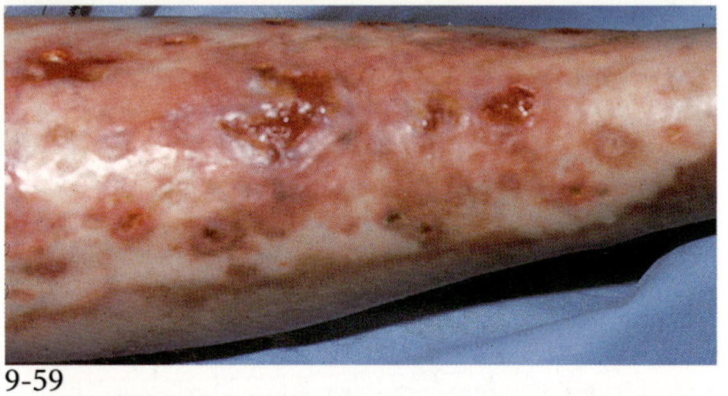

9-59

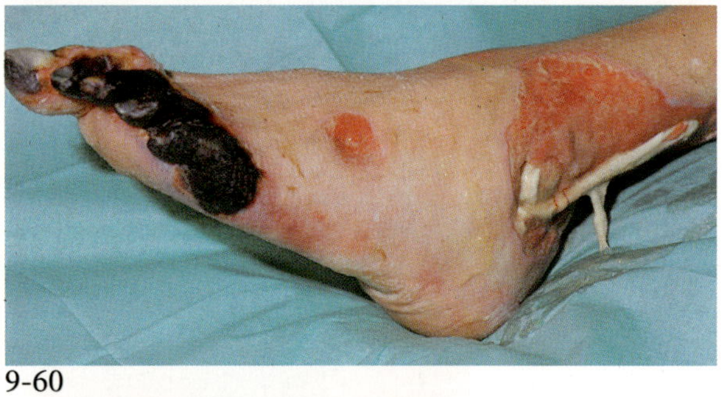

9-60

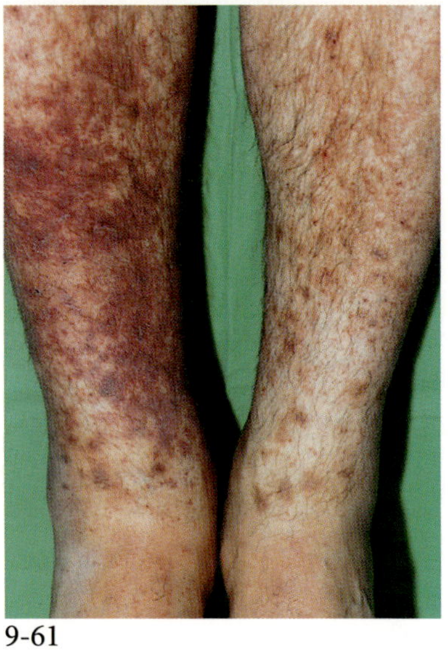

9-61

Fig. 9-58. Rheumatoid ulcer in a 72 year old woman with a long history of rheumatoid arthritis. Note the typical changes of the hands. The ulcerations look like ischemic ulcers and heal poorly. Histologically there is usually a lymphocytic vasculitis of the small distal vessels

Fig. 9-59. Leukocytoclastic angiitis in a 45 year old women. This is a poorly defined group of diseases that primarily affect the skin and are presumably caused by immune complex deposits. A variety of foreign antigens may stimulate the immune reaction; often the trigger is not found

Fig. 9-60. Severe acral necrosis in a 33 year old women with a poorly defined vasculitis. The necrosis is too severe for leukocytoclastic angiitis; her Achilles tendon is exposed. She previously had marked livedo reticularis

Fig. 9-61. Leukocytoclastic angiitis in a 52 year old woman. The palpable purpura cannot be made to disappear with diascopy. This was localized cutaneous vasculitis without evidence of systemic involvement. Cutaneous leukocytoclastic angiitis may be triggered by infections or medications and usually heals spontaneously. Patients with WEGENER's granulomatosis, HENOCH-SCHÖNLEIN purpura, essential cryoglobulinemic vasculitis and many other forms of systemic vasculitis can present with cutaneous lesions. Thus, cutaneous leukocytoclastic angiitis is a diagnosis of exclusion

Criteria of the American College of Rheumatology for the Diagnosis of Cutaneous Leukocytoclastic Angiitis

1. Age at onset >16 years
2. Ingestion of medication at time of first symptoms
3. Palpable purpura
4. Maculo-papular exanthem
5. Biopsy demonstration of leukocytoclastic angiitis

Not all patients have a history of recent use of medication. In many instances, no cause is found. The therapy is based on the underlying disease, if any is identified. The prognosis is good. On rare occasions low-dose systemic corticosteroids are employed

Figs. 9-62 – 9-67. Pseudoxanthoma elasticum (synonym: GRÖNBLAD-STRANDBERG syndrome; E.E.GRÖNBLAD, Swedish ophthalmologist; J.V. STRANDBERG, Swedish ophthalmologist) in a 39 year old female. Pseudoxanthoma elasticum (PXE) is an uncommon genodermatoses, usually inherited in an autosomal dominant pattern. There are abnormalities in the elastic fibers which calcify rapidly. The so-called xanthomatous changes in the skin are typically seen on flexor areas, such as the nape, axilla and inguinal area, as well as the antecubital and popliteal fossae. The retinal changes, known as angioid streaks, represent defects in the elastic fibers of Bruch's membrane. There may also be hemorrhage, ischemia and macular degeneration. Cardiovascular involvement is a major problem for many patients. About 30% – 50% have symptoms of impaired arterial circulation in the legs; the number with asymptomatic arterial stenoses and occlusions is much higher, perhaps as high as 80%. The diagnosis is made on the clinical findings and can be confirmed by a skin biopsy. There is no specific therapy

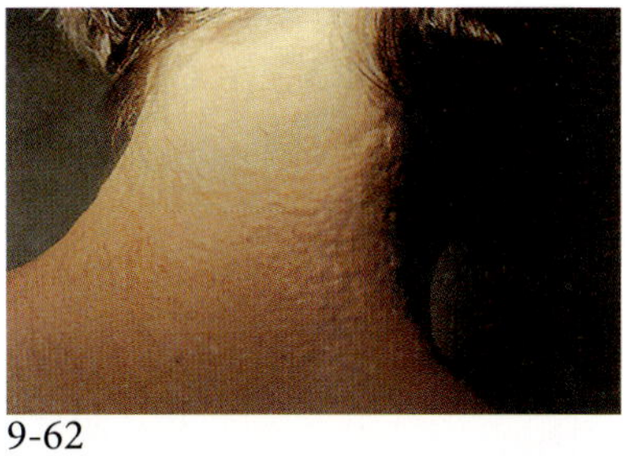

9-62

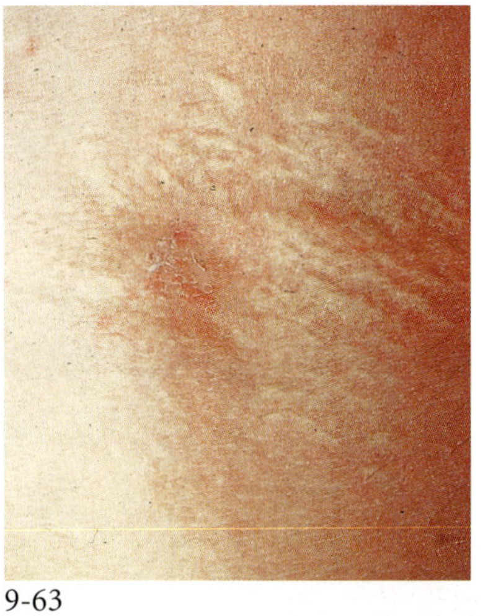

9-63

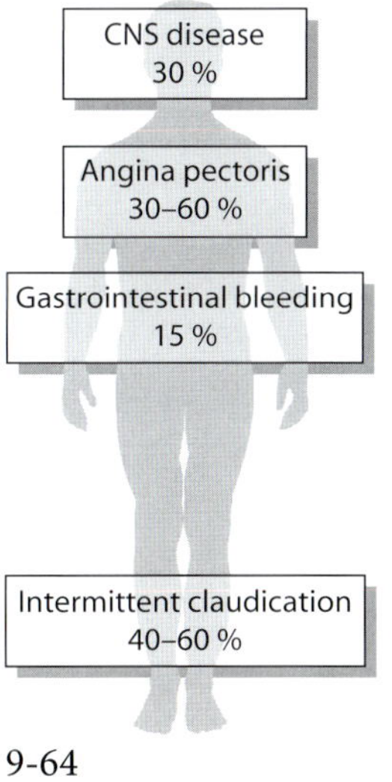

9-64

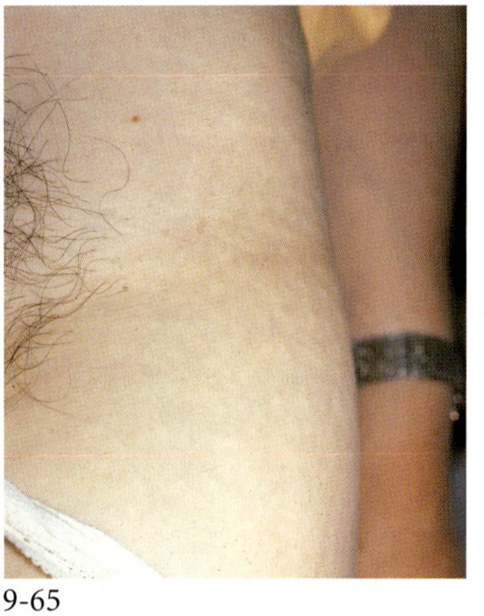

9-65

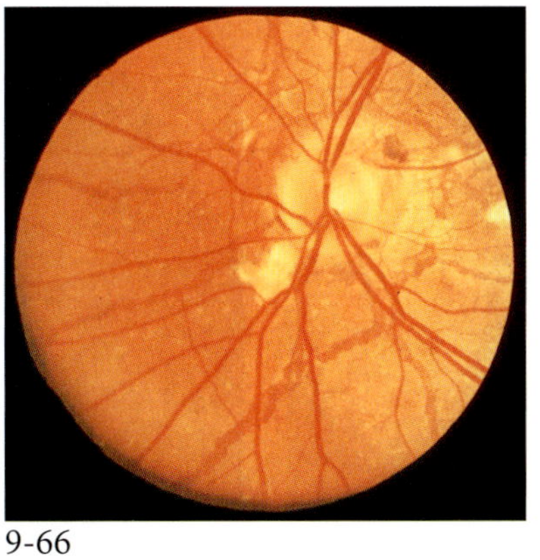

9-66

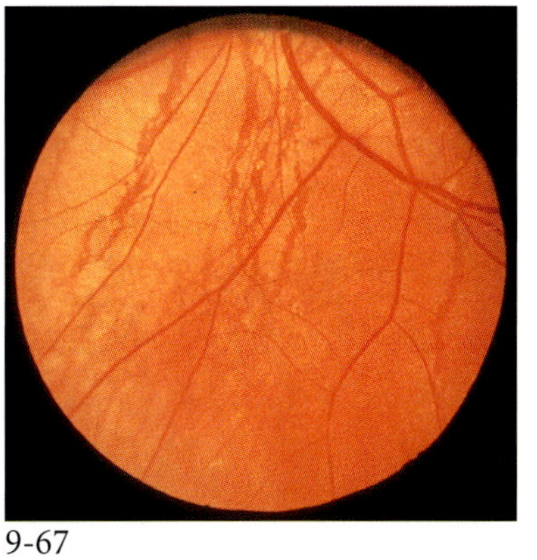

9-67

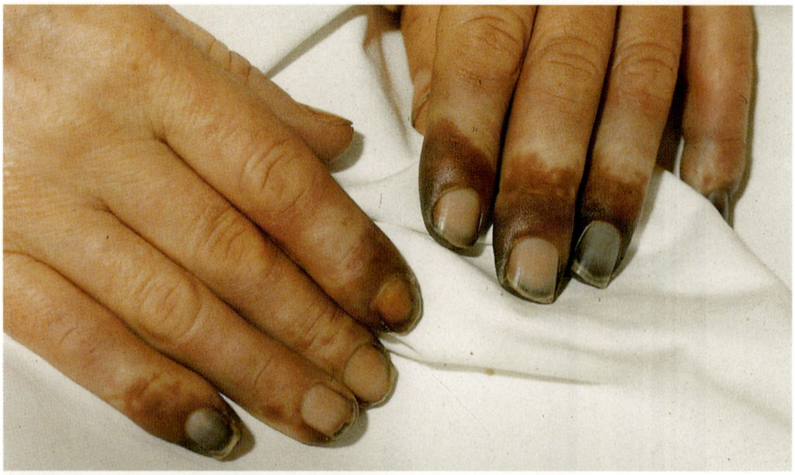

9-68

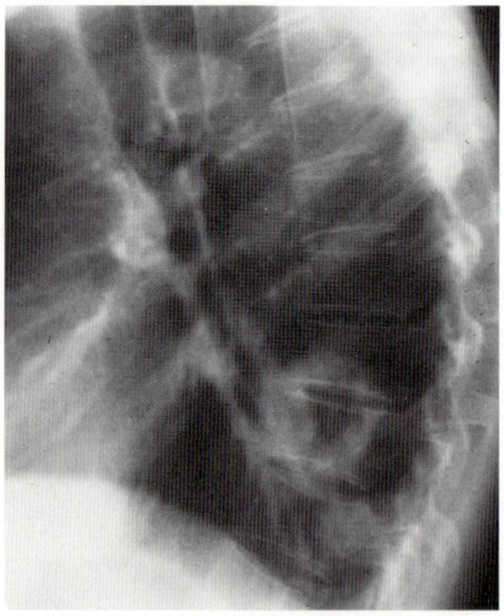

9-69

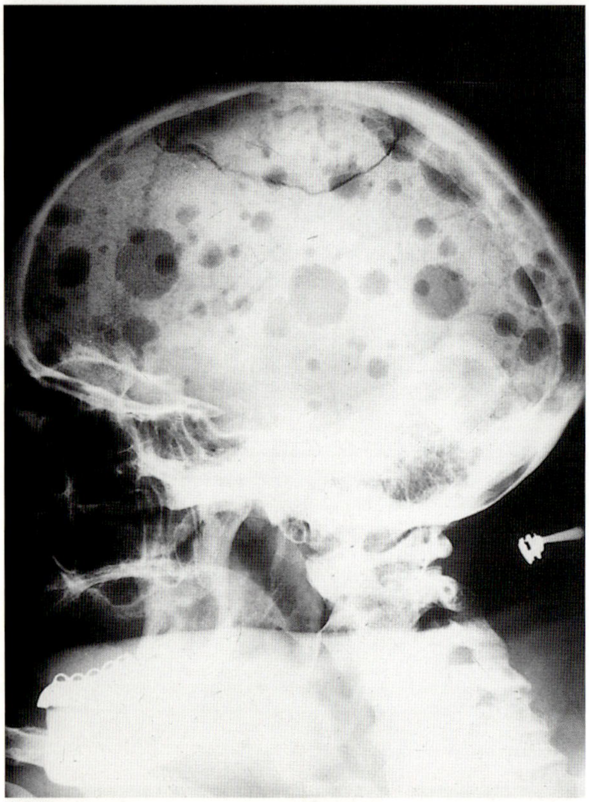

9-70

Fig. 9-68. Severe acral circulatory problems in a 55 year old patient with a bronchial carcinoma. Despite aggressive intervention, finger necrosis could not be avoided. There may be paraneoplastic tendency to thrombosis with elevated fibrinogen and α_2-macroglobulins leading to hyperviscosity

Fig. 9-69. Chest X-ray from the same patient

Fig. 9-70. Skull X-ray of a patient with multiple myeloma showing multiple osteolytic lesions

Figs. 9-71, 9-72. A 52 year old patient with multiple myeloma and hyperviscosity syndrome, showing marked ischemia especially of the second to fourth toes on the left

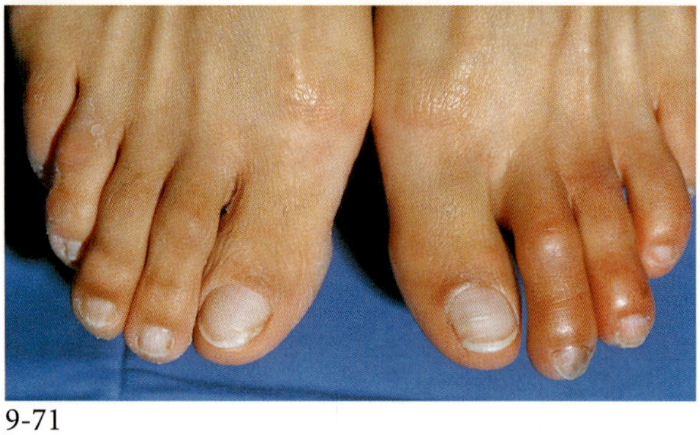

9-71

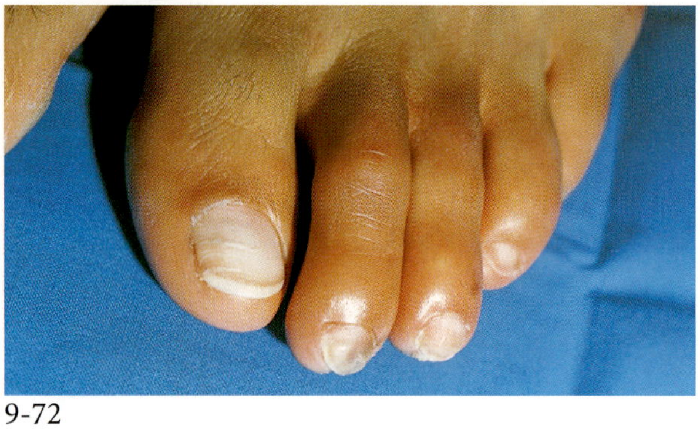

9-72

Figs. 9-73, 9-74. Atrial myxoma demonstrated with magnetic resonance imaging. The left atrium was almost entirely filled by the tumor. The 56 year old patient had experienced multiple emboli in arteries of the lower leg. The transesophageal echocardiogram showed a large myxoma in the left atrium. The diagnosis was confirmed on operation. Smaller myxomas are often asymptomatic and detected on routine examinations; they are often calcified. Myxomas are primarily intravascular tumors of endothelial origin. They can develop in any heart chamber or on a valve. Most atrial myxomas arise from the septum. Women are more often affected than men (3:1 ratio). The first symptoms usually arise between 30 and 60 years of age. While most myxomas are sporadic, some may be familial and others associated with CARNEY's syndrome (cutaneous myxomas, testicular tumors, CUSHING's syndrome)

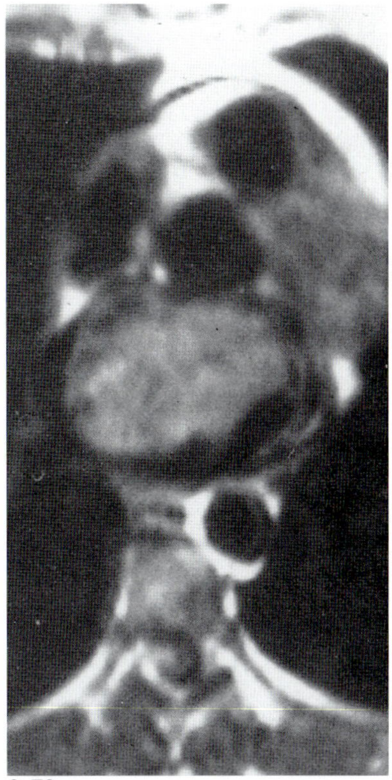

9-73

Figs. 9-75, 9-76. Operative specimen of a large atrial myxoma

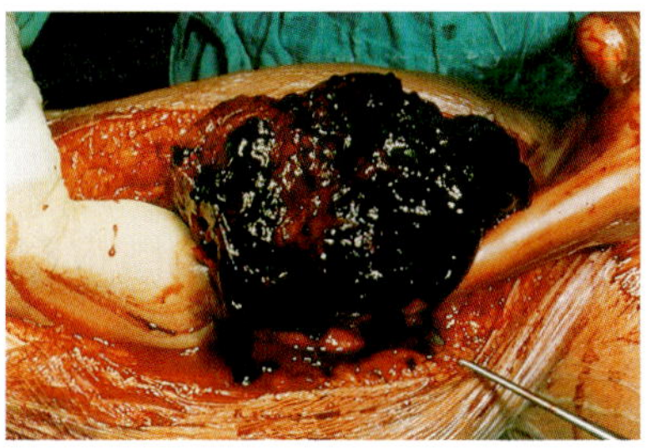

9-75

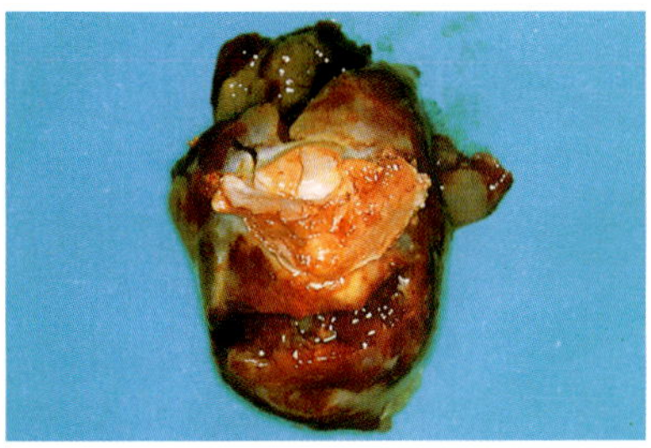

9-76

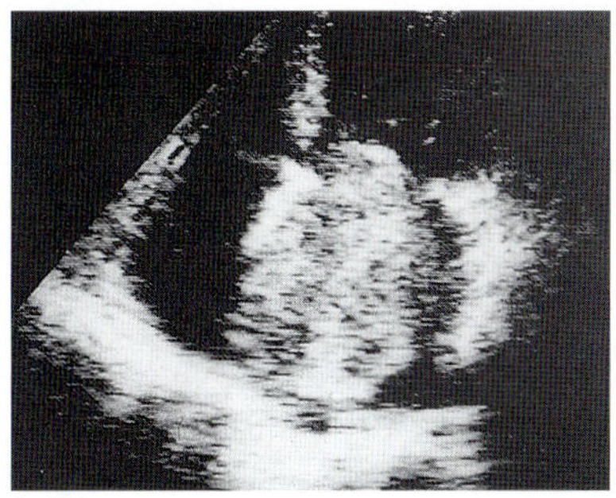

9-74

Fig. 9-77. Bullous pemphigoid. This 73 year old patient suddenly developed tense subepidermal blisters on an erythematous base. There was no obvious trigger. Some of the blisters ruptured, but a large intact one about the ankle is shown. Extensive evaluation revealed no underlying malignancy, although bullous pemphigoid can occasionally be a paraneoplastic marker. The typical auto-antibodies against the bullous pemphigoid antigens in the basement membrane zone were demonstrated. She had an elevated IgE level and eosinophilia. The lesions healed without scarring when she was treated with systemic corticosteroids

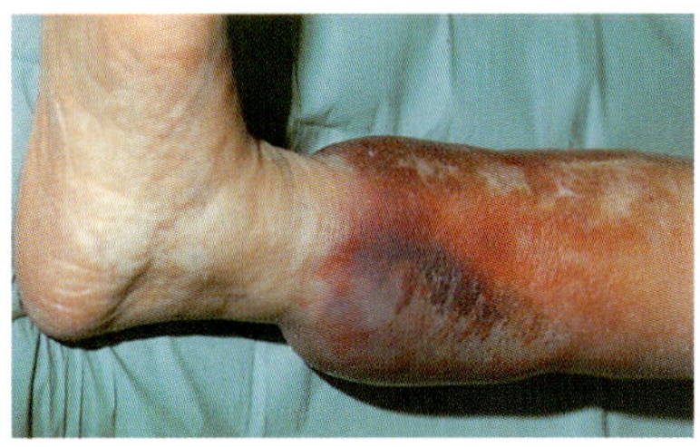

9-77

Part B: Venous System

Chapter 10: Diseases of Veins

Contents

A: Introduction

1. Anatomy of the Pelvic and Leg Veins

The veins of the extremities are divided into a superficial and a deep vein system. The superficial system is subcutaneous and separated from the deep system by the fascia. Connecting or perforating veins run through the fascia joining the two systems.

The deep veins accompany the main arteries and are often paired. Under normal conditions 80% of the venous drainage of the leg transported in the deep veins and 20% in the superficial veins.

The venous valves aid the return of blood to the heart and protect the venules and capillaries against excessively high pressures during muscular activity or prolonged standing. Except for the inferior vena cava, all the pelvic and leg veins have a varying number of valves (Table 10-1).

Greater Saphenous Vein

The greater saphenous vein arises from the superficial venous arcade on the dorsal aspect of the foot, runs along the inner aspect of the calf and thigh and joins the femoral vein in the inguinal region. There is always an effective valve at the point where the two vessels join, and two to three additional distal valves. In 20% of individuals the greater saphenous vein is duplicated; the two trunks join just distal to the fossa ovalis

Lesser Saphenous Vein

The lesser or small saphenous vein begins behind and just beneath the lateral malleolus and runs along the back of the calf. The exact site

Table 10-1. Number of venous valves

Vein	Number of valves	
	Average	Range
Superficial femoral	4	1–9
Popliteal	2	1–5
Posterior tibial	10	7–20
Anterior tibial	10	9–12
Peroneal	10	6–12
Greater saphenous	10	7–20
Lesser saphenous	8	5–15

where it joins the popliteal vein is highly variable. In more than 50% of individuals, the junction is located 1–4 cm proximal to the knee joint.

The femoro-popliteal vein approaches the lesser saphenous vein from a cranio-medial direction. This vein lies in an epifascial position and also shows a wide anatomic variation. Of clinical importance is its ability to serve as a communication between the great and lesser saphenous veins when the latter has incompetent valves (the GIACOMINI anastomosis – CARLO GIACOMINI, 1840–1898, Italian anatomist). This can cause distal greater saphenous varicosities.

Deep Subfascial Veins

The deep leg veins are named after the accompanying artery. In the calf the posterior tibial, peroneal and anterior tibial veins are usually paired. They have a large number of valves, as required by the marked hydrostatic pressure. They all join the popliteal vein just below the knee; V. poplitea then passes with the popliteal artery through the popliteal space.

The muscular veins are another distinct vein group. They too have a large number of valves. The soleus veins join the peroneal vein in the lower part of the calf. The gastrocnemius veins join the popliteal vein just above the knee joint. The superficial and common femoral veins run parallel to the femoral arteries until the inguinal ligament where the common femoral vein becomes the external iliac vein.

Perforating Veins

The perforating veins pass through the fascia connecting the superficial and deep veins. They are of great importance both in the development of venous disease of the legs and in its surgical treatment. Their valves direct the blood flow from the surface into the deep system. Especially important are the perforating veins on the medial side of the calf that join the posterior tibial vein. They are found along LINTON's line, a vertical line just posterior to the medial malleolus and are known as the COCKETT group of perforating veins (I–II–III) and SHERMAN's vein.

Pelvic Veins

The blood from the legs goes via the external and common iliac veins into the inferior vena cava. The common iliac vein is formed by the joining of the external and internal iliac veins at about the level of the sacro-iliac joint. Intimal proliferation in the left common iliac vein at its junction with the inferior vena cava is a risk factor for the development of leg and pelvic vein thromboses. The left common iliac vein is crossed at this point by the right common iliac artery and the arterial pulsations may play a role in causing the endothelial proliferation and left ilio-femoral thrombophlebitis (MAY-THURNER syndrome).

Inferior Vena Cava

The valveless inferior vena cava passes through the diaphragm on the right just anterior to the vertebral column. It receives blood from the renal and adrenal veins, the right ovarian vein, the hepatic veins and many parietal veins. In about 1% of individuals, there is a double infrarenal inferior vena cava.

Morphology of the Vein Wall

The diameter of the veins varies from less than1 cm to 4 cm. The wall is made up of a variety of mesenchymal elements. Elastin allows distensibility; collagen offers support, and the proteoglycans help modulate vessel permeability and have a sieve effect. The veins of the legs are somewhat thicker and stronger because of the increased pressures to which they are routinely exposed.

The three layers of the venous wall are somewhat different from those of arteries. The intima consists of a basement membrane covered by luminal endothelial cells. It is joined to the media by collagen fibers. The media is made up of coiled or corkscrew collagen and elastic fibers admixed with smooth muscle bundles. In the adventitia, the fiber network is bound to the interstitium, stabilizing the vein.

2. Physiologic Basis of Venous Stasis

Low Pressure System and Venous Return

In contrast to the arterial system, the venous system is highlighted by:

- Low intraluminal pressure
- Slower blood flow and thus greater blood volume

The main physiologic tasks of the veins are to transport blood centripetally, to store blood modulating blood volume and to adjust the pressure in the venules. The elasticity, valve system and superficial–deep networking accomplish this normally. This low pressure system contains about 80% of the entire blood volume. Its compliance is about 200 times that of the arterial system. The arteries only have about 15% of the blood volume.

The return of the blood to the heart is regulated through three different mechanisms, depending on the position of the body and venous load.

Abdominal Suction Pump

The abdominal-thoracic two-phase pump is an important factor in returning venous blood to the heart. During inspiration, the intra-abdominal pressure is raised, which compresses the veins in the retroperitoneal space and produces a brief centrifugal blood flow. Normally the valves in the peripheral veins close; if they are incompetent, then reflux occurs with increased peripheral venous pressure. In expiration the diaphragm rises and the intra-abdominal pressure drops. As a result there is a negative pressure exerted on the venous system, encouraging blood flow to the heart as the valves open.

Color duplex ultrasonography can demonstrate these breathing-related variations, in a study of the common femoral vein. Figure 10-1 shows the frequency-time spectrum in the inspiratory and expiratory phases. The abdominal suction pump system is most important in individuals who are lying down and at rest. In a standing or walking person, the effects of gravity and the muscle pump are more important.

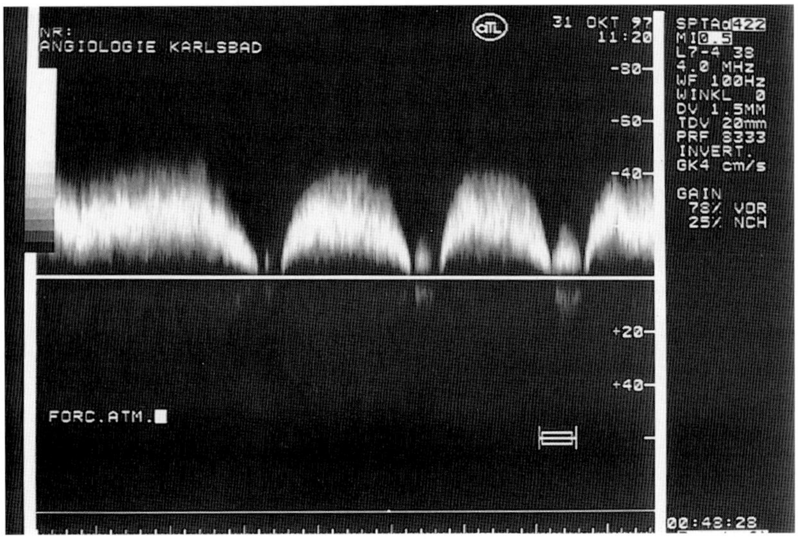

Fig. 10-1. Frequency-time spectrum showing the inspiratory stoppage and expiratory flow in the common femoral artery

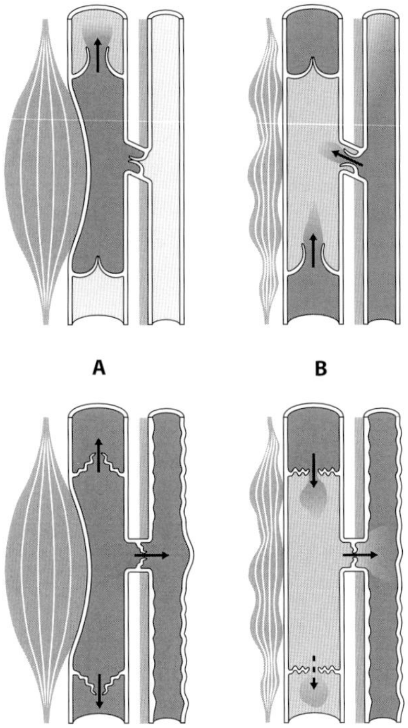

Fig. 10-2 A, B. The muscle-fascia pump. The physiological condition is shown *above*. Muscle contraction and valve closure (**A**), followed by relaxation (**B**) drive the blood towards the heart. In the *lower drawings*, venous insufficiency is shown, as the incompetent valves allow blood to flow centrifugally and back into the epifascial compartment

Muscle-Fascia Pump

The pumping action of the muscles combined with the valve-like action of the fascia plays a major role in venous return from the extremities when an individual is walking or otherwise active. This mechanism has several different aspects (Fig. 10-2).

(a) The subfascial veins running through the muscles are squeezed like a sponge by the contraction of the muscles. This is the main stimulus to venous blood flow in the legs.
(b) The larger veins running adjacent to the muscles are also compressed by the muscle contraction. Because of their valve network, blood is directed centripetally. As the muscles relax and the fascial space expands, a suction effect is created pulling more blood into the system. One can view the system as moving the blood step-by-step from one valve to another.
(c) The perforating veins offer a site where blood can be sucked from the epifascial layer into the deeper system. They are closed when the muscles contract as the fascial slits serve as valves. Significant pressure does not normally develop in these short thin paired veins.

The action of the muscle pump of the legs in exercise is comparable to that of the heart at rest. The firmness of the skin increases the extrafascial play of the pumping, while the fascia and muscles work against each in the deep space.

Arterio-venous Pressure Difference

While the thoraco-abdominal pressure difference and the muscle-fascia pump play the major role in adjusting the venous return to the degree of activity, the arterio-venous pressure difference is decisive when the individual is at rest. Variations in blood pressure, blood flow and arterio-venous shunting can regulate this pressure.

3. Epidemiology

- Some 70% of the population in Western societies have pathologic changes in their leg vein system.
- Women are more often affected than men.
- About 20% have significant varicosities of a superficial vein.
- About 10% have chronic venous insufficiency.
- More than 1% have a stasis ulcer.
- About 0.02% of patients die yearly from pulmonary embolus.

4. Diseases of Leg Veins

4.1 Varicose Veins

Definition

Varicose veins are permanently dilated, cylindrical or saccular epifascial or perforating veins damaged as a result of chronic high pressure and degenerative changes. One distinguishes between primary (idiopathic or congenital) varicosities and secondary or acquired forms. The term varicose is taken from the Latin varicosus and means knotted. The venous dilation can be focal or lengthy and is often combined with coiling, lengthening or tangling.

Etiology and Pathogenesis

The following factors are responsible for primary varicosities:

- Familial predisposition; it is estimated that about 75% of varicosities are genetically determined.
- Increasing age.
- Congenital absence of the venous valves.
- Vein wall weakness caused by mechanical or hormonal factors.
- Obesity (perhaps more of a factor in women).
- Pregnancies (21% of childless women have varicosities; 34% of those with one child, and 42% of those with two)

Varicose veins are associated with a reduction in the muscular and elastic fibers in the wall of the vein. Both structural defects in the fibers and proteins of the venous wall and increased activity of lysosomal enzymes play a role. The venous valves also tend to weaken with increasing age.

Most primary varicosities begin in the distribution of the greater saphenous vein (>75%). Secondary varicosities are usually associated with post-thrombotic events, but may reflect an arterio-venous fistula.

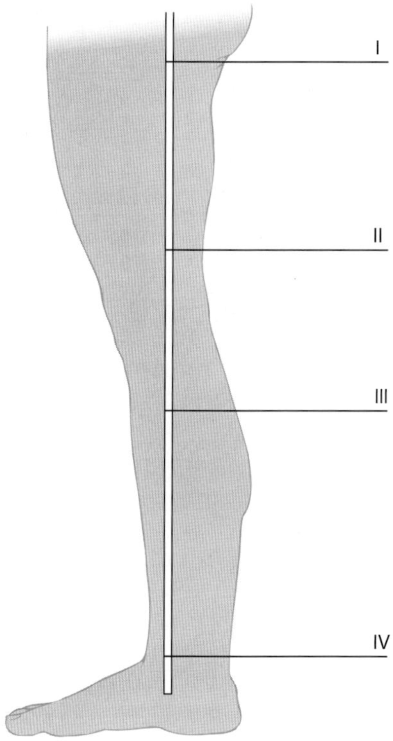

Fig. 10-3. Stages of varicosities of the greater saphenous vein.

Clinical Features

Varicosities of the major epifascial veins alone usually cause few symptoms. Over years, the patients may complain of a heavy or tired feeling in their legs following prolonged sitting or standing. Pains, cramps and edema are uncommon. The main symptoms are:

- Heavy feeling in legs, which improves with walking or running
- Tired legs
- Pain in the area of the varicosities, especially when standing

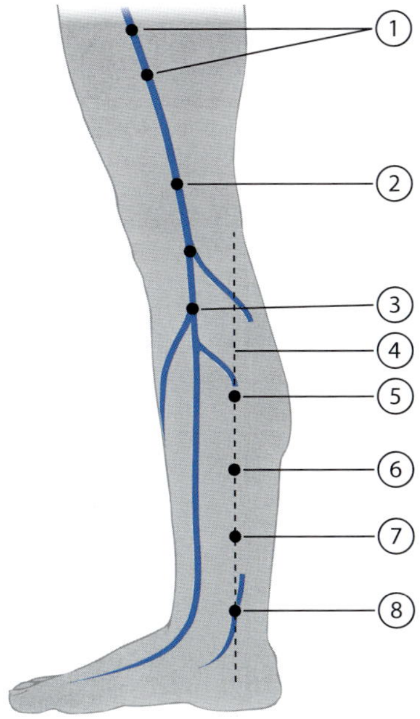

10-4

- Premenstrual pain around the varicosities, as well as over reticular and star-burst veins
- Ankle edema, especially in the evening
- Increased symptoms when warm
- Improvement when the leg is elevated
- Rarely cramps in the foot or leg at night

1a. Varicosities of the Greater Saphenous Vein

The varicosities of the greater saphenous vein arise because of an incompetent valve at the sapheno-femoral junction and spread distally.

Stages of Greater Saphenous Vein Varicosities

Stage I: Incompetent valves in the sapheno-femoral junction (no clinical findings)

Stage II: Incompetent valves between the inguinal area and one hand-breadth above the knee (minimal clinical changes, scattered star-burst veins and reticular varicosities)

Stage III: Incompetent valves from the inguinal region to below the knee

Stage IV: Incompetent valves from the inguinal region to the medial malleolus

1b. Varicosities of the Accessory Veins

There are four major types of varicosities involving accessory or collateral veins that feed into the greater saphenous vein.

- Varicosities of the accessory lateral vein that runs from the anterio-lateral aspect of the thigh distally often over the knee to reach the greater saphenous vein
- Varicosities of the medial accessory vein that runs on the anterio-medial aspect of the thigh
- Varicosities of the dorsal venous arch that runs on the anterio-lateral aspect of the lower leg
- Varicosities of the posterior crural venous arch that runs on the medial aspect of the lower leg; this is also the origin of the Cockett veins

1c. Varicosities of the Lesser Saphenous Vein (Fig. 10-5)

- Stage I: Incompetent valves at the junction with the popliteal vein
- Stage II: Incompetent valves from the knee to mid-calf
- Stage III: Incompetent valves from the knee to the lateral malleolus

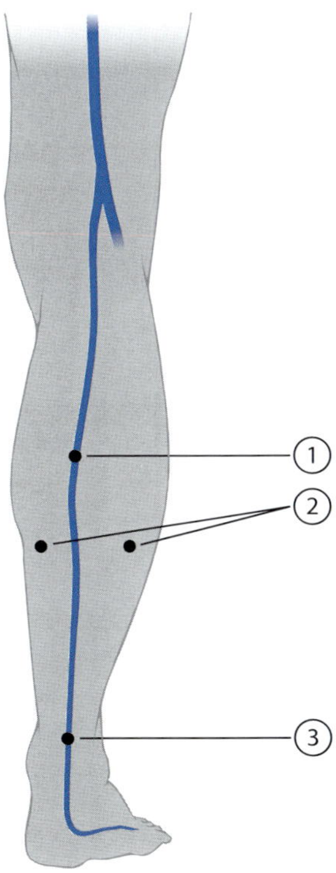

10-5

Fig. 10-4. Location of the most important perforating veins associated with the greater saphenous vein. ① Dodd group; ② Hunter; ③ Boyd; ④ Linton line; ⑤ Sherman (24 cm); ⑥ Cockett III (18 cm); ⑦ Cockett II (13.5 cm); ⑧ Cockett I (6.7 cm)

Fig. 10-5. Location of the most important perforating veins associated with the lesser saphenous vein. ① gastrocnemius point (May); ② lateral perforating veins; ③ 12 cm perforating vein

1d. Other Types of Varicosities

Reticular Varicosities. Small matted or net-like collection of veins, of no hemodynamic importance, often seen without insufficiency of the major veins.

Spider Varicosities. These tiny intradermal micro- varicosities arise from larger veins. They may have an arterial – capillary component and be red, or be primarily venous and thus blue. They are most commonly seen on the medial aspect of the thigh, and on the medial and lateral aspects of the foot where they may have a wreath-like appearance. In contrast to telangiectases, they cannot be completely emptied by pressure.

Canyon Varicosities. Patients with advanced chronic venous insufficiency and phlebosclerosis may have superficial thin-walled, membrane-like veins which appear to lie in chiseled paths or canyons in the sclerotic dermis.

Juvenile Varicosities. Juvenile varicosities can arise because of incompetent valves in epifascial veins where they penetrate the fascia. They can also be associated with deep vein insufficiency.

Recurrent Varicosities. Recurrent varicosities may develop following sclerotherapy or an operation. In the latter case, branches are often left behind as the junction between an accessory vein and a trunk vein was tied off.

Diagnosis

History

A positive family history is common. More than 70% of varicosities can be attributed to genetic predisposition.

Inspection and Palpation

A varicosity of the superficial system is most easily recognized when the patient is standing. Simple inspection allows one to identify most types of varicosities. Palpable holes in the fascia often help to identify incompetent perforating veins.

Tests

The many standard functional tests (TRENDELENBURG, PERTHES, SCHWARTZ, PRATT and LINTON) play no role today, as they have been replaced by reliable non-invasive ultrasonography.

Diagnostic Procedures

Doppler Ultrasonography and Color Duplex Ultrasonography. Continuous wave Doppler ultrasonography or color duplex ultrasonography can be used to identify incompetent valves in the superficial and deep venous systemic and document the extent of insufficiency (stages I–IV) with the help of the Valsalva maneuver.

Phlebomanometry (Vein Pressure Measurement). Measuring the venous pressure before and after a fixed amount of exercise was formerly an important way of measuring the capacity on demand of the venous system (dynamic venous return flow). These studies were time-consuming and invasive; today they are rarely used except for very complex cases or when trying to assess the degree of severity of an advanced post-thrombotic syndrome, such as in a disability evaluation.

Photoplethysmography/Light Reflection Rheography (LRR). This technique is based on measuring the changes in a reflected ray of light as caused by flowing erythrocytes. While the procedure is popular, it is rarely of help in distinguishing between various venous diseases, but may be useful as a means of following changes in venous flow.

Phlebography. Phlebography may be a useful alternative to ultrasonography when planning surgical procedures. Its main advantage is a more extensive and permanent documentation of the changes. Phlebography is very dependent on the skills of the examiner, just as is Doppler or duplex ultrasonography.

Therapy

Varicosities should not be ignored. They should be treated if they are causing the patient problems or if there is any sign of chronic venous insufficiency. Additional indications include recurrent superficial thrombophlebitis or rupture of a varicosity. In younger patients, treating varicosities may be viewed as a prophylactic measure in some instances.

General Measures

Practical steps include weight loss and regular physical activity (walking, swimming, bicycling). Individuals with a job where they are sitting or standing for long periods should be encouraged to interrupt this position frequently. If possible, elevating the legs occasionally during the day is often helpful.

Surgical Removal

If the great or lesser saphenous veins or perforating veins require treatment, the only treatment is surgery. In addition to the standard vein ligation and stripping, microsurgical techniques have been developed.

Sclerotherapy

Injection of sclerosing agents is useful for small diameter vessels and to treat residual or recurrent varicosities after the removal of major veins. Attempts to use sclerotherapy to treat the major veins, the larger accessory veins or large perforating veins are usually doomed to failure.

Compression Therapy

Regular compression therapy is the conservative alternative approach for varicosities and chronic venous insufficiency. In addition, it is the most important step following sclerotherapy or vein stripping. Compression is also required to treat complications such as phlebitis or a ruptured varicosity. Optimal compression can be achieved with compression bandages (either changed frequently or left on for a longer period) or compression stockings.

4.2 Thrombophlebitis

Definition

Superficial thrombophlebitis is a non-infectious, limited inflammation of an epifascial vein with luminal occlusion caused by a thrombus.

Etiology and Pathogenesis

Superficial thrombophlebitis of the legs is often associated with preexisting varicosities and then trauma or immobilization. On the arms, it is often iatrogenic, following an injection or infusion. Thrombophlebitis can also develop spontaneously or be associated with a severe underlying disease but without an obvious trigger.

Clinical Features

The characteristic features can usually be identified clinically. The affected vein produces a red, warm, tender cord.

Special Types of Thrombophlebitis

Superficial Migratory Thrombophlebitis

Synonyms. Thrombophlebitis migrans

This variant tends to involve clinically normal veins, either spreading from a single focus along a vein or jumping from one vein to another. Typically there are coin-sized erythematous nodules along an otherwise normal vein. Usually younger patients are affected. Superficial migratory thrombophlebitis can be idiopathic (primary) but may also be associated with various types of vasculitis (thromboangiitis obliterans, BEHÇET's disease, WEGENER's granulomatosis, lupus erythematosus, polymyalgia rheumatica, polyarteritis nodosa), coagulation disorders or as a paraneoplastic marker (especially with carcinoma of the pancreas).

MONDOR's Syndrome
Synonyms. Mondor's phlebitis (HENRI MONDOR, 1885–1962, French surgeon)

Mondor's syndrome is a superficial thrombophlebitis of the superficial thoracic veins, producing a painful or tender cord along the anterior rib line. The cause is unknown. While the pain can occasionally be severe and the changes look dramatic, the course is usually uneventful. Occasionally the inflammation can extend onto the arm.

Diagnosis

The distinctive findings can be identified by inspection and palpation. Duplex sonography is useful to identify extension into the deep venous system. Important differential diagnostic consideration include:

- Paraneoplastic syndrome
- Borreliosis
- BEHÇET's syndrome
- Thromboangiitis obliterans (BUERGER's disease)
- Erythema nodosum, sometimes a marker for underlying disease

Therapy

- Mobilization! Bed rest is undesirable; it increases the risk of the thrombosis spreading into the deep vein system.
- Cold packs along with compression.
- Systemic non-steroidal anti-inflammatory drugs (indomethacin, ibuprofen), or other pain-relieving agents
- If there is extensive thrombophlebitis involving the sapheno-femoral junction or the sapheno-popliteal junction, then heparinization for 1–2 weeks (low molecular weight heparin is very suitable) or an emergency ligature of the sapheno-femoral junction should be considered.
- If there is recurrent thrombophlebitis, then varicosities should be treated surgically.

4.3 Deep Vein Thrombosis (DVT)

Synonyms. Thrombophlebitis, phlebothrombosis, venous thrombo embolism

Definition

Acute complete or incomplete thrombotic closure of the deep infrafascial veins, primarily of the leg, pelvis, vena cava and veins of the neck. The venous clots tend to grow and release emboli to the lungs.

Epidemiology

Thrombophlebitis or phlebothrombosis is the third most common acute cardiovascular disease, following myocardial infarctions ad strokes. It has an incidence about three per 1000. Over 90% of the thromboses arise in the vena cava or the pelvic and leg veins; only 1.5% in the veins of the arms.

The exact frequency of deep vein thromboses in a general population is hard to determine, because many thrombi are clinically silent. The modern peri-operative thrombosis prophylaxis has reduced the incidence of post-operative thromboses and emboli which formerly was about 10% for small procedures, 25% for abdominal operations and up to 50% for orthopedic and neurosurgical procedures. (Table 10-2).

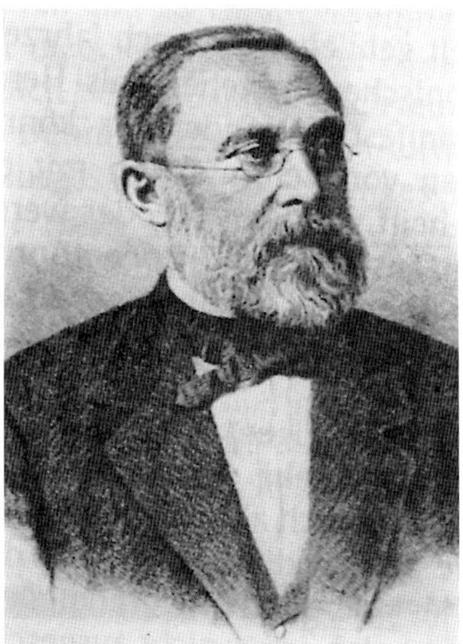

Fig. 10-6. Rudolf Virchow (October 13, 1821 – September 5, 1902). German pathologist who directed the famous Institute of Pathology in Berlin, starting in 1845

Etiology and Pathogenesis

Virchow in 1856 (Fig. 10-6) described a triad of pathogenic factors for the development of deep vein thrombosis. They are still valid today.

- Vessel wall or endothelial alterations (inflammatory, degenerative, traumatic, allergic)
- Reduced blood flow velocity (immobilization, varicosities, paraplegia, local blockage, fractures, right heart failure)
- Changes in the blood (hyperviscosity, hyperfibrinogenemia, altered platelet function, congenital abnormalities in platelets or coagulation factors)

Thromboses of the legs are most common, and the left is more often involved than the right. Both reduced flow in the left common iliac vein where it crosses the right common iliac artery and in 20% of patients endothelial changes just before it joins the inferior vena cava help explain this predilection.

Table 10-2. Incidence of thromboembolic events in relationship to various diseases or events

Disease or event	Low risk	Medium risk	High risk
General surgery	Age < 40 years; length of operation < 60 min	Age >60 years; length of operation >60 min	Age > 60 years; length of operation > 60 min and additional risk factors
Orthopedic surgery	–	–	Elective knee and hip replacement surgery
Trauma	–	–	Multiple trauma, fractures of large bones, soft tissue damage
Accompanying diseases or conditions	Pregnancy	Myocardial infarction, cardiac failure, post-partum, previous deep vein thrombosis or pulmonary embolus	Stroke
Incidence of thromboemboli with prophylaxis (%)			
Distal DVT: calf	2	10–40	40–80
Proximal deep vein thrombosis: popliteal, femoral, iliac veins	0.4	2–8	10–20
Symptomatic pulmonary embolus	0.2	1–8	5–10
Fatal pulmonary embolus	0.002	0.1–0.4	1–5
Recommended Prophylaxis	Compression stockings, early mobilization	Heparin 5000 IU subcutaneously 2×, then low molecular weight heparin; intermittent external pneumatic leg compression	Heparin 7500 IU subcutaneously 3×, then low molecular weight heparin, coumarin; intracaval filter; intermittent external pneumatic leg compression

From Diehm, Deutsches Ärzteblatt, 1997.

The cause of deep vein thrombosis remains unknown in 30% – 40% of cases. the major risk factors are shown in Table 10-3.

Both thrombophlebitis and phlebothrombosis should be regarded as potential paraneoplastic markers when they occur without any obvious risk factors. The presence of an underlying tumor should be assumed until it is proven otherwise.

Clinical Features

- Dull tugging pain in the entire leg (usually improves with horizontal positioning)
- Pain in the calf resembling a pulled muscle
- Heavy feeling in leg
- Acute edema formation, initially about the ankle but later involving the entire leg and thigh if the iliac veins are affected
- Cyanosis of the limb
- Inflamed veins on the dorsal surface of the foot

Table 10-3. Risk factors for venous thromboemboli

Risk factor	Comments
Advanced age	Exponential increase after age 50 years
Sex	Healthy young women have three times the risk of age-matched young men, no sex differences in the elderly
Immobilization	Increased risk in paralyzed limb following stroke or paraplegia, also during long trips (economy class syndrome)
Previous DVT	40–60-fold increased risk
Anesthesia	Greater risk with general as compared to local or regional anesthesia
Type of operation	Higher risk with abdominal, orthopedic and neurological surgery
Pregnancy	Risk not increased during pregnancy, clearly increased in post-partum period
Malignancy– known or occult tumor, chemotherapy, radiation therapy	Thromboses in up to 30% of cases. Risk of occult malignancy with idiopathic thrombosis 2.7 times the general population, with recurrent idiopathic thromboses, risk increased up to 20-fold
Platelet dysfunction	The incidence of thromboses in thrombocythemia is disputed
Hypercoagulable states:	
Acquired:	
Antiphospholipids	
polycythemia vera	
Other types of polycythemia	
Elevated levels of plasminogen activator- inhibitor	
Inherited:	Account for 50% of hereditary thromboses
APC resistance (Factor V-Leiden)	
AT-III defects	
Protein S or C defects	
Hyperhomocystinuria	
Trauma	Thromboses with severe head injury, 54%; pelvic fracture, 61%, femur or tibia fractures, 80% or 77%
Other disorders	Myocardial infarction, cardiac failure, peripheral arterial disease, nephrotic syndrome, cirrhosis, fever, hyperviscosity; obesity is a controversial risk factor
Medications and drugs:	
Heparin	Incidence of heparin-associated thrombocytopenia type II between 0.5–2.7%
Oral contraceptives	Increased risk, about fourfold; when combined with smoking, sevenfold. Risk not eliminated with low-estrogen compounds (<50 g)
Cocaine, heroin	

Diagnosis

The clinical symptoms and signs of deep vein thrombosis are fairly sensitive but very non-specific and therefore not very useful (Table 10-4). The clinical diagnostic accuracy for deep vein thrombosis is approximately 50%. The absence of clinical signs of thrombophlebitis does not exclude the diagnosis. It is therefore essential to perform some type of vascular imaging study to confirm or exclude the presence of a thrombus.

The two most useful studies are duplex ultrasonography and phlebography which are contrasted in Table 10-5. While phlebography was long considered the gold standard, today duplex ultrasonography in the hands of an experienced examiner is preferable. If it is not available, then phlebography is the method of choice.

Table 10-4. Important signs of thrombosis

Sign	Location of pain
Payr	Pain in sole both with tapping but also when bearing weight
Bisgaard	Tenderness in the retro-malleolar area
Homan	Calf pain with plantar flexion
Lowenberg	Calf pain with blood pressure cuff; difference between left and right
Meyer	Tender pressure points along the deep veins
Pratt	Pain with pressure in the popliteal space

Table 10-5. Advantages and disadvantages of duplex ultrasonography vs phlebography

Advantages	Disadvantages
Better visualization of the sapheno-femoral junction, deep femoral vein, muscular veins and parallel veins	Poor documentation
More precise differential diagnostic aid (hematoma, Baker's cyst, arterio-venous fistula) and better view of vein wall (tumor)	Difficult study in obese patients and those with extensive edema
Assessment of characteristics of thrombus	Long examination time (20 min/leg)
Non-invasive and equally accurate	Long learning curve for examiners
Repeatable as often as needed	Dependent on skills of examiner
Bedside monitoring	Not all areas visualized
	Pulmonary embolus from compression during examination possible

Continuous wave Doppler ultrasonography is a simple method to search for proximal thromboses. Plethysmography is less sensitive and specific than the imaging techniques. Computerized tomographic phlebography and magnetic resonance phlebography are becoming increasingly important especially for proximal thromboses such as those of the vena cava (Tables 10-6, 10-7).

Table 10-6. Differential diagnosis: thrombophlebitis versus phlebothrombosis

Thrombophlebitis	Phlebothrombosis
Signs of inflammation: erythema, warmth, pain, localization	Cyanosis of leg, especially when standing
Usually localized edema, although can be diffuse	Diffuse swelling of limb (difference in circumference compared to normal limb, firmer consistency)
Painful inflamed superficial venous cord	No visible or palpable thrombosis Dull pain in entire leg Filled "sentinel veins" on back of foot, over tibia Positive signs (see Table 10-4)

Table 10-7. Diagnostic approach for deep vein thrombosis

	Symptomatic DVT		Asymptomatic DVT		Location	Comments
	Sensitivity	Specificity	Sensitivity	Specificity		
Phlebography	Gold standard	Gold standard	Gold standard	Gold standard	Iliac, femoral, popliteal, lower leg	Invasive, hard to interpret with recurrences
Vein closure plethysmography	92%	95%	22%	98%	Femoral, popliteal	Not sensitive for lower leg and non-occlusive proximal thrombi, comparison of sides needed
Compression ultrasonography	97%	97%	59%	98%	Femoral, popliteal	Sensitive test for symptomatic DVT
Continuous wave Doppler ultrasonography	88%	88%	–	–	Femoral, popliteal	Interpretation subjective, doubled veins often misinterpreted
Color duplex ultrasonography	95%	97%	92%	96%	Iliac, femoral, popliteal, lower leg	Can be repeated as often as needed, requires experienced examiner and lengthy exam; adjacent vessels seen

Measuring the levels of D-dimers is another useful procedure. Unfortunately the specificity of the D-dimer level is poor. The main role of the D-dimer test is in recurrent thromboses and when screening for pulmonary embolus.

The benefits of primary thrombosis prophylaxis are well-documented. Physical measures include early ambulation, use of compression stockings and intermittent pneumatic compression. The major medication is subcutaneous unfractionated heparin in low doses; i.e., 5000–7500 IU every 8–12 h. Such regimens have been shown effective in many high risk situations and also protect against pulmonary embolus. Low molecular weight heparin is more convenient, and is also widely used for pre- and post-operative prophylaxis.

Therapy

See Tables 10-8 and 10–9.

Table 10-8. Recommended duration of oral anticoagulation (OA) with deep vein thromboses

Type of thromboses	Duration	Intensity of OA (INR)
Thrombus ± pulmonary embolus with associated risk factor (post-operative)	6 weeks	2–3
Initial thrombus in calf without risk factor ± pulmonary embolus	3 months	2–3
Initial multi-level thrombus without risk factor ± pulmonary embolus	6 months	2–3
Initial secondary thrombus ± pulmonary embolus without permanent risk factor	6 months	2–3
Recurrent multi-level thrombus without risk factors	12 months	2–3
Recurrence of a primary multi-level thrombus while being anticoagulated with INR of 2.0–3.0	Long term	3.0–4.5
Recurrence of secondary thrombus with a time-limited risk factor (immobilization, curable malignancy)	For the period of the increased risk	2.0–3.0
Initial diagnosis of APC resistance, protein C, protein S or AT-III deficiency without thrombus	No therapy, prophylaxis in risk situations	
Initial thrombus with APC resistance and other risk factors	6 months	2.0–3.0
Initial or recurrent thromboses in hereditary platelet disorders without other risk factors	Long term	2.0–4.5
Recurrent thromboses in anti-phospholipid syndrome	Long term	3.0–4.5

INR, International Normalized Ratio.

Table 10-9. Treatment of deep vein thrombosis

Conservative (heparin)	Thrombolysis	Thrombectomy
Standard therapy for every thrombosis	*Careful indications, exclusion of many contraindications*	*Rarely indicated*
Limited calf thrombosis	Multi-level thrombosis or recurrent thrombosis, in which the localization and size make a post-thrombotic syndrome likely	Definite indication: phlegmasia cerulea dolens
Older (>7 days) multi-level thrombosis	Thrombosis <7–10 days old	In special cases: descending pelvic vein thrombosis in pregnancy; ascending superficial thrombophlebitis, which involves deep vein system
Thrombosis in patient with life expectancy <10 years	Phlegmasia cerulea dolens prior to thrombectomy	
Axillary-subclavian vein thrombosis (Paget-von Schrötter syndrome)	With or without first rib resection if symptoms are marked	
Thrombosis in pregnancy		

General Measures

Patients with new isolated lower leg or calf thromboses should not be immobilized. In contrast, new thromboses in the popliteal, thigh or iliac veins require hospitalization for 5–7 days with bed rest. Optimal compression therapy consists of daily application of compression bandages during the acute phase and then use of custom-fitted compression stockings once swelling has subsided.

There are three basic therapy schemes:

1. Conservative treatment with heparin, trying to keep the PTT 1.5–2.5 times the normal value, or using low molecular weight heparin.
2. Fibrinolysis with streptokinase (conventional or anisoylated), urokinase or tPA (tissue plasminogen activator) can be used systemically or infused locally. Fibrinolysis should be employed as early as possible.
3. Operative thrombectomy can be used for fresh (less than 5–8 days old) proximal thromboses. In some centers the procedure is performed via the femoral vein with a balloon catheter. Temporary adjunctive arteriovenous fistulas have also been advocated in this setting.

Oral anticoagulant therapy with coumarin derivatives should be employed for 4–6 months; if there has been a simultaneous pulmonary embolus, then the anticoagulation should be used for one year. Patients with congenital deficiencies in protein C, protein S, and anti-thrombin III as well as APC resistance require life-long anticoagulation. The trend today is towards early usage of oral anticoagulants. If there are contraindications (hemorrhagic diathesis, bleeding, gastrointestinal ulceration, poorly controlled hypertension, pregnancy and others), then either subcutaneous heparin or low molecular heparin therapy must be carried out for the recommended period. Alternatively an inferior vena cava filter can be placed.

Adjuvant Therapy

Pain and marked swelling are best treated by compression therapy with elevation of the leg. Absolute immobilization is not required. This therapy can be carried either in the hospital or on an outpatient basis. Compression stockings should be worn for 6 months following a distal thrombosis; in the case of proximal or multi-level thromboses, 2 years of compression stocking use is suggested.

4.4 Post-thrombotic Syndrome and Chronic Venous Insufficiency

Definition

This clinical constellation arises in association with alteration of the vein system on account of various chronic venous diseasis. The unifying factor appears to be an ambulatory venous and capillary hypertension. There are typical changes on phlebography and with duplex ultrasonography including incompetent valves, reflux in the deep vein system, impaired cutaneous lymphatic drainage, chronic-progressive impairment of the microcirculation, more easily damaged skin and restricted mobility in the ankle joint.

Epidemiology

- One of the most common vascular diseases seen in a clinical practice.
- Prevalence over 10%.
- Women affected three times as often as men.
- Some 10% of these individuals (1% of population) have a leg ulcer secondary to their venous disease.

The combination of venous and cutaneous changes with constant venous hypertension is known as chronic venous insufficiency (CVI). The most common type of secondary CVI is the post-thrombotic syndrome.

Clinical Features

Chronic venous insufficiency is usually divided into three stages:

Stage I: Corona phlebectatica paraplantaris (filling and ectasia of small veins on the lateral and medial aspects of the foot, forming a wreath or crown), minimal edema

Stage II: Additional cutaneous findings including stasis dermatitis, hypo- and hyperpigmentation, atrophie blanche and induration (dermatoliposclerosis)

Stage III: Healed (IIIa) or active (IIIb) stasis ulcer

Diagnosis

Clinical inspection and palpation usually allows a diagnosis. Assessment of the aterial status is also to perform in assessing the arterial status. The mobility of the ankle joint should be assessed and a directed neurological examination performed. Doppler and duplex ultrasonography and plethysmography are needed, as well as phlebodynamometry, to assess the pumping function of the leg muscles and the general adequacy of the valves.

Therapy

The therapy should be adjusted to the current complaints of the patient. The overall goal is to reduce the ambulatory venous and capillary hypertension. Possibilities include:

- Regular compression therapy with either compression stockings or elastic bandages.
- In more advanced cases, intermittent pneumatic compression.
- Diuretics are only useful early in the treatment and for a short period of time.
- Physical therapy (cold showers, exercise with special attention to ankle joint).
- Sclerotherapy of varicosities.
- Surgical procedures:
  1. Ligation of incompetent perforating veins (often associated with ulcers)
  2. Removal of varicosities (for example, accessory veins)
  3. Special ulcer surgery (excision, split thickness grafting)
- Medications (systemic antibiotics, various topical medications).

4.5 Phlegmasia Cerulea Dolens

Definition

Sudden and rapidly progressive thrombosis blocking all the veins of a limb.

Clinical Features

In a short period of time extreme swelling of the limb appears, along with a deep livid color. The swelling is tender and painful. The venous pressure points are extremely tender. The arterial pulses are reduced or absent, because obstruction of the capillary and arteriolar circulation. Hypesthesia, paresthesia and motor impairment of the limb all appear.

- Complications: Hypovolemic shock, gangrene, pulmonary embolus
- Mortality as high as 50%
- Therapy
  a. No compression!
  b. Anticoagulation with heparin, volume replacement, thrombectomy or fibrinolysis

5. Axillary and Subclavian Venous Thrombosis

Synonyms. PAGET-VON SCHRÖTTER syndrome, effort thrombosis

Definition

Thrombosis of the axillary or subclavian vein.

Etiology and Pathogenesis

The site of predilection is a narrowing in the thoracic outlet region where the vessels pass between the clavicle and the first rib. Some authors classify the Paget-von Schrötter syndrome as part of the thoracic outlet syndrome.

Major risk factors include sports such as baseball, handball, basketball, tennis and swimming. Chopping and splitting wood is another potential cause.

Clinical Features

The arm is swollen and has a livid mottled appearance. The collateral veins on the anterior thorax are filled and visible. The patients have a dull pain and heavy feeling in their arm.

Diagnosis

History, inspection, palpation, Doppler or duplex ultrasonography, phlebography.

Differential Diagnosis

- Tumors of the mediastinum, less often the axilla or supraclavicular space
- Callus formation after clavicular fracture
- Iatrogenic injury from catheter or pacemaker

Therapy

Acute anticoagulation with heparin with the patient hospitalized for 5–7 days. Fibrinolysis, either systemic or local, with our without first rib resection, should only be performed in some cases (professional athlete, concert pianist), since permanent disability does not always develop in the arm. Oral anticoagulation for 3–4 months is suggested.

B: Supplementary Figures and Legends

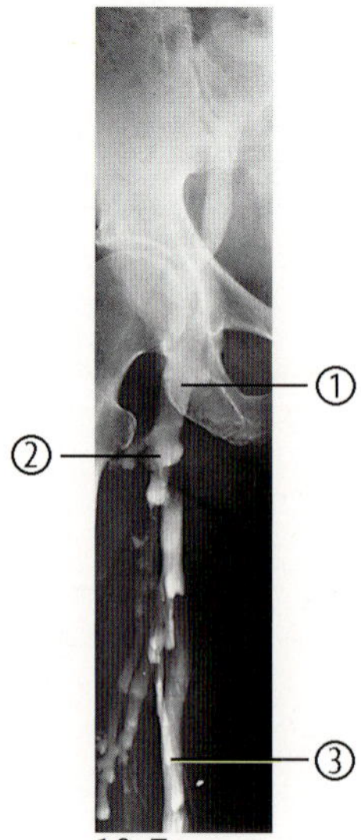

10-7

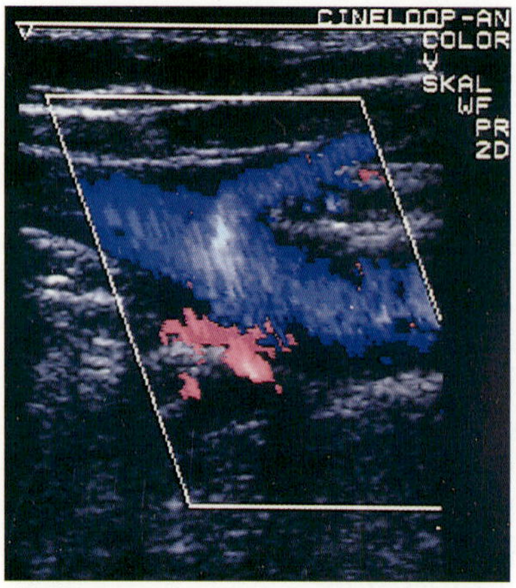

10-8

Fig. 10-7. Phlebography showing the right external iliac, common femoral, superficial femoral and deep femoral veins. The common femoral vein arises 5–10 cm below the inguinal ligament from the joining of the superficial and deep femoral veins.
① Common femoral vein
② Deep femoral vein
③ Superficial femoral vein

Fig. 10-8. Color duplex ultrasonography, showing the normal appearance of the sapheno-femoral junction during expiration. Blood is flowing into the junction via the greater saphenous vein and the epigastric veins from the abdominal wall

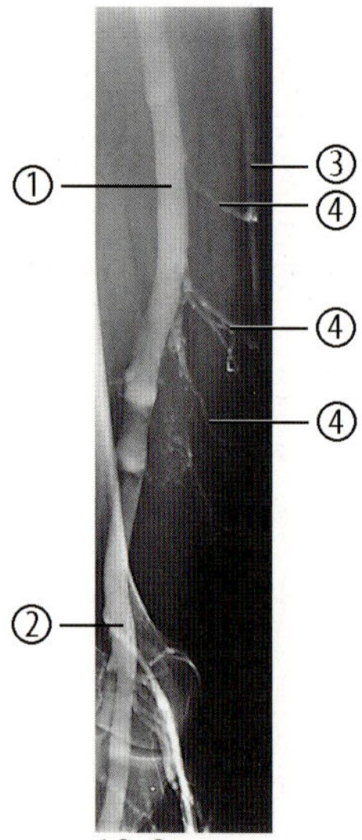

10-9

Fig. 10-9. Phlebography showing the superficial femoral, popliteal and greater saphenous veins, as well as the group of DODD perforating veins. The superficial femoral vein begins in the adductor canal as a continuation of the popliteal vein. The greater saphenous vein courses from the medial edge of the foot and along the medial aspect of the calf, draining numerous superficial veins. These accessory veins usually become visible when varicosities develop.
① Superficial femoral vein
② Popliteal vein
③ Greater saphenous vein
④ DODD perforating veins

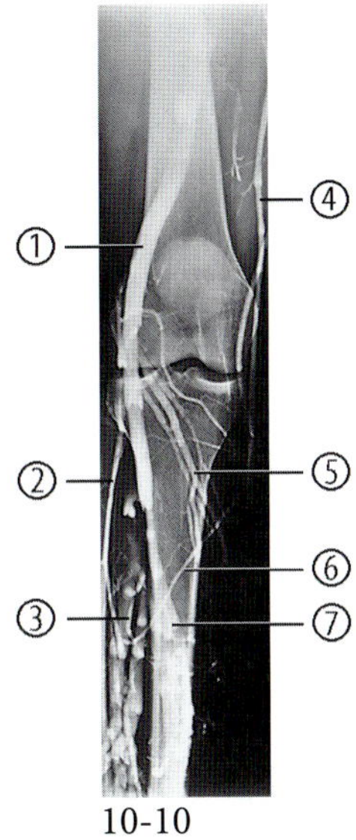

10-10

Fig. 10-10. Phlebography showing the popliteal vein, as well as the veins of the gastrocnemius, tibial and peroneal groups, along with the greater saphenous vein with its anterior arch and the lesser saphenous vein. The popliteal vein arises from the joining of the anterior and posterior tibial veins. In the popliteal space, the vein usually runs postero-lateral to the popliteal artery. The lesser saphenous vein runs along the lateral border of the foot, behind the lateral malleolus and then up the posterior aspect of the calf to join the popliteal vein in the vicinity of the knee. ① popliteal vein; ② lesser saphenous vein; ③ peroneal veins; ④ greater saphenous vein; ⑤ gastrocnemius veins; ⑥ anterior arch of the greater saphenous vein; ⑦ tibial veins

Figs. 10-11, 10-12. Color duplex ultrasonography showing the anterior tibial artery with the two accompanying anterior tibial veins both in longitudinal and cross-section

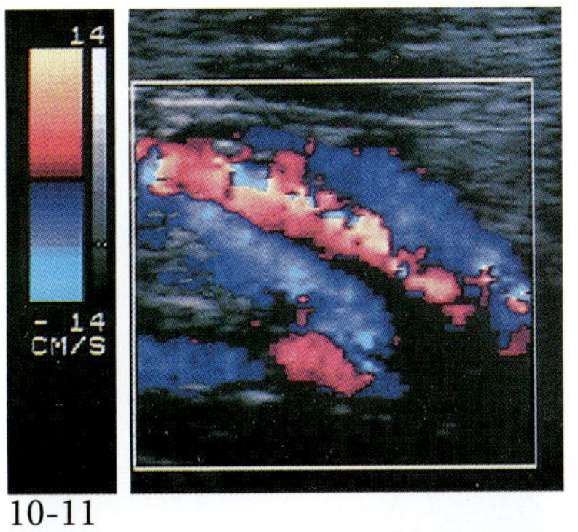

10-11

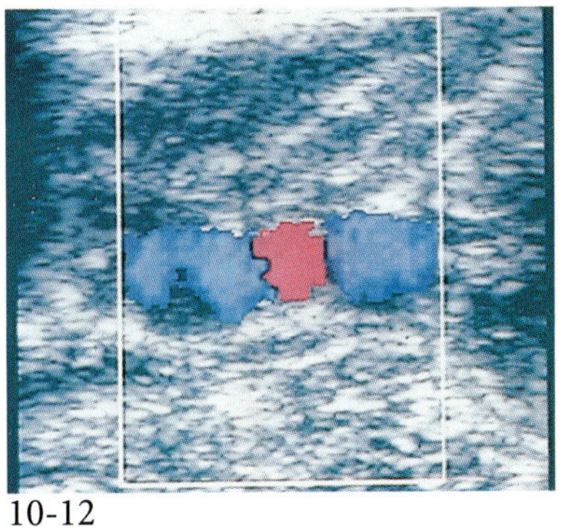
10-12

Fig. 10-13. Phlebography showing bilateral inferior vena cavas with bifurcation at the level of L2. The ontogenic development from paired vessel precursors is responsible for the large number of anatomic variants and abnormalities. In the third embryonic week the paired cardinal veins and then the subcardinal veins begin to form. The vena cava develops out of the fusion of various segments. The most common variant is a paired infrarenal vena cava, seen in 1% of individuals. A single vena cava on the left occurs in 0.2% of individuals

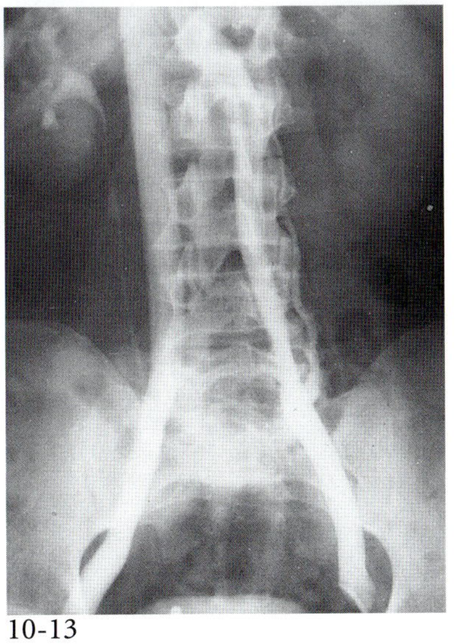
10-13

Fig. 10-14. Phlebography showing doubled superficial femoral veins, as well as the greater saphenous vein with Dodd perforating veins and the lesser saphenous vein. A doubled superficial femoral vein is common, seen in about 20% of individuals.
① Superficial femoral vein, doubled
② Greater saphenous vein
③ Dodd perforating veins
④ Lesser saphenous vein

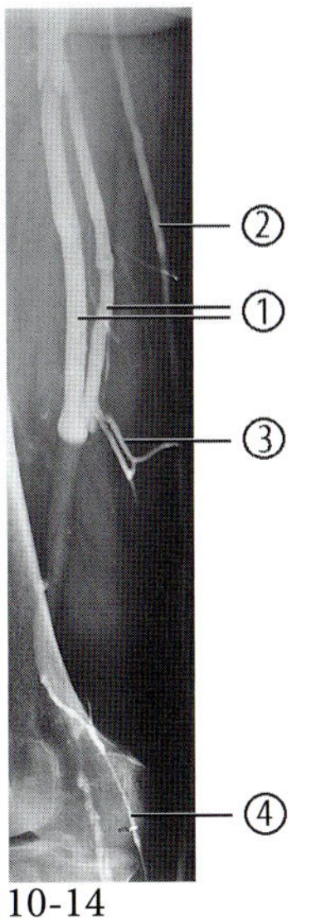

10-14

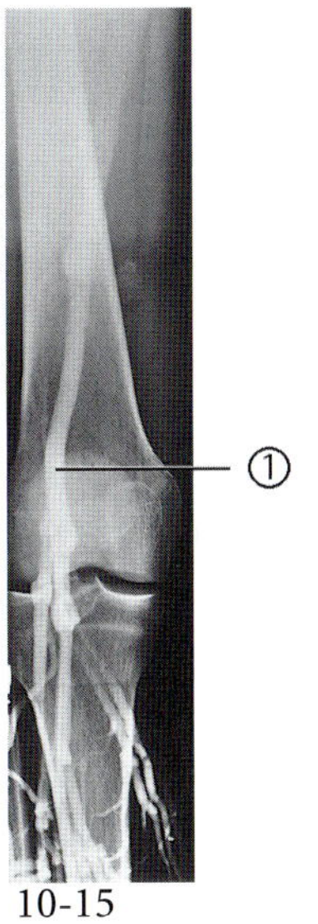

10-15

Fig. 10-15. Phlebography. In about 40% of individuals, the lesser saphenous vein and the popliteal vein join above the knee, resulting in doubled veins in the popliteal space.
① More proximal junction

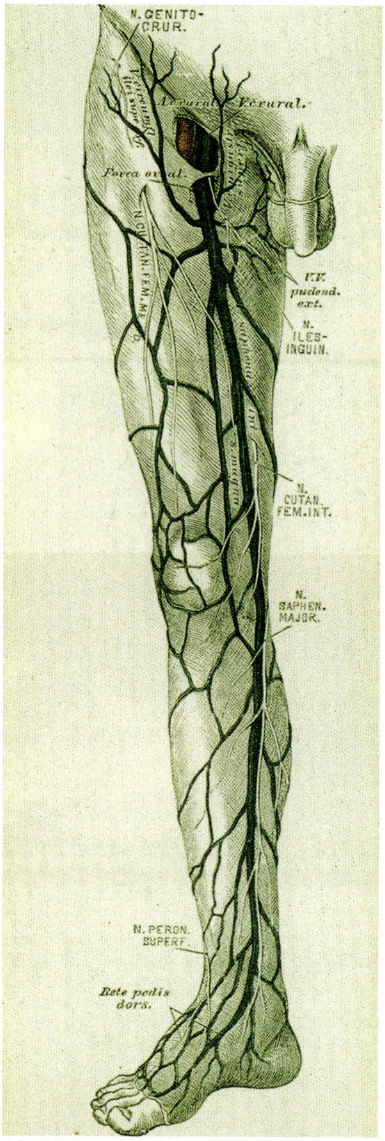

10-16

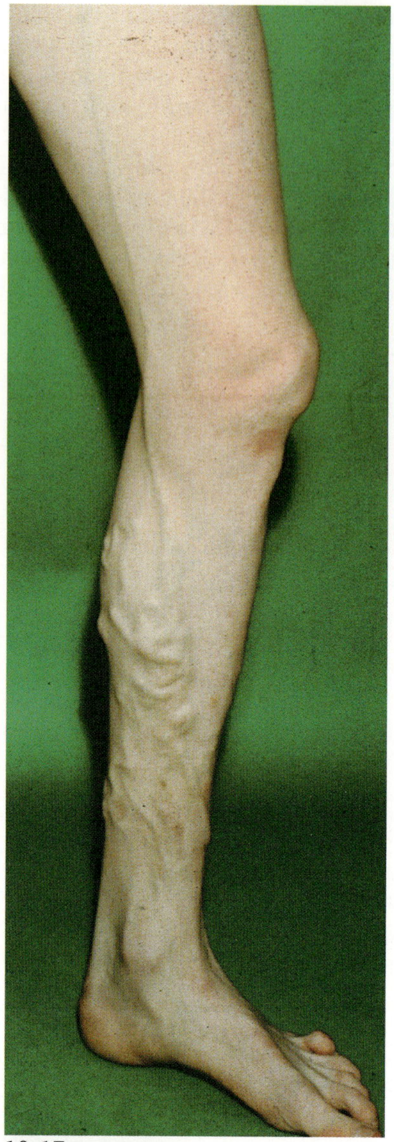

10-17

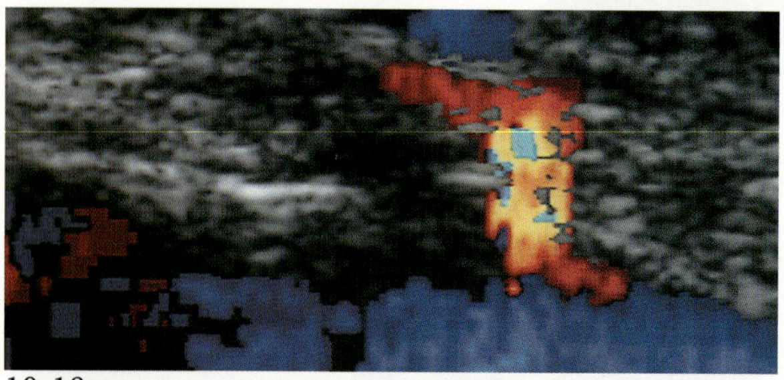

10-18

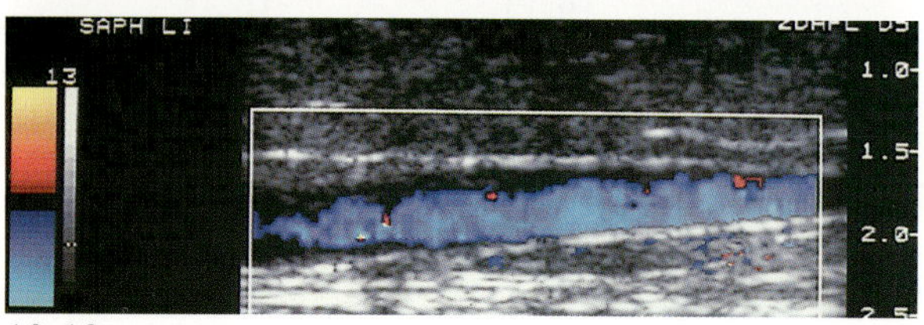

10-19

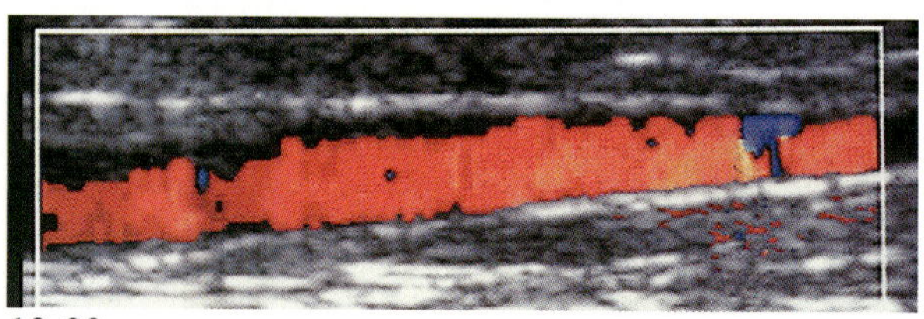

10-20

Fig. 10-16. Superficial veins of the leg. (From C. HEITZMANN, *Deskriptive und topographische Anatomie der Menschen*, 1893)

Fig. 10-17. Stage IV varicosity of the greater saphenous vein caused by an incompetent sapheno-femoral junction. Varicosities of the larger superficial limb veins always develop proximally and extend distally (groin to foot). One distinguishes between primary varicosities caused by congenital vein valve or wall defects and secondary varicosities usually related to the post-thrombotic syndrome. In this picture, a cylindrical varicosity courses across the thigh. The calf shows marked varicosities with coiling; the defect extends to the level of the malleolus, making this stage IV

Fig. 10-18. Color duplex ultrasonography showing incompetent sapheno-femoral junction valves with a bruit. By using manual compression or the Valsalva maneuver, the function of the greater saphenous vein in the inguinal region can be checked. If reflex is identified, showing an inadequate valve at the junction, then the varicosities are traced distally

Fig. 10-19. Color duplex ultrasonography of the greater saphenous vein showing flow towards the heart in expiration

Fig. 10-20. Same section of the greater saphenous vein with Valsalva maneuver. The reversal of flow indicates incompetent venous valves

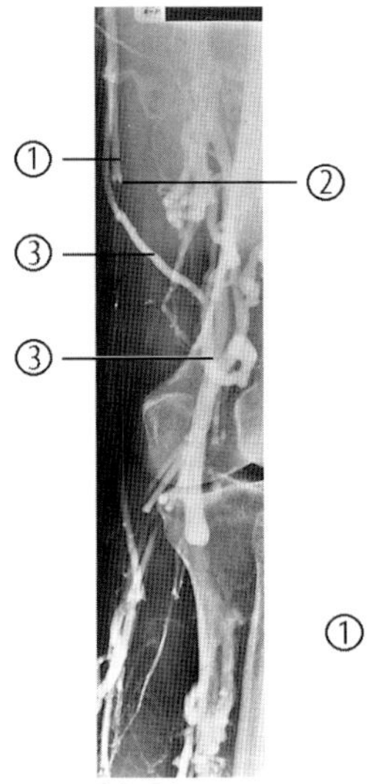

10-21

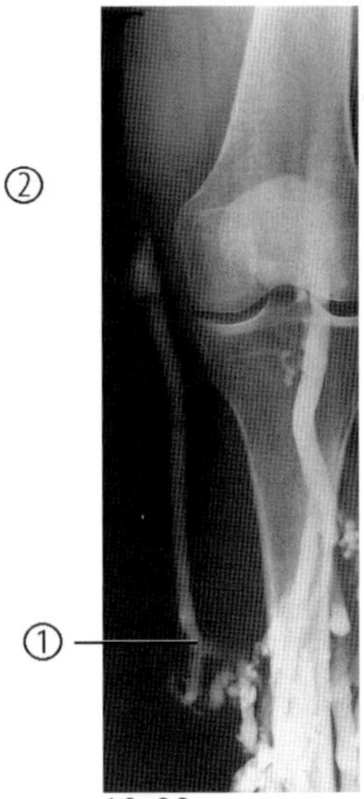

10-22

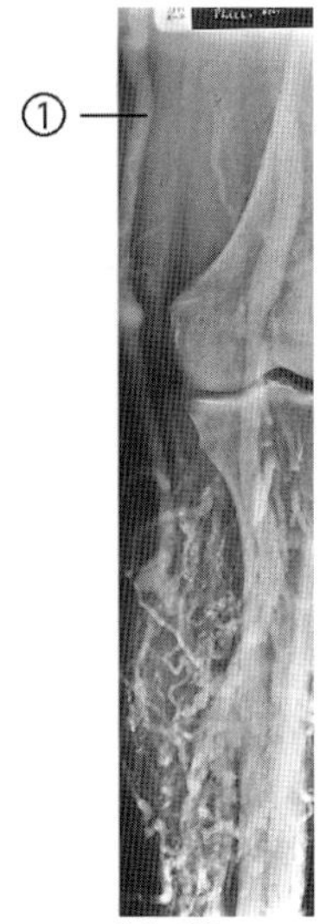

10-23

Fig. 10-21. Phlebography showing a varicosity of the greater saphenous vein reaching from the sapheno-femoral junction to the distal calf, thus a stage II lesion. In addition, the GIACOMINI vein (CARLO GIACOMINI, 1840–1898, Italian anatomist) is incompetent (stage II: incompetent valves from the inguinal area to one handbreadth above the knee).
① Greater saphenous vein
② Distal extent of incompetent valves
③ Giacomini anastomosis

Fig. 10-22. Phlebography showing a stage III varicosity of the greater saphenous vein, extending to the calf and also involving some of the accessory veins (stage III: incompetent valves extending to one handbreadth below the knee).
① Greater saphenous vein

Fig. 10-23. Phlebography showing a stage III varicosity of the greater saphenous vein with involvement of the accessory veins.
① Greater saphenous vein

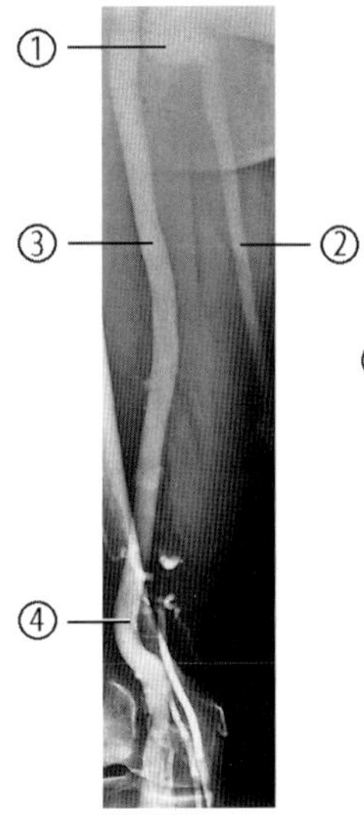

10-24

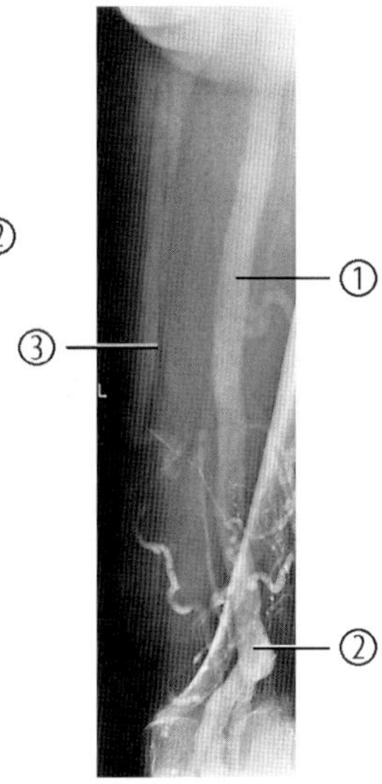

10-25

Fig. 10-24. Phlebography showing massive varicosities of the greater saphenous vein with aneurysmal enlargement in the proximal thigh.
① aneurysm of the greater saphenous vein; ② greater saphenous vein; ③ superficial femoral vein; ④ popliteal vein

Fig. 10-25. Phlebography showing complete stage IV varicosities of the greater saphenous vein. The accessory veins are widened and the valves incompetent. These changes in the accessory veins are an integral part of varicose changes; they have been described as atony of the veins.
① atony of the superficial femoral vein; ② atony of the popliteal vein; ③ greater saphenous vein

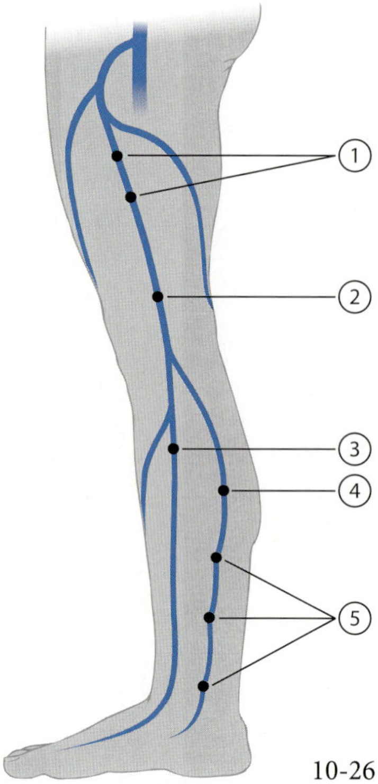

10-26

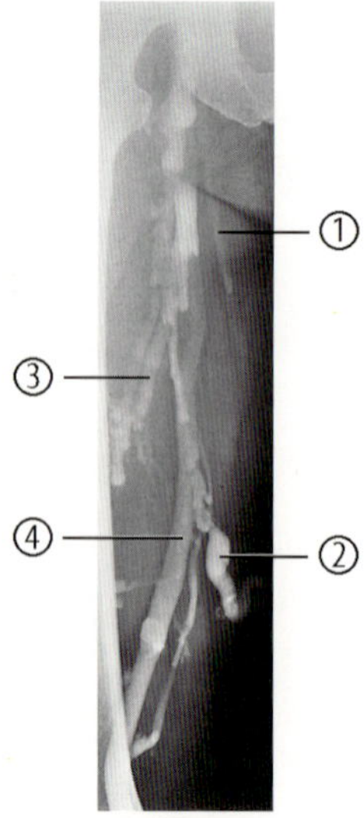

10-27

Fig. 10-27. Phlebography showing widened perforating veins of the greater saphenous vein. In a complete varicosity, the sapheno-femoral junction valves are incompetent. In an incomplete varicosity, the problem begins with the perforating veins and accessory veins. Here the perforator is in the middle of the thigh and is a DODD vein.
① Greater saphenous vein
② Dilated DODD perforating vein
③ Deep femoral vein
④ Superficial femoral vein

Fig. 10-26. The clinically important perforating veins on the medial aspect of the leg. The perforating veins are the veins that connect the deep and superficial veins, passing through the fascia. There are more than 100 perforating veins in each leg. In a healthy leg, the flow goes from the superficial to the deep venous system. (After HACH-WUNDERLE 1997)
① DODD veins, ② HUNTER vein, ③ BOYD veins, ④ SHERMAN vein, ⑤ COCKETT veins

Figs. 10-28 – 10-30. Various degrees of severity of incomplete varicosity of the greater saphenous vein with DODD perforating veins

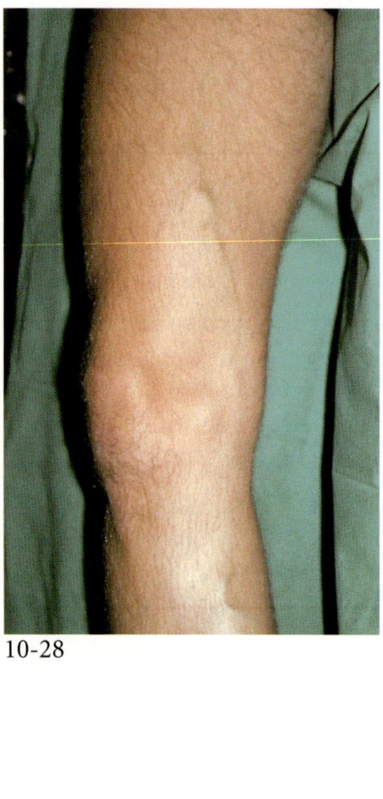

10-28

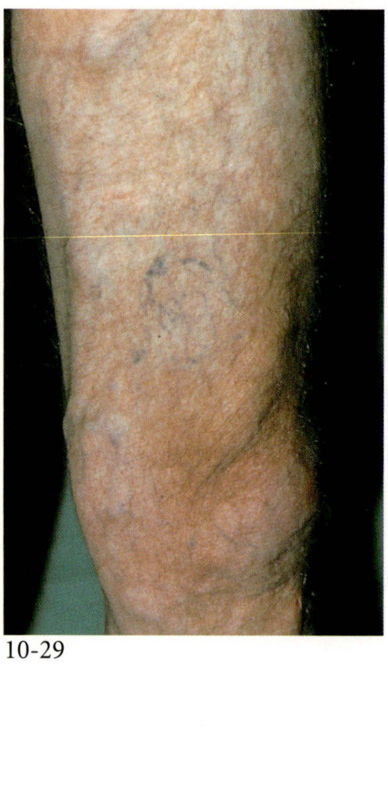

10-29

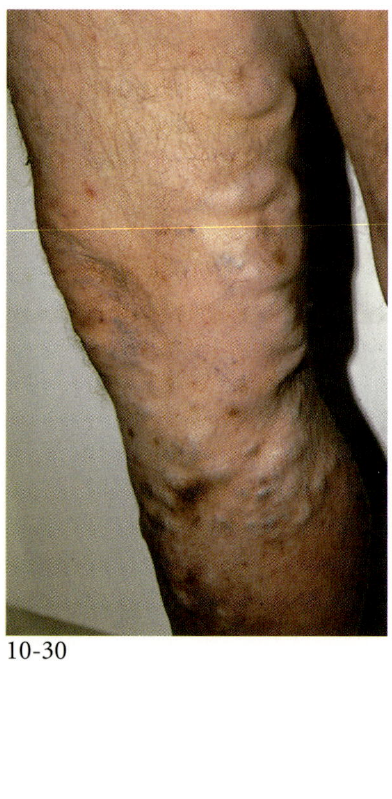

10-30

Fig. 10-31. Incompetent HUNTER vein with varicosities of the accessory veins following removal of the greater saphenous vein. The distal perforating veins of the DOFF group, are found at the end of the adductor or HUNTER's canal (JOHN HUNTER, 1728–1793, British anatomist and surgeon) and are thus called HUNTER veins

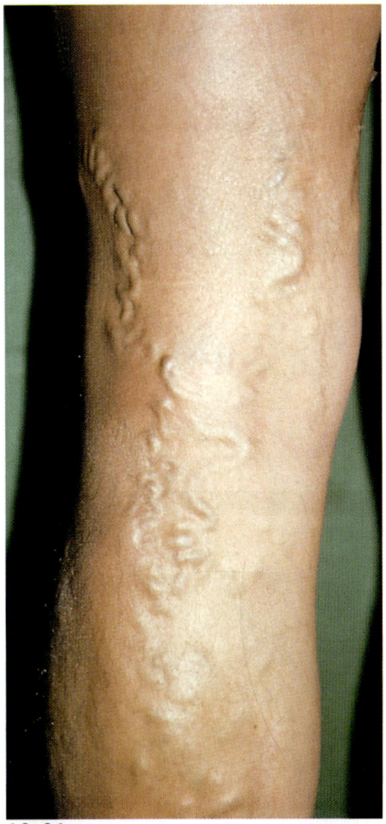

10-31

Figs. 10-32, 10-33. Atypical course of an incomplete varicosity of the greater saphenous vein with a blow-out aneurysm on the anterior surface of the thigh

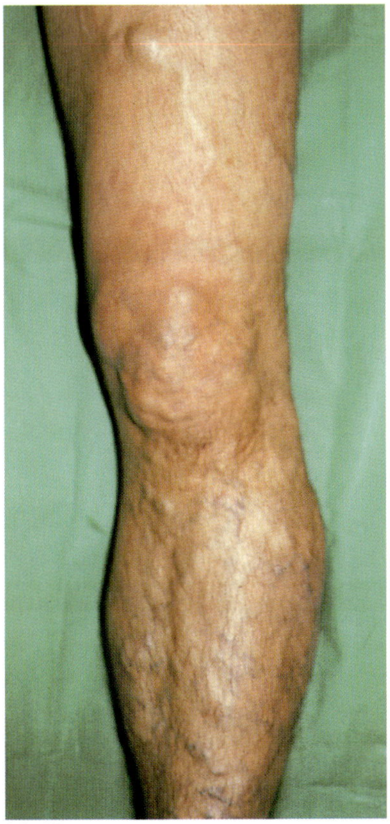

10-32

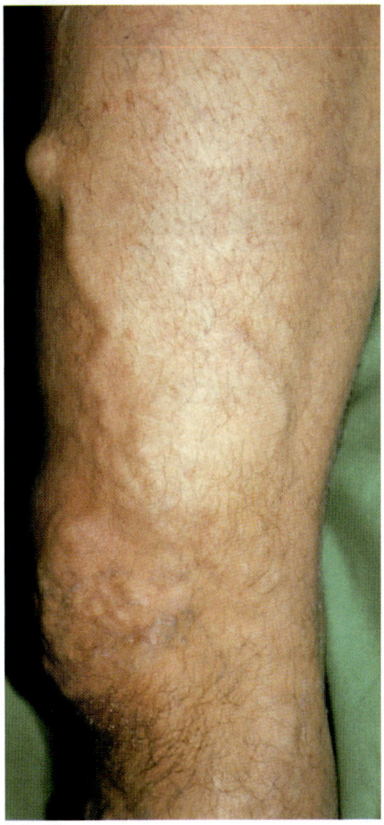

10-33

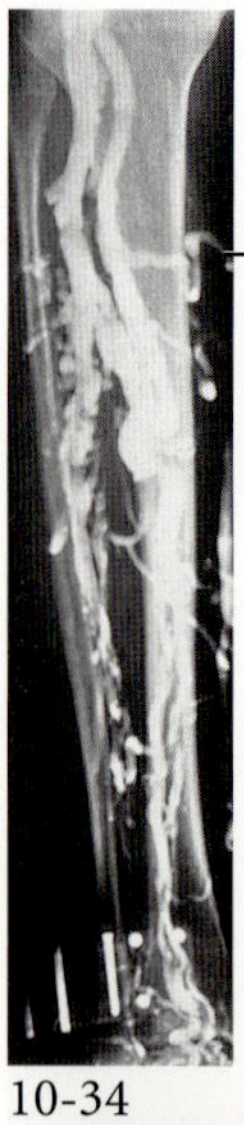

10-34

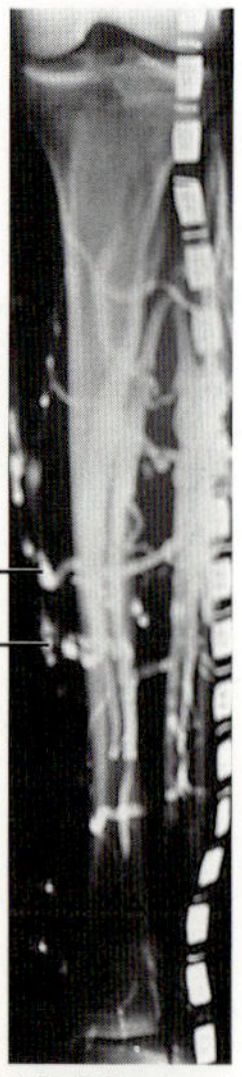

10-35

Fig. 10-34. Phlebography showing incompetent perforating vein on the medial aspect of the lower leg and ankle ①. The BOYD (A.M. BOYD, contemporary British phlebologist) perforating veins connect the greater saphenous vein with the posterior tibial veins at the level of the tibial tuberosity

Fig. 10-35. Phlebography showing the COCKETT veins along LINTON's line. They connect the dorsal venous arch with the posterior tibial veins.
①, ② COCKETT perforating veins

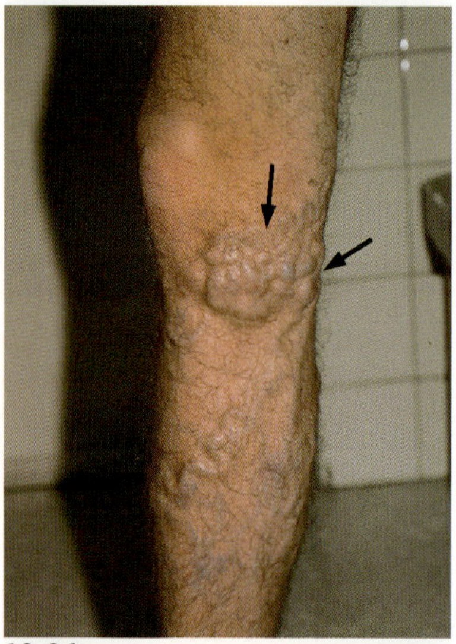

10-36

Fig. 10-36. Clinical appearance of an incompetent BOYD perforating vein with varicosities of the accessory veins

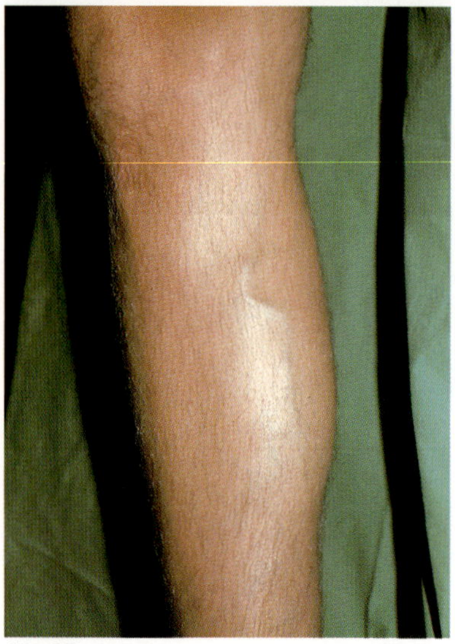

10-37

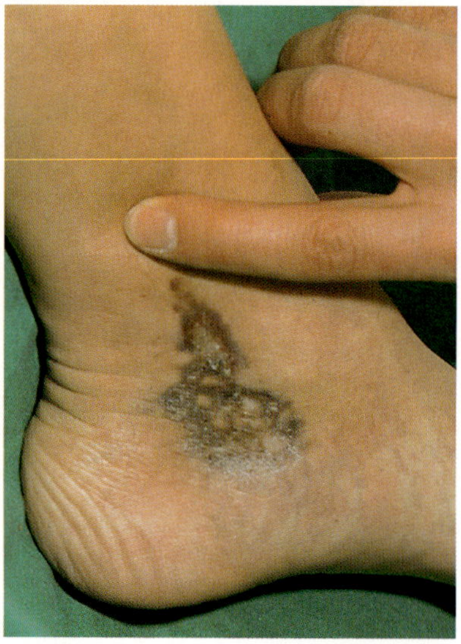

10-38

Fig. 10-37. Moderate incompetence of the SHERMAN perforating vein

Fig. 10-38. Incompetent COCKETT veins with signs of chronic venous insufficiency over the medial malleolus, including hyperpigmentation and focal areas of atrophie blanche.
The defect in the fascia is easily palpated with the finger

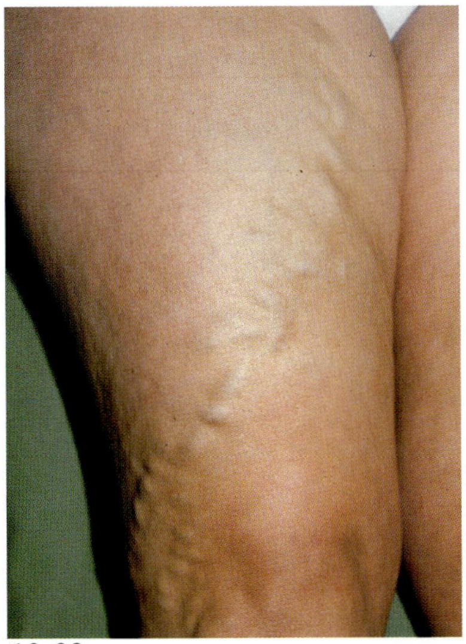

10-39

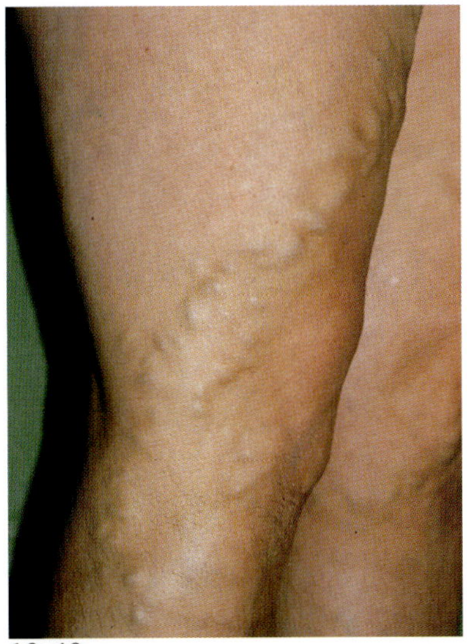

10-40

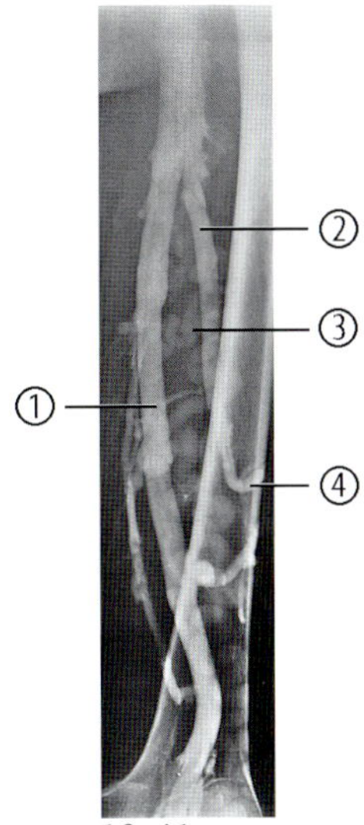

10-41

Figs. 10-39, 10-40. Varicose changes in the accessory veins draining into the right greater saphenous vein. Varicosities of the lateral accessory saphenous vein are easily identified clinically. On the lateral side of the calf they join the other accessory varicosities. More than half the accessory varicosities of the greater saphenous vein involve the lateral accessory saphenous vein

Fig. 10-41. Phlebography showing grade III varicosities of the accessory lateral saphenous vein extending distal to the knee joint. There is no sign for a varicosity of the greater saphenous vein and the sapheno-femoral junction is intact.
① Superficial femoral vein
② Deep femoral vein
③ Lateral accessory saphenous vein
④ Muscular veins

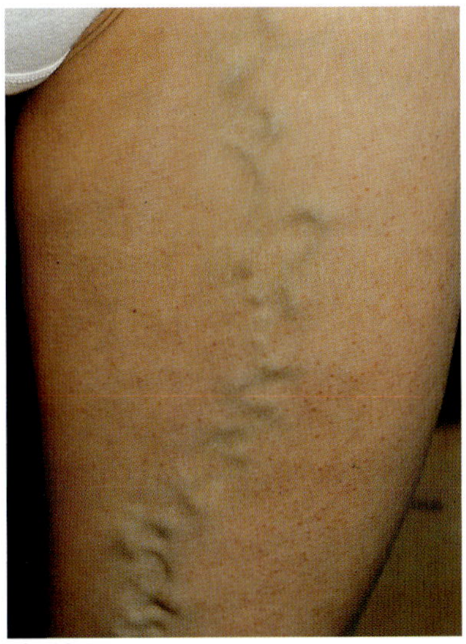

10-42

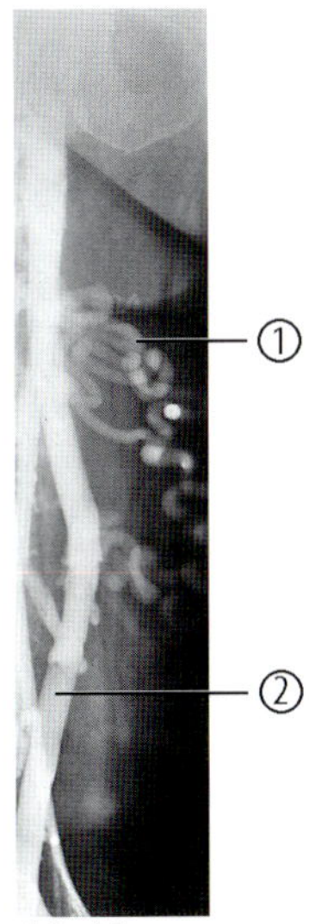

10-43

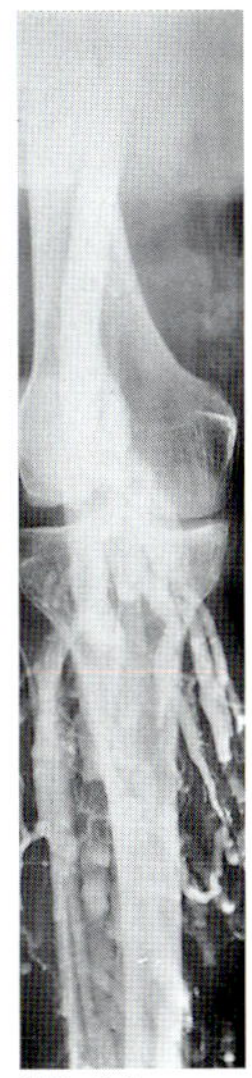

10-44

Fig. 10-42. Varicosity of the medial accessory saphenous vein

Figs. 10-43, 10-44. Phlebography showing marked varicosity of the medial accessory saphenous vein. The vessel can be followed in retrograde fashion to the knee joint
① Medial accessory saphenous vein
② Superficial femoral vein

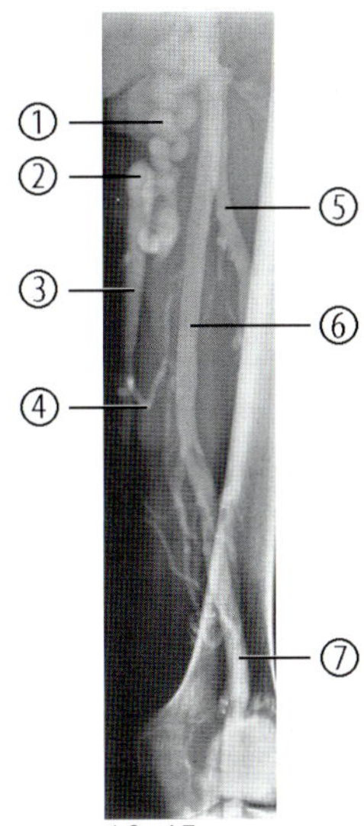

10-45

Fig. 10-45. Phlebography showing a varicosity of the greater saphenous vein also involving an accessory vein which enters in the sapheno-femoral junction region.
① Accessory saphenous vein
②, ③ Greater saphenous vein
④ Dodd perforating vein
⑤ Deep femoral vein
⑥ Superficial femoral vein
⑦ Popliteal vein

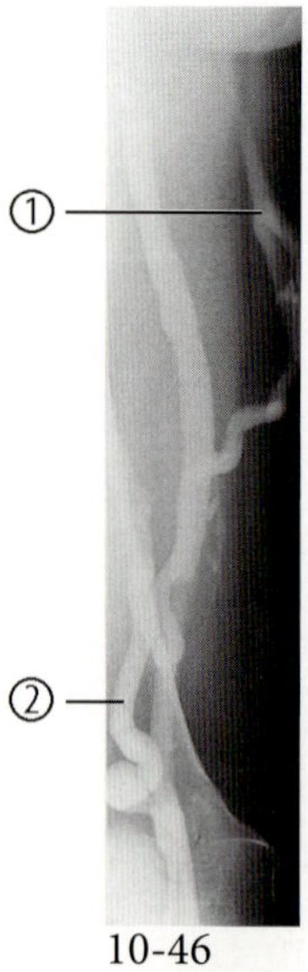

10-46

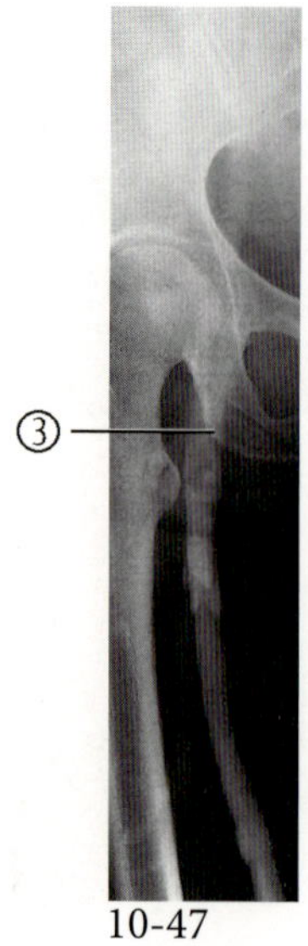

10-47

Figs. 10-46, 10-47. Phlebography showing incomplete greater saphenous vein varicosity of the dorsal type, caused by an incompetent GIACOMINI anastomosis. Varicosities of the medial accessory saphenous vein are often associated with incompetent femoro-popliteal vein and their GIACOMINI anastomosis. In this way, connections between varicosities of the greater saphenous vein and lesser saphenous vein can develop.
① Proximal level of incompetent valves
② Giacomini anastomosis
③ Intact sapheno-femoral junction

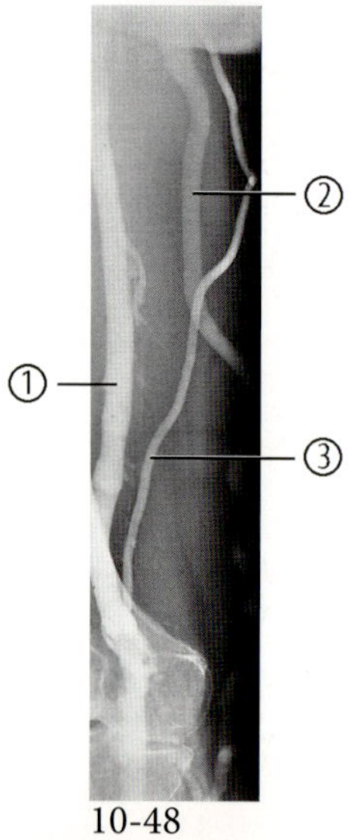

10-48

Fig. 10-48. Phlebography showing complete greater saphenous vein varicosity of the dorsal type, caused by an incompetent GIACOMINI anastomosis.
① Superficial femoral vein
② Greater saphenous vein
③ GIACOMINI anastomosis

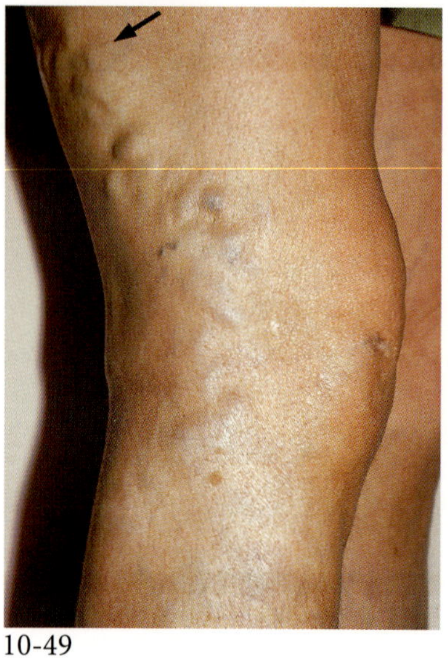
10-49

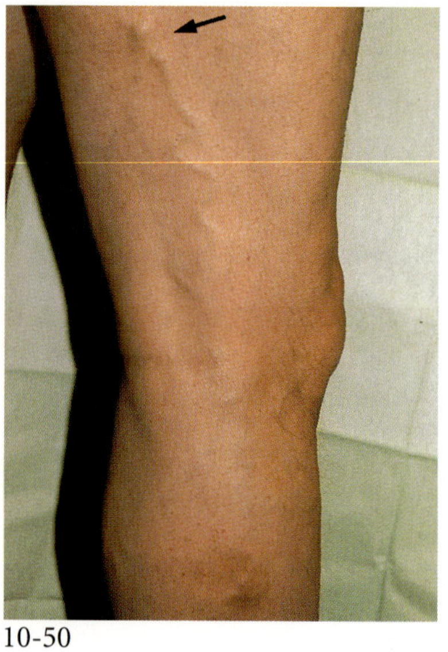
10-50

Figs. 10-49, 10-50. Varicosities of the deep perforating veins (after HACH). Because of the incompetent perforating veins to the deep femoral artery, varicosities develop on the lateral surface of the proximal thigh.
The fascial defect is easily seen (*arrows*)

Fig. 10-51. Phlebography showing a complex developmental anomaly of the deep and superficial veins in a 21 year old woman. A vessel is seen running from the lateral aspect of the thigh dorsally and then dropping down to join an anomalous superficial femoral vein. The junctional valve is incompetent. The superficial femoral vein describes an arch curving anteriorly and following a path where the greater saphenous vein usually runs. It is possible that during embryological development parts of this vessel were incorporated into the aberrant one. Finally there is an additional rudimentary vein

Figs. 10-52, 10-53. Clinical appearance of the same patient with anomalous accessory vein varicosities

Fig. 10-54. Dilated skin capillaries on the buttock of the same patient, seen in the *upper left* part of the figure

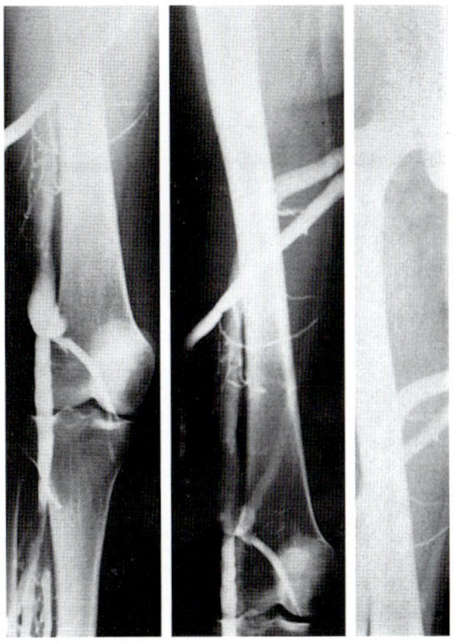

10-51

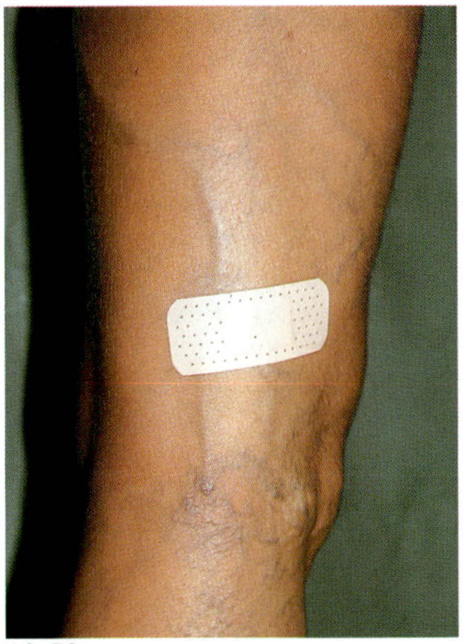

10-52

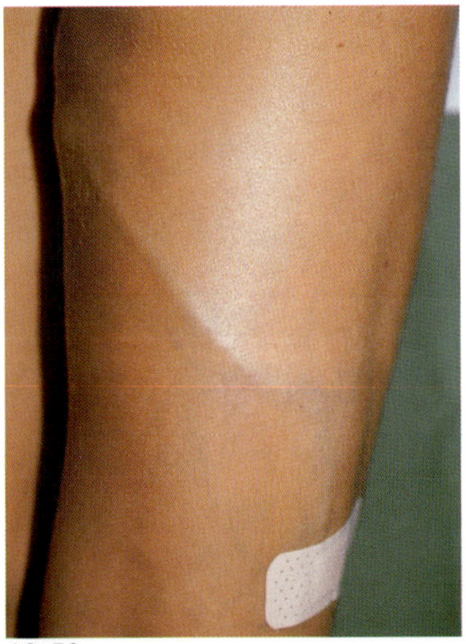

10-53

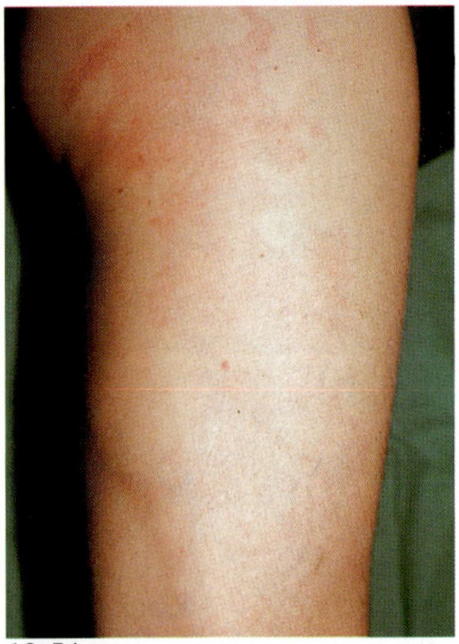

10-54

Figs. 10-55, 10-56. Clinical appearance of persisting marginal veins in a 33 year old man. Some persisting marginal veins (lateral posterior veins) are associated with KLIPPEL-TRENAUNAY syndrome. Other such veins drain directly into the superior gluteal veins and thus into the pelvic veins

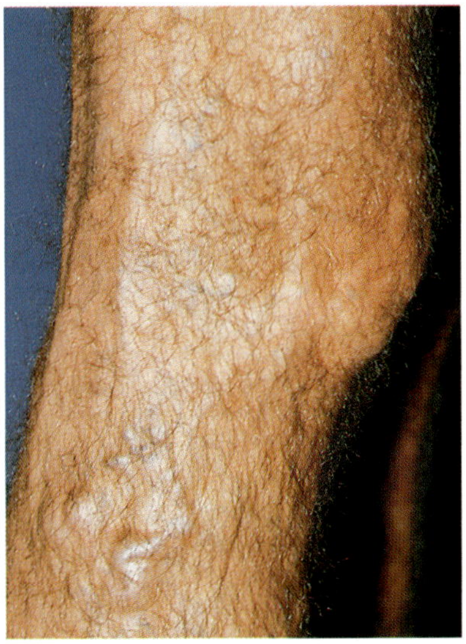

10-55

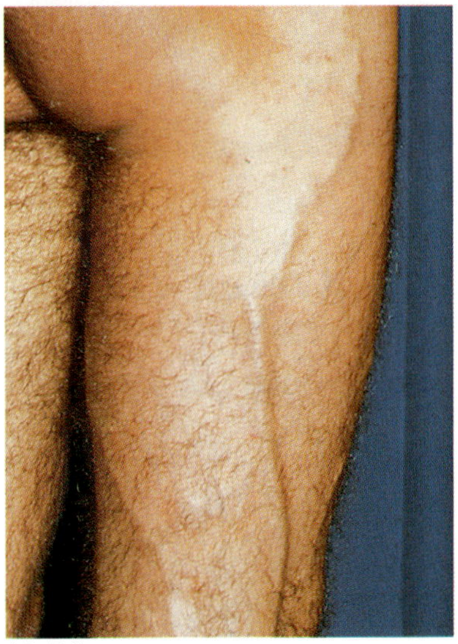

10-56

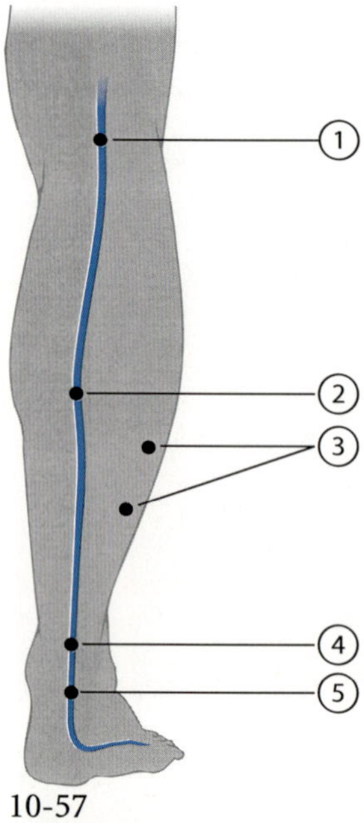

10-57

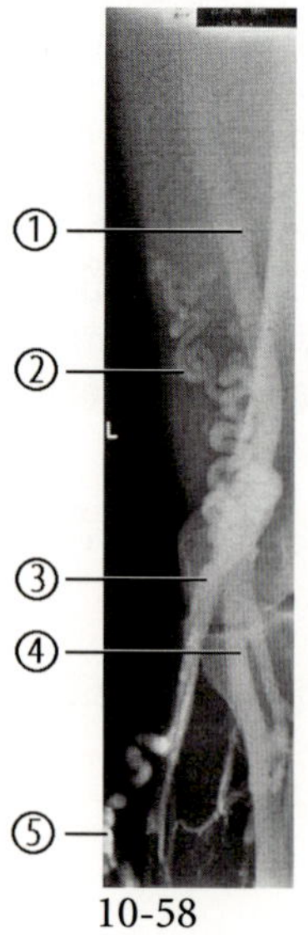

10-58

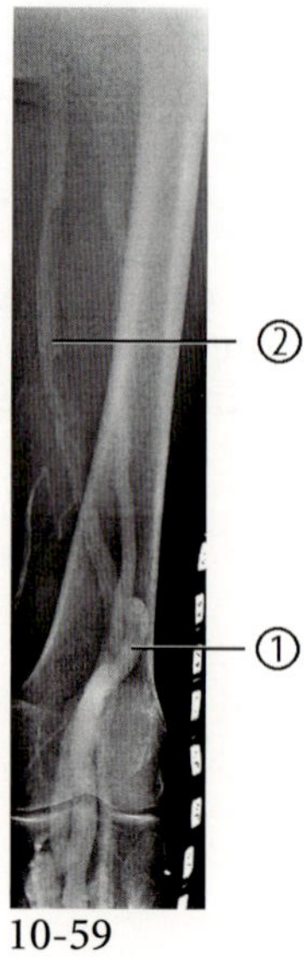

10-59

Fig. 10-57. The lesser saphenous vein and the clinically important perforating veins on the latero-dorsal aspect of the calf (after HACH and HACH-WUNDERLE 1997). The MAY (ROBERT MAY, 1914–1984, Austrian phlebologist) perforating vein connects the lesser saphenous vein and the gastrocnemius veins in the middle of the calf. The connections between the lesser saphenous vein and peroneal veins occur at the level of the lateral malleolus as BASSI (GLAUCO BASSI, born 1914, Italian phlebologist) perforating veins at 9 cm, as well as at 12 cm.
① popliteal perforating vein;
② May perforating vein;
③ lateral perforating vein;
④ 12 cm perforating vein;
⑤ Bassi perforating vein (9 cm)

Fig. 10-58. Phlebography showing stage II varicosities of the lesser saphenous vein with involvement of an accessory vein. In addition, an accessory vein is seen extending cranially from the junction.
① Superficial femoral vein
② Accessory vein varicosities
③ Lesser saphenous vein
④ Popliteal vein
⑤ Accessory vein varicosities

Fig. 10-59. Phlebography showing a stage III varicosity of the lesser saphenous vein with marked dilatation of the vessel.
An unusual flow phenomenon can be send in the superficial femoral vein, as contrast material is mixed with blood entering from the accessory veins. This has been called the "chimney smoke" sign.
① Lesser saphenous vein
② Flow phenomenon

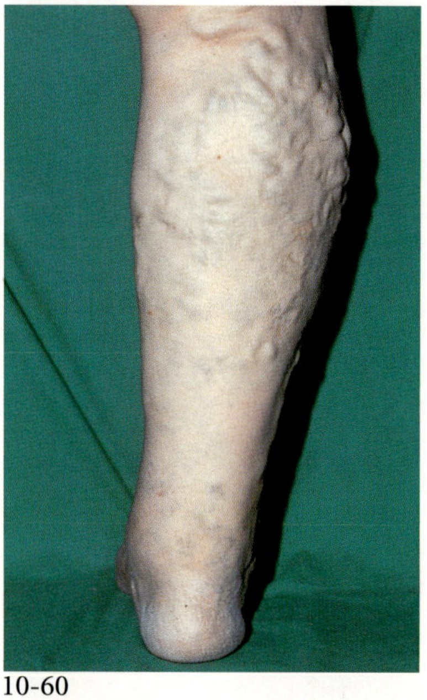

10-60

Fig. 10-60. Clinical appearance of varicosities of the lesser saphenous vein with additional varicosities of the accessory veins. Clear swelling of the ankle is present with chronic venous insufficiency

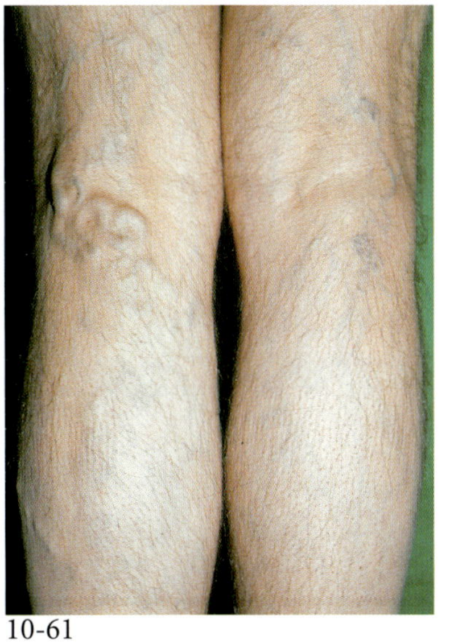

10-61

Fig. 10-61. Incompetent valve at the junction of the lesser saphenous vein and popliteal vein with varicosities of the accessory veins.

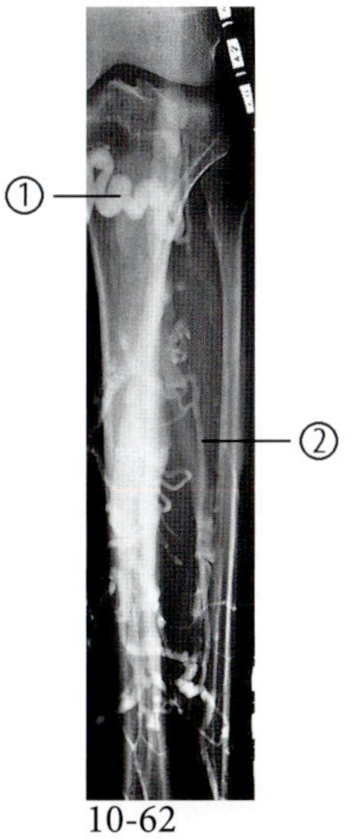

10-62

Fig. 10-62. Phlebography showing incompetent perforating vein in the popliteal space. Via an accessory vein, this has caused distal dilation and insufficiency of the lesser saphenous vein.
① Popliteal perforating vein
② Lesser saphenous vein

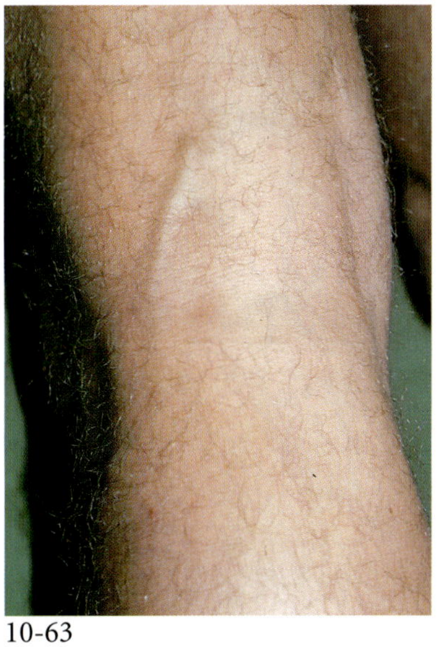

10-63

Fig. 10-63. Relatively high popliteal perforating vein with varicosity of an accessory vein. The perforating vein is just about at the level of the termination of the lesser saphenous vein, so that it is difficult to exclude a varicosity of the lesser saphenous vein clinically

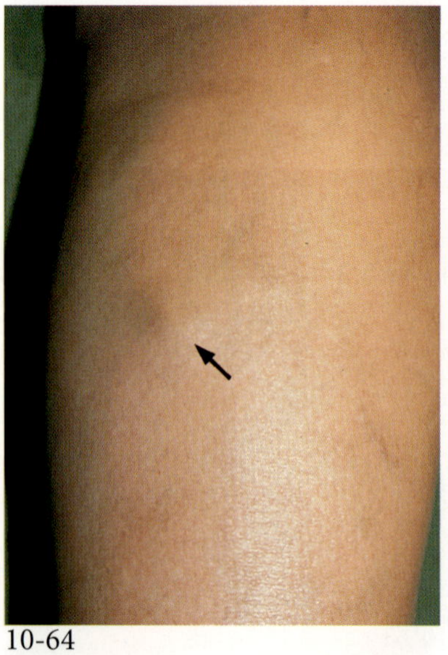

10-64

Fig. 10-64. Incompetent perforating vein of the calf with blow-out (*arrow*) that is easily seen

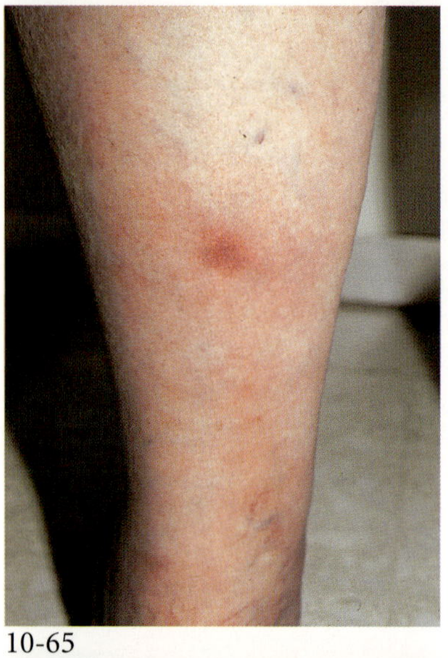

10-65

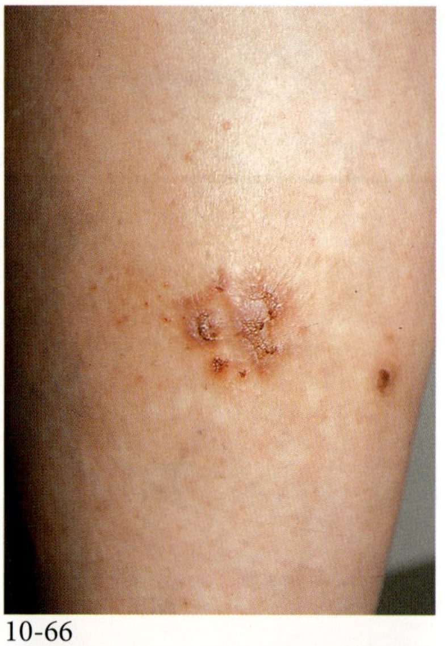

10-66

Fig. 10-65. Thrombosis of a perforating vein with local phlebitis at the pressure point of the soleus veins

Fig. 10-66. A focal area of chronic dermatitis directly over an incompetent perforating vein of the calf

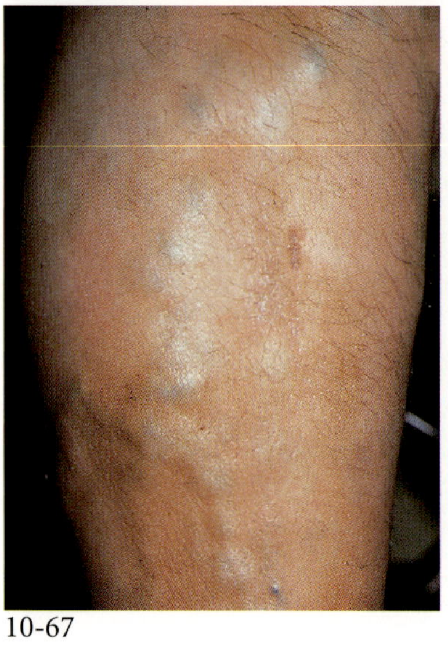

10-67

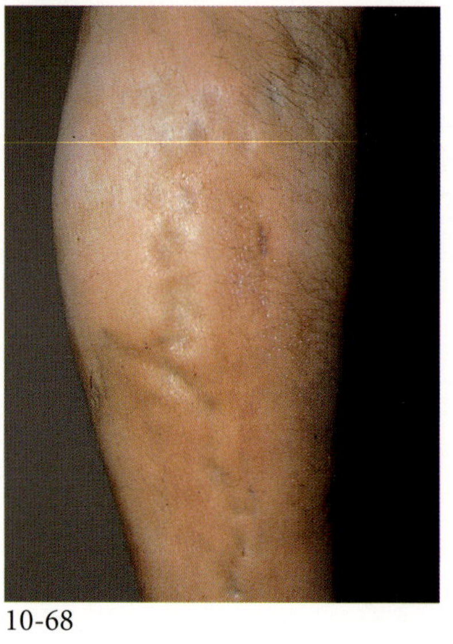

10-68

Fig. 10-67. Filled canyon varicosity

Fig. 10-68. Empty canyon varicosity, showing the derivation of the name: A canyon varicosity is a thin-walled superficial vein which makes a dent or canyon in the sclerotic dermis associated with chronic venous insufficiency. They are difficult to treat, as both surgery and sclerotherapy yield poor results

Fig. 10-69. Pretibial varicosity, involving the dorsal venous arch, an accessory vein of the greater saphenous vein. These varicosities are prominent over the tibia and often painful or easily injured

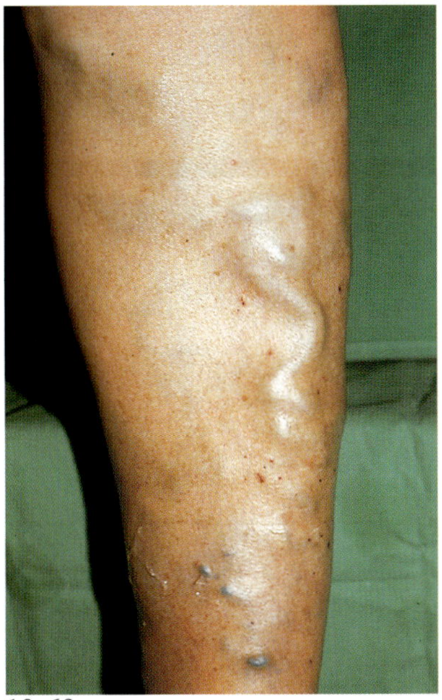

10-69

Fig. 10-70. Ruptured varicosity with bleeding is a feared complication for patients with varicose veins. Here is a bleeding lesion following injury to the tibial surface. Often the bleeding does not stop spontaneously and a firm compression bandage and elevation of the leg are required

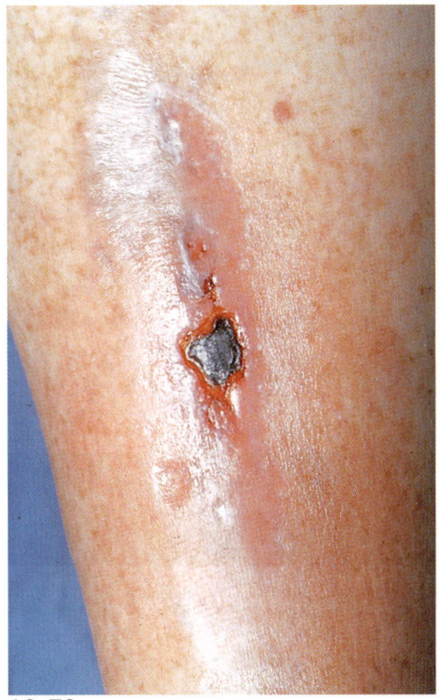

10-70

Fig. 10-71. Perforating veins about the ankle. The KUSTER perforating veins are found about the medial and lateral malleoli and along the edge of the foot. (After HACH und HACH-WUNDERLE 1997)

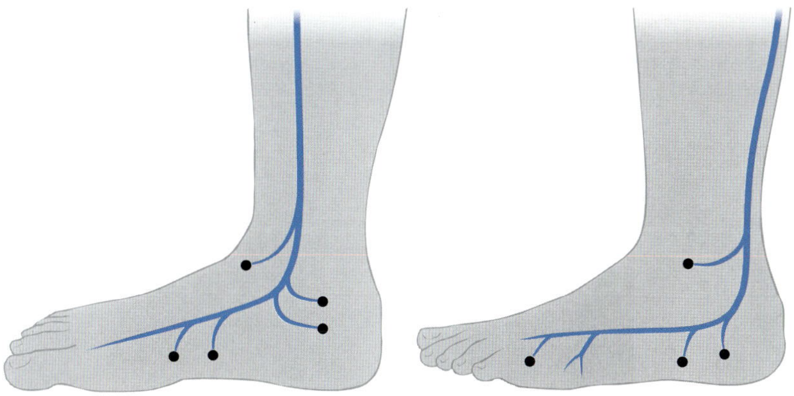

10-71

Fig. 10-72. Varicosity of accessory vein on dorsal aspect of ankle with pretibial varicosity

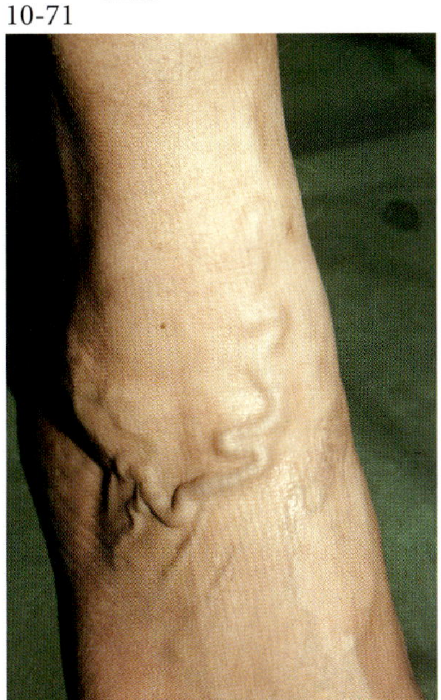

10-72

Fig. 10-73. Scratch marks over a distal varicosity of the lesser saphenous vein. In the early stages of stasis dermatitis, pruritus is often a complaint

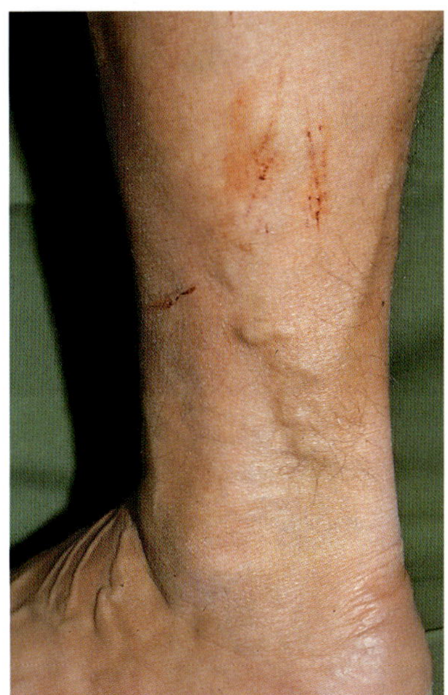

10-73

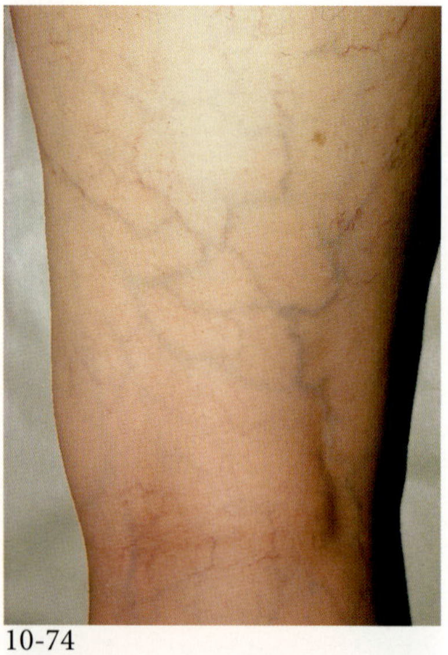
10-74

Fig. 10-74. Reticular varicosities on the dorso-medial aspect of the thigh. These dilated veins lie in the uppermost layers of the subcutaneous layer and show through the skin, with a net-like pattern. They have no direct connection to the infrafascial venous system. Although reticular varicosities have no hemodynamic significance, they are a cosmetic problem. Sclerotherapy is the treatment of choice

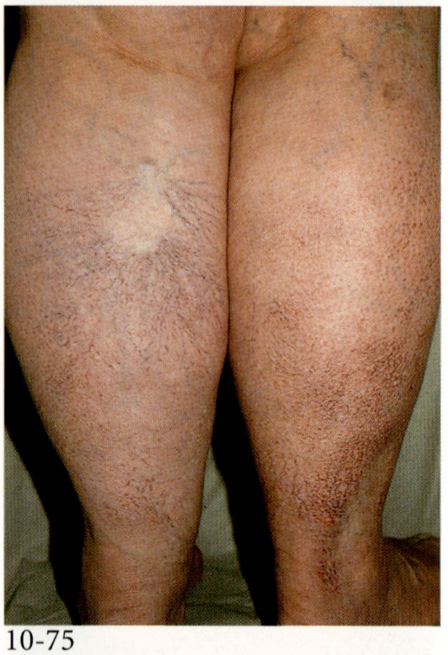
10-75

Fig. 10-75. Numerous spider veins on both legs of a 41 year old woman. These lesions are tiny intradermal micro-varicosities. They can be single, multiple or confluent. In extreme cases, wide areas of the skin are covered. Again spider veins have no hemodynamic significance. Some patients complain of pain and heavy legs, especially in the premenstrual phase

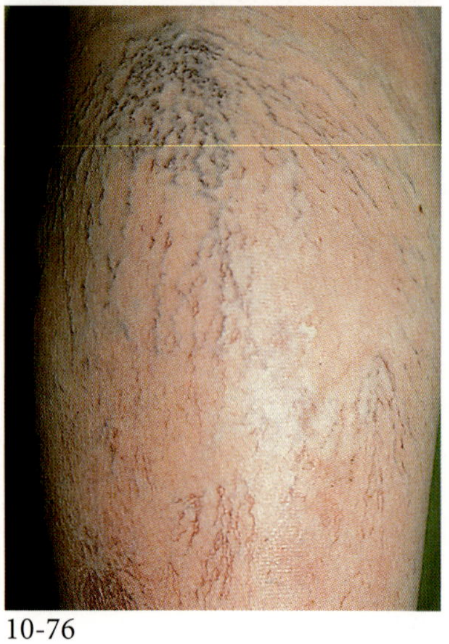
10-76

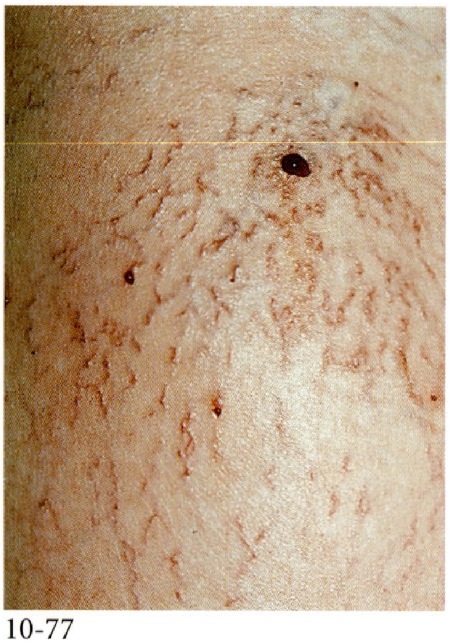
10-77

Fig. 10-76. Both red and blue spider veins in the same patient. The blue lesions are best treated with sclerotherapy, while a variety of laser systems seem best for the red variant

Fig. 10-77. Rupture of a spider vein in the same patient.

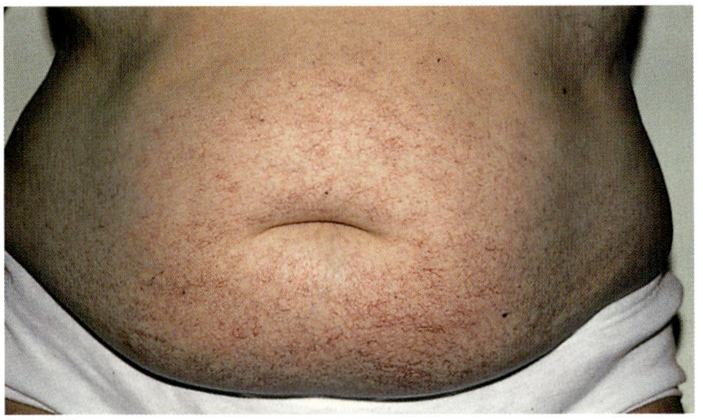

10-78

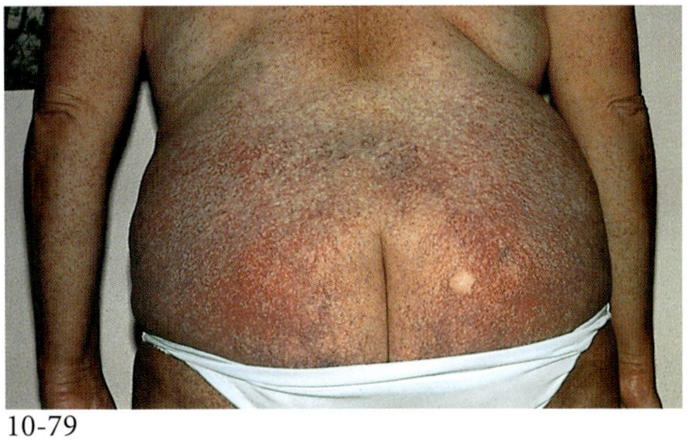

10-79

Figs. 10-78–10-82. A 64 year old women with widespread telangiectases which began after 35 years of age and are most prominent on the legs. The nasal, ocular and vaginal mucosa are all affected. Phlebography showed incompetent perforating veins on the lower legs, but the pathogenesis of the widespread proliferation is unclear

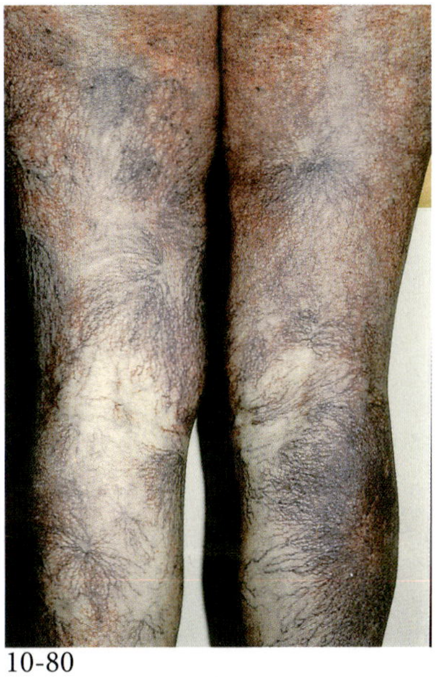

10-80

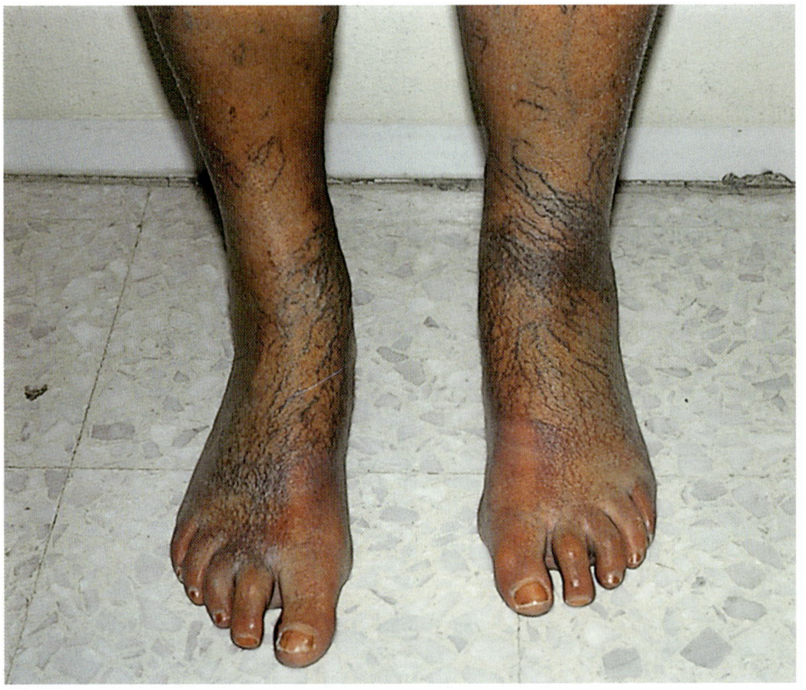

10-81

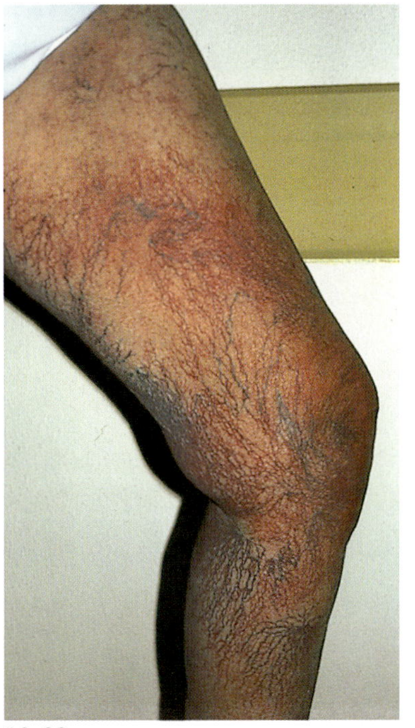

10-82

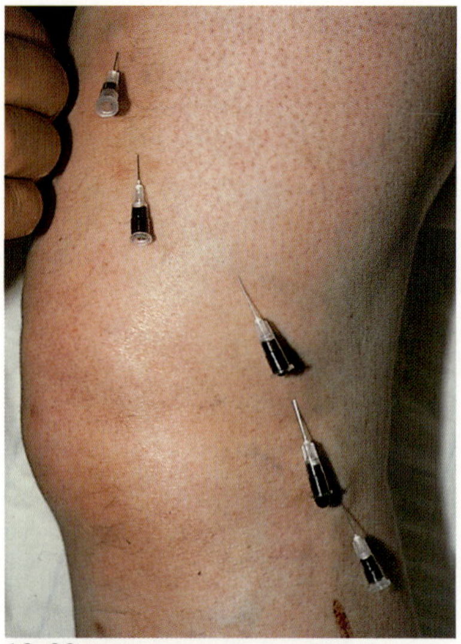

10-83

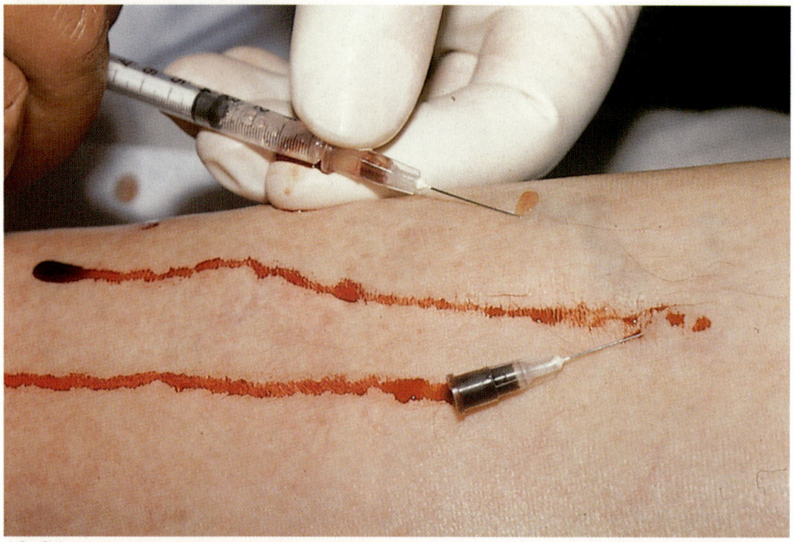

10-84

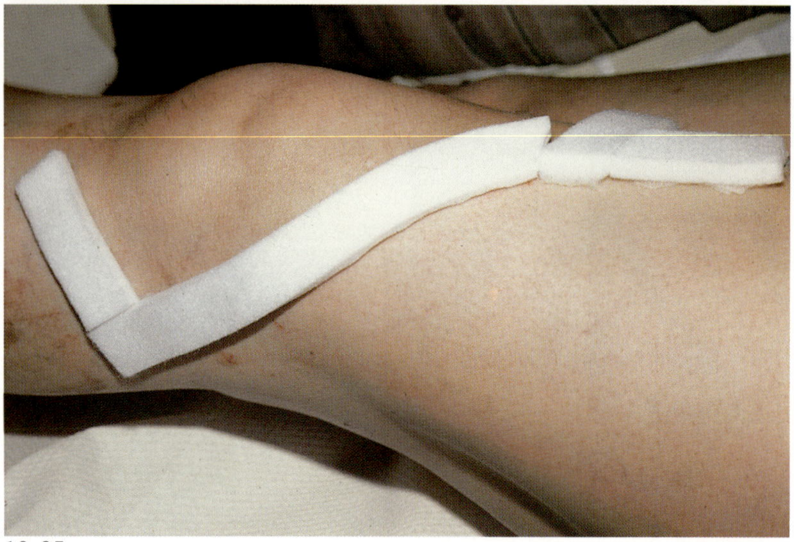

10-85

Figs. 10-83 – 10-85. Sclerotherapy for a varicosity of the lateral accessory saphenous vein. According to the SIGG (KARL SIGG, Swiss phlebologist) technique:

- Venipuncture is performed with multiple fine needles not attached to syringes. The patient stands for this part of procedure.
- Injection of the sclerosing material is performed when the patient is lying down. Not more than 1.0 ml should be injected at any site.
- For larger varicosities, the air block technique can be used, injecting 0.5 ml of air prior to the sclerosing material.
- Immediately after injection, the varicosities are compressed, here with adhesive felt strips.
- At the conclusion of the injections, a compression dressing is applied.

Fig. 10-86. Necrosis following para-venous injection. Such a lesion heals slowly and leaves a scar. If one notices that the injection has been para-venous, the injection of physiologic saline to dilute out the sclerosing material generally prevents necrosis

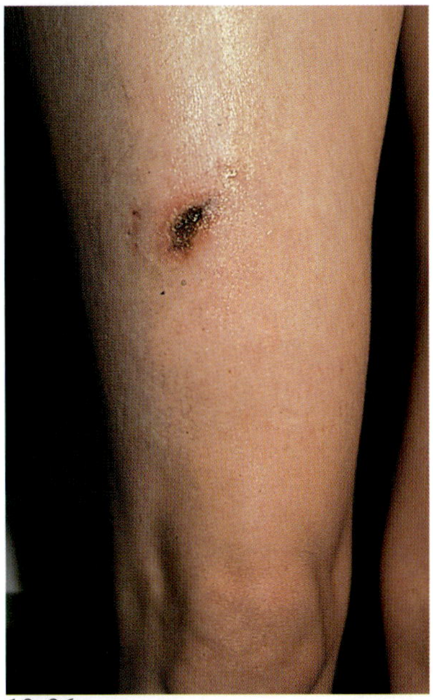

10-86

Fig. 10-87. Scarring following sclerotherapy

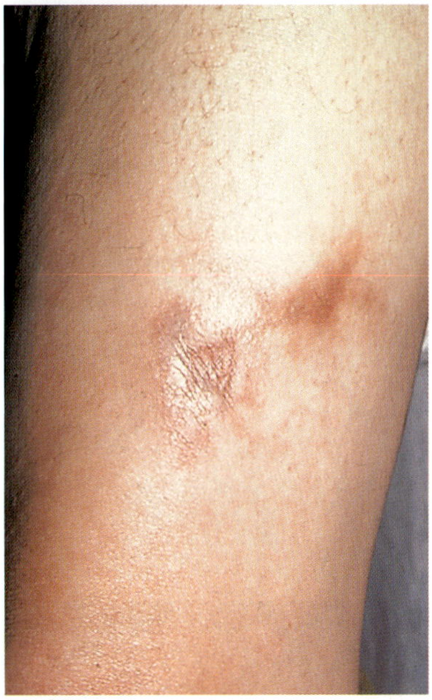

10-87

Fig. 10-88. Hyperpigmentation is a most uncommon complication of sclerotherapy

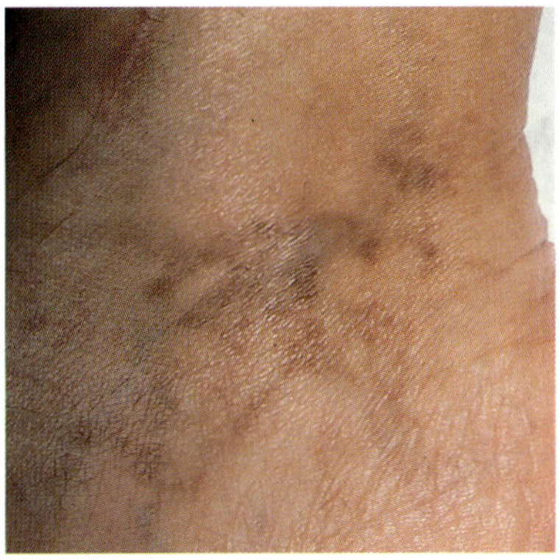

10-88

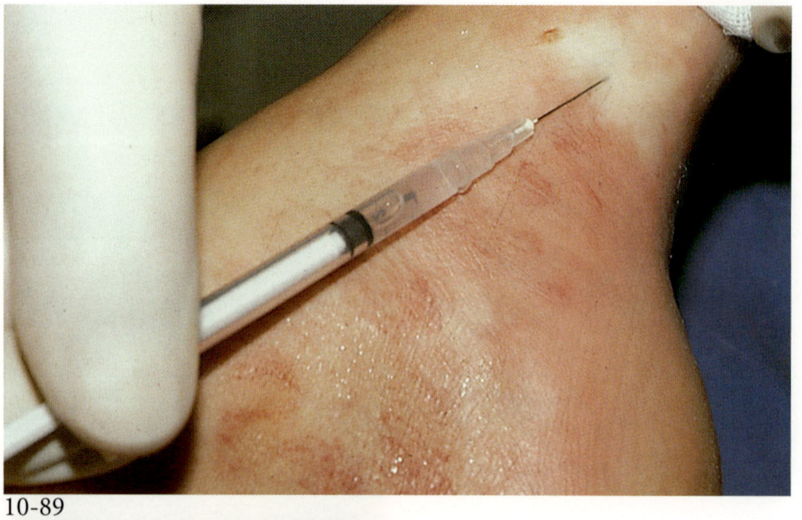

10-89

Fig. 10-89. Sclerosing spider veins requires a very fine needle, usually 30- or 32-gauge. While larger varicosities should be injected intravascularly, sometimes smaller ones, which are hard to canulate, can be eliminated by injection of a minute amount of dilute sclerosing agent in a para-vascular position

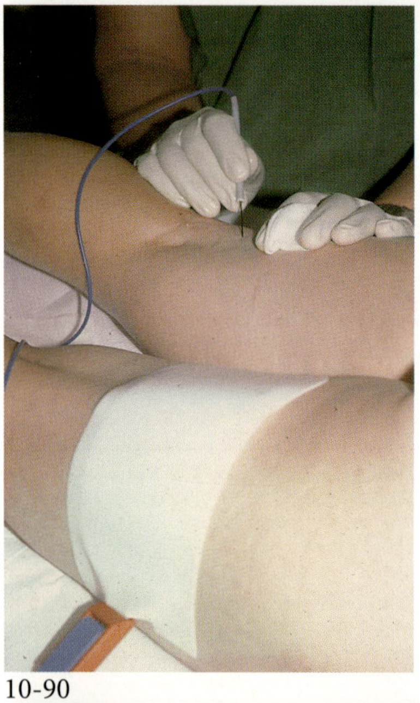

10-90

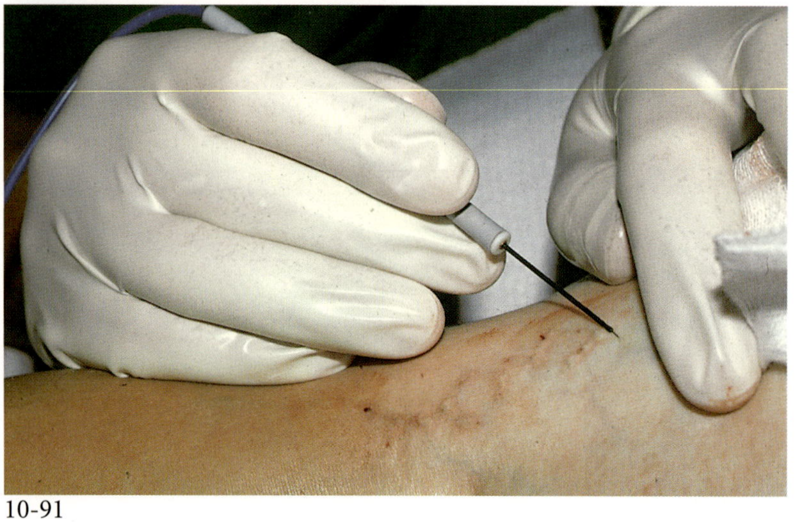

10-91

Figs. 10-90, 10-91. Electrotherapy of spider veins in the popliteal space. A very fine needle and high frequency alternating current are usually employed, although a number of systems can be used

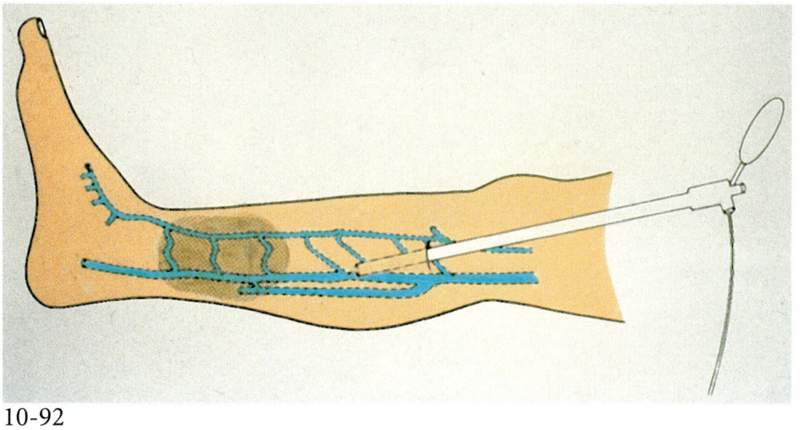

10-92

Fig. 10-92. Endoscopic subfascial dissection of perforating veins. This method of interrupting incompetent perforating veins is often used when dermatoliposclerosis or an ulcer are present. The entry site is an area of healthy skin, usually the proximal calf. The perforating veins of the calf (COCKETT, SHERMAN, BOYD, MAY and soleus) are all accessible. In the direct technique (FISCHER) the vein is dissected and clipped. In the indirect technique (HAUER) the perforating vein is coagulated following the procedure with a video monitor

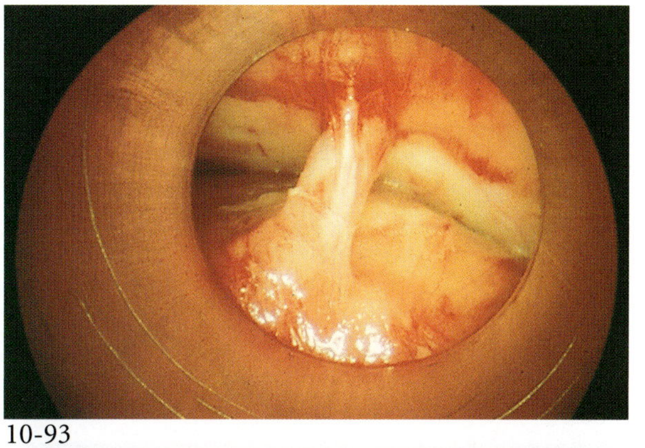

10-93

Fig. 10-93. Perforating vein with accompanying artery. The fascia is at the top and the slit for the vein can be seen. Muscles are seen at the bottom

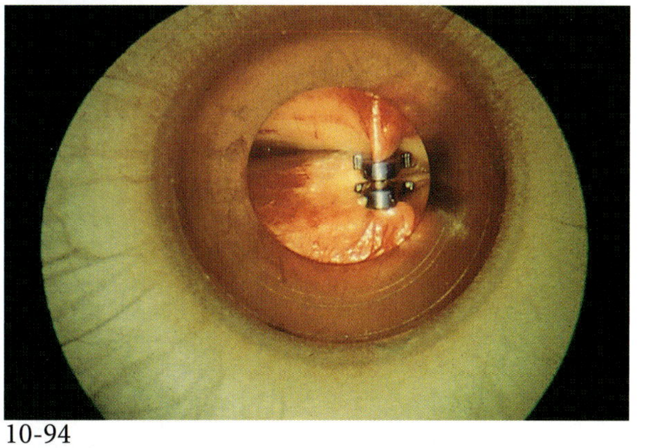

10-94

Fig. 10-94. Absorbable clips are used to block off the perforating vein

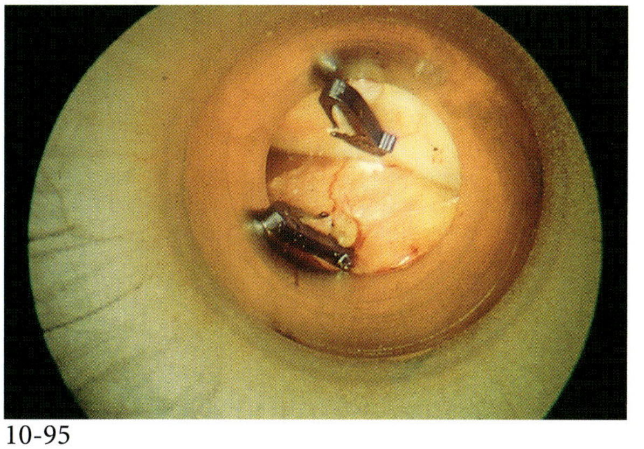

10-95

Fig. 10-95. Once it has been clipped, the vein is cut in between the two clips

In the Varady technique, a tiny 1.5 mm incision is made. Using special instruments the varicosity is exposed, tracked and removed.

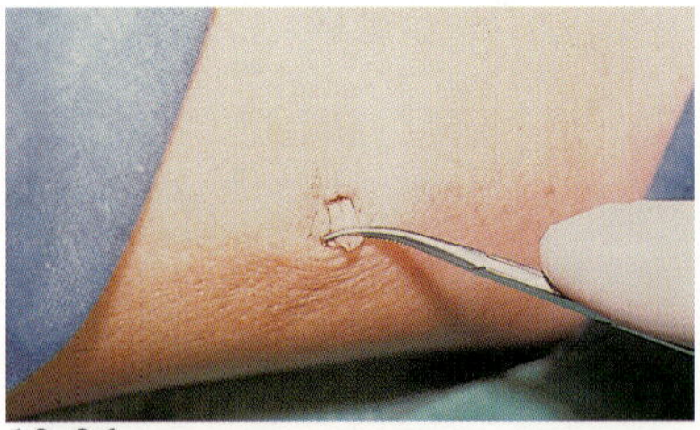
10-96

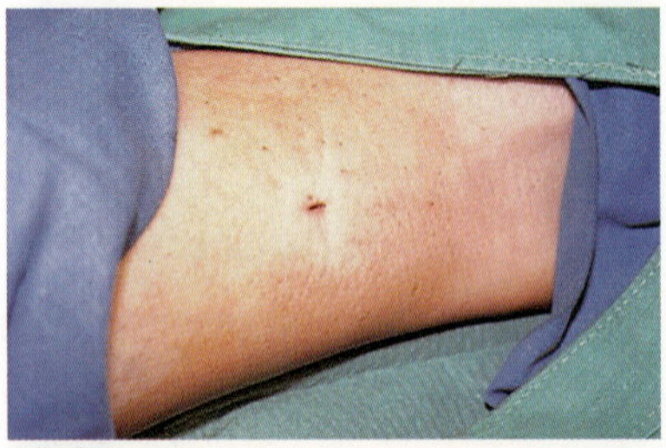
10-97

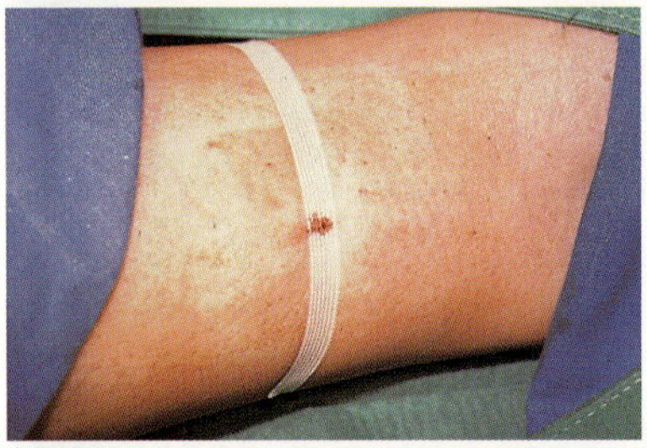
10-98

Fig. 10-96. After exact localization with Doppler ultrasonography, the perforating vein (here Cockett II) and the accessory vein are exposed

Fig. 10-97. Appearance following removal of varicosity

Fig. 10-98. The incisions are closed with adhesive strips, followed by a compression dressing

Removal of an Accessory Vein Varicosity of the Ventral Plantar Arch

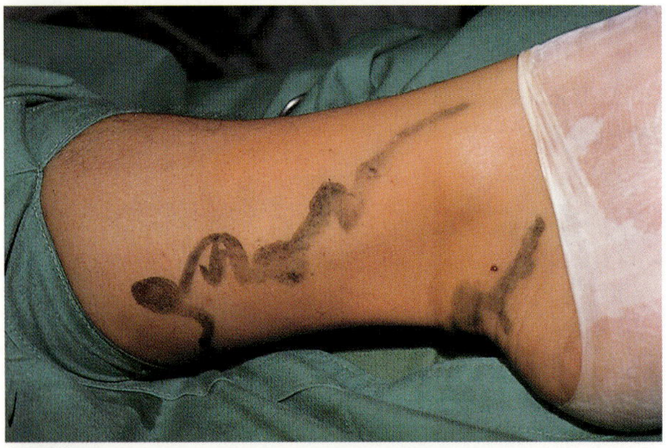
10-99

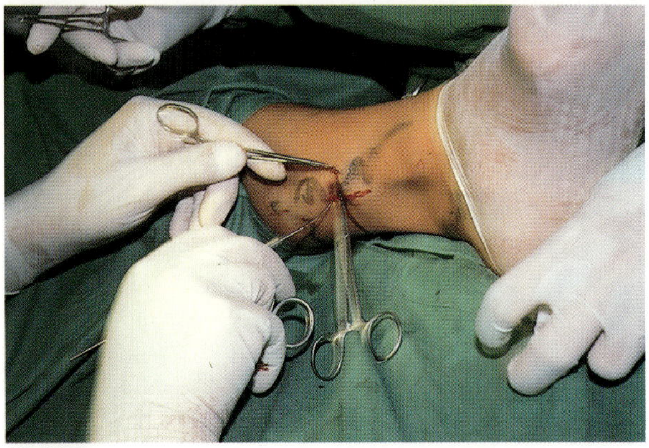
10-100

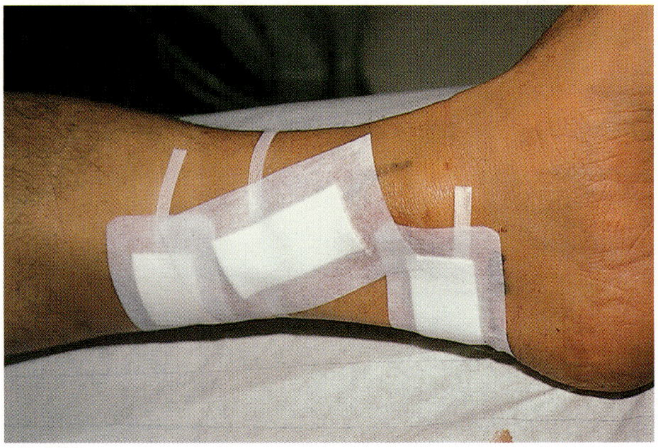
10-101

Fig. 10-99. The varicosity is marked

Fig. 10-100. Removal of the varicosity through multiple incisions

Fig. 10-101. Wound closure with pressure tape dressings

Figs. 10-102–10-104. Partial removal of the greater saphenous vein from the HUNTER to the COCKETT perforating veins. Along the course of the stripped greater saphenous vein, a pressure bandage is applied

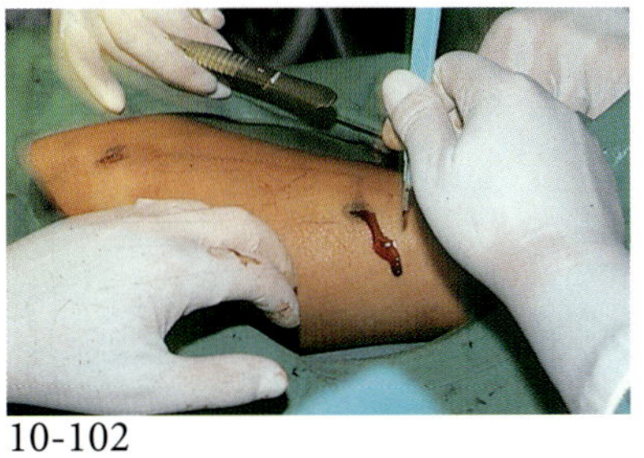
10-102

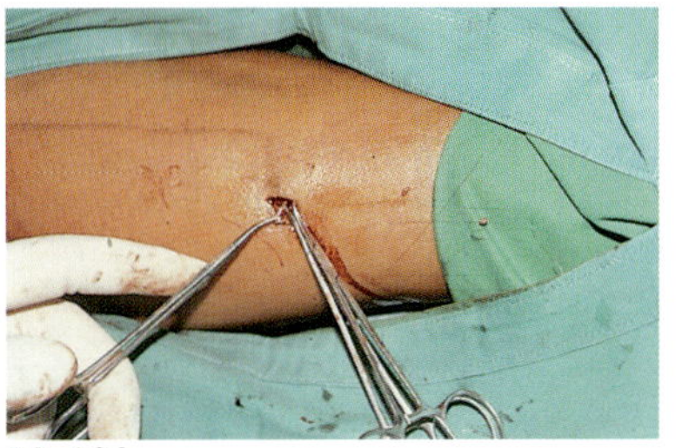
10-103

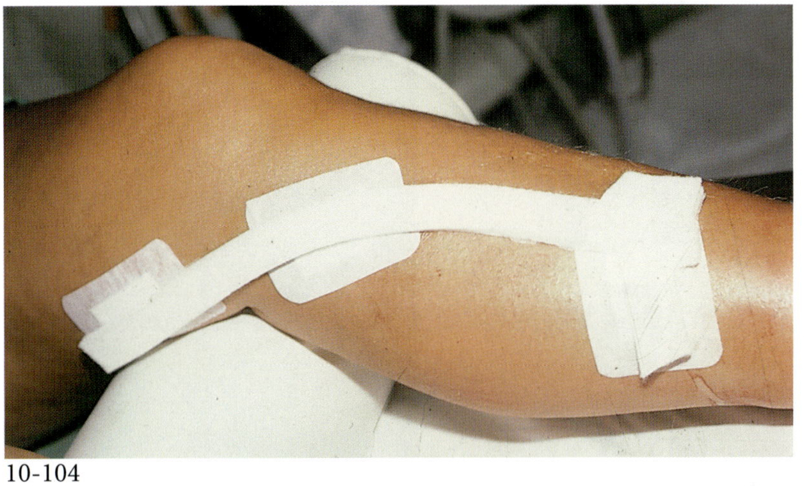
10-104

Figs. 10-105, 10-106. Partial removal of the lesser saphenous vein in the popliteal space. The proximal portion of the vein is exposed and then an 8 cm long varicose vein removed

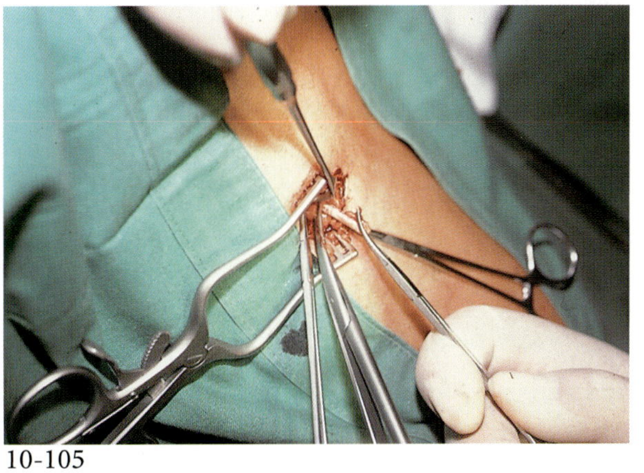
10-105

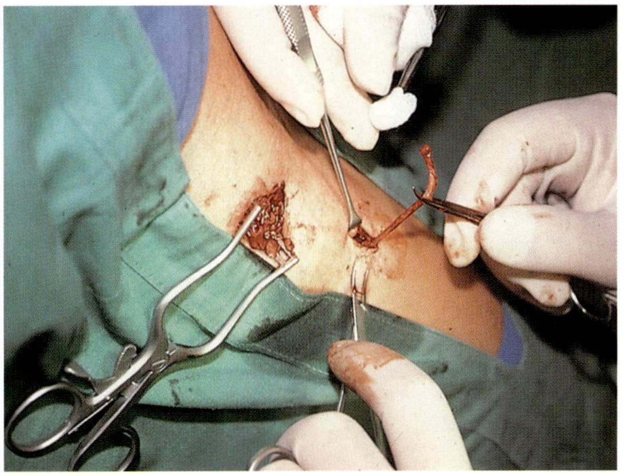
10-106

A 21 year old woman had a complex developmental anomaly of the venous system of her right leg (KLIPPEL-TRENAUNAY syndrome)

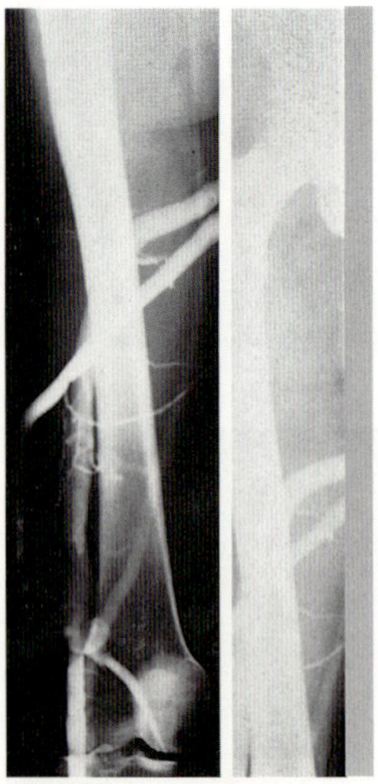

10-107

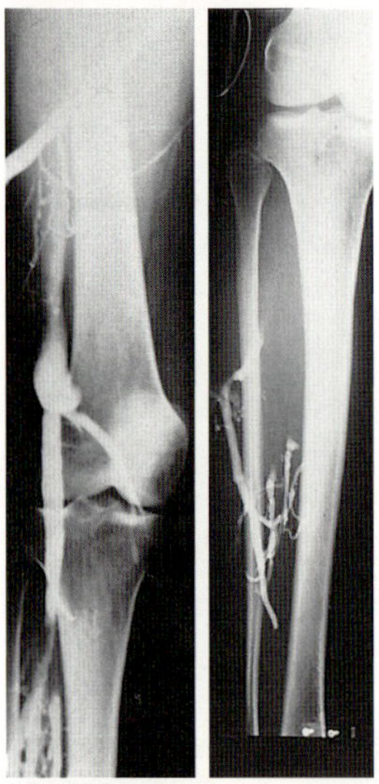

10-108

Figs. 10-107, 10-108. Phlebography showing varicosities on the lateral surface of the thigh. The valves of this anomalous vein on the postero-lateral aspect of the thigh are incompetent. The superficial femoral vein also has an aberrant course, running in an epifascial plane proximally. In the same area is another vessel which can be followed to the calf in the usual course of the superficial femoral vein, but does not have the usual divisions at its distal end

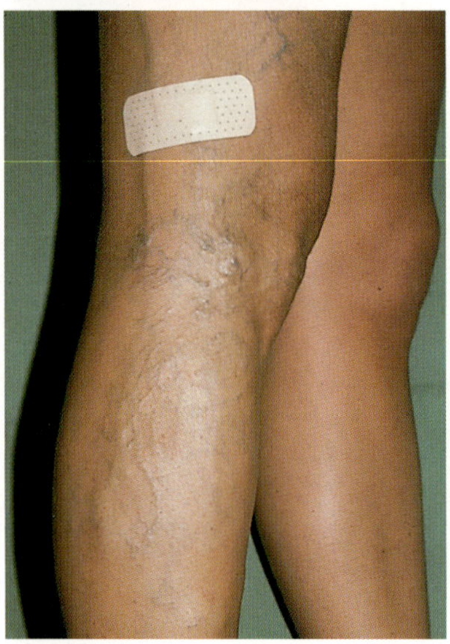

10-109

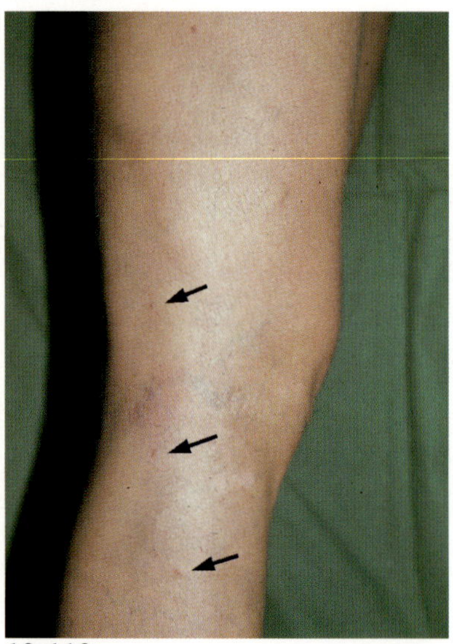

10-110

Fig. 10-109. Pre-operative appearance

Fig. 10-110. Appearance following mini-incision approach with very good cosmetic result. The tiny scars are shown (*arrows*)

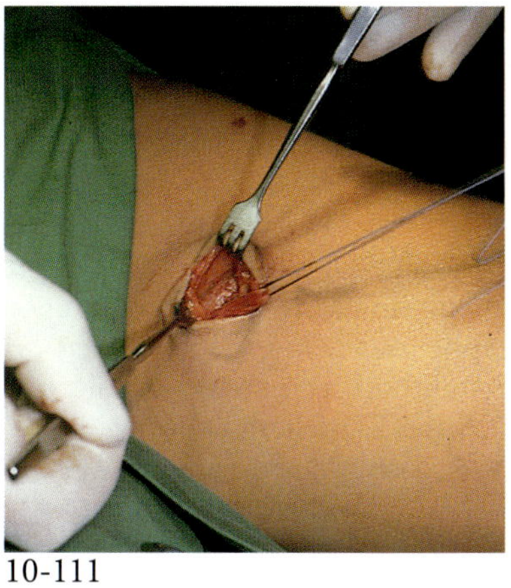
10-111

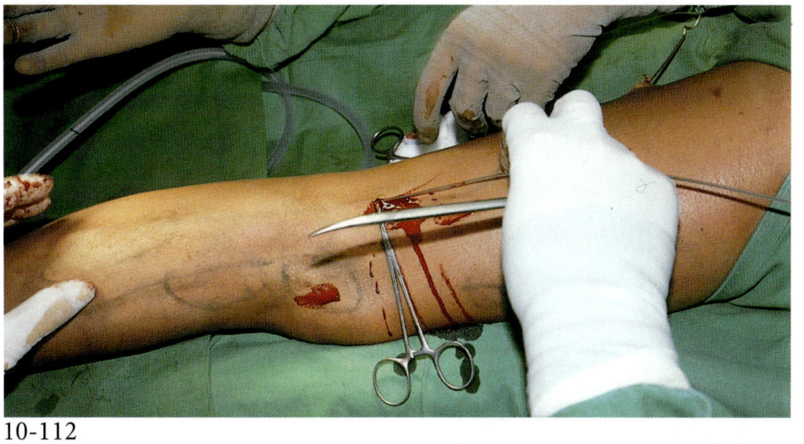
10-112

In the same patient as shown on the previous page, the Babcock (William Wayne Babock, 1872–1963, American surgeon) operation was performed.

Fig. 10-111. Exposure of the proximal level of incompetence of the marginal vein

Fig. 10-112. Introduction of a probe into lateral accessory saphenous vein

Fig. 10-113. Exposing the probe at the distal level of incompetence at the lateral malleolus.

Fig. 10-114. Exposure of the large accessory varicosity

Figs. 10-115, 10-116. Stripping the veins

Fig. 10-117. Closing the skin with intracutaneous sutures

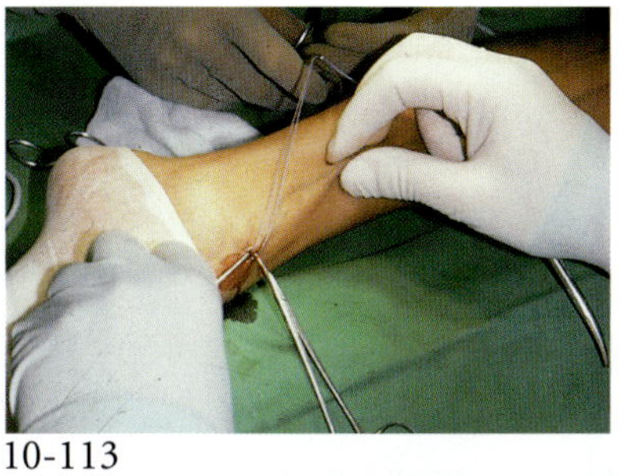
10-113

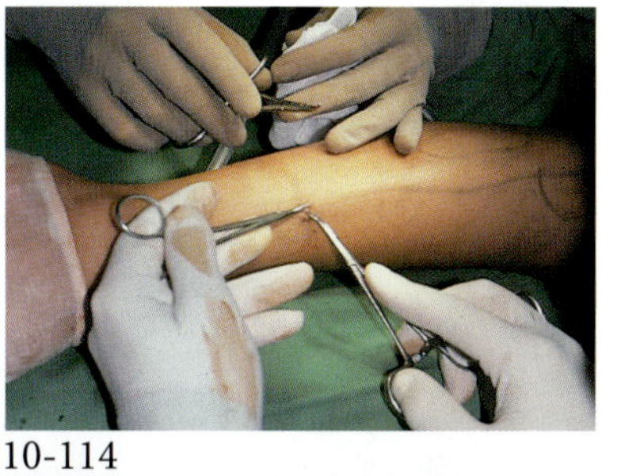
10-114

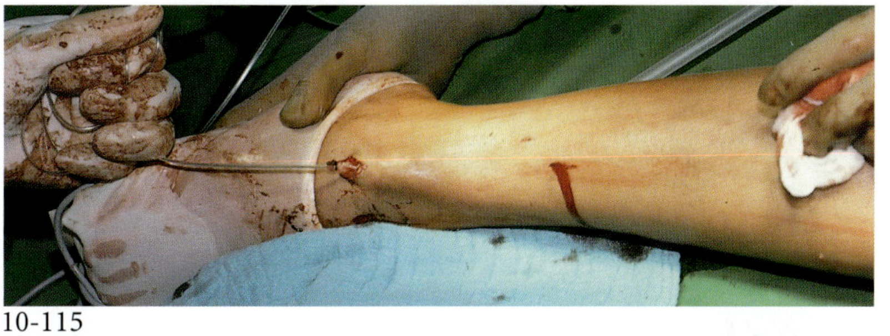
10-115

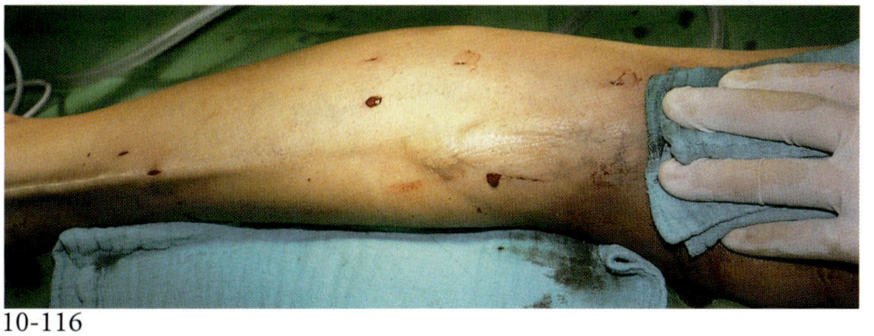
10-116

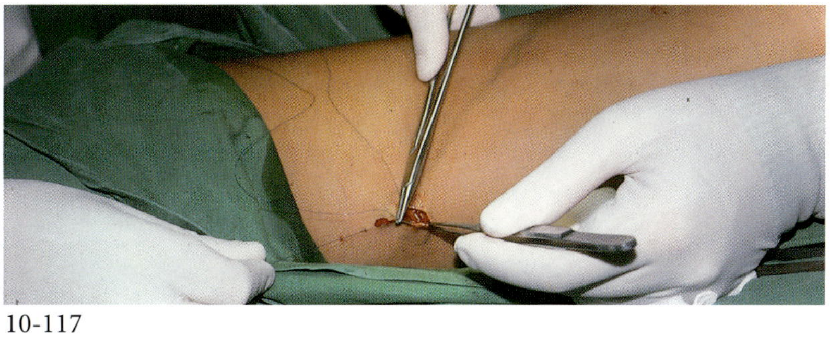
10-117

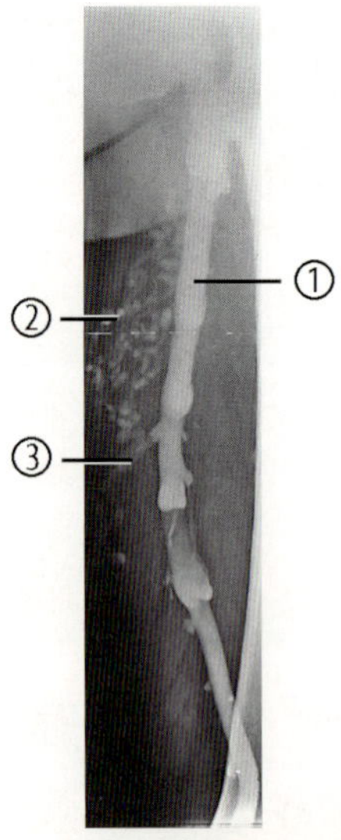

10-118

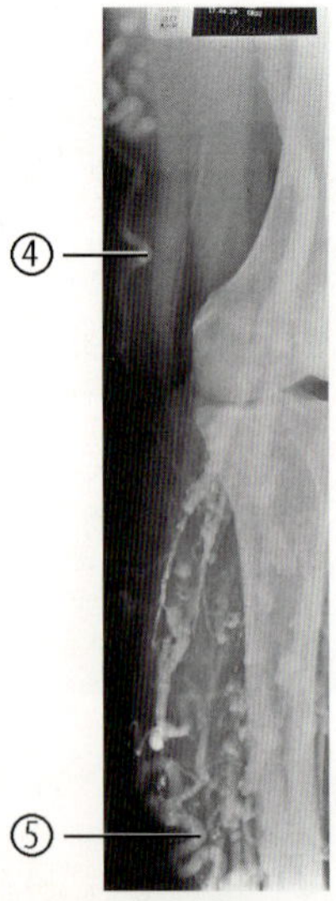

10-119

Figs. 10-118, 10-119. Phlebography showing recurrence of a varicosity of the greater saphenous vein because of side branches at the ligated sapheno-femoral junction and an incompetent perforating vein in the mid-thigh. The main branch of the greater saphenous vein is shown in the distal thigh and proximal calf.
① Superficial femoral vein
② Branches at the sapheno-femoral junction
③ Incompetent perforating vein
④ Greater saphenous vein
⑤ Accessory branch of the greater saphenous vein

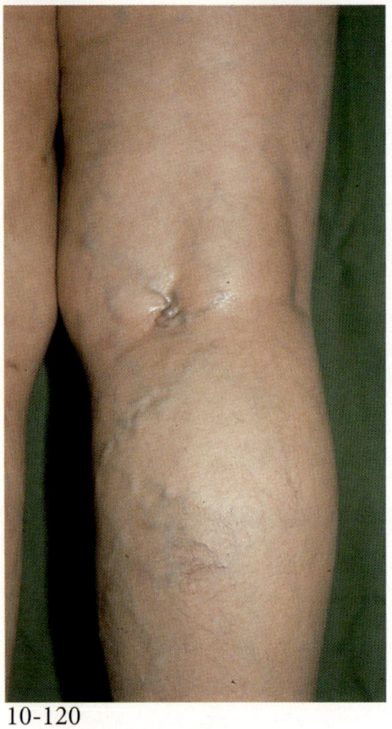

10-120

Fig. 10-120. Appearance following removal of the greater and lesser saphenous veins. Post-operative varicosities of multiple accessory veins on the dorso-medial aspect of the leg

"Recurrent varicosities": The operative scars on the leg give clues as to what procedure was originally performed. In the area of the greater saphenous vein there are two possibilities:

- Babcock procedure, with high ligation with or without stripping
- Moszkowicz (Eli Moszkowicz, 1879–1964, American pathologist) procedure, which is no longer done, but which combined a high ligation with retrograde sclerotherapy

Usually the explanation is an inadequate initial operative procedure. Sometimes the sapheno-femoral junction is not adequately exposed and branches or segments of the vein are left behind that are later fed by perforating veins, causing varicosities.

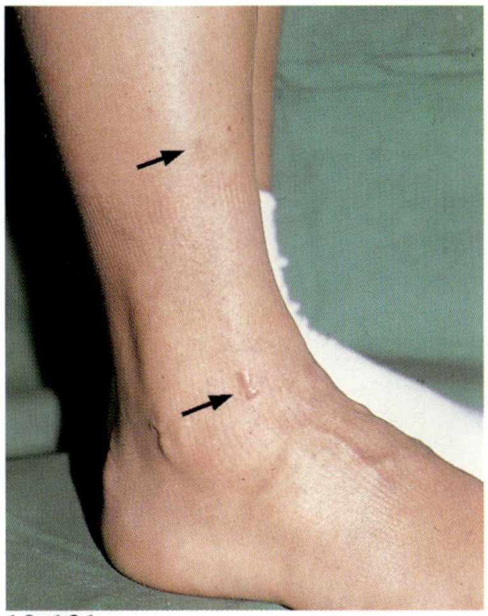

10-121

Fig. 10-121. Modest keloid formation over distal incision (*arrow*); keloids are relatively common in the tight skin about the ankle

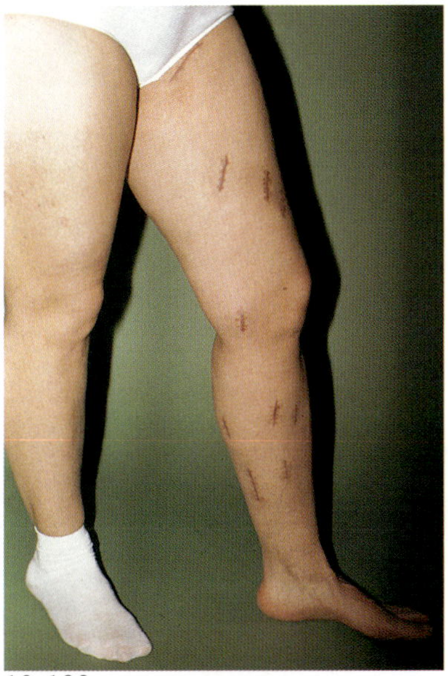

10-122

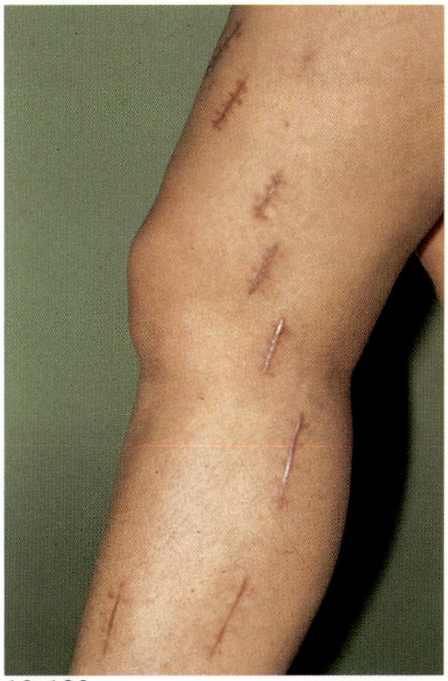

10-123

Figs. 10-122, 10-123. A 32 year old woman following removal of the greater saphenous vein. The cosmetic results are unsatisfactory and do not reflect the current state of surgical skills. Both the medial and lateral aspects of the leg show multiple keloidal scars

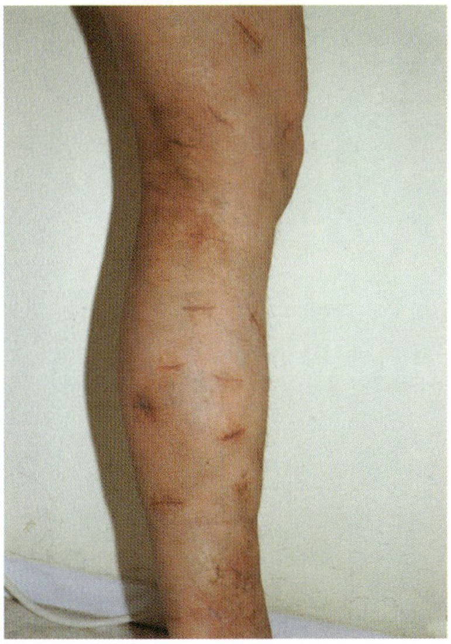

10-124

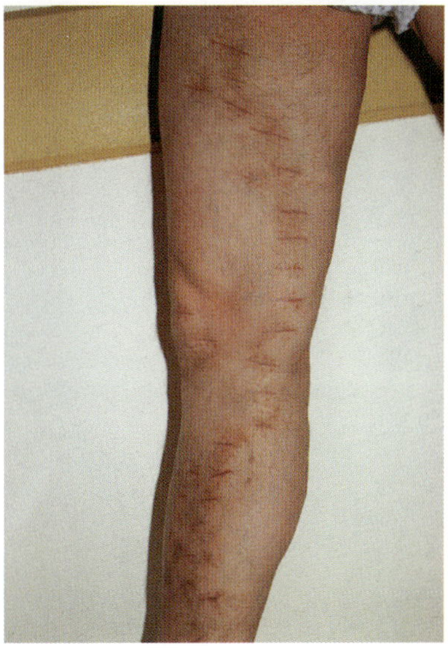

10-125

Figs. 10-124, 10-125. Scarring following a stripping operation done years ago. Once again, the cosmetic results are unsatisfactory

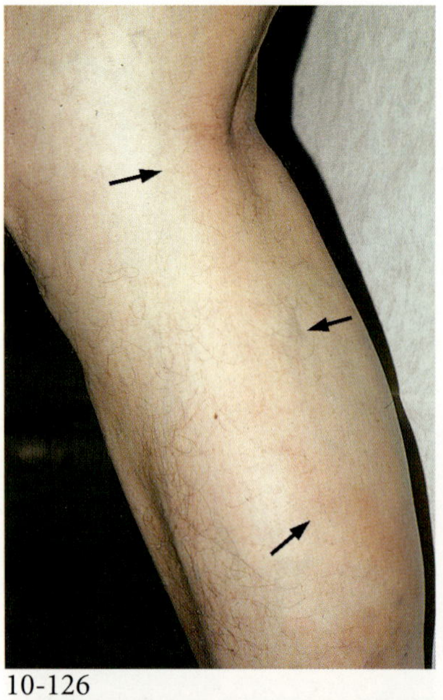
10-126

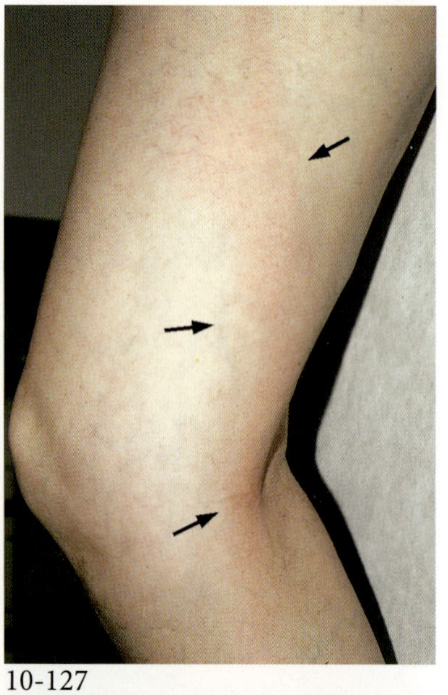
10-127

Figs. 10-126, 10-127. A 34 year old man with acute thrombophlebitis (*arrows*) from the calf ascending almost to the inguinal ligament. The cause was never determined. A paraneoplastic phenomenon was excluded and there was no evidence for BEHÇET's syndrome, other forms of vasculitis, or thromboangiitis obliterans

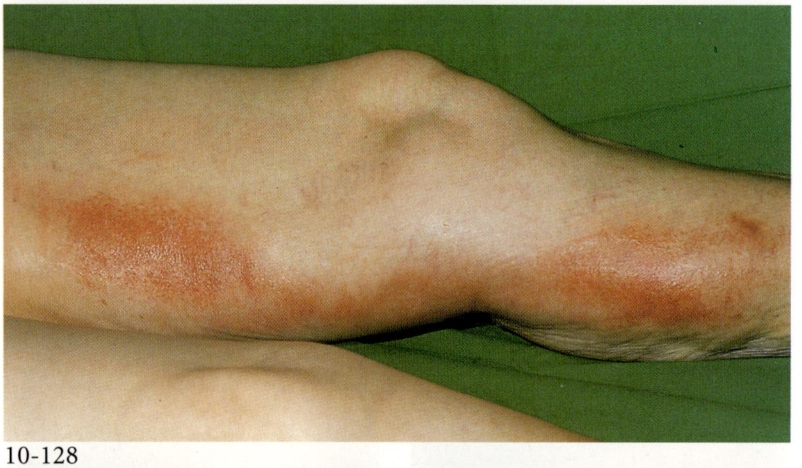
10-128

Fig. 10-128. Massive thrombophlebitis in pre-existing varicosities

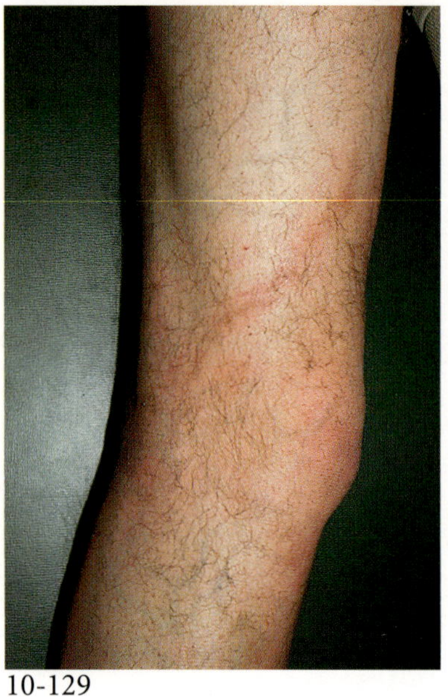
10-129

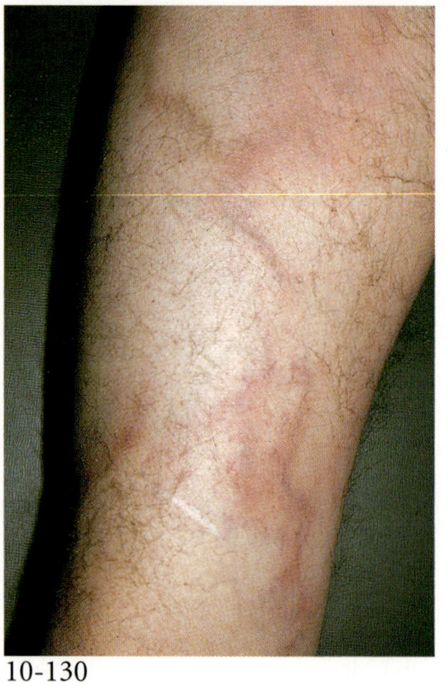
10-130

Figs. 10-129, 10-130. Prominent long segment of thrombophlebitis in a 30 year old man with a past history of inferior vena cava thrombosis and bilateral iliac vein thrombosis. The nature of the underlying clotting defect was never identified

Figs. 10-131, 10-132. Acute thrombophlebitis in the thigh. The fluctuant nodule can be incised and the thrombus removed. Generally the pain and inflammation will then resolve rapidly. A compression dressing should be applied from the foot to past the site of the thrombosis. If there are incompetent perforating veins or if the thrombosis is near a junction, one should be more cautious since bleeding can occur

Fig. 10-133. Recurrent thrombophlebitis in a patient with thromboangiitis obliterans (BUERGER's disease). The 38 year old man had segmental occlusion of the arteries of the lower legs bilaterally. He had already had migratory thrombophlebitis at 21 years of age. The patient had continued to smoke. There are discrete erythematous area on the medial aspect of the leg (*arrows*)

Figs. 10-134, 10-135. Acute thrombophlebitis (*arrows*) on the back of the foot in a patient with thromboangiitis obliterans. The acral ischemia is also obvious

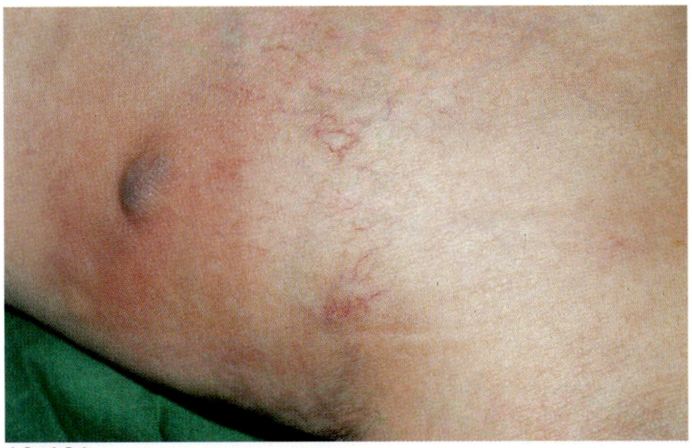

10-131

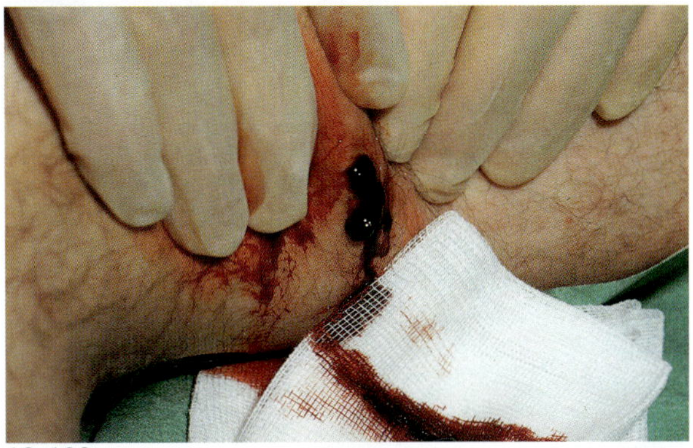

10-132

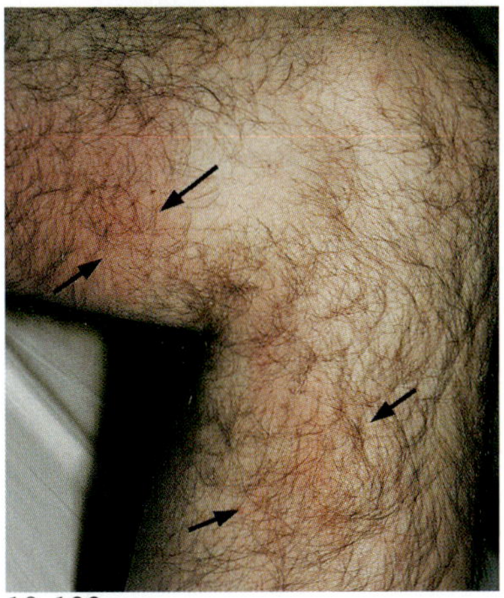

10-133

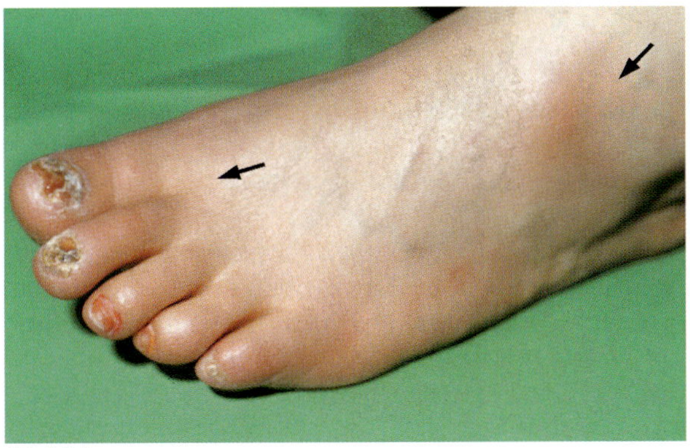

10-134

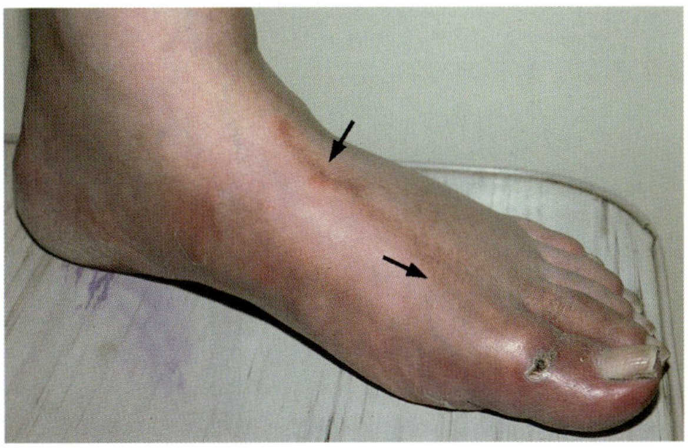

10-135

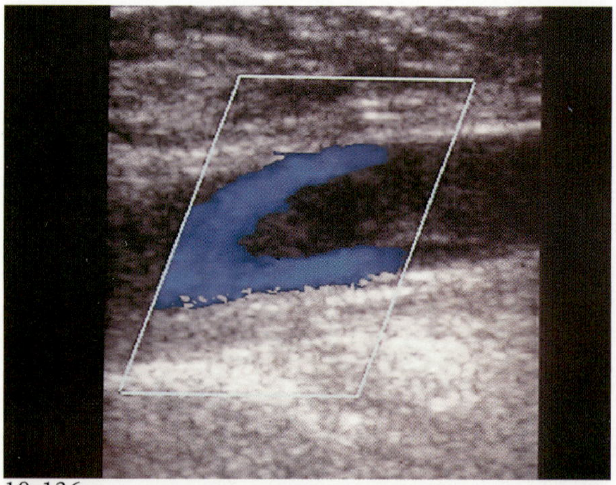

10-136

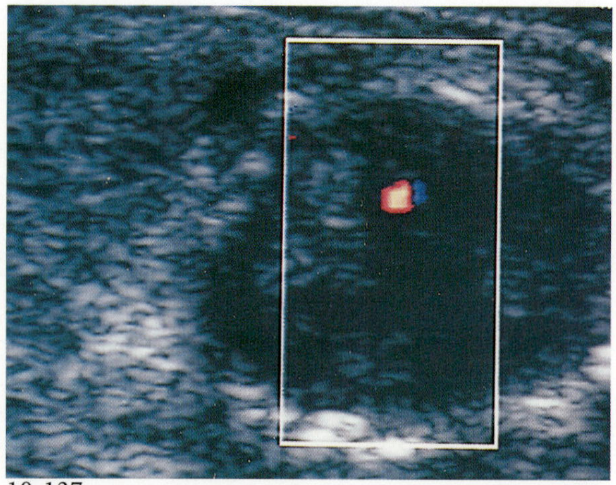

10-137

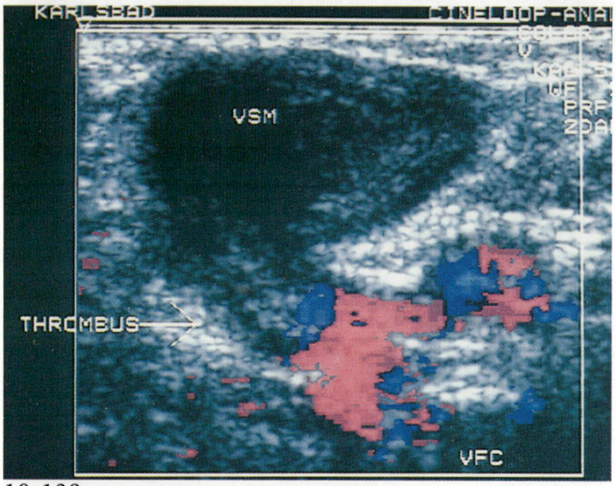

10-138

Fig. 10-136. Color duplex sonography showing a fluttering or unstable thrombus in the external iliac vein of a 36 year old paraplegic

Fig. 10-137. Color duplex sonography showing an extensive thrombus in the common femoral vein. There is a tiny residual lumen in the center. The thrombus was not compressible

Fig. 10-138. Color duplex sonography showing acute thrombophlebitis in a varicose greater saphenous vein which is almost completely occluded. The thrombus extends into the common femoral vein (collar button thrombosis)

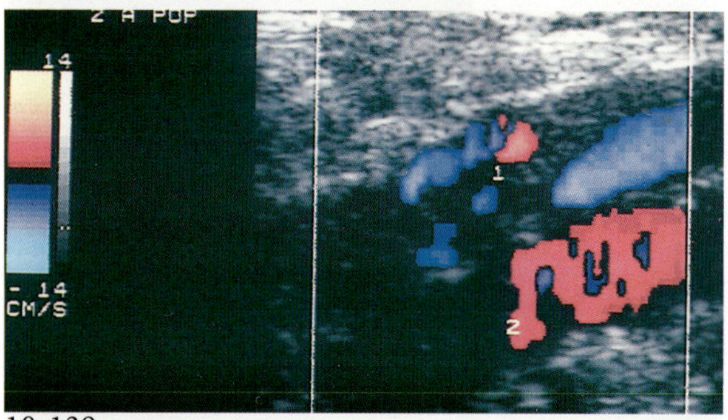

10-139

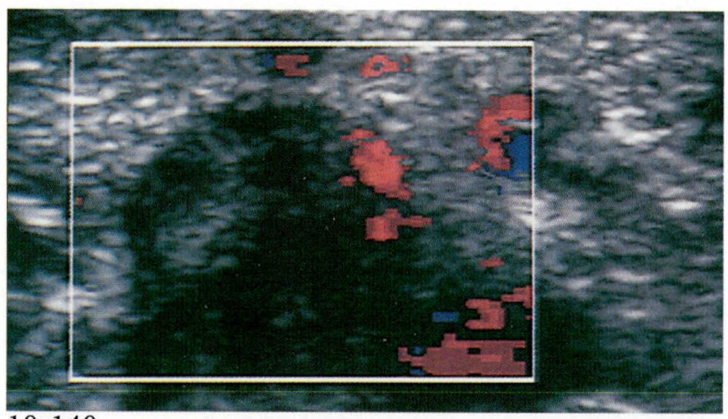

10-140

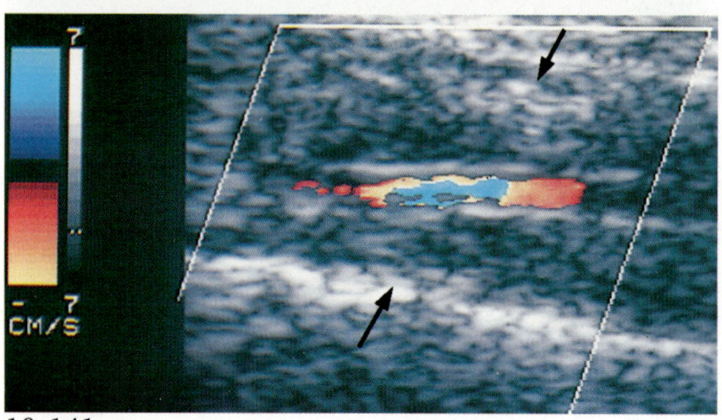

10-141

Fig. 10-139. Color duplex sonography showing recanalization of an old thrombus in the popliteal vein

Fig. 10-140. Same lesion in cross-section

Fig. 10-141. Color duplex sonography showing thrombosis of the posterior tibial group. The examination was performed with compression. The painful dilated calf veins (*arrows*) are not compressible. Normal flow is seen in the posterior tibial artery

Fig. 10-142. Color duplex sonography showing the femoral vein and sapheno-femoral junction. The junction is clearly widened because a number of collateral veins join the greater saphenous vein at this level. The patient has occlusion of the iliac vein on the other side

Fig. 10-143. A 25 year old man with iliac vein thrombosis following radiation therapy for seminoma. Prominent suprapubic varicosities through collateral formation

Fig. 10-144. Occlusion of the inferior vena cava. The superficial epigastric veins are enlarged and provide collateral circulation. They may anastomose with the periumbilical veins near the umbilicus

Fig. 10-145. The patient in Fig. 10-143 developed thrombophlebitis in veins collateral

Fig. 10-146. Phlebography showing a suprapubic varicosity, similar to the patient above

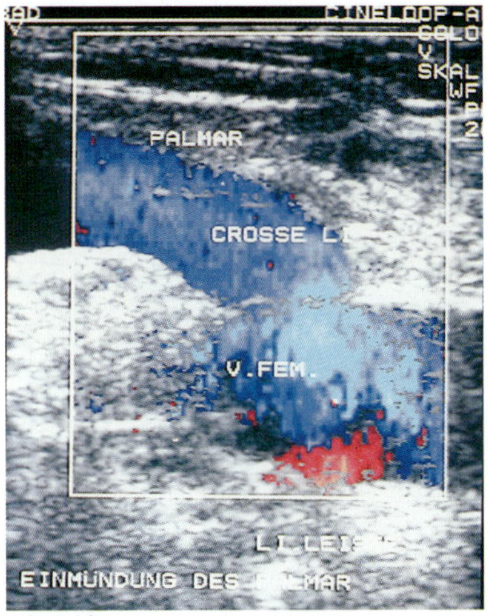

10-142

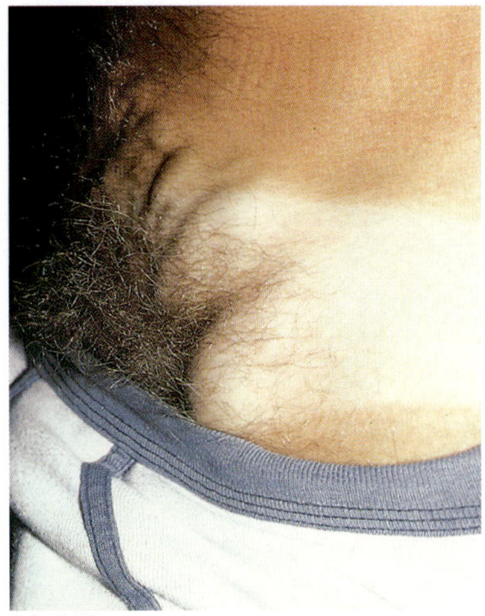

10-143

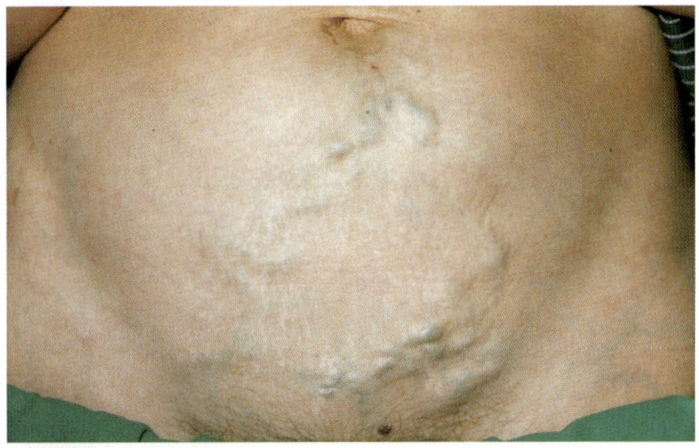

10-144

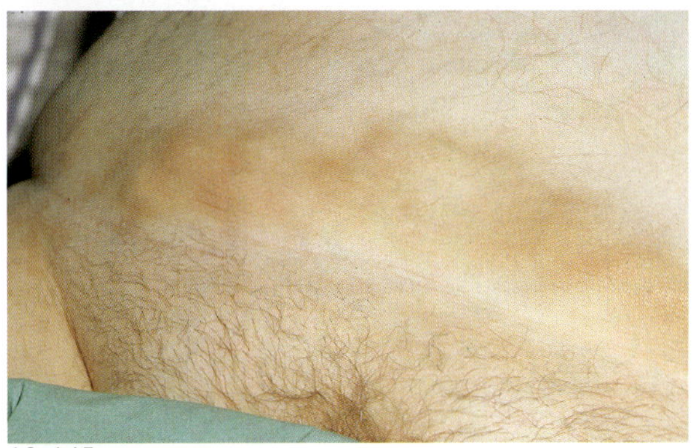

10-145

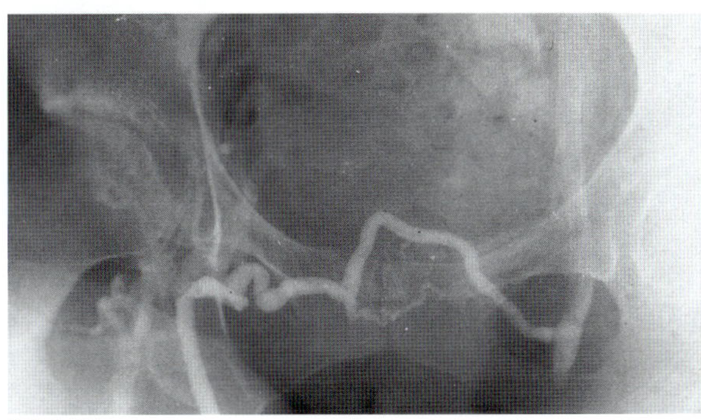

10-146

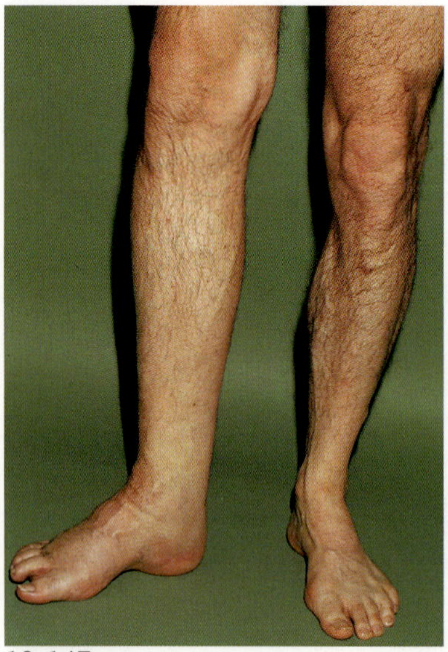

10-147

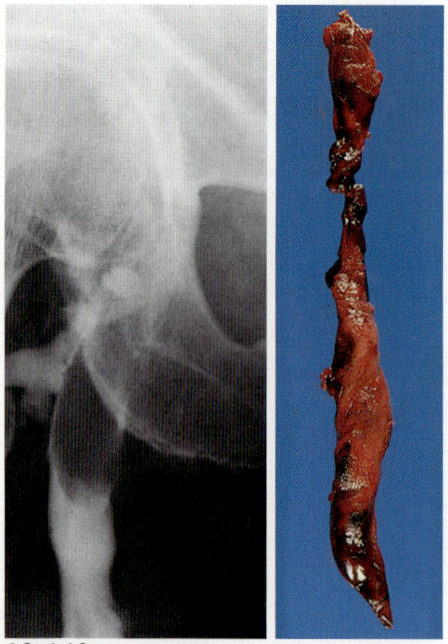

10-148

Fig. 10-147. Pre-operative appearance of an acute thigh vein thrombosis.

Fig. 10-148. Phlebogram and the operative specimen from the same came.

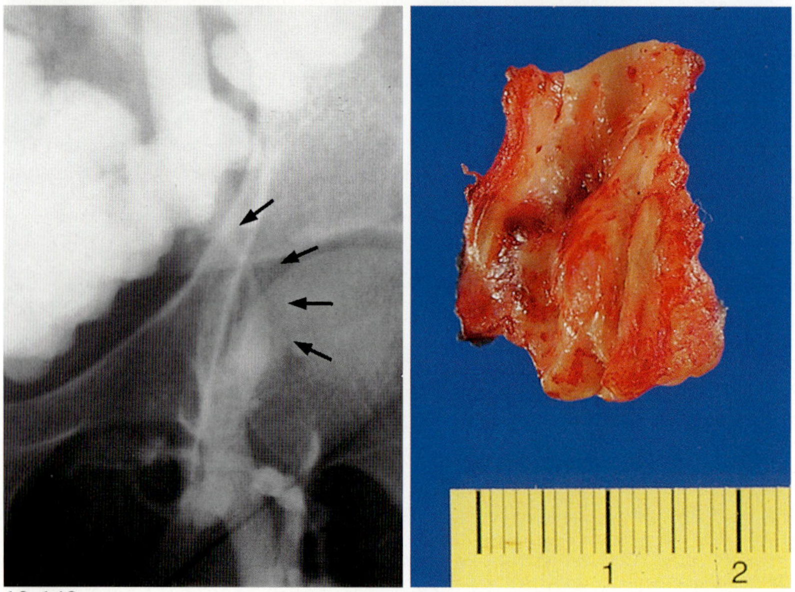

10-149

Fig. 10-149. Phlebography showing a scarring stenosis of the femoral vein (*arrows*) following thrombectomy. The scarred section was excised (specimen at *right*) and replaced with a section from a duplicated greater saphenous vein

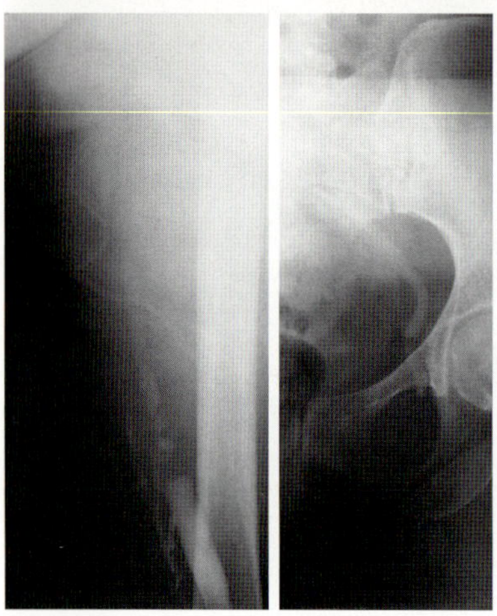

10-150

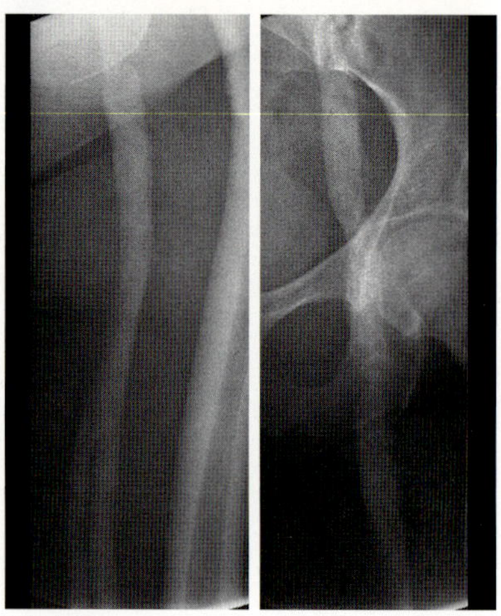

10-151

Fig. 10-150. Phlebography showing an acute thrombosis of the iliac, thigh and leg veins without collateral formation, indicating that the lesion is relatively new

Fig. 10-151. Control phlebogram after thrombectomy through the femoral vein; there are no residual signs of thrombosis

Figs. 10-152, 10–153. Venous thrombosis of the thigh and iliac veins. An arterio-venous fistula was created in the inguinal region because the thrombi had been firmly adherent. The post-operative angiogram shows the fistula and a stenotic but patent iliac vein (*arrows*)

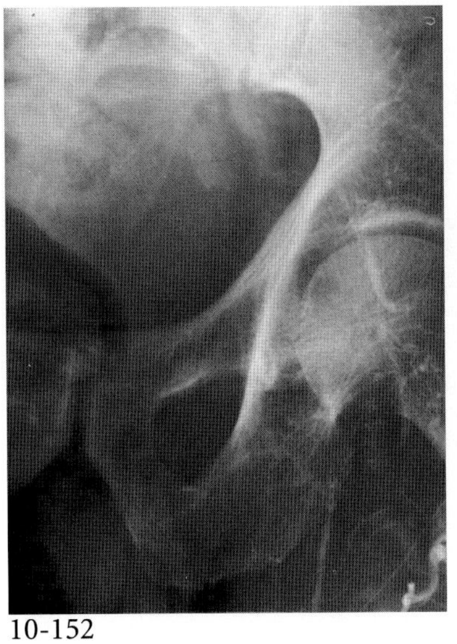

10-152

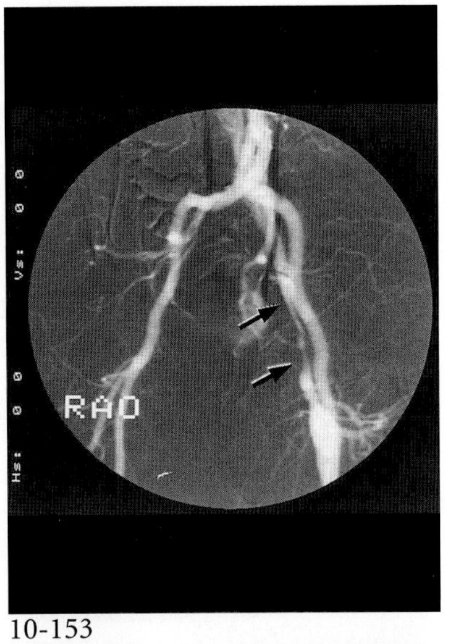

10-153

Fig. 10-154. Phlebography showing acute thrombosis of the femoral vein as well as the entire iliac system and the inferior vena cava at the level of the bifurcation

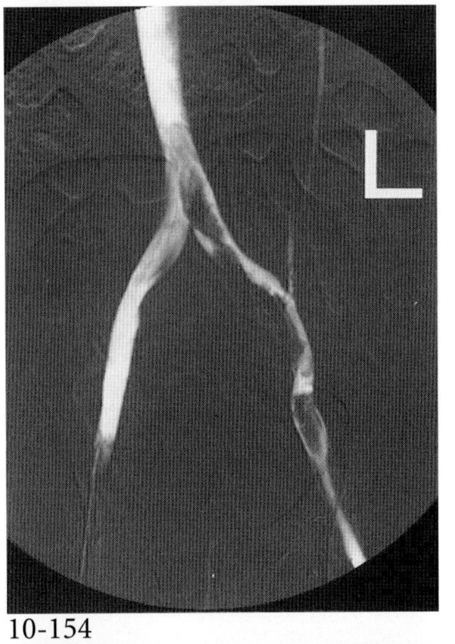

10-154

Fig. 10-155. A thrombectomy was attempted, but residual thrombi were still present. The catheter was accidentally passed into the ascending lumbar vein; in the past incomplete thombectomies were often the result of improper placement of the catheter. Today intra-operative control phlebography or fluoroscopy eliminates this possibility

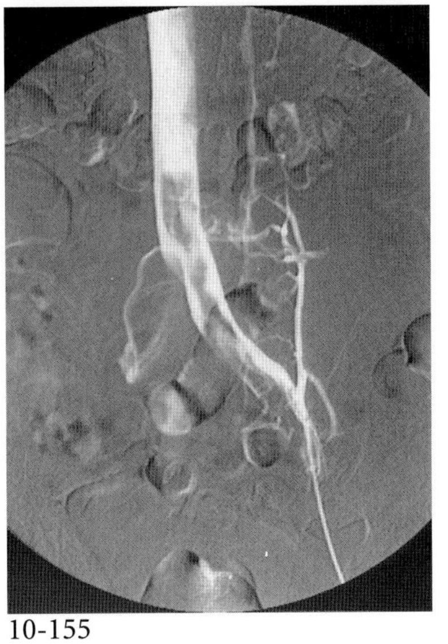

10-155

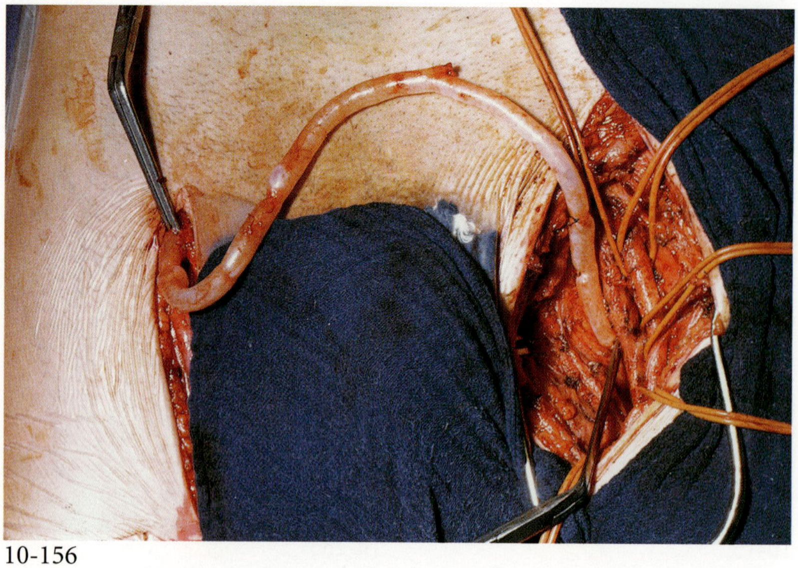

10-156

Fig. 10-156. The PALMA operation is designed to provide collateral circulation following iliac vein occlusion. In this case, the right greater saphenous vein was attached to the left femoral vein because the patient had a left-sided iliac vein thrombosis

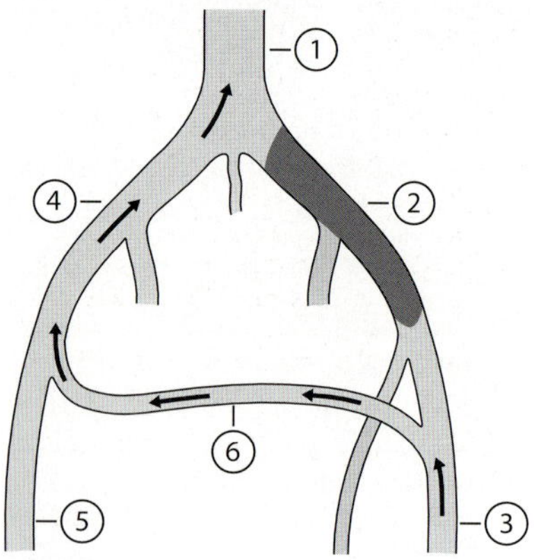

10-157

Fig. 10-157. The PALMA operation:
① Inferior vena cava
② Occlusion of the left common and external iliac veins
③ Left femoral vein
④ Right common iliac vein
⑤ Right femoral vein
⑥ Right greater saphenous vein

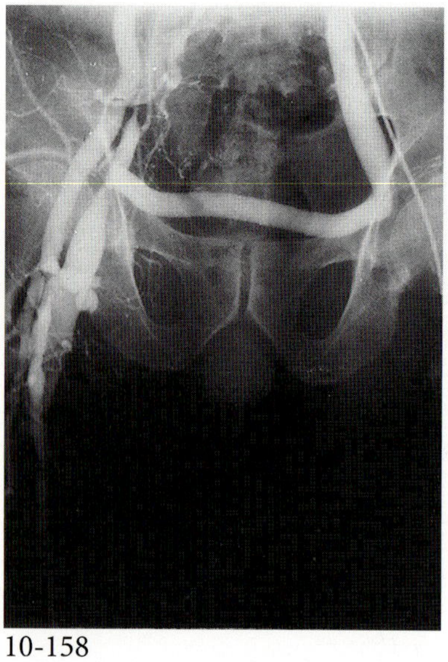

10-158

Fig. 10-158. Tumor-related occlusion of the left common and external iliac veins. Phlebography showing results after inserting a high iliaco-iliac cross-over bypass (12 mm PTFE) with creation of an arterio-venous fistula. The angiogram was performed via the right femoral artery. This procedure has been called a "high PALMA" operation

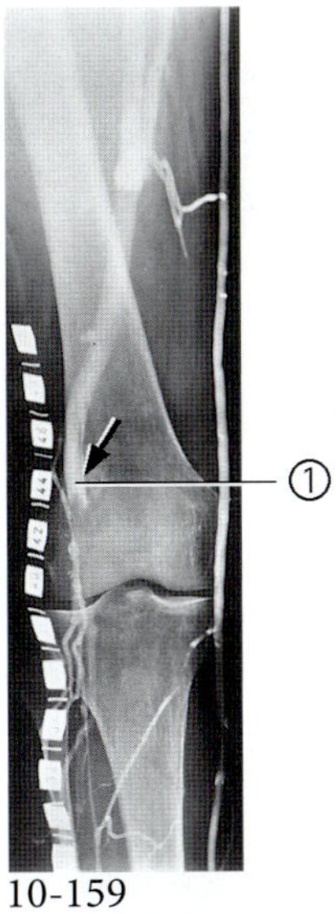

10-159

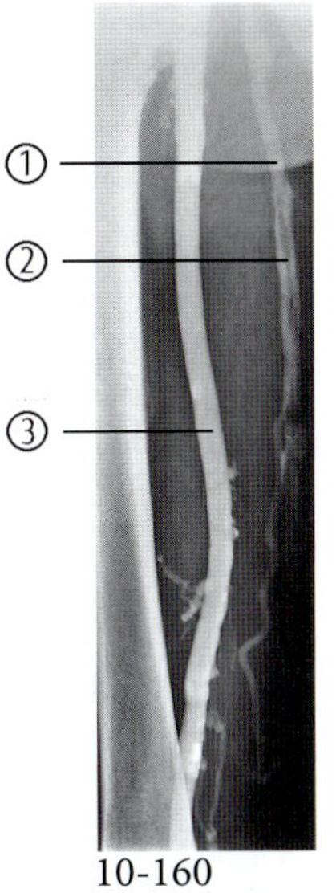

10-160

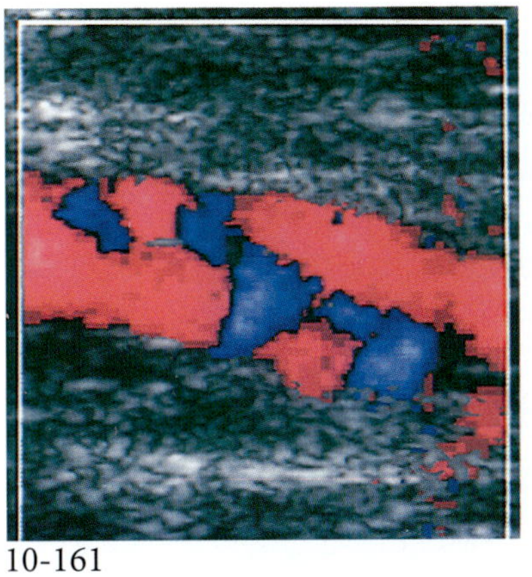

10-161

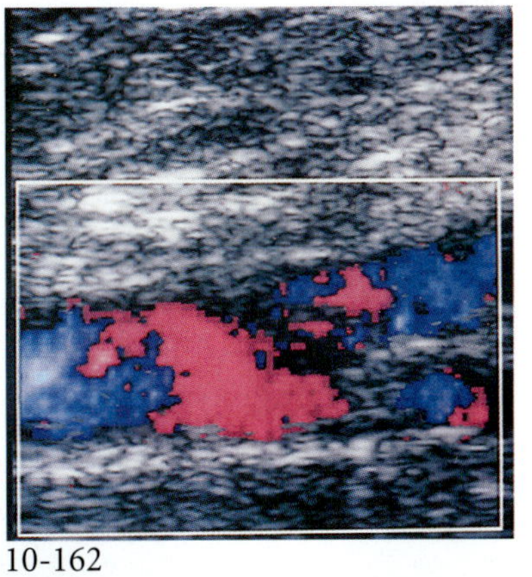

10-162

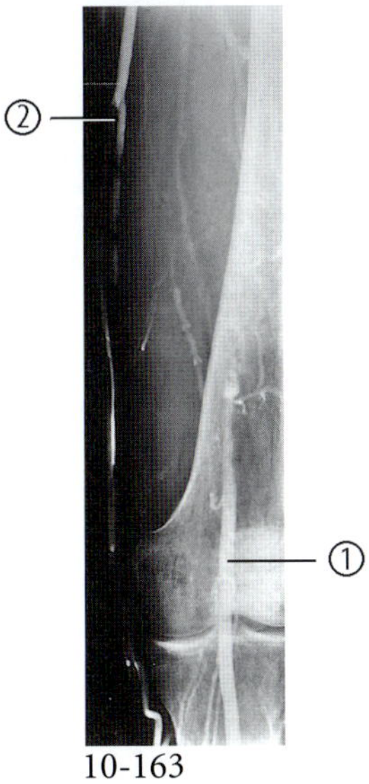

10-163

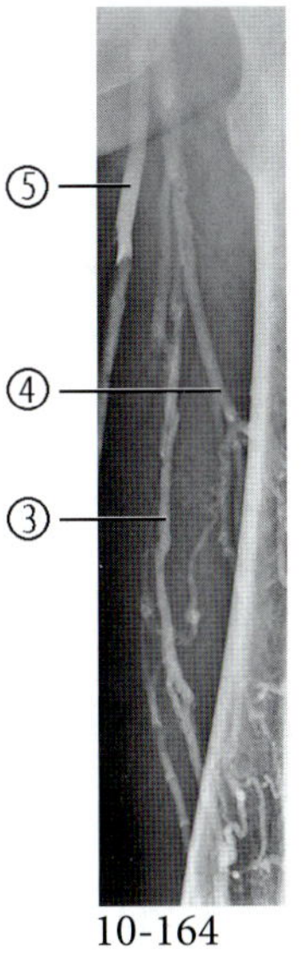

10-164

Fig. 10-159. Phlebography showing complete occlusion of the lower leg and popliteal veins. The epifascial veins provide collateral circulation. The dome-shaped projection into the vascular lumen ① and *arrow* pointing in the direction of the heart indicates an ascending thrombus

Fig. 10-160. Phlebography showing varicose enlargement of the greater saphenous vein with complete thrombosis. In the proximal part of the vessel a fresh thrombus is surrounded by contrast material.
① greater saphenous vein,
② thrombus,
③ superficial femoral vein

Fig. 10-161. Color duplex sonography showing appearance following phlebothrombosis of the popliteal vein with post-thrombotic syndrome. There has been partial recanalization. The findings are best explained by the development of a septum in the vein during partial recanalization. Phlebography cannot achieve this detail

Fig. 10-162. Color duplex sonography showing recanalization following thrombosis of superficial femoral vein

Figs. 10-163, 10-164. Phlebography showing acute thrombosis of the superficial femoral vein and appearance 8 months later. The patient has the post-thrombotic syndrome (grade I–II) with evidence of recanalization of the vein, but complete destruction of the valves and collateral circulation via the perforating veins to the greater saphenous vein and the deep femoral vein.
① Popliteal vein
② Greater saphenous vein
③ Recanalized superficial femoral vein
④ Deep femoral vein
⑤ Greater saphenous vein

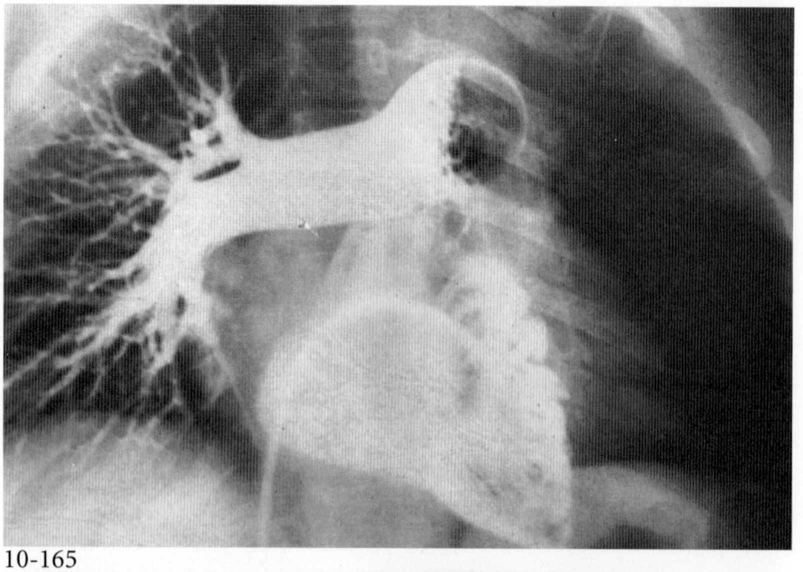

10-165

Fig. 10-165. Pulmonary arteriogram showing a massive pulmonary embolus which has interupted the entire pulmonary flow to the left lung

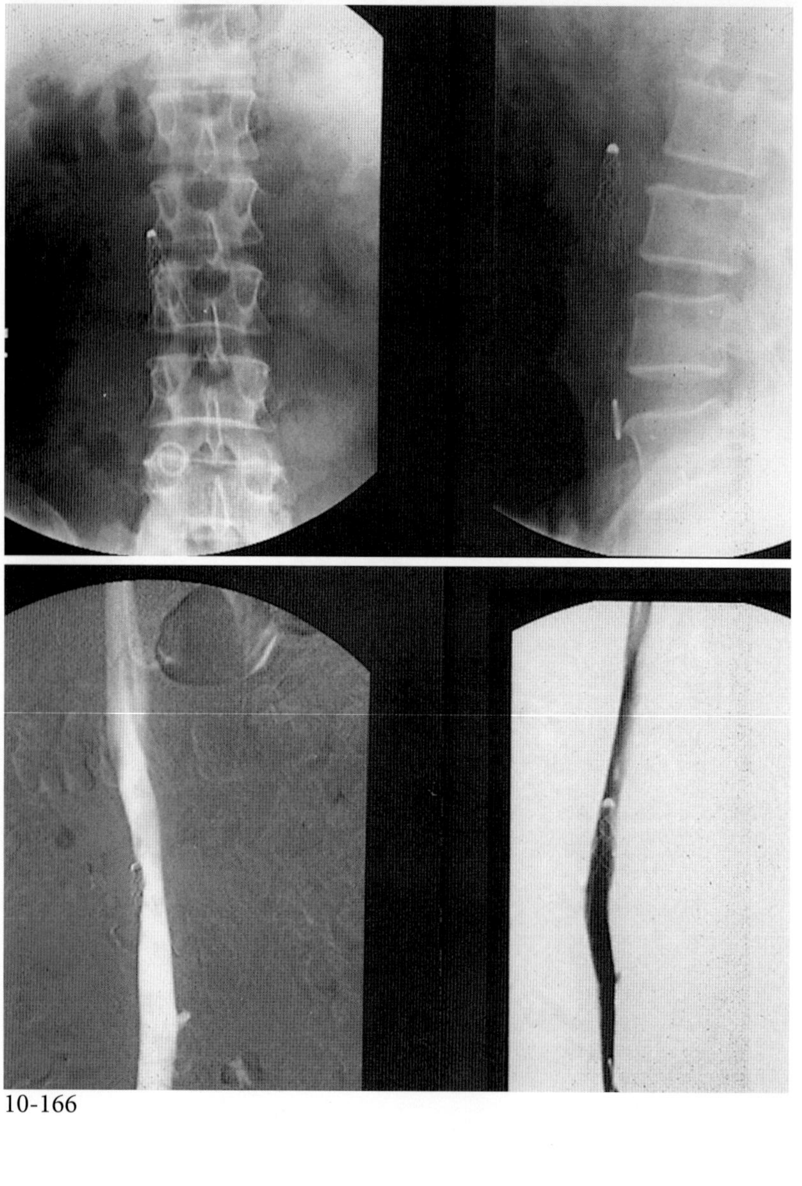

10-166

Fig. 10-166. Appearance following insertion of an inferior vena cava filter. Such filters are used to prevent recurrent pulmonary emboli which can develop despite anticoagulation. They are designed not to interfere with blood flow but to trap emboli. One side-effect is an increased rate of vena caval occlusion. The best known vena cava filters are:

- Mobin-Uddin umbrella filter (now obsolete)
- Kimray-Greenfield filter

Figs. 10-167 – 10-170. Various degrees of severity of phlegmasia cerulea dolens are shown. The underlying problem is complete sudden occlusion of the entire venous drainage of a limb. The lack of capillary circulation and the compression of small arteries and arterioles by the blocked fluid leads to peripheral arterial occlusion.
Treatment consists of restoring fluid, treating shock and providing pain relief. If the thrombi can be partially removed operatively, that is the usual approach.
If an operation is not possible, systemic fibrinolysis is the next step. Any delay in instituting therapy leads to marked irreversible tissue damage and often amputation

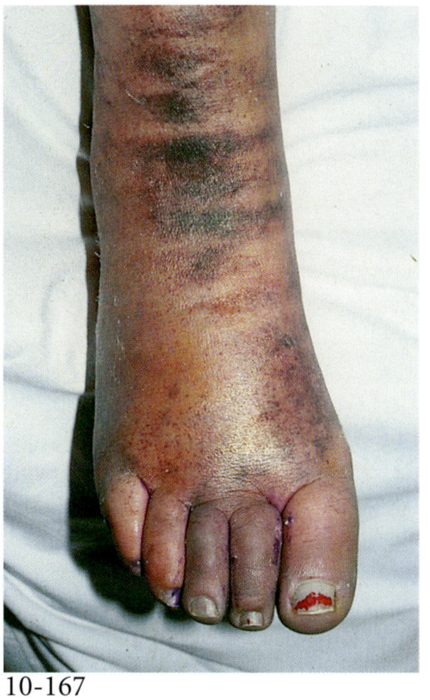

10-167

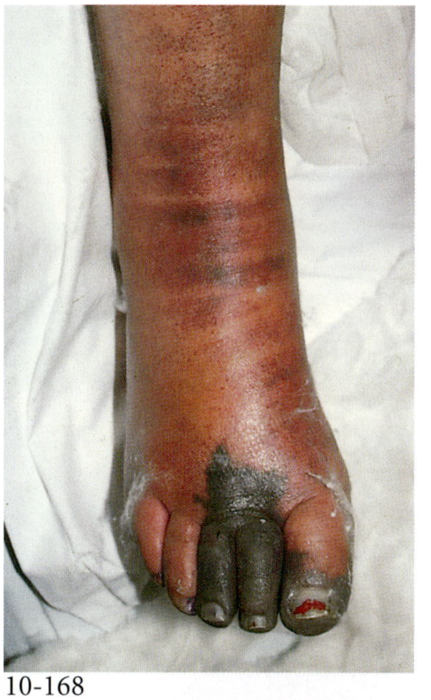

10-168

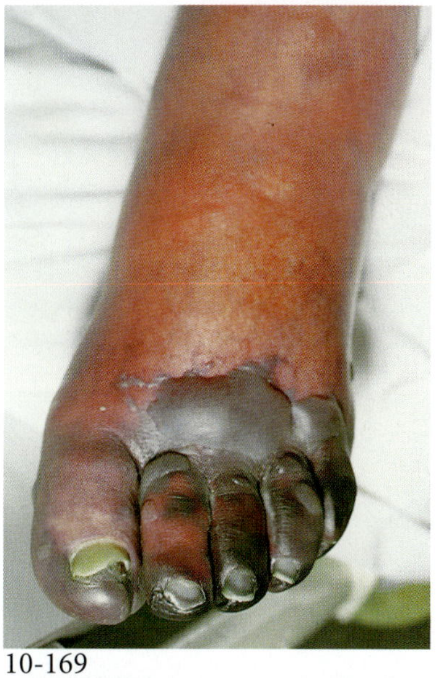

10-169

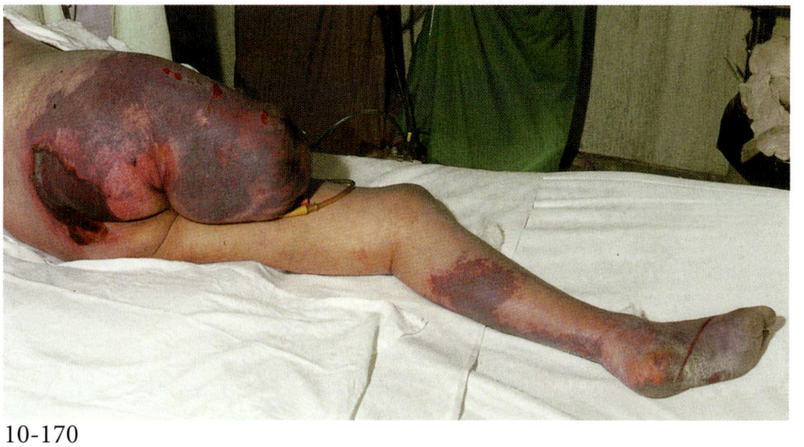

10-170

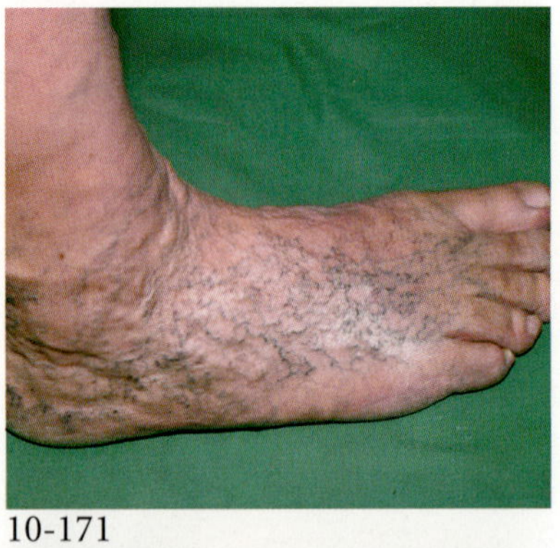

10-171

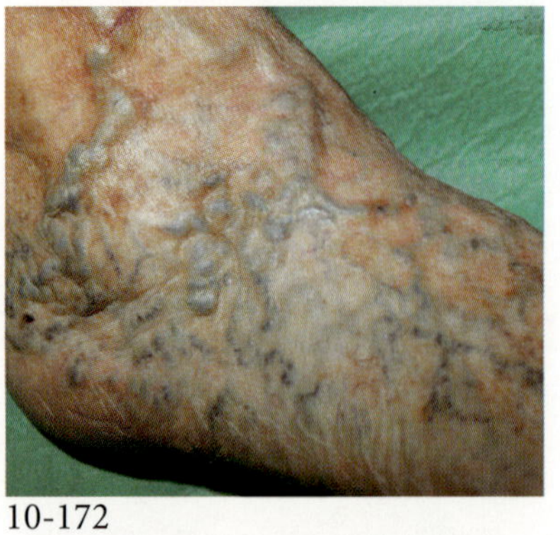

10-172

Figs. 10-171, 10-172. Corona phlebectatica paraplantaris in CVI. The blue network of overfilled veins about the ankle and the dorsal surface of the foot is a sure sign of CVI

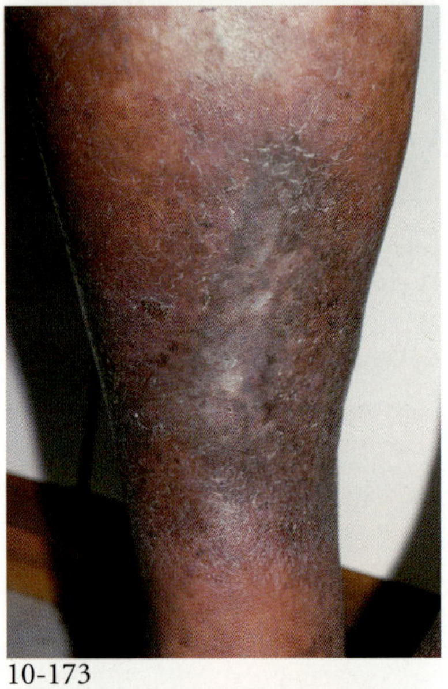

10-173

Fig. 10-173. Typical skin changes in CVI. The initial erythematous patches of stasis dermatitis have become hyperpigmented and lichenified (chronic inflammation with increased skin markings, often smoother surface and decreased flexibility). Small fine scales may also be seen

Figs. 10-174, 10-175. Atrophie blanche describes the white porcelain-like irregular areas that reflect obliterated lymphatics and capillaries because of increased pressure in an inadequate venous system. The red spots are dilated coiled capillaries. Atrophie blanche is common about the ankle and on the back of the foot in CVI

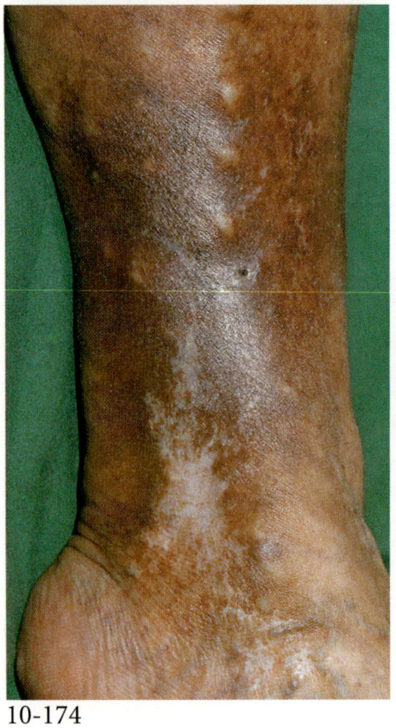

10-174

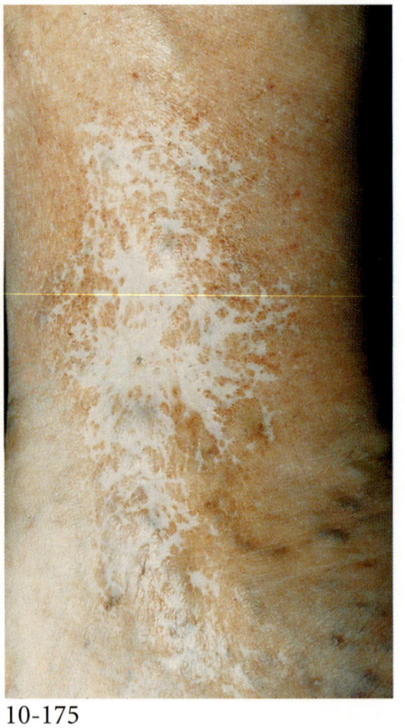

10-175

Fig. 10-181. The spirochete *Borrelia burgdorferi* is the causative agent of Lyme disease and other forms of borreliosis

Fig. 10-182. The hard-bodied tick *Ixodes ricinus* transmits both *Borrelia burgdorferi* and viral encephalitis.

Fig. 10-176. Recurrent stasis ulcer in typical location near the medial malleolus with induration, hyperpigmentation, atrophie blanche and venous ectasias

Fig. 10-177. Chronic therapy-resistant stasis ulcer which has been present for months. The skin is hyperpigmented with the sharp border probably determined by the distribution of an incompetent perforating vein. The ulcer is clearly secondarily infected.

Fig. 10-178. Incompetent perforating veins are a common cause of ulceration. Often there is a second factor, such as poorly fitting shoes or trauma. While perforating veins associated with the greater saphenous vein are most often affected, explaining the medial location of most ulcers, the lesser saphenous vein can also be affected, as shown here

Figs. 10-179, 10-180. Acrodermatitis chronica atrophicans (Pick-Herxheimer) is an uncommon late manifestation of borreliosis. In this relatively early stage, the erythematous patches and plaques about the ankles, often with cyanosis, can be mistaken for vascular lesions. Later there is marked atrophy with clearly visible veins (cigarette paper skin)

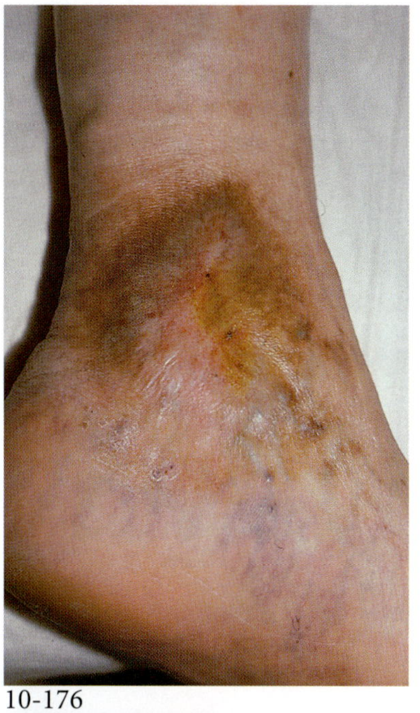
10-176

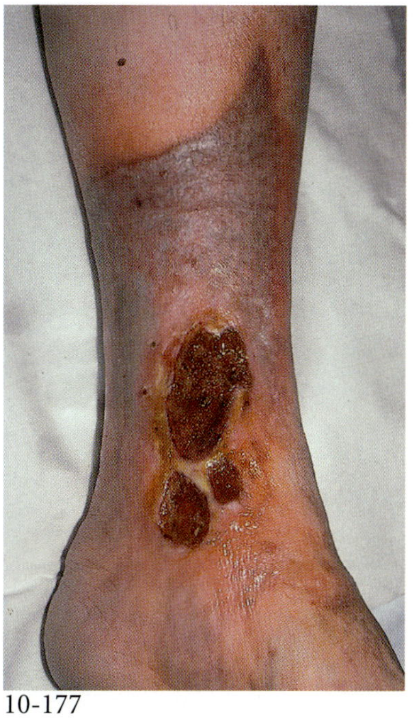
10-177

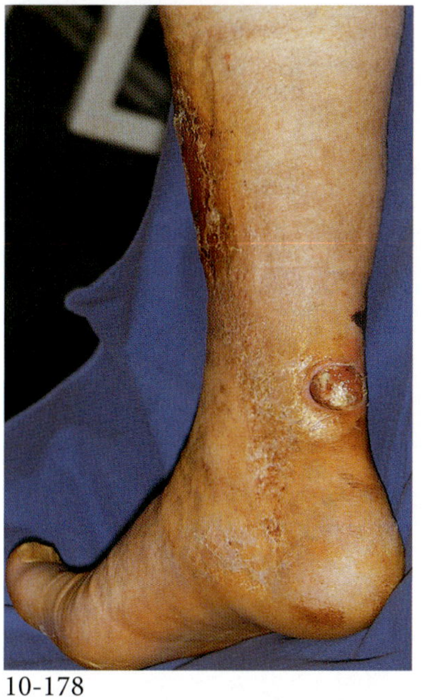
10-178

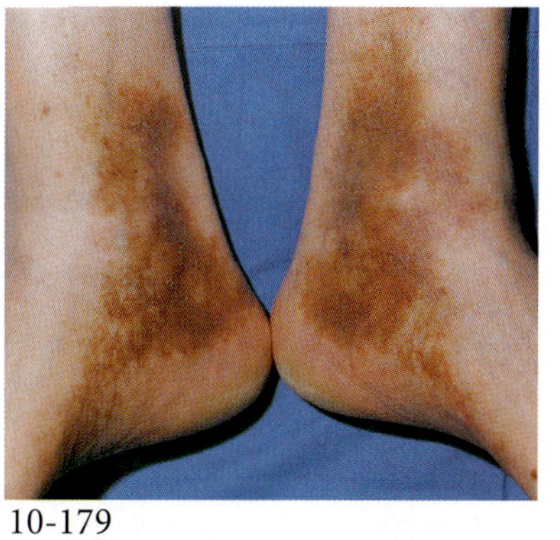
10-179

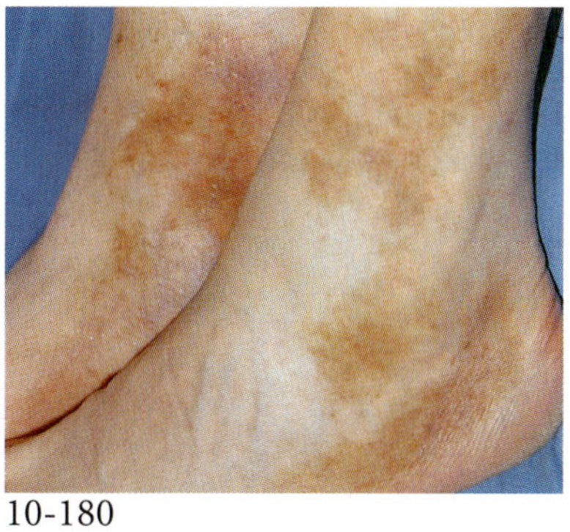
10-180

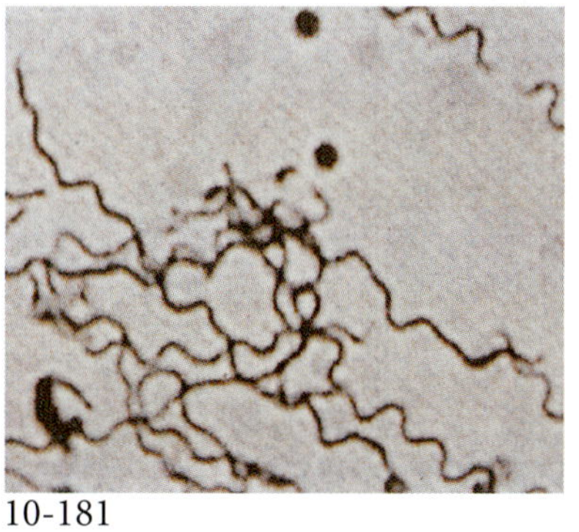
10-181

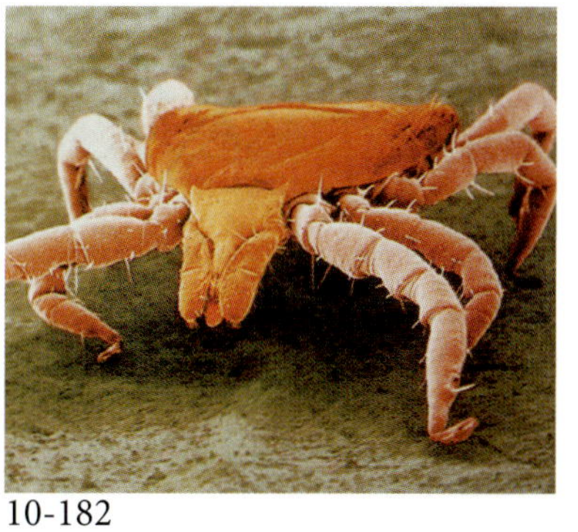
10-182

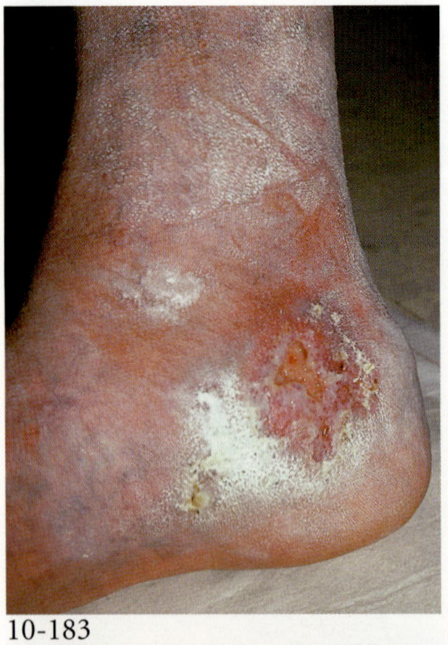
10-183

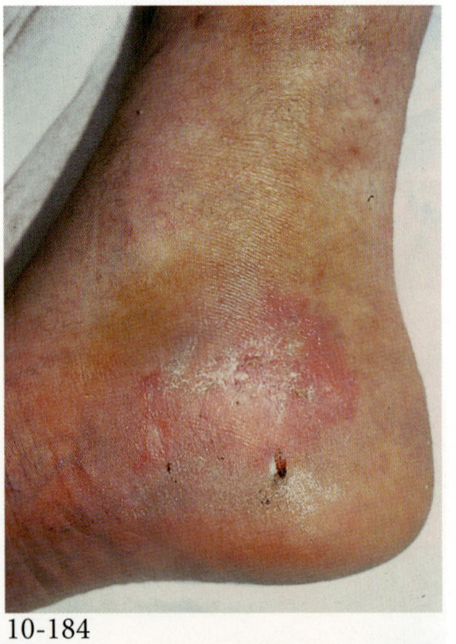
10-184

Fig. 10-183. Weeping stasis ulcer on inner aspect of ankle. The use of a variety of different creams and ointments over many years predisposed patients with stasis ulcers to allergic contact dermatitis, frequently from topical antibiotics or anesthetics. The allergic contact dermatitis further delays healing of the ulcer

Fig. 10-184. Appearance following regular compression therapy

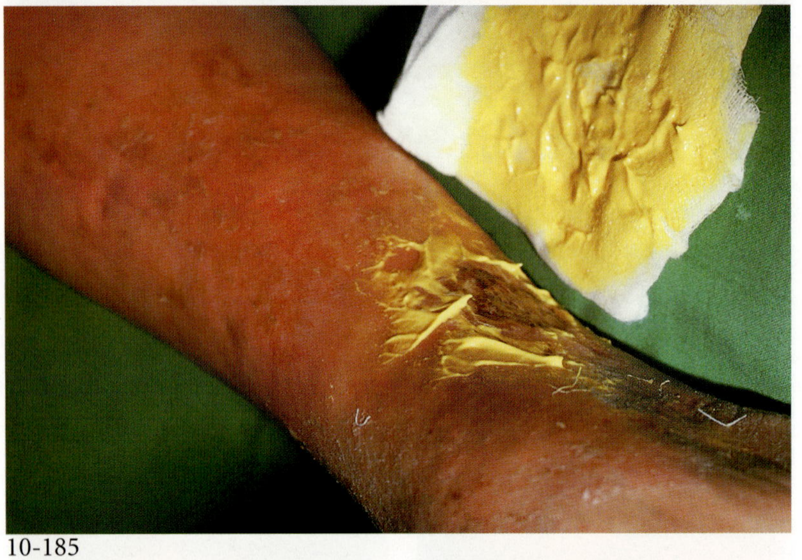
10-185

Fig. 10-185. Frustrated patients frequently try unusual products on their stasis ulcers. This individual showed up with a mustard dressing

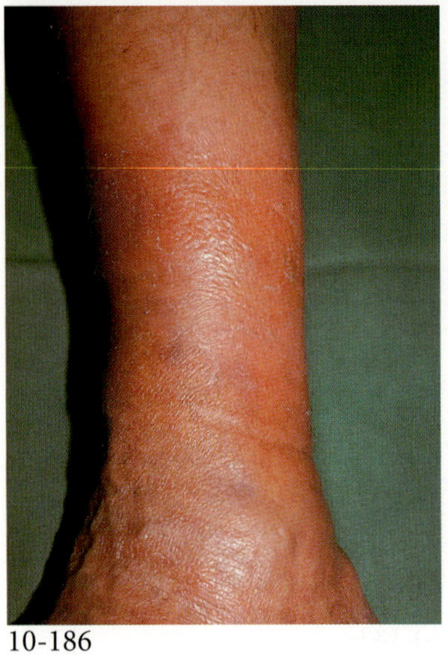
10-186

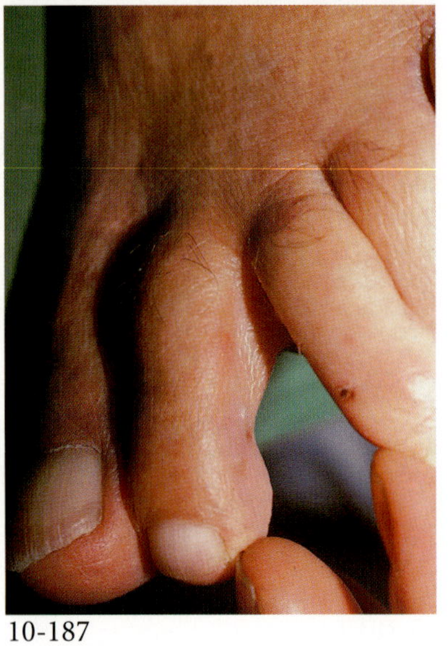
10-187

Fig. 10-186. This individual developed erysipelas in a leg with CVI.

Fig. 10-187. Interdigital tinea pedis is often the entry point for the streptococci which cause erysipelas, as well as for other bacteria. The feet in CVI are more susceptible to fungal infections, but regular use of topical antifungal creams is usually effective

Fig. 10-188. When stasis ulcers involve the entire circumference of the leg just above the ankle, they are described as spats-like ulcers. There is diffuse impairment of the superficial vascular network, leading to extensive but superficial necrosis

Fig. 10-189. The same patient 6 months later with complete healing of the extensive ulcer. The contour of the leg is usually altered, with a sclerotic constriction at the ulcer site, with a thickened calf. The term "inverted wine bottle" leg has been used to describe this distinctive picture Series of pictures showing the surgical treatment of a large deep stasis ulcer

Fig. 10-190. Pre-operative appearance

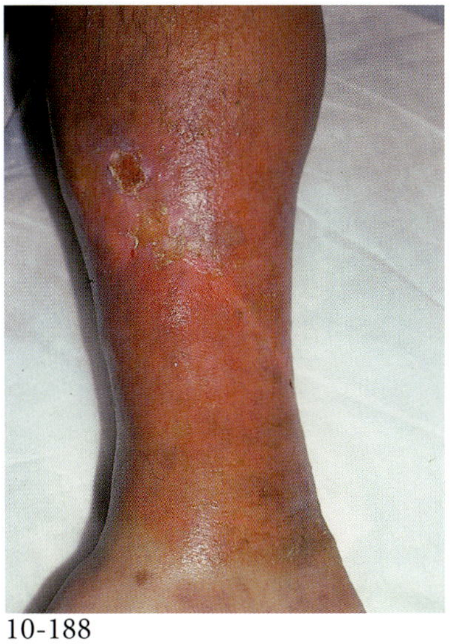

10-188

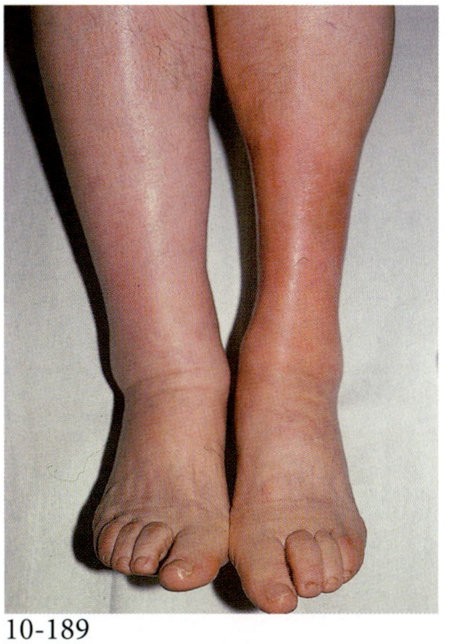

10-189

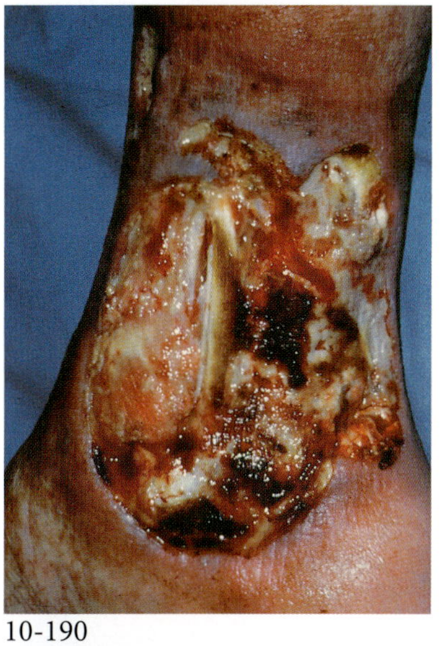

10-190

Fig. 10-191. After wound cleaning and aggressive debridement, a mesh graft was applied over good granulation tissue

Fig. 10-192. Good healing 4 weeks later

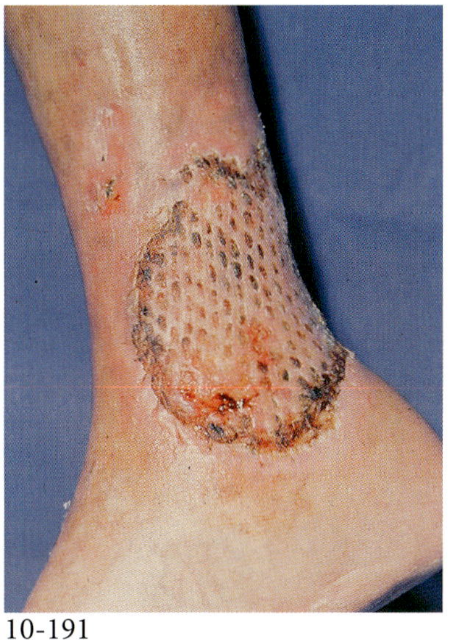

10-191

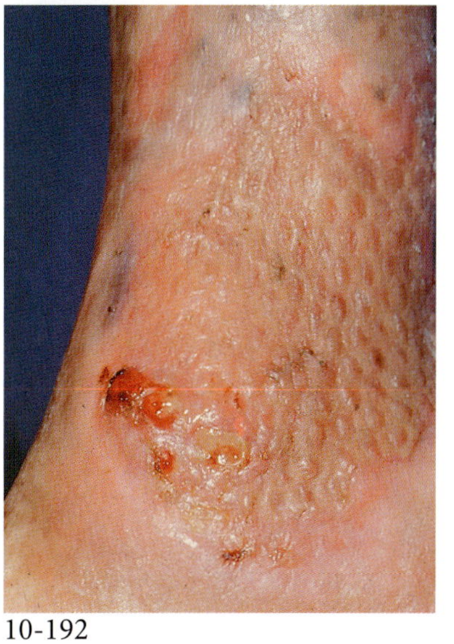

10-192

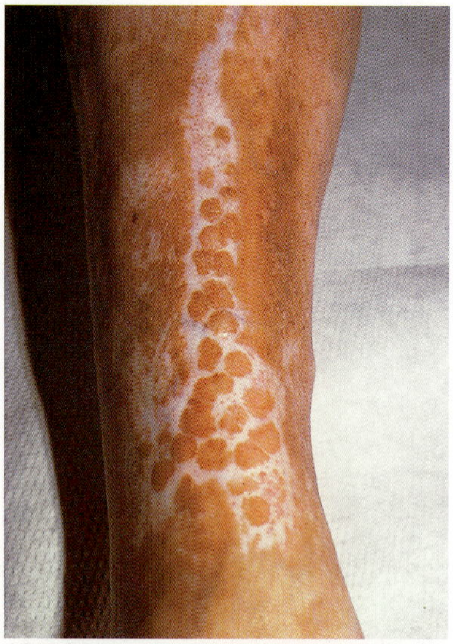

10-193

Fig. 10-193. REVERDIN (JACQUES-LOUIS REVERDIN, 1842–1908, Swiss surgeon) or pinch grafts are tiny pieces of epidermis and upper dermis that are applied to a wound with good granulation tissue at the base. They can be quite effective in stasis ulcers

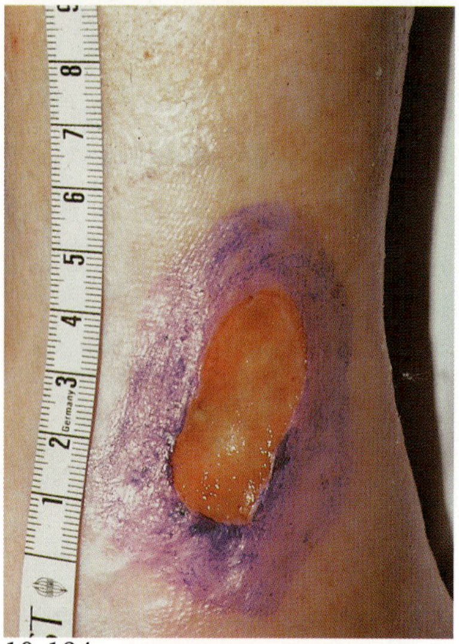

10-194

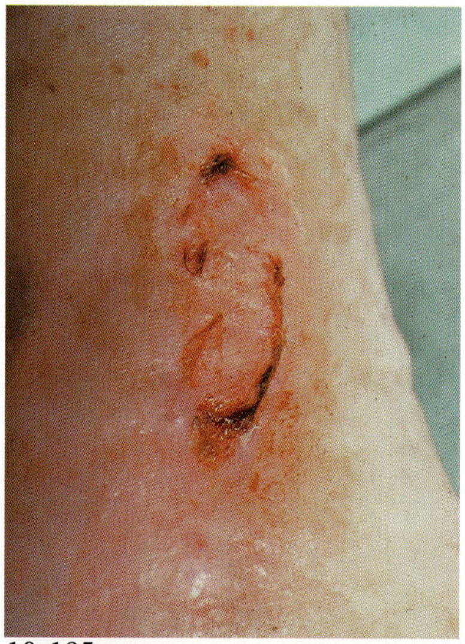

10-195

Figs. 10-194, 10-195. Superficial but chronic stasis ulcer over the medial malleolus. After removal of the greater saphenous vein and skin grafting, the ulcer healed quickly

Figs. 10-196–10-198. Large but superficial stasis ulcer with *Pseudomonas aeruginosa* infection. A skin graft led to good healing

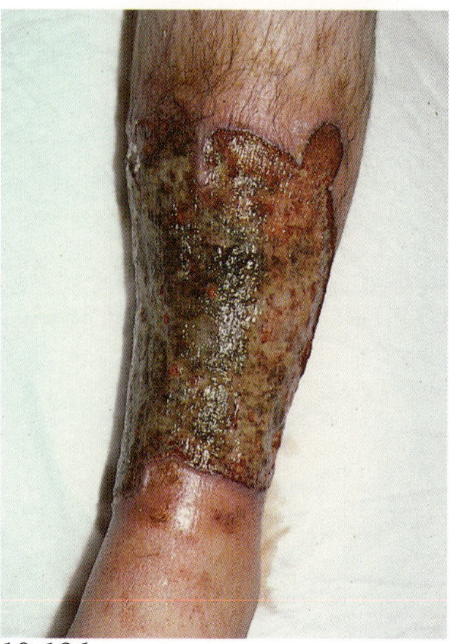

10-196

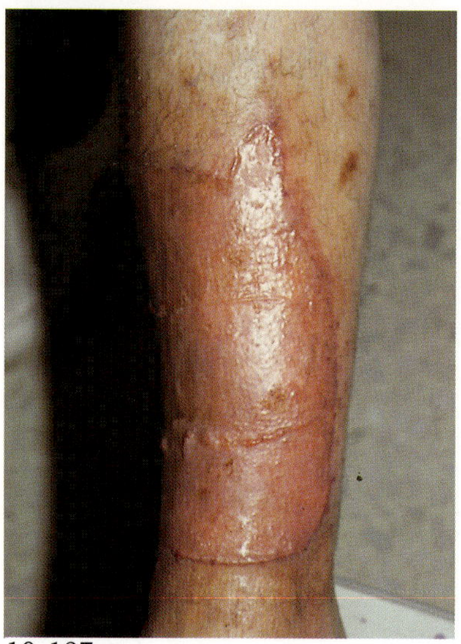

10-197

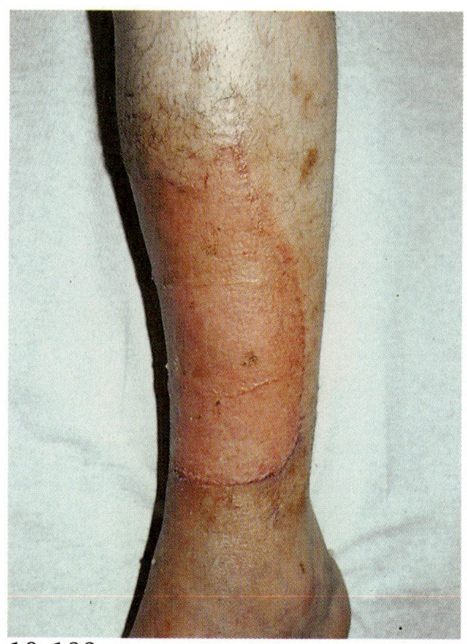

10-198

Figs. 10-199, 10-200. Iatrogenic friction blisters developed at the edge of compression bandages in an older patient. There was no underlying arterial disease

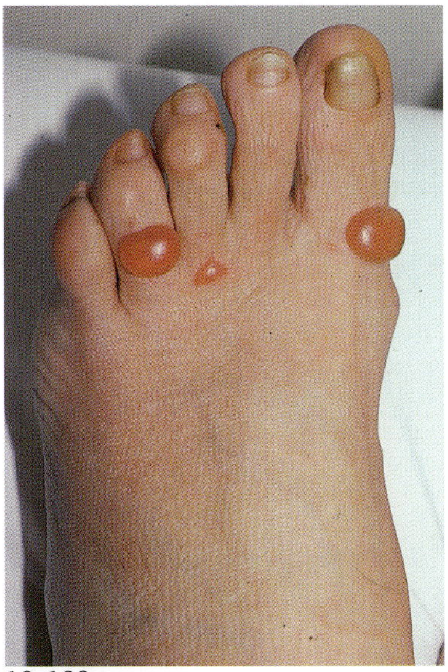
10-199

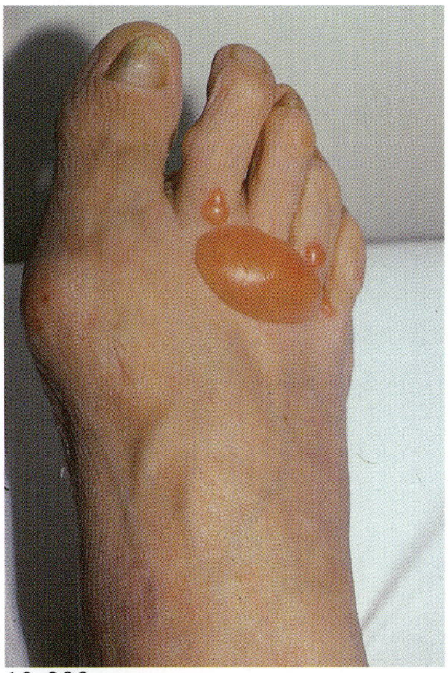
10-200

Figs. 10-201, 10-202. Superficial blisters and erosions secondary to pressure dressings in 67 year old women. The lesions healed when pressure and friction were reduced

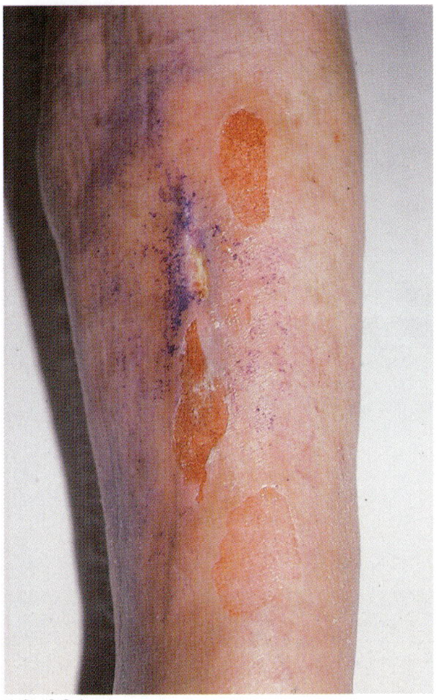
10-201

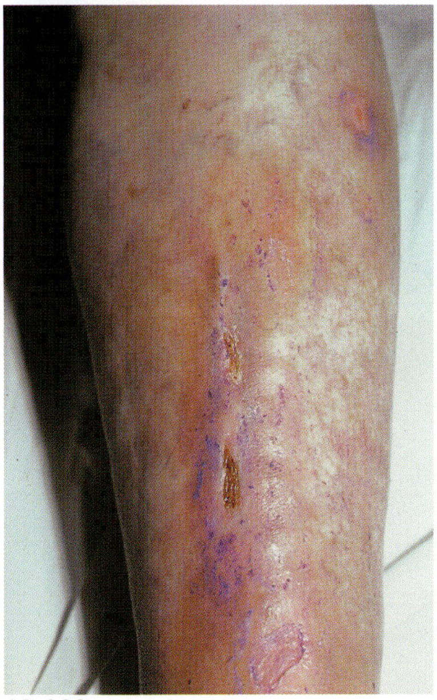
10-202

Fig. 10-203. Necrosis following extravasation of contrast material; this accident occurred before the introduction of milder, water-soluble agents

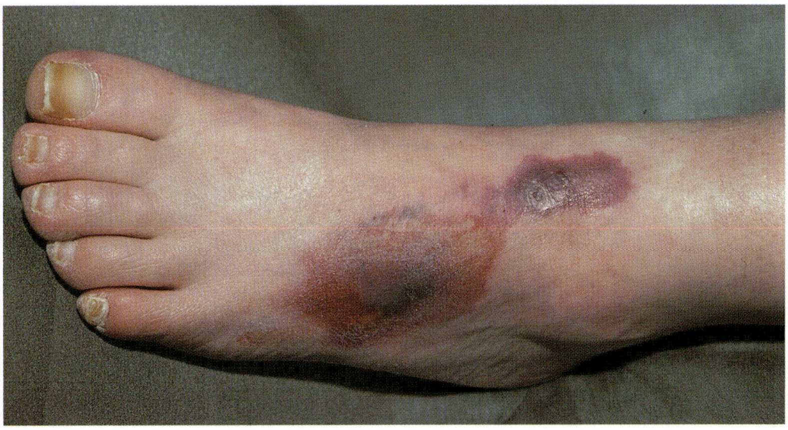
10-203

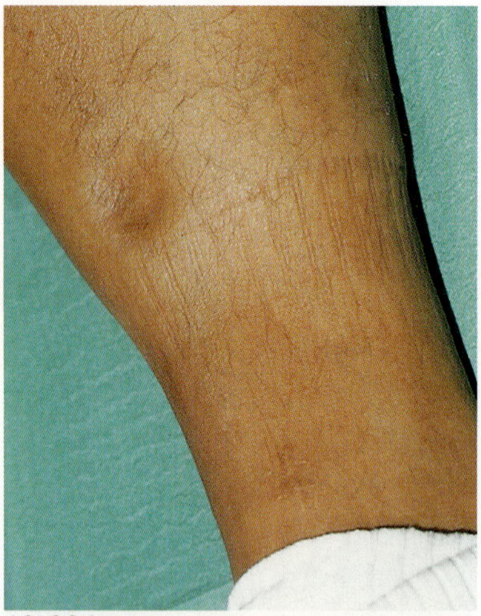
10-204

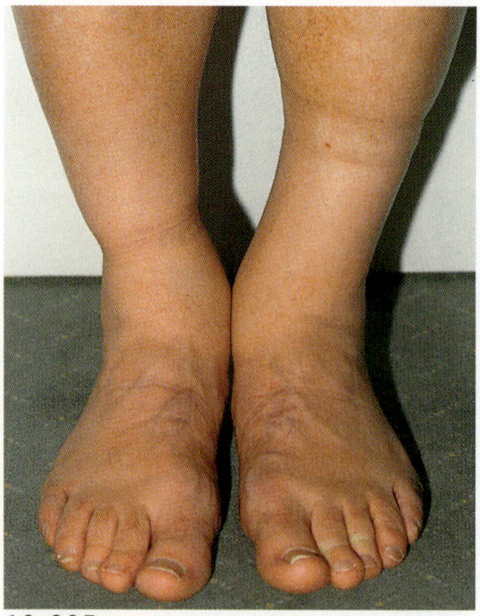
10-205

Fig. 10-204. Pitting edema secondary to cardiac failure is usually bilateral and most often pre-tibial, as shown here

Fig. 10-205. Peripheral edema as a complication of nifedipine therapy for hypertension. Diuretics do little to help this transudation edema and the calcium channel blockers must be stopped

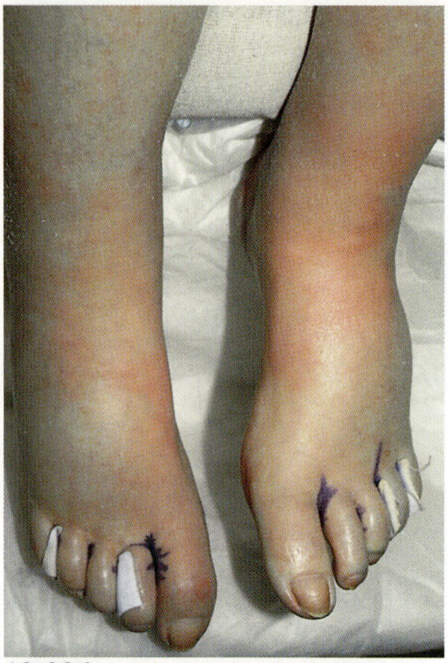
10-206

Fig. 10-206. Leg edema in a terminally ill patient with cardiac failure, renal failure and peripheral arterial disease

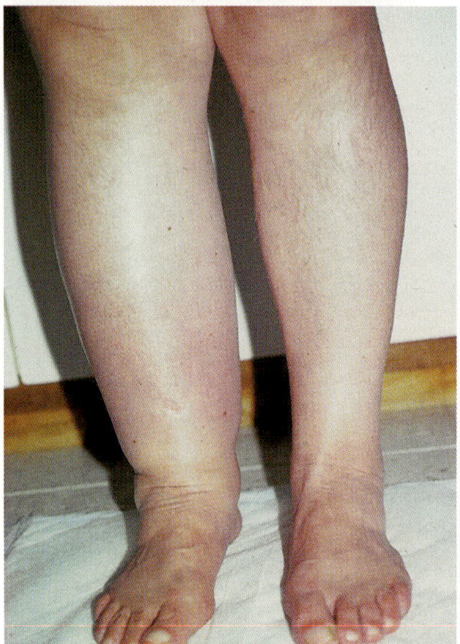
10-207

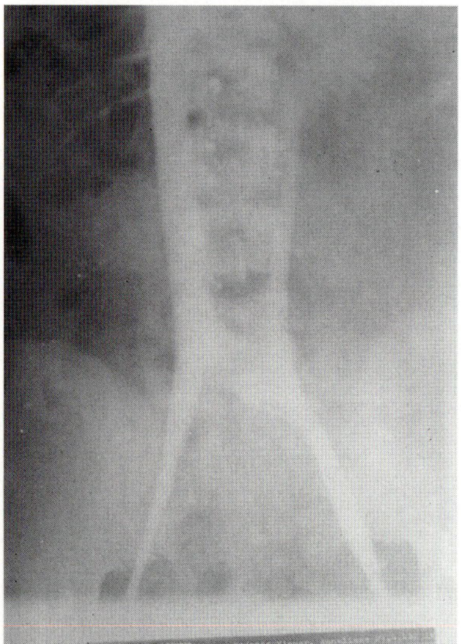
10-208

Figs. 10-207, 10-208. A 43 year old female with an exudative enteropathy and hypoproteinemia with markedly reduced IgG levels. Phlebography showed a persistent left inferior vena cava with the common iliac vein. showing both segments, While the edema in the buttocks and legs can be explained by both the hypoproteinemia and the aberrant venous return, the reason for the disproportionate changes in the right leg is unclear

Fig. 10-209. Ruptured Baker's (Morant Baker, 1839–1896, English surgeon) cyst on the *right* in a patient with arthritis of the right knee. Baker's cysts are extensions of the synovium that generally balloon out posteriorly. They can reach a sufficient size to impinge upon the nerves. If they rupture, a thrombophlebitis of the calf can be mimicked (pseudo-thrombophlebitis syndrome). Baker's cysts can develop in association with a wide variety of knee problems, especially if there is hemorrhage or accumulation of fluid in the joint. They are often seen with rheumatoid arthritis, but less frequently with Reiter's syndrome, Sjögren's syndrome and lupus erythematosus. They also develop in traumatic and degenerative joint disease

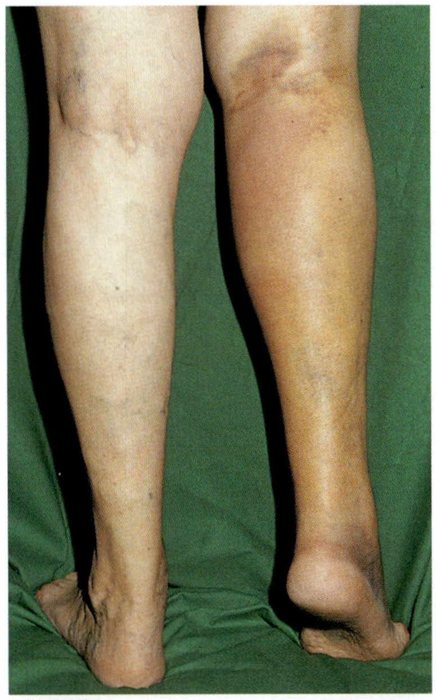

10-209

Fig. 10-210. Compression of the popliteal vein by a Baker's cyst. The main differential diagnostic consideration is a phlebothrombosis

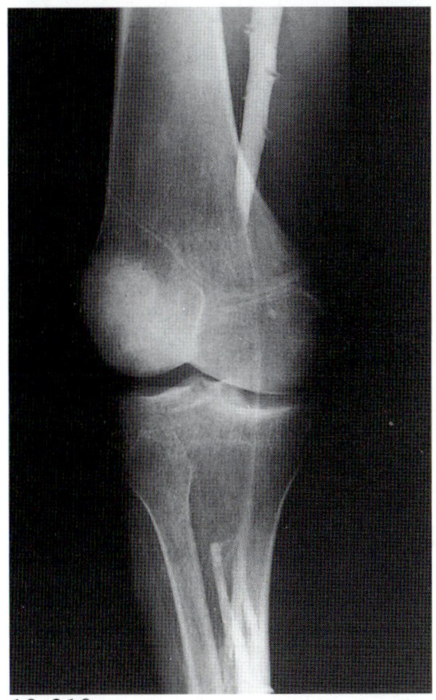

10-210

Fig. 10-211. Color duplex sonography showing a large Baker's cyst in the popliteal fossa. The popliteal vein is completely blocked, showing no blood flow. The popliteal artery is partially occluded and shows increased blood flow velocity just as with other stenoses

Fig. 10-212. Color duplex sonography showing another large Baker's cyst and its relationship to the nearby vessels.

1 Popliteal artery
2 Popliteal vein
3 Baker's cyst

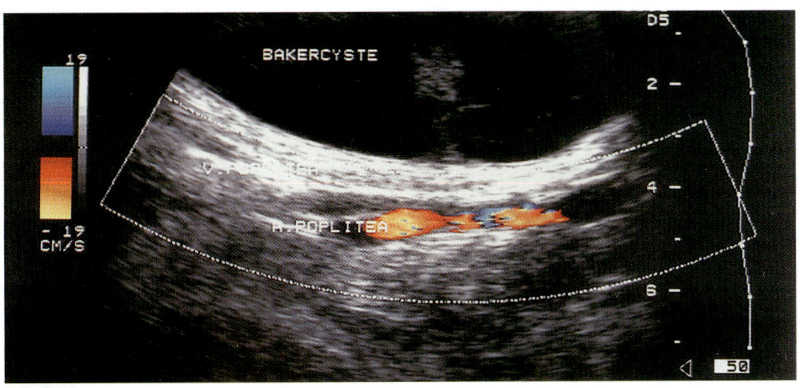

10-211

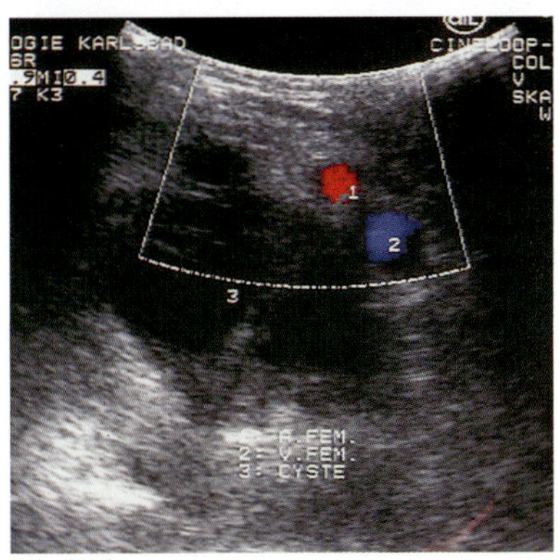

10-212

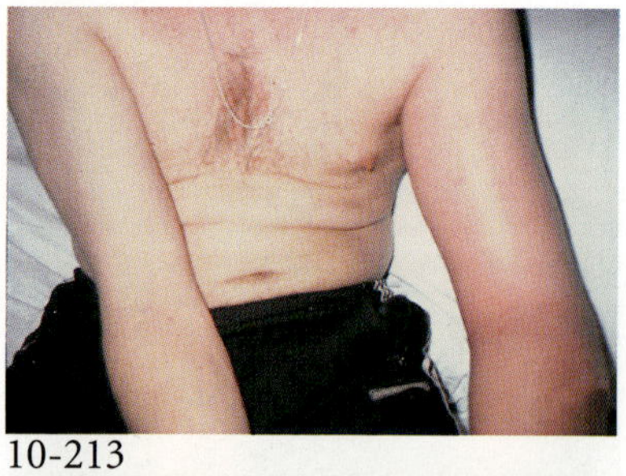

10-213

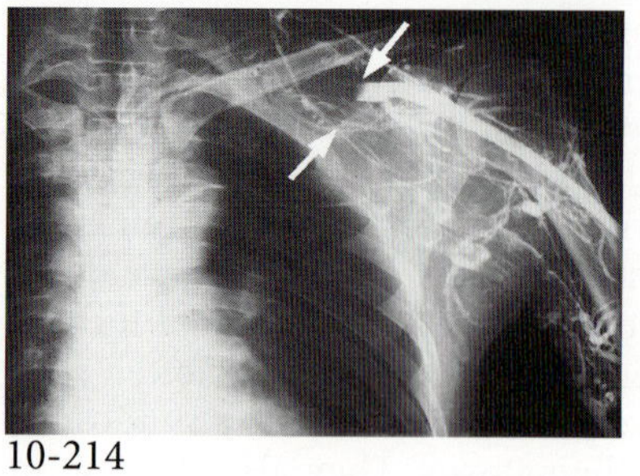

10-214

Fig. 10-213. Left subclavian vein thrombosis in a 46 year old man. The left arm is swollen and livid with clear widening of the veins on its upper aspects (warning veins)

Fig. 10-214. Phlebogram from the same patient showing complete occlusion of the subclavian vein (*arrow*) with many collaterals

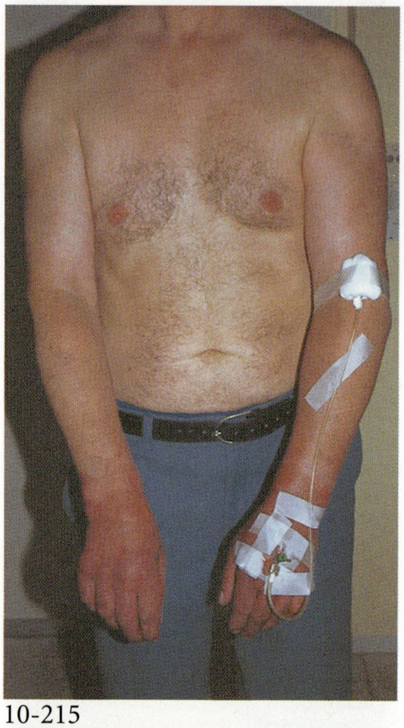

10-215

Fig. 10-215. A 51 year old man with acute left subclavian vein thrombosis. The arm is swollen and livid, while collateral veins can be seen on the left chest wall. Local fibrinolysis with urokinase was carried out

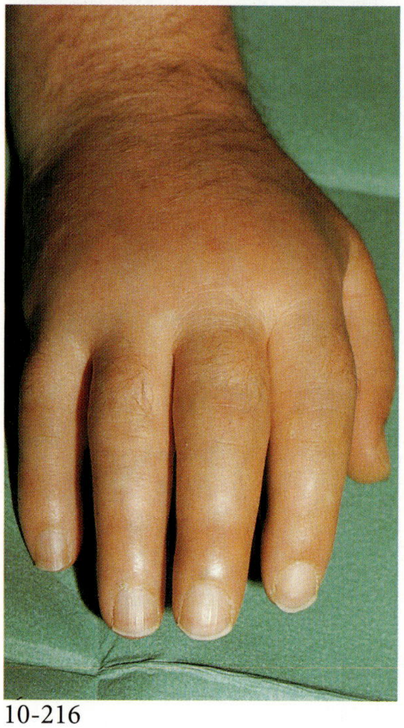

10-216

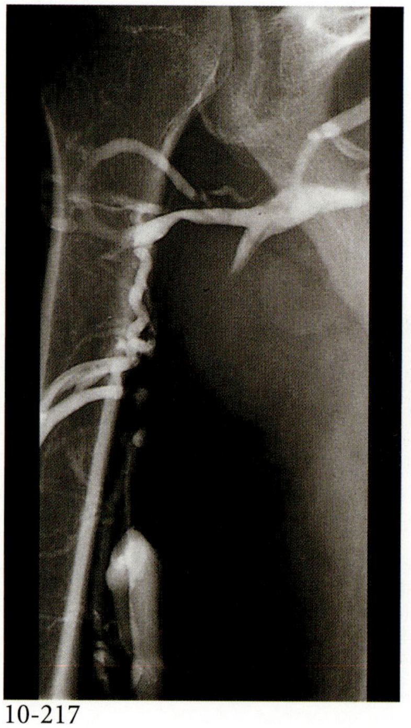

10-217

Fig. 10-216. Massive edema of the back of the hand and forearm in a patient with acute axillary vein thrombosis

Fig. 10-217. Phlebogram from the same patient showing complete occlusion of the axillary vein

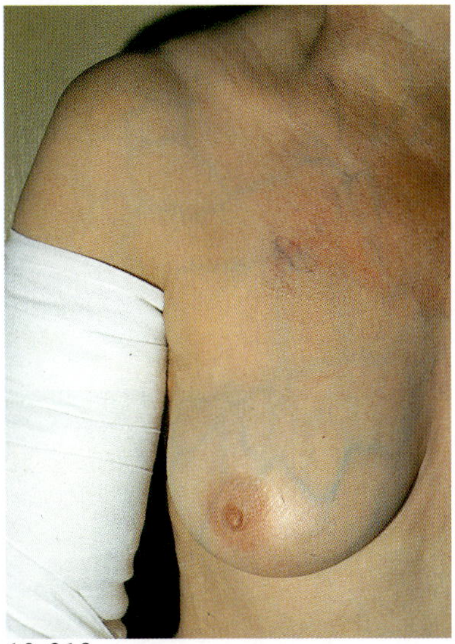

10-218

Fig. 10-218. Collateral veins on the chest wall of a 52 year old woman with a subclavian vein thrombosis

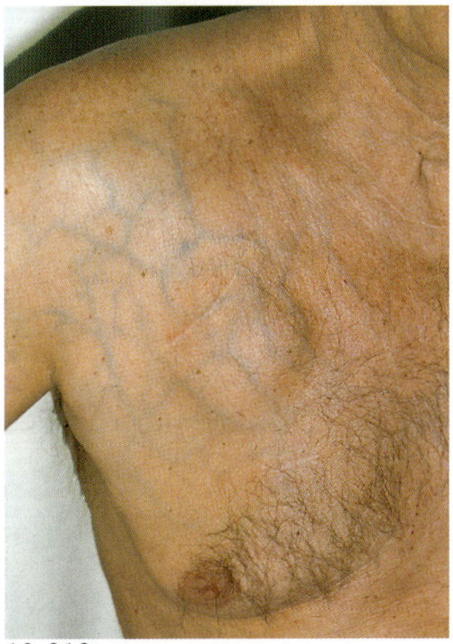

10-219

Fig. 10-219. Paget-von Schrötter syndrome following insertion of pacemaker using subclavian vein. Numerous collateral veins are seen

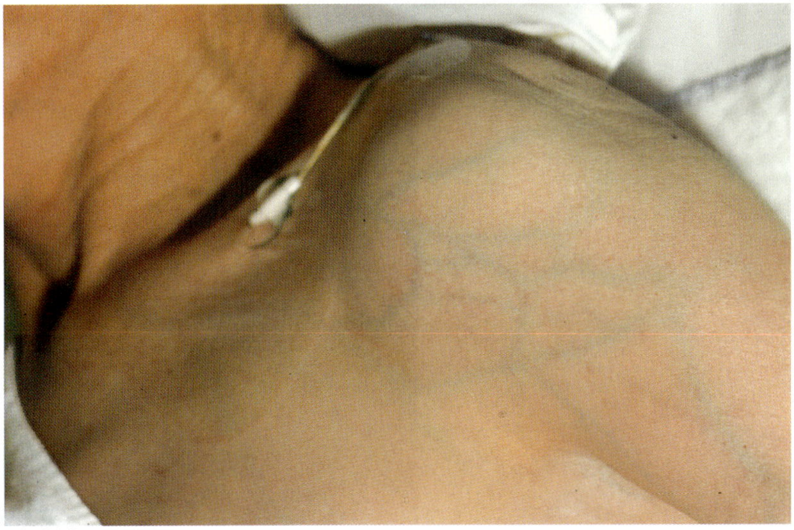

10-220

Fig. 10-220. Subclavian vein thrombosis following insertion of a central venous line

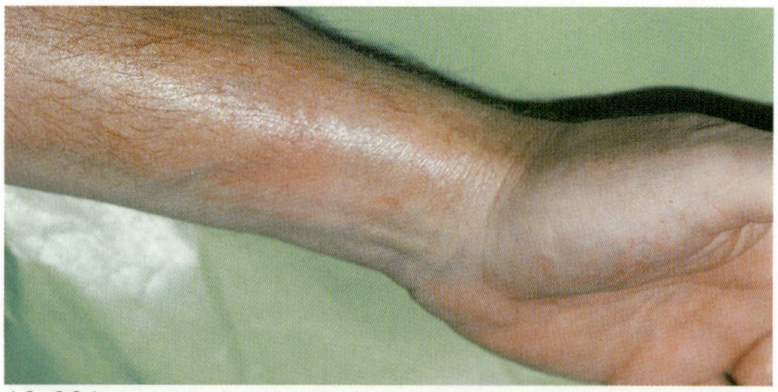

10-221

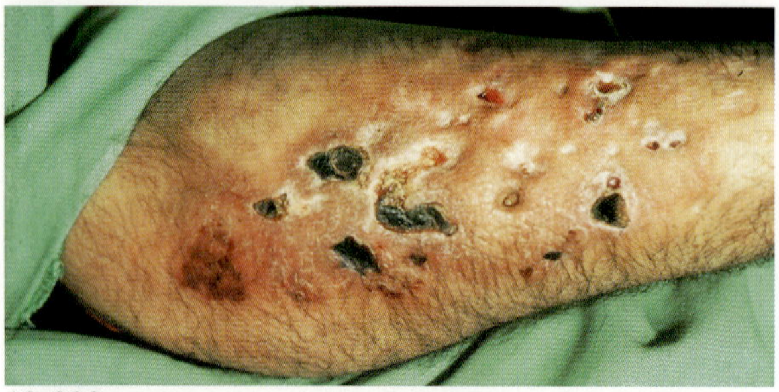

10-222

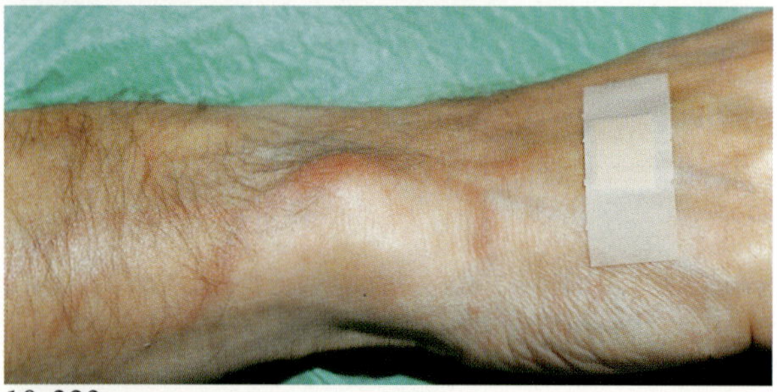

10-223

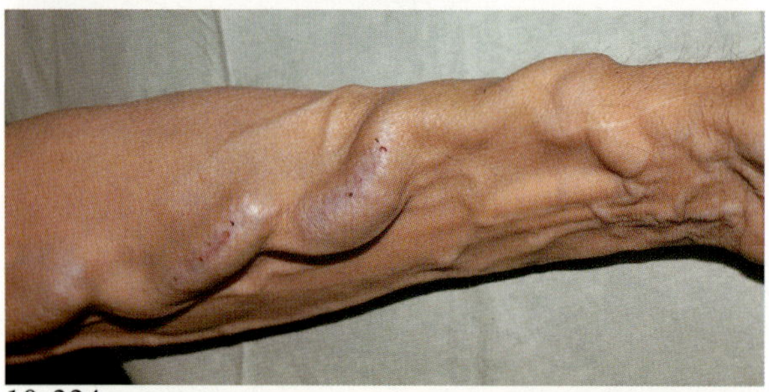

10-224

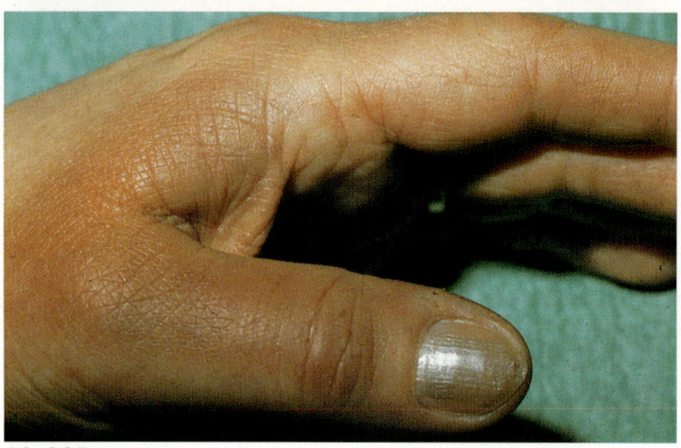

10-225

Fig. 10-221. Superficial migratory thrombophlebitis of the forearm in a 24 year old patient with thromboangiitis obliterans

Fig. 10-222. A similar patient with thromboangiitis obliterans and superficial migratory thrombophlebitis of the arm but with marked necrosis

Fig. 10-223. Inflammation of a vein during infusion of prostaglandin E_1. This is not a true irritant phlebitis because the erythema and swelling disappear soon after the infusion is stopped. There appears to be a hyperemia of the vessel wall

Fig. 10-224. Hemodialysis shunt (Brescia-Cimino type). In this procedure the radial artery is joined to a large adjacent vein producing an arterio-venous shunt with sufficient flow (150 – 200 ml/ min.) for hemodialysis. Large veins develop on the forearm, often with visible vibration (thrills) and loud bruits

Fig. 10-225. Paroxysmal hematoma of the finger in a 40 year old woman. Apparently minor trauma leads to rupture of a digital vein producing a sudden painless swelling and discoloration of the digit. Resolution is spontaneous and rapid; occasionally cold compresses are required

Fig. 10-226. Swelling of hand following strangulation of forearm

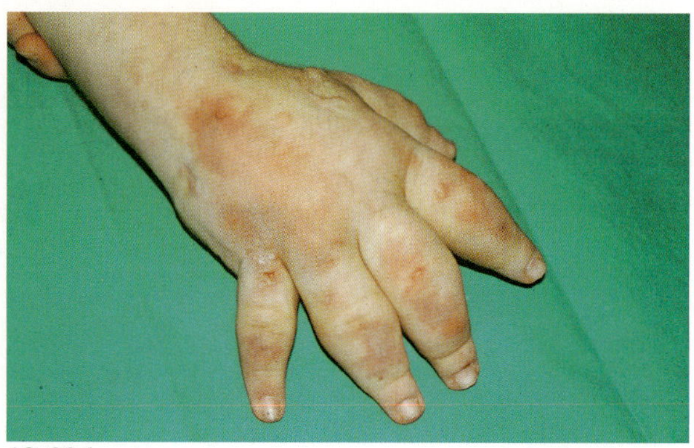

10-226

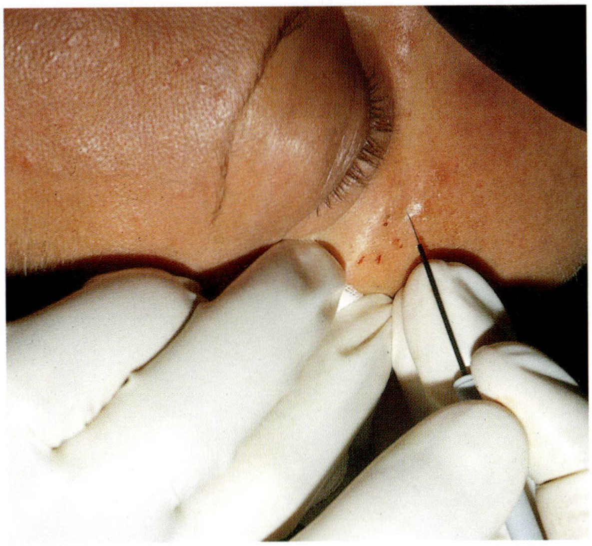

10-227

Fig. 10-227. Electrocautery therapy of fine facial telangiectases

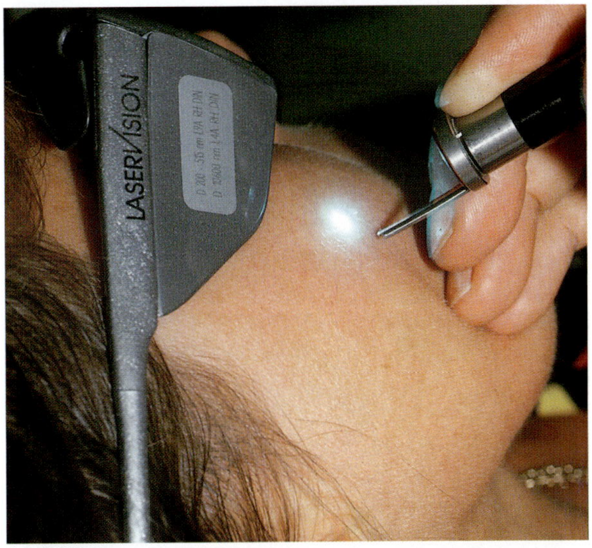

10-228

Fig. 10-228. Removal of facial telangiectases using a pulsed dye laser. Two laser systems offer the best promise for small vascular lesions and pigmentary changes – pulsed dye lasers and Q-switched ruby lasers. For vascular lesions the pulsed dye laser is more often used. Lesions which respond well include nevi flammei, hemangiomas and telangiectases

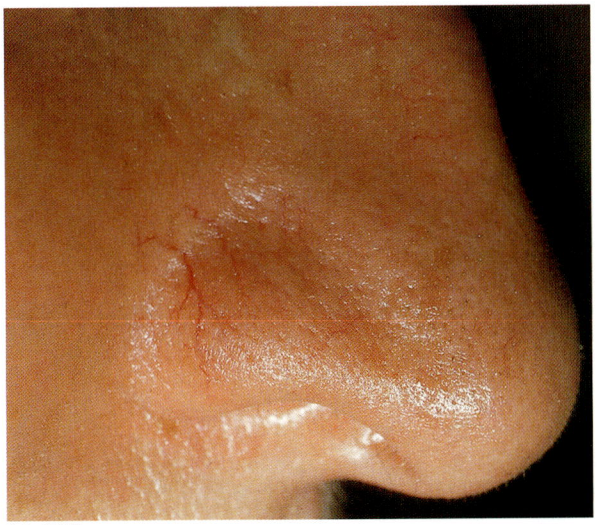

10-229

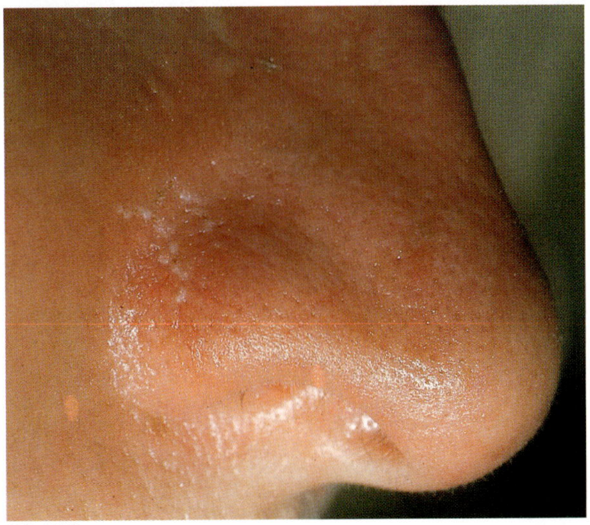

10-230

Figs. 10-229, 10-230. Before and after pictures, using a tunable dye laser to treat telangiectases

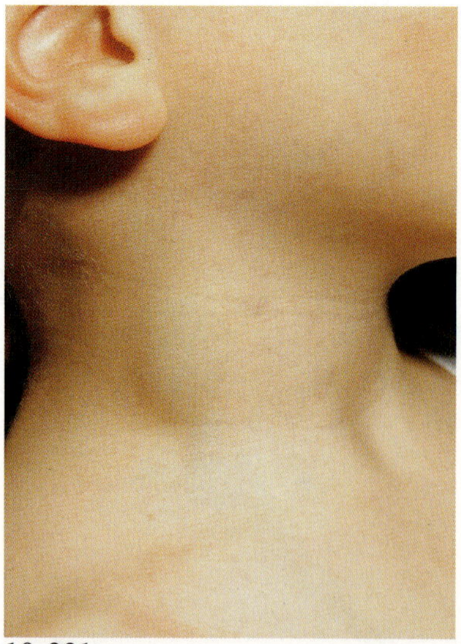
10-231

Fig. 10-231. Asymptomatic swelling on right side of the neck of a 10 year old boy. He had a congenital dilatation of the internal jugular vein which became apparent with straining or when the head was in a dependent position. The lesion is of no clinical significance

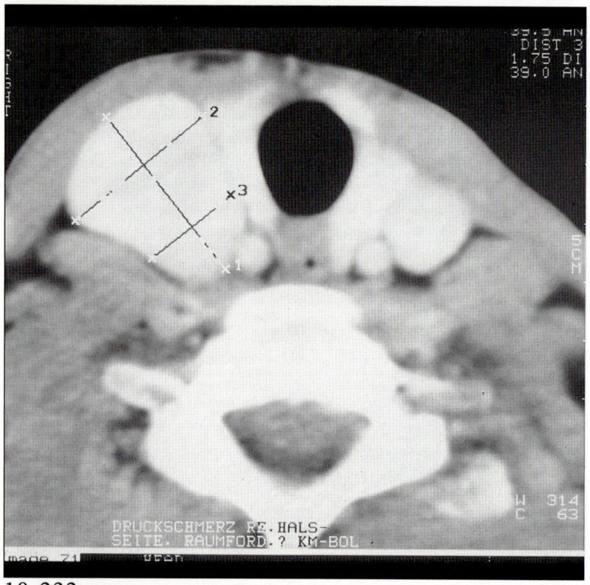

10-232

Fig. 10-232. Computerized tomography showing an aneurysm of the internal jugular vein in a 70 year old woman who became dizzy when she bent over. As she changed position, venous return was impaired leading to symptoms

Figs. 10-233, 10-234. Pre- and post-operative views following correction of jugular vein aneurysm using a running suture to oversew the vein and reduce the size of the lumen

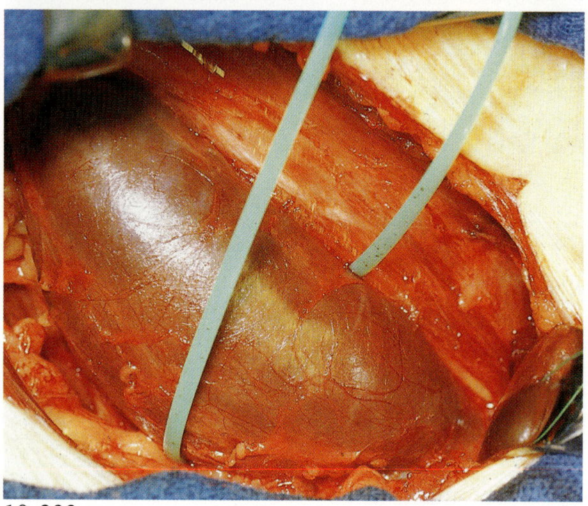
10-233

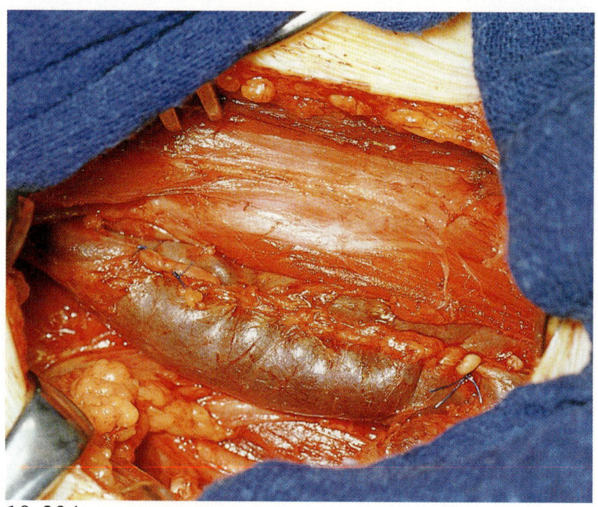
10-234

Fig. 10-235. Varicocele in a 48 year old man. A varicocele is an enlargement and lengthening or coiling of the section of the internal spermatic vein which forms the pampiniform plexus about the spermatic cord. The internal spermatic (or testicular) vein has a long course from the testes to the level of the kidney. The right internal spermatic vein enters the inferior vena cava while the left joins the left renal vein. Most varicoceles appear in young (15–25 years old) men and are on the left. The vein can be tied off using a variety of approaches (pararectal, inguinal or lumbar incisions) or reached and occluded with a catheter. If asymptomatic, no treatment is necessary

Figs. 10-236, 10-237. Angiography of a varicocele. The right femoral vein is entered and the catheter advanced to the left renal vein. The contrast material is injected during a Valsalva maneuver. Further injections with the catheter advanced to the level of S1 show a compromised vessel with a marked varicocele.
Distal occlusion was achieved by the insertion of three coli emboli and injection of a sclerosing material. In addition, coil embolization of the branches at the level of the iliac crest was performed

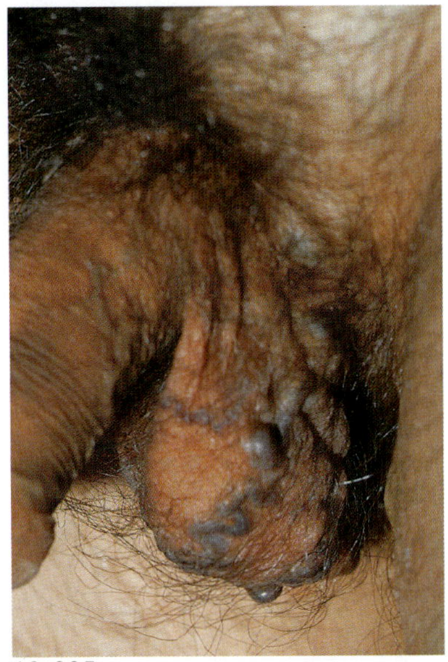

10-235

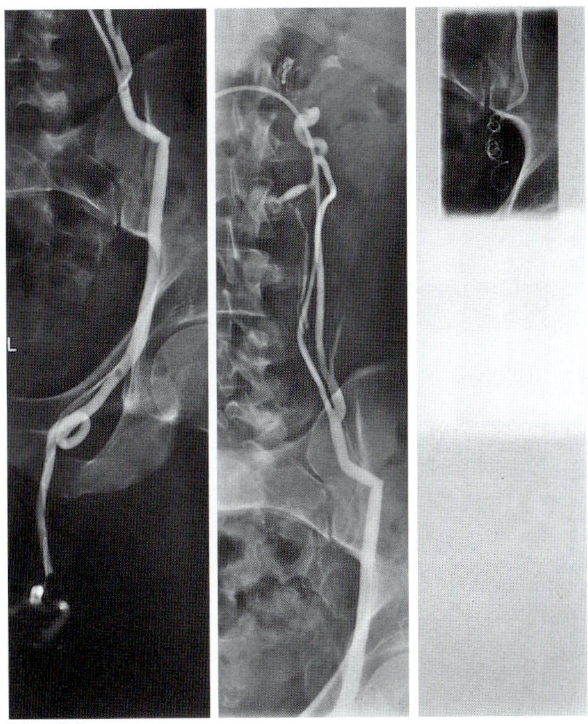

10-236

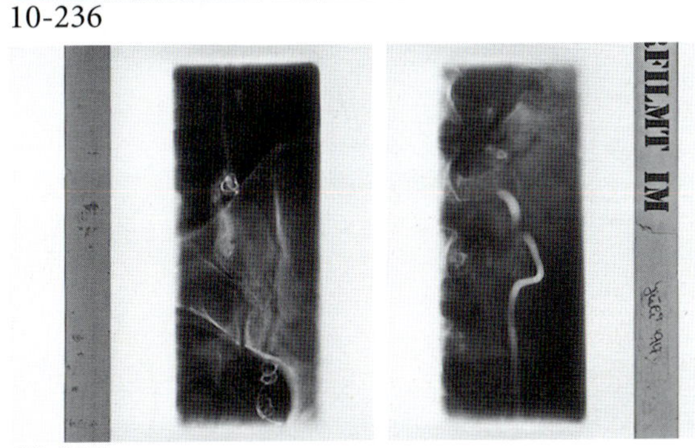

10-237

Part C: Lymphatic System

Chapter 11: Diseases of the Lymphatics

Contents

A: Introduction

Lymphedema

Definition

Lymphedema is the result of a disturbance in lymphatic transport, resulting in an accumulation of lymph in the extremities. The legs are involved about three times as frequently as the arms.

Etiology

There is both primary (congenital) and secondary (acquired) lymphedema. The main causes of primary lymphedema include:

- Hypoplasia of the lymphatic vessels (most common)
- Hypoplasia of the lymphatic collecting system
- Aplasia of the lymphatic channels
- Lymph node hypoplasia with fibrosis
- Hereditary hypo- and aplasia of the lymphatic vessels in small children (Milroy disease)

The main causes of secondary lymphedema are:

- Trauma (such as post-operative changes)
- Tumors (carcinoma of the breast or prostate, Kaposi's sarcoma and many others)
- Chronic inflammation (recurrent erysipelas)
- Artifactual changes (Secrétan syndrome)
- Radiation therapy
- Borreliosis
- Filariasis

Pathogenesis

Lymphedema develops when the transport capacity of the lymphatic system is no longer sufficient to satisfactorily maintain the extravascular circulation of plasma proteins. The main causes are either developmental or functional disturbances in the lymphatic system or excessive demands made upon a normal system.

Primary Lymphedema

Primary lymphedema may be familial or sporadic. Lymphatic hypoplasia means that the lymphatic vessels are too few in number and too narrow. In aplasia, lymphatic channels are either partially or completely missing. Lymphangiectasis refers to dilated lymphatics with inadequate valves.

If the age of onset is less than 35 years, one speaks of lymphedema praecox, while with later onset, the preferred term is lymphedema tardum.

Secondary Lymphedema

Most lymphedema is secondary, caused by compression or interruption of lymphatic channels or damage to lymph nodes. In tropical lands, filariasis is probably the most common cause, but in North America and Western Europe most lymphedema can be blamed on cancers and their treatment (surgery, ionizing radiation).

Clinical Features

Nine-tenths of all patients are women. The legs are affected about three times as often as the forearms and arms. At a glance, the legs have a pole- or column-like appearance with obliteration of the contours around the ankle. The natural skin folds over the metatarsal-phalangeal joint, the anterior aspect of the ankle, the popliteal space and even the groin may be exaggerated. In contrast to cardiac or venous edema, the toes are typically swollen. The skin folds on the back of the toes are hard to pick up or squeeze because of the dermal fibrosis (STEMMER sign, Fig. 11-1). There may also be interdigital dermatophyte infections. Edema sacs may develop behind the malleoli. The back of the foot is thickened and there may be focal induration. The edema has a rubbery consistency, while the skin color is normal. In advanced stages, there may be a reactive papillomatosis of the skin.

Lipedema is a similar disorder. There is an abnormality of the subcutaneous fat with marked thickening. Often there is a familial predisposition to the disorder. Only women are affected. The legs are typically symmetrically swollen, with a sharp collar just above the uninvolved malleoli. The inelegant term of piano legs has been used. The areas are painful. The back of the foot is normal and the Stemmer sign is negative. A definite disturbance in the lymphatics has not been demonstrated.

Diagnosis

The diagnosis of lymphatic diseases is usually made based on the history and the clinical evaluation with inspection and palpation.

Fig. 11-1. STEMMER sign (*arrow*)

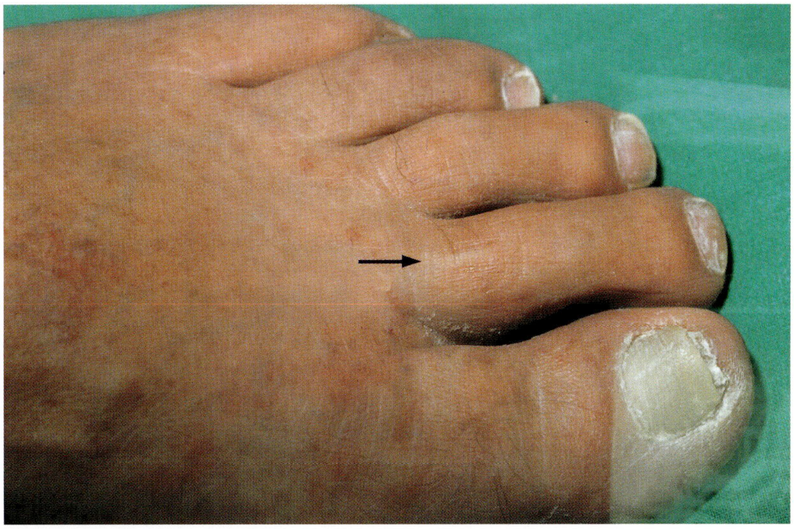

Clues for primary lymphedema include:

- Gradual onset
- Slowly progressive swelling
- Ascending spread
- The dorsal surface of the foot is swollen and the skin of the toes often can not be pinched up into folds (STEMMER sign).

The spread of secondary lymphedema is often descending. Edema of the foot, deep folds at the anterior aspect of the ankle joint and retromalledar edema all appear late.

Lymphedema is divided into three stages, regardless of its cause.

Stage I: Soft, puffy reversible pitting edema
Stage II: Spontaneously reversible edema, but pitting is difficult to elicit
Stage III: Chronic irreversible edema (lymphostatic elephantiasis)

Table 11-1. Differential diagnosis of lymphedema

Types	*Cause*	*Diagnosis*	*Localization*
Venous (phlebedema)	Acute and chronic venous insufficiency	Clinical features	Unilateral
Cardiac edema	Cardiac failure, especially right-sided	Clinical features	Bilateral
Lipedema	Unknown	Painful	Bilateral
Local edema			
Traumatic	Fractures, soft tissue injury, reflex sympathetic dystrophy	Clinical features	Unilateral
Artifactual	Dull trauma (persistent pounding on back of hand),	Clinical features	Unilateral
	restrictive clothing or bands	Clinical features	Unilateral
Rheumatic	Active arthritis, bursitis	Clinical features	Unilateral
Inflammatory	Skin, soft tissue infection	Clinical features	Unilateral
Premenstrual or pregnancy edema	Unknown (hormonal?)	History	Bilateral
Nephrotic syndrome	Hypoproteinemia	Clinical features	Bilateral
Myxedema	Hypothyroidism	Clinical features	Bilateral

Imaging Studies

If the clinical diagnosis is unclear, imaging studies can be performed (This should be very seldom by the case).

Indirect Lymphangiography with Water-Soluble Contrast Material

Indirect lymphangiography is a radiological method to demonstrate peripheral lymphatic vessels following the intradermal or subcutaneous infusion of an appropriate water-soluble contrast material. Normal lymphatic channels show a straight or curved course. If the drainage is abnormal, course reticular or flame-shaped accumulations of contrast material may be seen.

Direct Lymphangiography with Regular Contrast Material
This old method is contraindicated today. The oily contrast material simply caused too many foreign body reactions.

Functional Lymphoscintigraphy
^{99m}Technetium is injected subcutaneously in the second interdigital fold. The impulses are measured over a 2-h period as the radioactive substance is transported away. The exposure to radiation is minimal. A normal static and dynamic lymphoscintigram excludes damage to the lymphatics and lymph nodes as a cause for edema. A pathological pattern indicates either primary or secondary damage to the lymphatic system.

Fluorescent Microlymphography
This very specialized and expensive method is only used in a few centers. Fluorescent-labeled dextran (MW 150,000) is injected subepidermally, allowing visualization of the lymphatic capillary networks.

Therapy

The goal of therapy is to reduce the load on the lymphatics and to improve their transport capacity. All possible factors placing a burden on the system must be avoided or reduced, while at the same time attempts are made to improve its function.

A. General Measures

Every patient with lymphedema needs therapy. When there is massive or monstrous lymphedema with ulcers, fistulas and other complications, hospitalization is necessary. Erysipelas is a common complication which is also best treated in the hospital. All other types of lymphedema can be treated on an out-patient basis. Underlying disorders, such as tumors, heart disease or orthopedic problems, must also be approached aggressively.

The patient must be convinced of the importance of prophylactic measures to avoid secondary complications. Crucial are daily exercises, careful skin care, avoidance of tight clothing and limiting exposure to heat, cold and sunlight. Bacterial and fungal infections can be avoided or treated early if the skin is monitored closely.

In Stage I lymphedema the patient should wear moderate compression stockings. Those individuals with Stage II or III disease need a higher degree of compression. Often it is impossible to fit them with a stockings. Specially customized compression therapy are necessary.

B. Special Measures

The lymphatic transport capacity can be increased by complex physical therapy regimens which include manual lymph drainage and compression therapy. The program should be directed by a physical therapist. Such measures can halt the natural progression of the disease or even reverse it. Active physical therapy exercises can soften the lymphedema and increase central return. Depending on the severity of the lymphedema, the treatment can be provided daily or less frequently. One limb can be treated or a whole body regimen provided. The physical therapy can be directed towards troublesome swollen areas to make fitting with stockings easier.

Pressure can be applied by inflatable boots which can be used to provide intermittent pneumatic compression. This approach is a nice supplement to physical therapy. The initial treatment with mechanical intermittent compression alone should be avoided.

The first phase of the special lymphedema therapy usually lasts about 25 days. The patient receives lymphatic drainage physical therapy once or twice daily and wears firm compression bandages which are wrapped about the limbs to include the digits. In the second phase the lymphatic drainage is carried out several times a week and compression stockings are worn.

C. Medical Treatment

Diuretics are often prescribed for lymphedema but they are not effective and should be avoided. The treatment of choice for erysipelas is parenteral penicillin, usually penicillin G 2–6 million units daily. Once the acute infection has resolved, oral penicillin VK 1.0 g qid is recommended for a total treatment of at least two weeks. Recurrent erysipelas may require long-term antibiotic prophylaxis.

Filariasis must be treated with the appropriate antihelminthic agents; often diethylcarbamazine 2 mg/kg daily over four weeks is used.

D. Surgical Treatment

Operative procedures should only be considered if aggressive physical therapy fails. There are two basic approaches. The swollen damaged subcutaneous tissue can be excised, plastic skin closure performed and then physical therapy and compression re-instituted. If the venous flow is normal, then lympho-venous anastomoses can be attempted. Autologous lymphatic transplantation is a technically complex procedure only carried out in a few centers.

Course and Prognosis

A cure for lymphedema is not possible. The longer it is present, the less likely it is to respond to treatment. In secondary lymphedema following radical mastectomy, the early introduction of physical therapy and compression therapy is essential to produce long-term success.

Complications

Lymphangitis

Ascending lymphatic infections are of great concern to the patient. The erythematous fine subcutaneous cords disturb the patient more than the initial local infection, such as a furuncle, cellulitis, abscess or even secondarily infected tinea pedis. There is usually an associated lymphadenopathy of the associated axillary or inguinal nodes. The patient is usually febrile with an elevated erythrocyte sedimentation rate and leukocytosis. Treatment consists of appropriate, culture-directed systemic antibiotics as well as appropriate local care of the initial infection.

Erysipelas

Erysipelas is caused by group A streptococci that penetrate the skin through tiny areas of injury. In the case of lymphedema, the entry site is often an untreated interdigital tinea pedis. A rapidly expanding warm red patch with sharply defined borders spreads out from the initial infection site. Associated signs of sepsis, such as fever and chills, underline the need for parenteral antibiotics.

Lymphatic Fistula

Lymphatic fistulas may develop after injuries or operative procedures such as biopsies, lymph node excision, arterial operations or draining a lymphocele. The most common problem is secondary infection. The main therapy is the use of a firm compression dressing and patience, although occasionally operative exposure and ligation is necessary.

Lymphangiosarcoma (Stewart-Treves Syndrome)

Chronic lymphedematous changes may evolve into an angiosarcoma. The appearance of painless bruise-like patches and nodules within an area of lymphedema is always suspicious. A biopsy should be performed immediately. Lymphangiosarcomas have a poor prognosis, as both extensive local destruction and metastasis are likely. Often a limb amputation is required. The best approach is aggressive treatment of lymphedema, as malignant change is almost always limited to limbs with severe involvement.

Post-mastectomy Syndrome

About half the women who undergo a radial mastectomy some develop lymphedema of the arm. Both the surgical removal or the lymph nodes and ionizing radiation play a role. There may be a delay of months or years before the lymphedema becomes apparent. It is essential to exclude the presence of either a local recurrence or lymph node metastases as a contributive causative factor for the swelling.

Ten days after a mastectomy physical therapy as well as compression dressings should be instituted. Regular treatment over 3–4 years often is so effective that therapy can be stopped. If the lymphedema is already well established, then the special physical therapy measures discussed above are required. The initial treatment lasts about five weeks and in severe cases must be carried out in special clinics. In such instances, the life-long use of an upper extremity compressive device may be needed.

B: Supplementary Figures and Legends

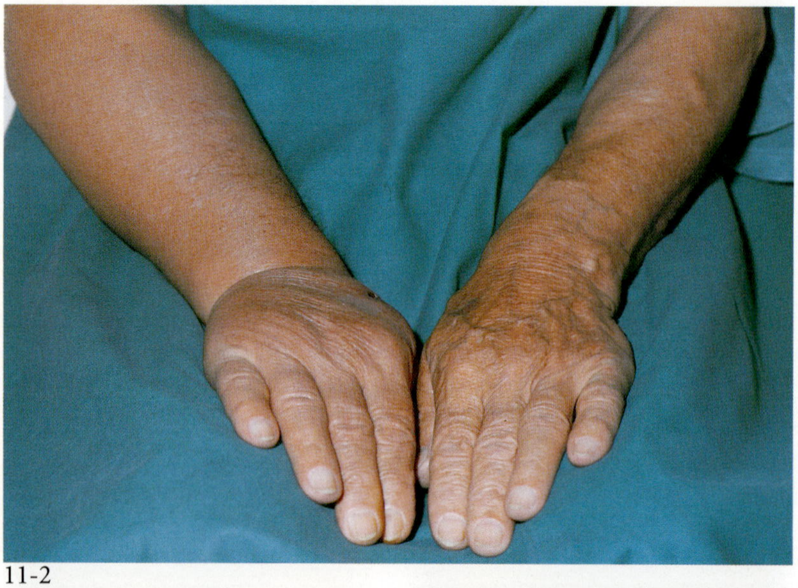

11-2

Fig. 11-2. Lymphedema of the right arm in a 58 year old woman following radical mastectomy for carcinoma of the breast

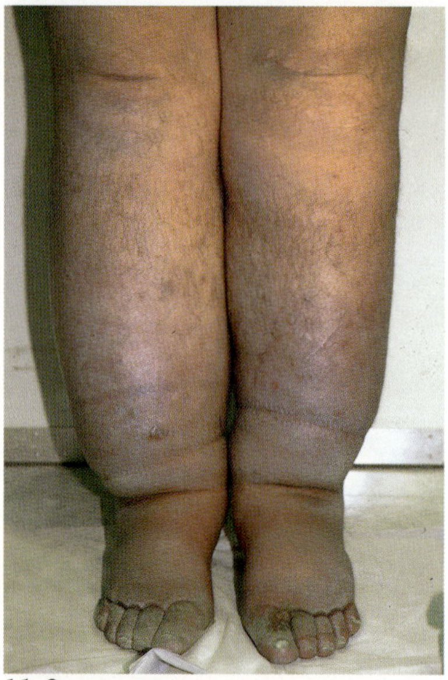

11-3

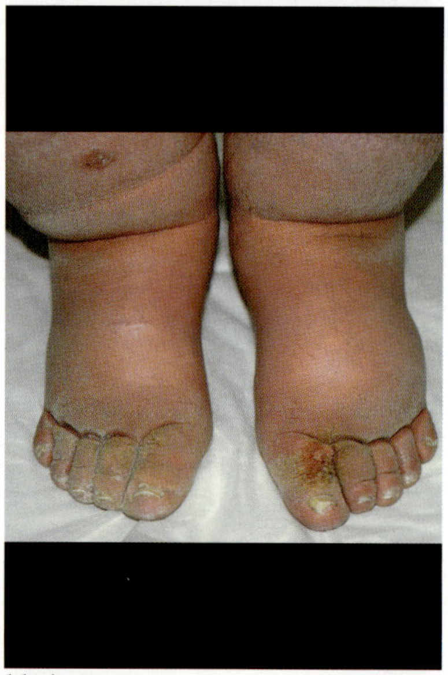

11-4

Figs. 11-3, 11-4. Severe lymphedema of both legs. The column- or pole-like profile of the legs is easily appreciated. Deep skin folds, swelling of the dorsal surface of the foot, localized changes in the retro-malleolar space and about the knees are all seen. The Stemmer sign is positive. The persistent lymphatic blockage leads to the development of tiny lymphangiomas or lymphatic cysts which are associated with verrucous skin changes and occasionally misdiagnosed as warts

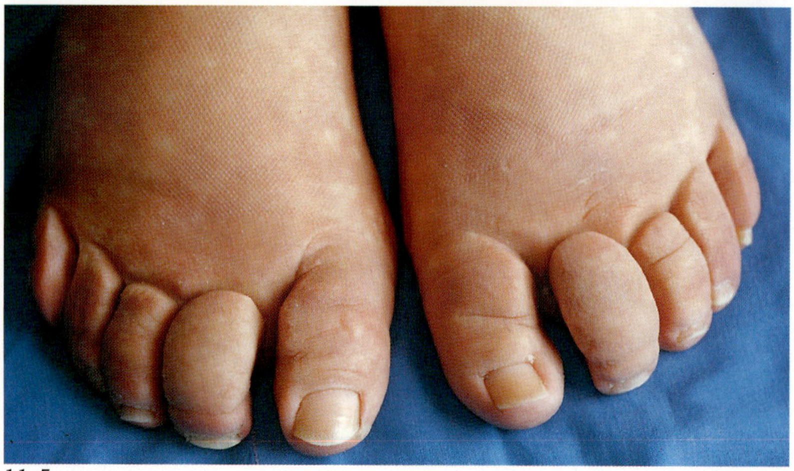

11-5

Fig. 11-5. Anterior part of foot and toes in 52 year old woman with primary lymphedema

Figs. 11-6 – 11-9. This 45 year old women had both lymphatic and venous edema. She had not had any compression therapy. After 2 months of physical therapy (manual lymphatic drainage) and compression therapy, her legs were markedly improved as shown in the second set of photos

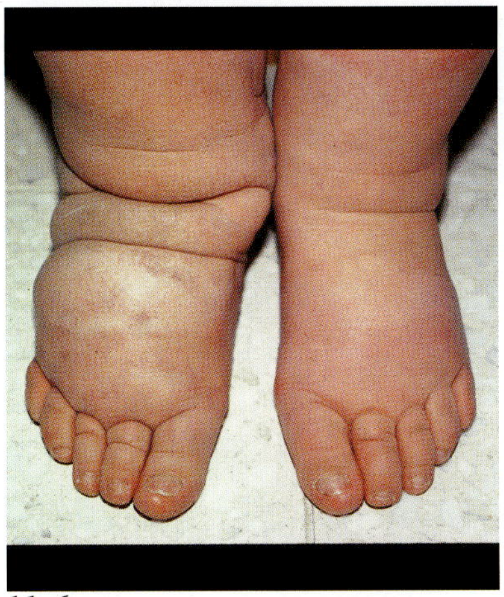

11-6

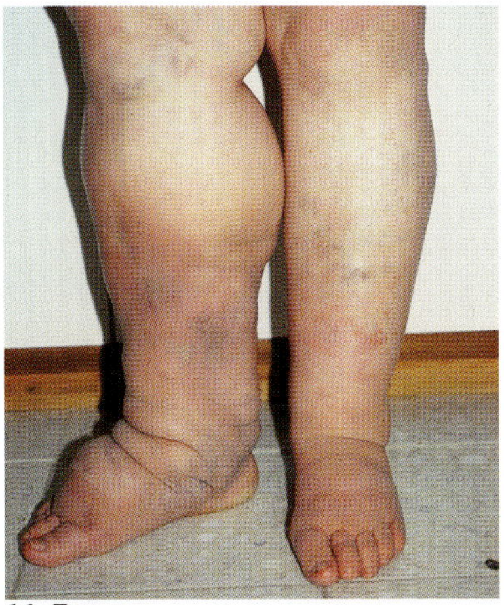

11-7

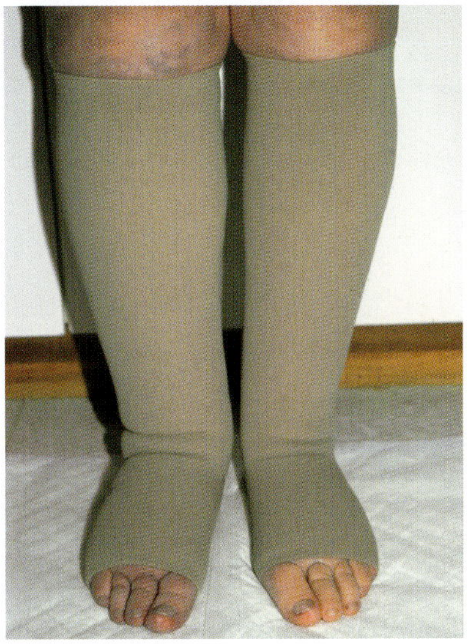

11-8

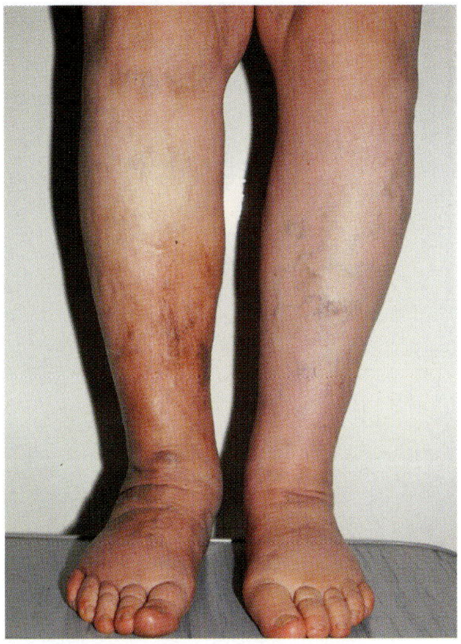

11-9

Fig. 11-10. As a result of multiple injuries to the thigh and lower leg, this patient developed severe secondary lymphedema

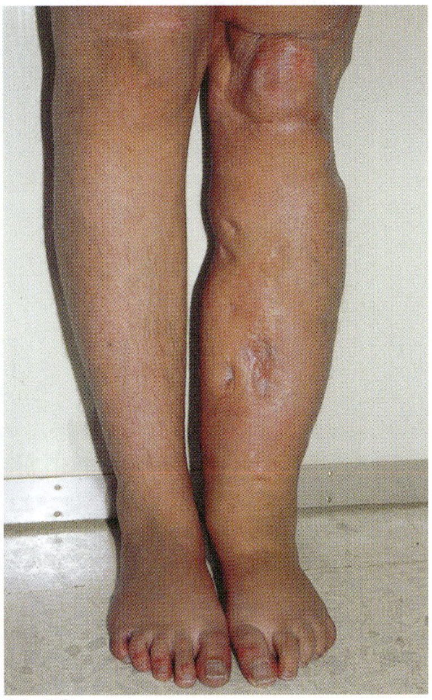

11-10

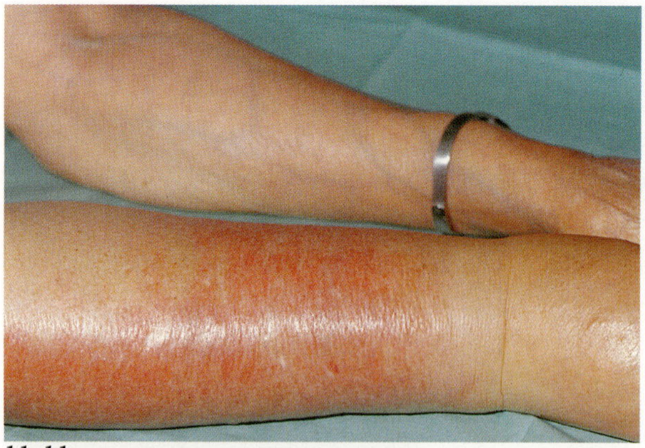

11-11

Fig. 11-11. Stewart-Treves syndrome (Fred W. Stewart, 1894–1970, American pathologist; Norman Treves, 1894–1964, American surgeon) in a 62 year old patient 10 years after radical mastectomy for carcinoma of the breast. The patient initially developed painless bruise-like lesions in her swollen forearm. The histological diagnosis was an lymphangiosarcoma

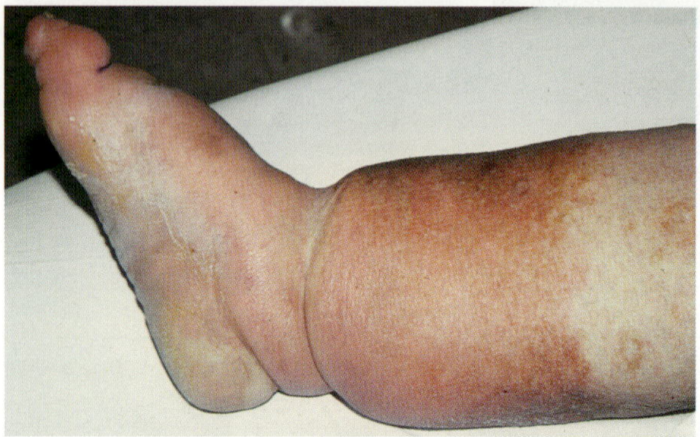

11-12

Fig. 11-12. Erysipelas in a 52 year old woman with diabetes mellitus who had both lymphatic and venous edema. The sharply-bordered, tender erythematous patch with peripheral spread is dramatic. The causative organisms are group A streptococci which enter through tiny skin defects, such as an interdigital tinea pedis

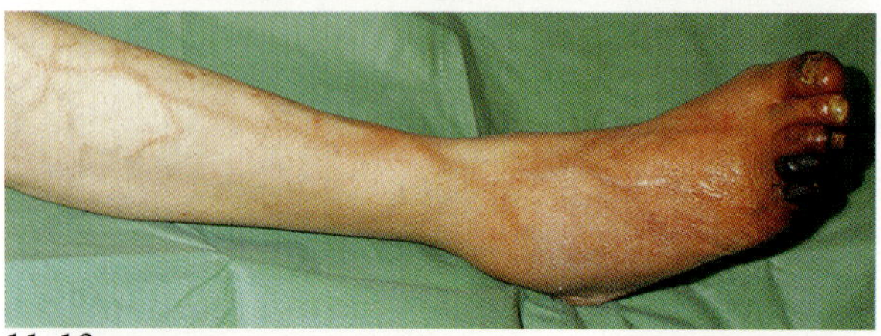

11-13

Fig. 11-13. Lymphangitis in a patient with diabetic foot syndrome (gangrene of the 4th and 5th toes). The red streaks of lymphangitis can be seen on the back of the foot and extending up the leg

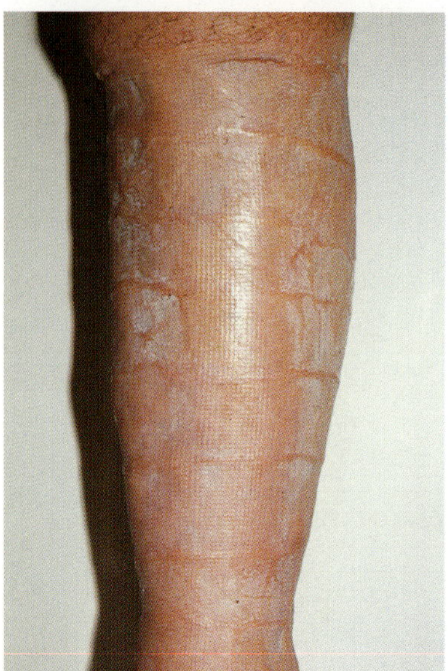

11-14

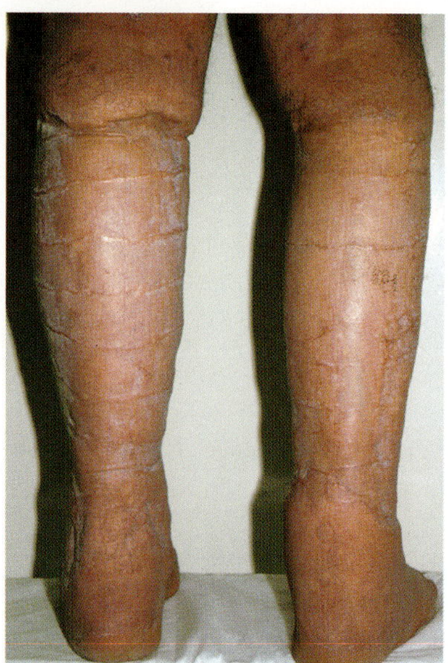

11-15

Figs. 11-14 – 11-15. Appearance following decortication operation in a 48 year old man. This technique is only employed for very severe lymphedema and is no longer extensively performed. The most radical method involves the complete excision of the skin and subcutaneous tissue including the muscle fascia. The defect is then covered either with the excised skin or with a split-thickness skin graft from another body site

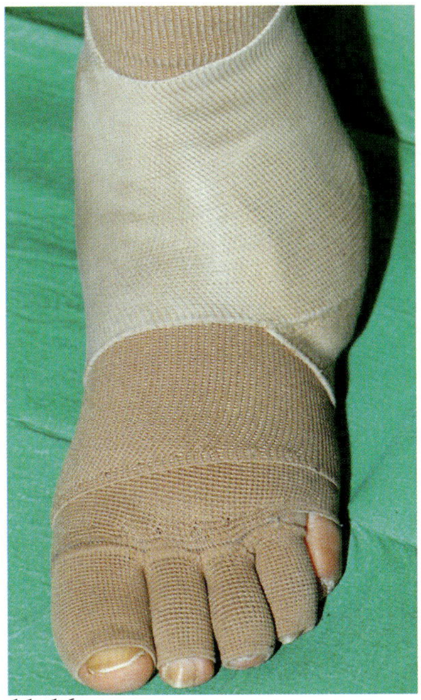

11-16

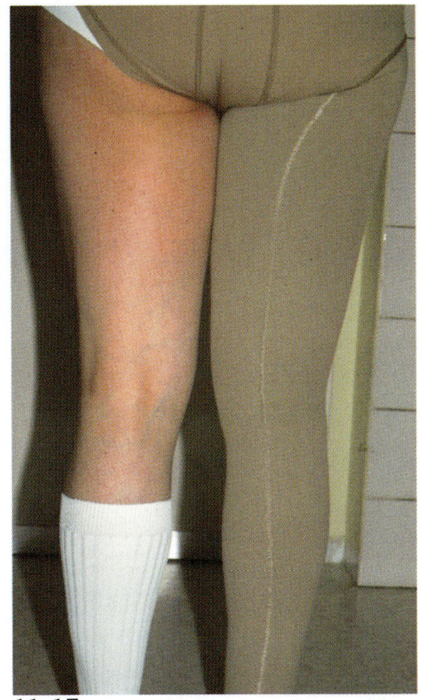

11-17

Fig. 11-16. Compression stocking with toes for optimal therapy of lymphedema. With this stocking, the toe edema can be effectively reduced. The best results are achieved when physical therapy is combined with compression therapy

Fig. 11-17. Custom-fitted compression stocking in a patient with unilateral lymphedema

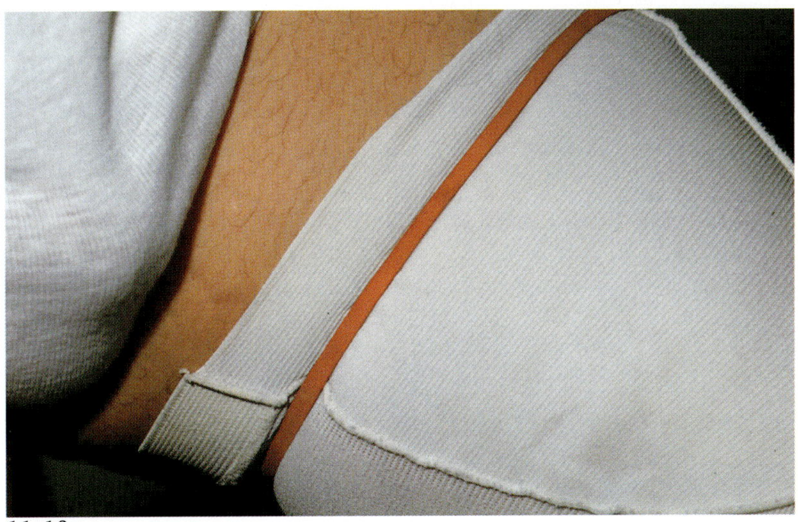

11-18

Fig. 11-18. Inadequate compression stocking in a 25 year old patient with primary lymphedema. Such a stocking is truly worthless. One must be sure that the patient's compression stockings are correctly fitted and replaced as they become stretched

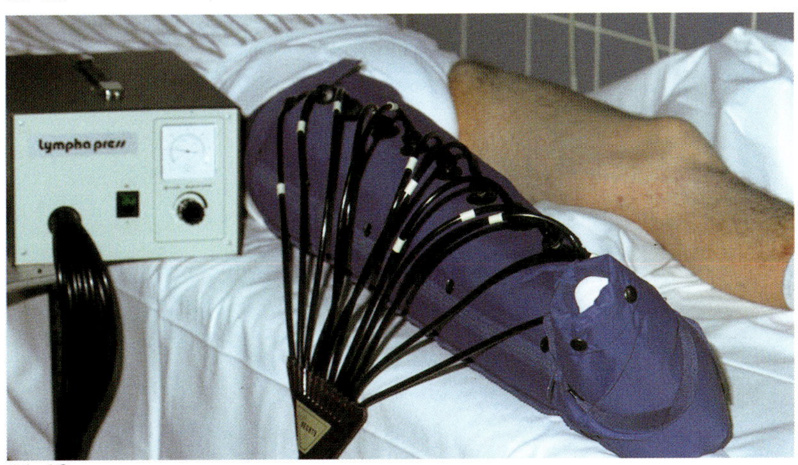

11-19

Fig. 11-19. Intermittent pneumatic compression should never be the primary therapy for lymphedema. In the second phase of the lymphedema therapy, this form of pneumatic therapy can be combined with physical therapy

Part D: Vascular Malformations

Chapter 12:
Congenital Malformations of Vessels

Contents

A: Introduction

Synonym. Angiodysplasia

Definition

Vascular malformations are congenital developmental errors in the vascular system. They can be solitary or occur in a variety of combinations.

History

Important events in the history of vascular malformations are shown in Table 12-1.

Table 12-1. Milestones in vascular malformations

Date	Physician	Malformation
129–199	Galen	Patent ductus arteriosus (The first detailed description was probably from Aranzio and not from Leonardo Botallo whose name is associated with the ductus arteriosus or ductus Botalli)
1707	Lealis-Lealis	Arterio-venous fistula (spermatic artery and vein)
1723, 1761	Stenzel, Morgagni	Aortic isthmus stenosis
1739	Winslow	Transposition of pulmonary veins
1777	Steidele	Aortic atresia
1830	Elliotson	Aorto-pulmonary fistula
1875	Gruber	Phlebectasia (aneurysm of jugular vein)
1900 1905	Klippel and Trénaunay	Angiodysplasia with tissue hyperplasia (original description actually 1869 – Trela and Monod)
1907	Munro	Suggested operation for patent ductus arteriosus
1913	Doyen	First attempt to repair patent ductus arteriosus
1928, 1930	Gsell, Erdheim	Cystic medial necrosis
1933	Oppenheimer	Dilated pulmonary artery
1939 1944	Gross and Hubbard	First successful repair of patent ductus arteriosus
1948 1968	Servelle and Trinquecoste	Venous malformations of the extremities

Epidemiology

About 1.5% of newborns have a vascular malformation. Two-thirds of these are peripheral, primarily venous malformations. The clinically most important lesions are arterio-venous fistulas and arterial malformations. More arterio-venous malformation are congenital than acquired.

Etiology and Pathogenesis

Angiogenesis begins in the third embryonic week. The earliest vascular system is a plexus. The expansion and differentiation of the vascular channels is accomplished by the fusion of adjacent vascular spaces, often coupled with enlargement of capillaries. The complicated development of the arterial, venous and lymphatic systems occasionally goes astray, leading to congenital malformations.

- An aplasia arises either because the embryological precursors are not present (agenesis) or fail to develop. Disturbances in organ differentiation early in development can cause a hypoplasia, in which case a stenosis or obliteration of a vessel can occur. In addition stenoses can result from dysplasia of the vessel wall (fibromuscular dysplasia).
- Congenital dilatations and aneurysms are characterized by hypoplasia of the smooth muscle of the media and adventitia. Elongation of the vessels is usually caused by weak elastic fibers. In contrast to changes caused by arteriosclerotic disease, congenitally elongated vessels typically show coiling or kinking.
- An arterio-venous fistula is a general term for all aberrant connections between veins and arteries. Some angiomas also contain arterio-venous fistulas. Congenital arterio-venous fistulas are more common (60% – 70% of total) than acquired lesions, especially in the head and neck region. On the extremities, traumatic and especially iatrogenic arterio-venous fistulas are more common.
- Telangiectases are small, permanently dilated bundles of vessels (capillaries and transitional vessels) found in the skin where they show an intradermal network. A common hereditary type of telangiectasia is OSLER-RENDU-WEBER disease (Fig. 12-1).
  Nevus flammeus is a congenital capillary malformation. In the KLIPPEL-TRÉNAUNAY syndrome, a unilateral nevus flammeus is combined with varicosities and hypertrophy of the soft tissue and bones.
- A cavernous hemangioma is a tumor-like proliferation with large primarily venous spaces. A racemose angioma is a congenital arterio-venous fistula in the skin, not a vascular proliferation. (Table 12-2, Fig.)

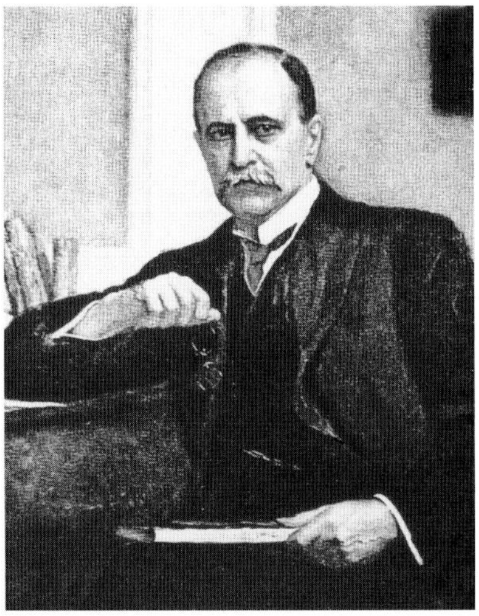

Fig. 12-1. Sir WILLIAM OSLER, 1849 – 1919, Canadian internist and pathologist, Johns Hopkins University, Baltimore. He was the first to describe hereditary telangiectases

Table 12-2. Types of congenital arterio-venous fistulas (after VOLLMAR)

	Type I-localized, direct shunt (patent ductus arteriosus)	Type II-generalized, complex shunt (KLIPPEL-TRÉNAUNAY)	Type III-localized tumor (angioma)
Morphology	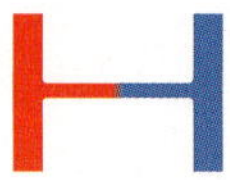	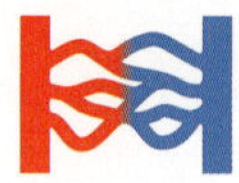	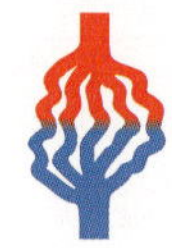
Frequency	Uncommon	Common	Uncommon
Location	Extremities, carotid artery	Extremities	Head, brain
Operability	Yes	Limited	Yes

After VOLLMAR.

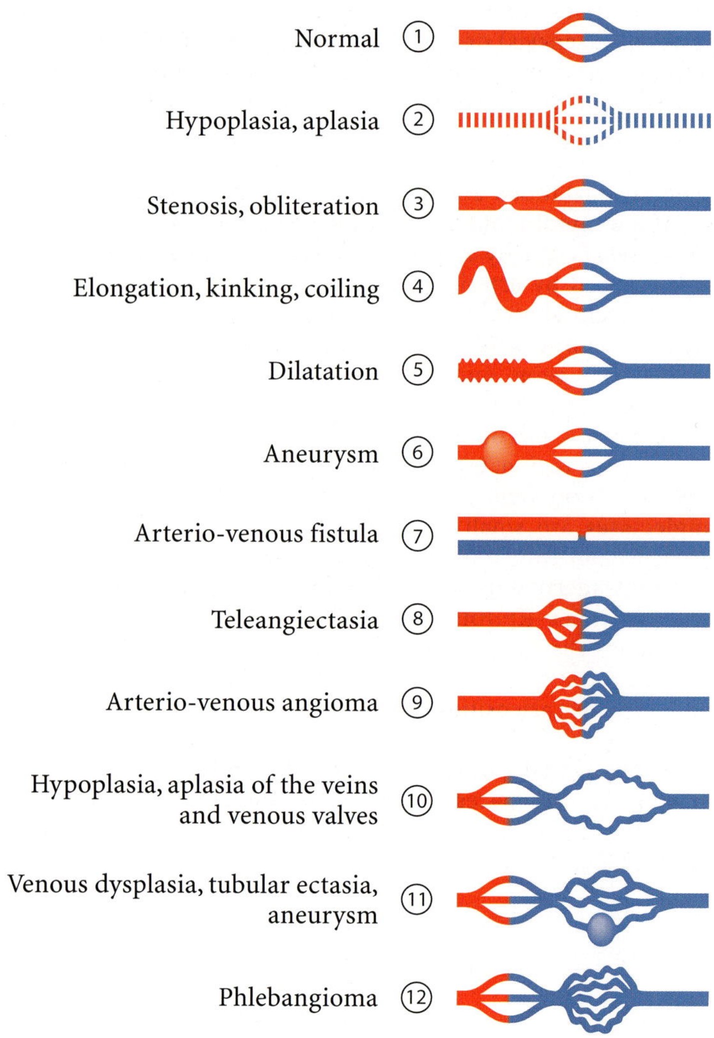

Fig. 12-2. The major vascular malformations

Topography

The most important locations of vascular malformations are shown in Fig. 12-3.

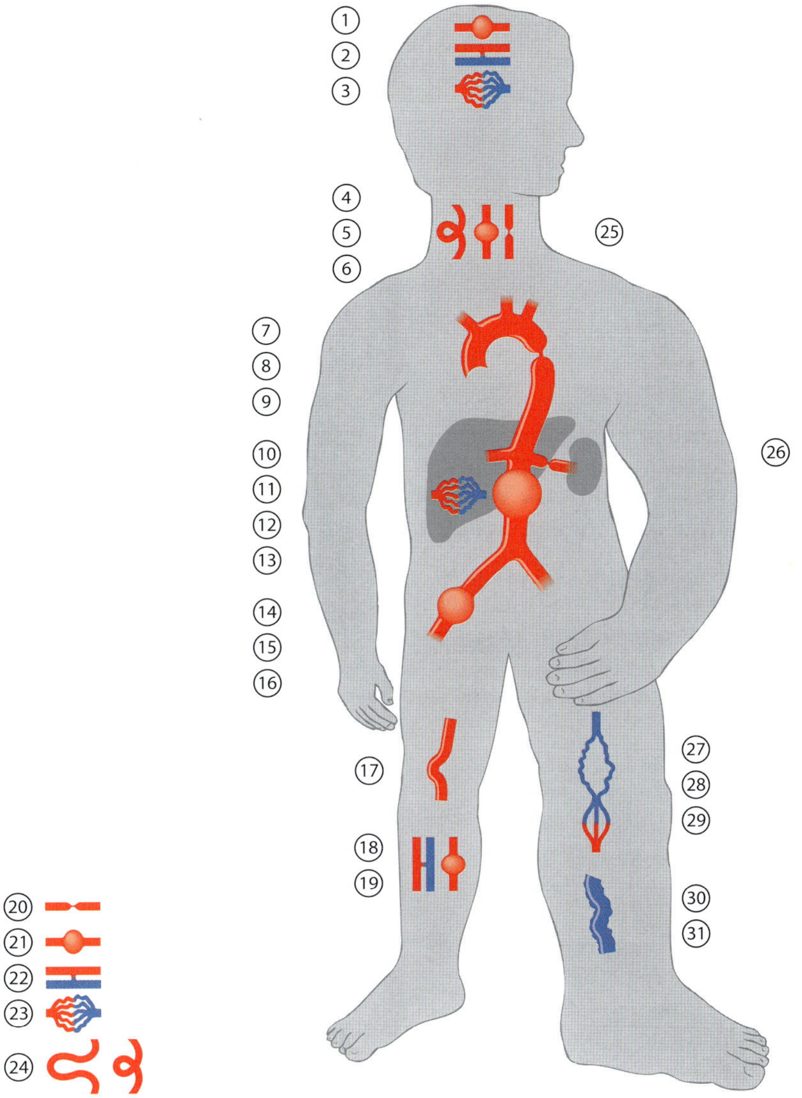

Fig. 12-3. Most important locations of vascular malformations

① Intracranial aneurysm (circle of Willis)
② Intracranial arterio-venous fistula
③ Angioma
④ Elongation of carotid artery
⑤ Fibromuscular dysplasia of carotid artery
⑥ Hypoplasia of vertebral artery
⑦ Coarctation of aorta
⑧ Aortic aneurysm
⑨ Aberrant supra-aortic branches
⑩ Arterio-venous fistula of visceral arteries
⑪ Fibromuscular dysplasia of renal artery
⑫ Accessory or polar renal arteries
⑬ Hepatic angioma
⑭ Aneurysms of iliac and leg arteries
⑮ Arterio-venous fistula
⑯ Angioma
⑰ Aberrant course of popliteal artery
⑱ Arterio-venous fistulas in leg and foot
⑲ Angioma
⑳ Stenosis
㉑ Aneurysm
㉒ Arterio-venous fistula
㉓ Angioma
㉔ Kinking, coiling
㉕ Aneurysm of jugular vein
㉖ Aberrant vena cava
㉗ Aberrant venous return
㉘ Aplasia, hypoplasia of veins, lymphatics
㉙ Aplasia of venous valves
㉚ Phlebectasia
㉛ Angioma with hypertrophy of tissue

Hemodynamics

The hemodynamics of congenital vascular obstruction and dilatation are similar to that of acquired arteriosclerotic and venous disorders. The so-called parasitic circulation refers to the problems associated with arterio-venous communications. The hemodynamic changes include:

Table 12-3. Hemodynamics of vascular malformations

Type of malformation	Arterial system	Venous system
Hypoplasia, obstruction	Reduced flow, peripheral hypoxia	Reduced flow, peripheral stasis
Dilatation, aneurysm	Turbulence, risk of thrombosis, bleeding, emboli	Centrifugal flow, peripheral stasis
A-V fistula		Parasitic circulation with cardiac load, trophic changes in tissue

- Reduced arterial blood pressure peripheral to the shunt
- Elevated venous blood pressure and stasis peripheral to the shunt
- Increased blood flow rate and thus increased perfusion volume, resulting in increased cardiac work load

Arterio-venous fistulas are often first discovered when complications occur. Pulsating masses of vessels may be noticed in the extremities. They can cause bleeding into joints or externally through the skin. Congenital arterio-venous fistulas rarely cause chronic cardiac failure, but this is more often seen in large traumatic fistulas.

Diagnosis

Clinical Evaluation

- History (personal and family)
- Inspection: tissue damage, stasis, tumors, growth disturbances
- Palpation of pulses
- Auscultation: turbulent flow with stenoses, bruits with arterio-venous fistulas

Diagnostic Procedures

- Ultrasonography
  - Continuous wave Doppler ultrasonography
  - B-mode duplex ultrasonography
- Angiography
  - Digital subtraction angiography, conventional angiography, computerized tomography, magnetic resonance imaging
- Other functional tests
  - EKG
  - Oscillography
  - Plethysmography
- Molecular genetic studies

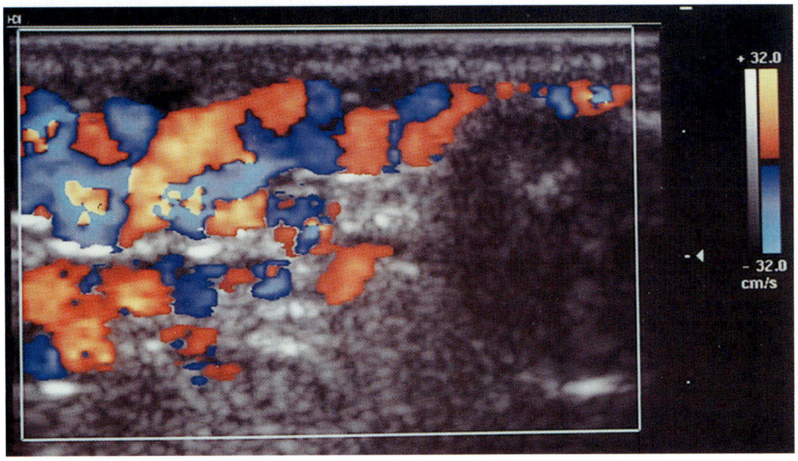

Fig. 12-4. Color duplex sonography showing a vascular malformation

Therapy

The treatment of vascular malformations is challenging. Invasive procedures such as catheter embolization or surgery should only be used in special circumstances. They are indicated when:

- Changes are localized and can be cured by treatment
- Complications develop such as severe hemodynamic features, growth disturbances or suspicion of malignant changes
- Cosmetic problems are marked

Arterio-venous Fistulas

Arterio-venous fistulas should be treated if their size suggests they are likely to have a negative effect on the heart or if hemodynamic abnormalities are already present. If the shunt volume is more than 25% of the total cardiac flow, there may be palpitations, tachycardia and increasing left-sided heart failure with exertional dyspnea. Other indications for therapy include local or regional problems, pressure on adjacent structures, local hypertrophy of tissues, venous stasis, and trophic changes in the skin and subcutaneous tissue. A tendency to bleeding with minor injuries and cosmetic importance are also considerations.

Therapeutic possibilities include ligation of a fistula and excision of circumscribed abnormal vascular tissue, as well as sclerosing approaches and compression therapy.

Angioma

Angiomas can be treated with a variety of lasers, as well as deep contact cryotherapy.

Generalized Vascular Malformations

Complex congenital malformations usually are very difficult to treat and usually require several different approaches, including surgery, catheter embolization and conservative measures. Care must be taken not to ligate a feeding vessel if subsequent embolization may become an important therapeutic option.

Venous Dysplasia

Phlebectasias and other venous malformations can be excised if their localization and size make it feasible.

B: Supplementary Figures and Legends

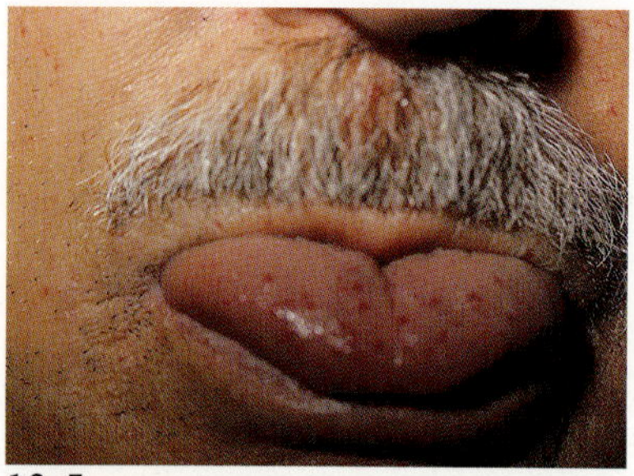
12-5

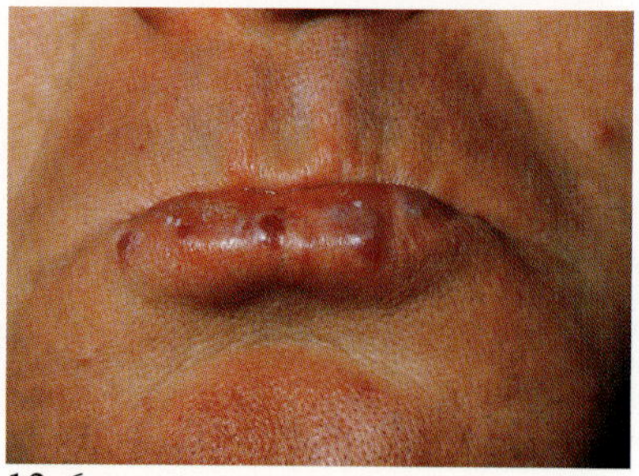
12-6

Fig. 12-5. A 60 year old patient with Osler-Rendu-Weber disease. Multiple telangiectases on the tongue

Fig. 12-6. A 55 year old patient with typical lip telangiectases

Fig. 12-7. A 40 year old man with telangiectases on nose

Fig. 12-8. A 45 year old woman with telangiectases about the ear

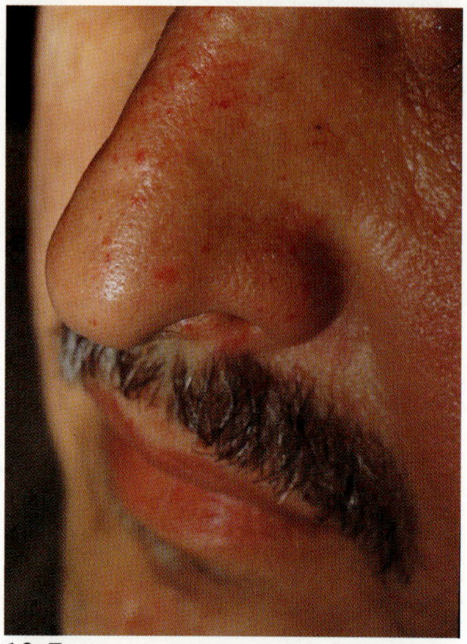
12-7

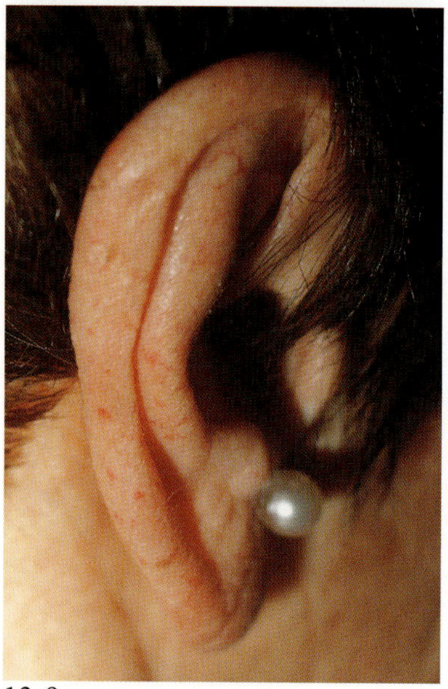
12-8

Osler-Rendu-Weber Disease

Synonym. Hereditary hemorrhagic telangiectasia

This disease is inherited in an autosomal dominant pattern. There is localized dilatation and convolution of venules and capillaries usually with a thinned vessel wall because of a defective or absent elastic lamina. The telangiectases can be found in all organs (mucosa of gastrointestinal tract, lungs and genitourinary tract, as well as brain, liver, spleen and bones). They are easily injured so that spontaneous bleeding is common. Nose bleeds are the most common presenting sign. Septic emboli from pulmonary a-v malformations are the leading cause of death. Only symptomatic therapy is possible.

Sir William Osler, 1849–1919, Canadian and American internist and pathologist;
Henri Rendu, 1844–1919, French internist;
Frederick Parkes Weber, 1863–1962, British physician

Figs. 12-9, 12-10. Congenital capillary-lymphatic malformation on the lateral aspect of the thorax in a 28 year old woman. The changes are sharply demarcated. The verrucous alterations are impressive. In the past such lesions were designated either as hypertrophic nevus flammeus or as verrucous hemangioma

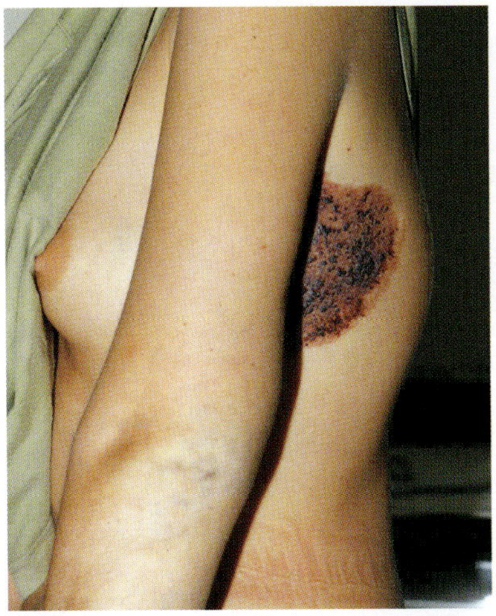

12-9

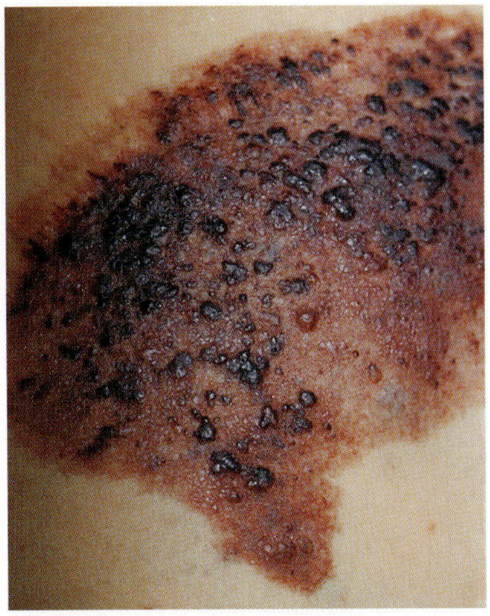

12-10

Figs. 12-11, 12-12. Multiple venous malformations about the knee and calf. The venous nodules are well-localized. Often there are associated changes in the deep venous system. In such cases, one should check for involvement of the bones and gastrointestinal tract

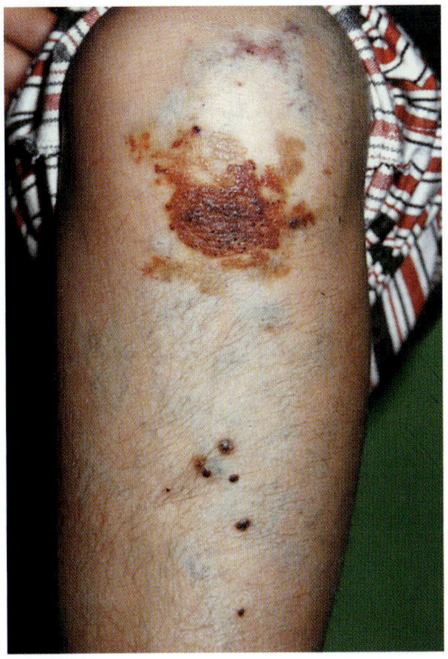

12-11

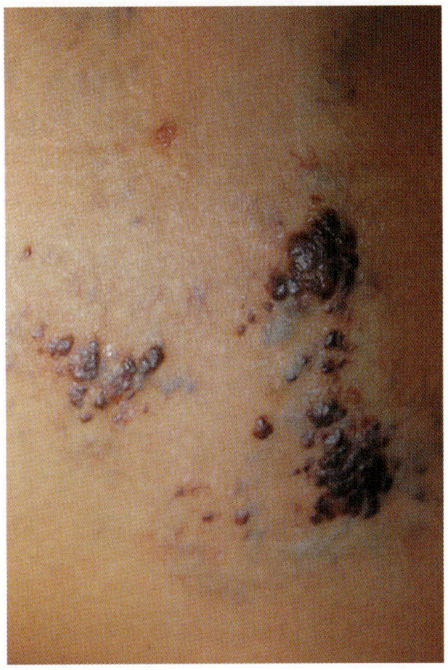

12-12

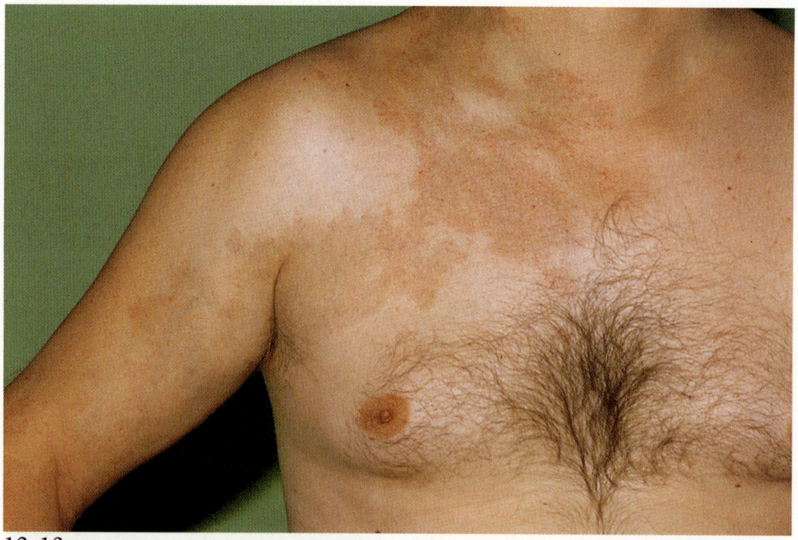

12-13

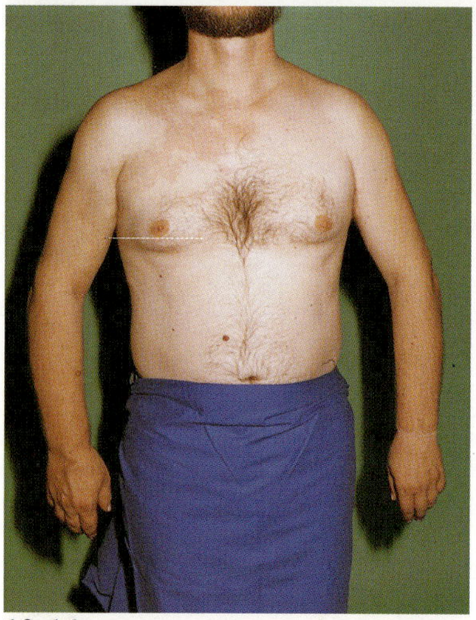

12-14

Figs. 12-13, 12-14. A 44 year old man with KLIPPEL-TRÉNAUNAY syndrome. There are telangiectases on the right arm and right side of the thorax, while the right arm is lengthened and shows increased venous filling

MAURICE KLIPPEL, 1858–1942, French neurologist
PAUL TRÉNAUNAY, 1875–1938, French physician

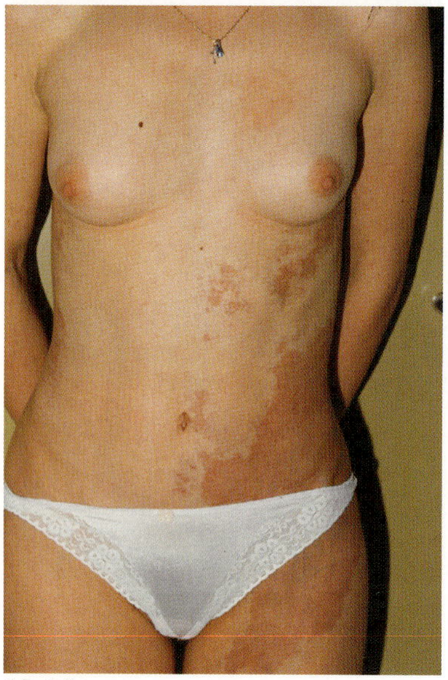

12-15

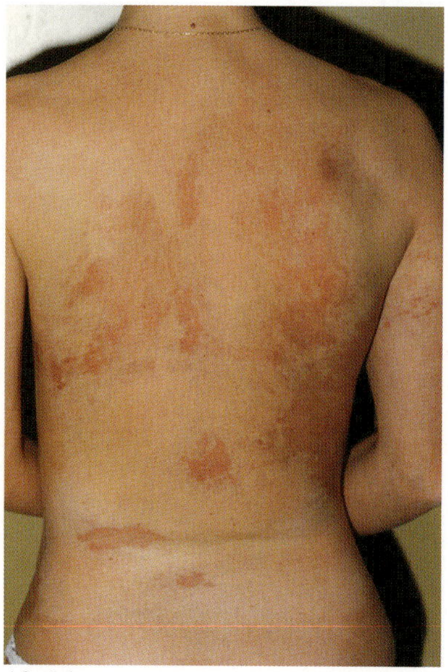

12-16

Figs. 12-15, 12-16. Capillary dysplasia in a 22 year old woman. The many tiny vascular nevi were present at birth

Figs. 12-17, 12-18. A 12 year old girl with Klippel-Trénaunay syndrome. The entire left side of her body has telangiectases. The left arm and leg are both enlarged and lengthened

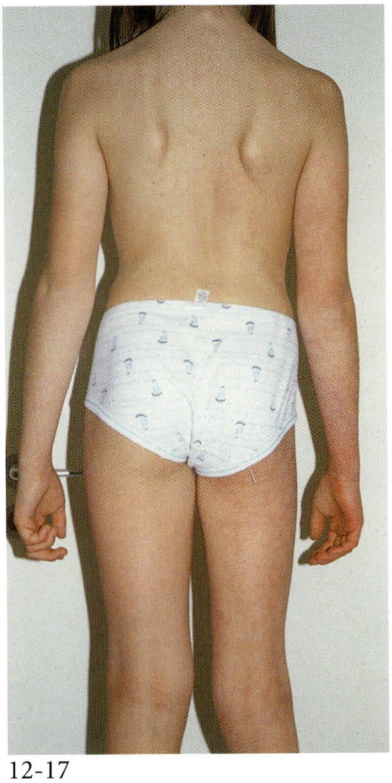

12-17

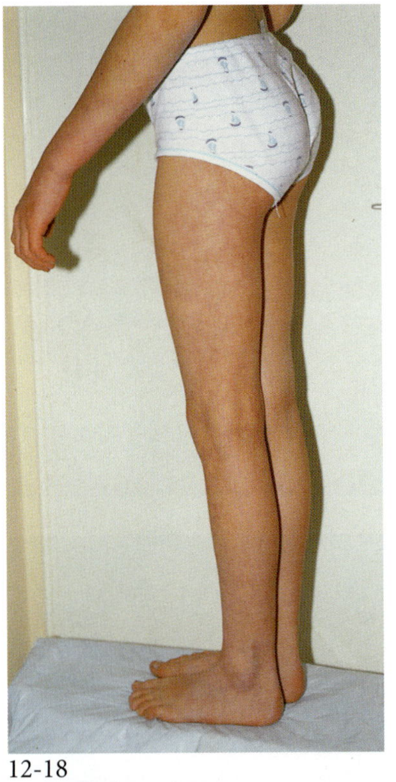

12-18

Figs. 12-19. 9 year old girl with Klippel-Trénaunay syndrome

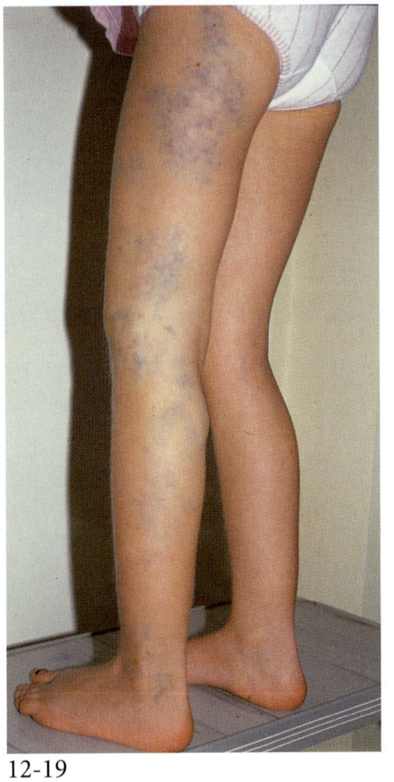

12-19

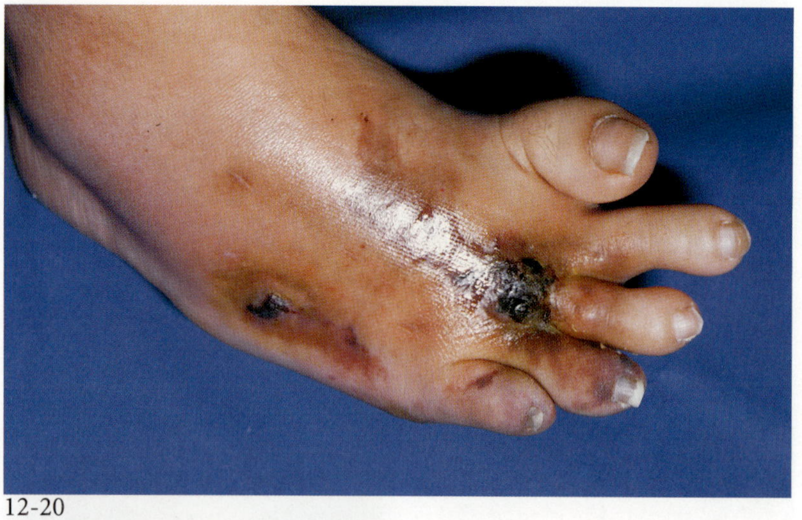

12-20

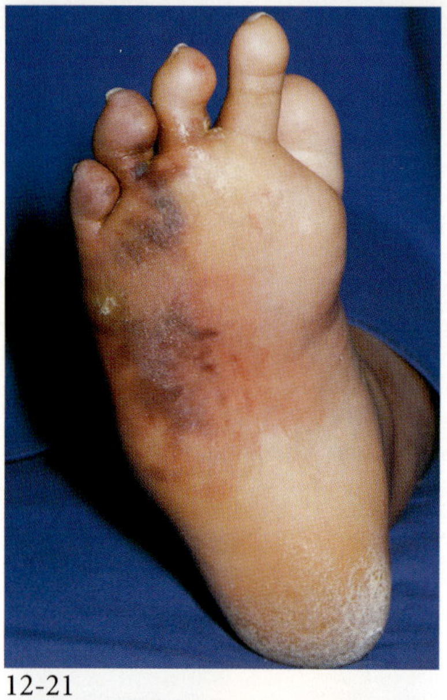

12-21

Figs. 12-20, 12-21. Plantar and lateral views of an arterio-venous fistula of the lateral aspect of the foot including the toes. The increased venous pressure is associated with necrosis and ulceration because of inadequate circulation

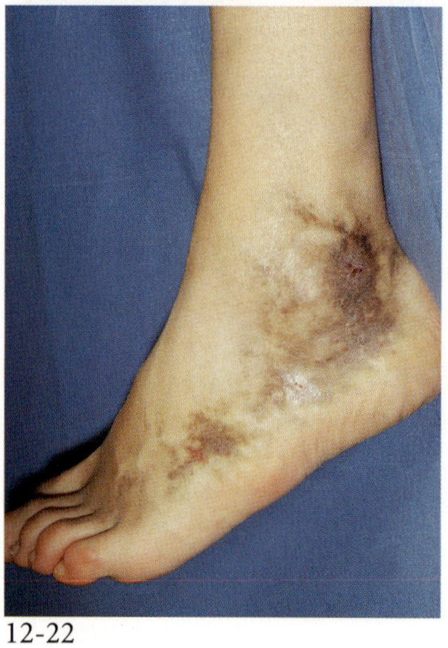

12-22

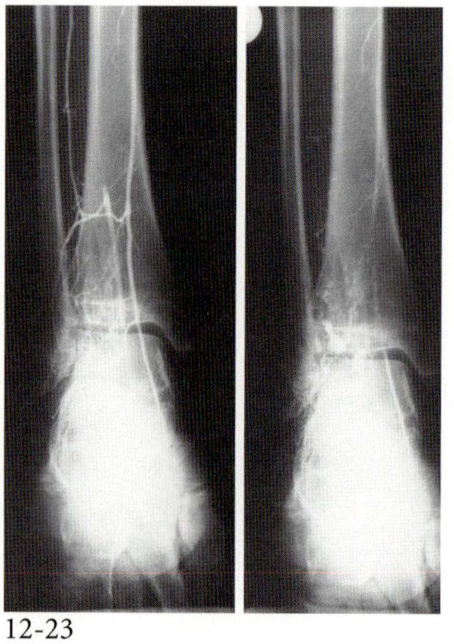

12-23

Figs. 12-22, 12-23. Arterio-venous fistula in a 30 year old man. One year after a soccer injury developed a leg ulcer as the first sign of the traumatic fistula

Figs. 12-24 – 12-26. Multiple arterio-venous fistulas or shunts in a 25 year old woman. Clinically erythematous nodules and ulcerations were present, while angiography showed multiple arterio-venous fistulas

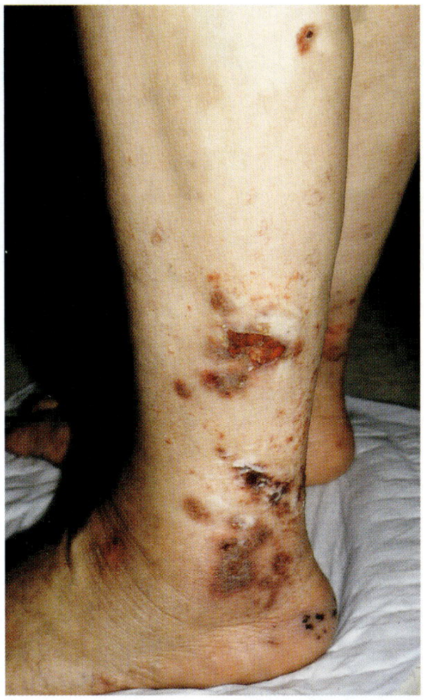

12-24

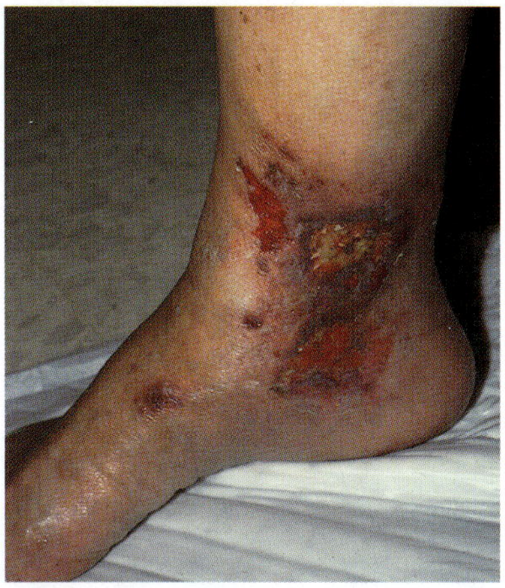

12-25

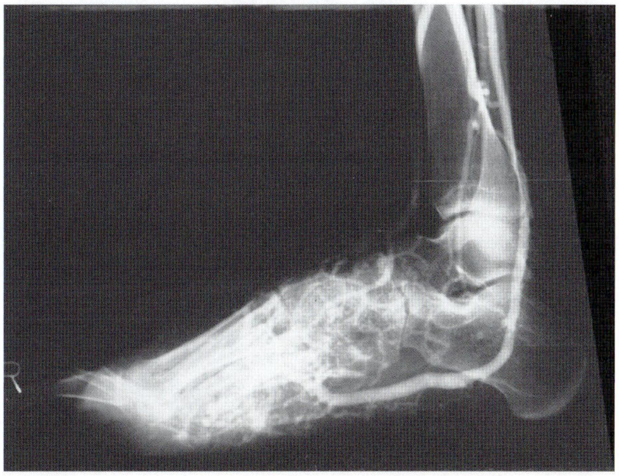

12-26

Figs. 12-27, 12-28. Arterio-venous malformation in the left index finger. The shunting leads marked venous filling of the dorsal surface of the hand. In the course of time, the patient required an amputation of the finger because of pain

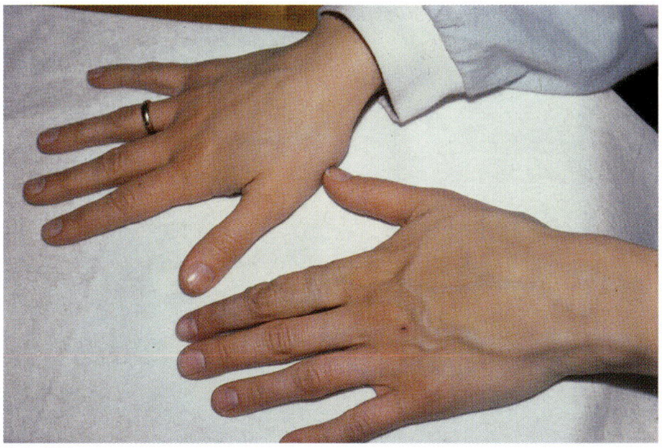

12-27

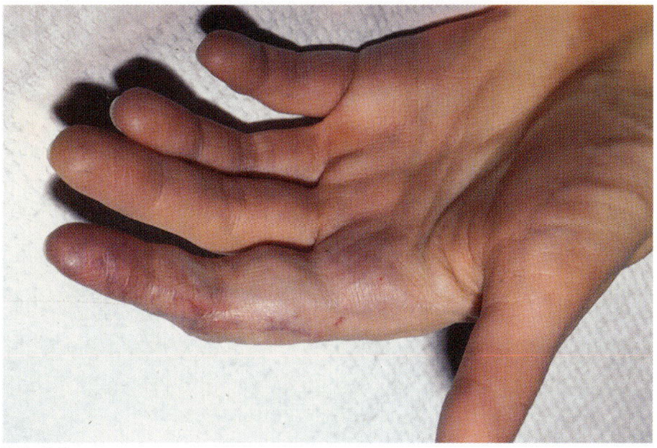

12-28

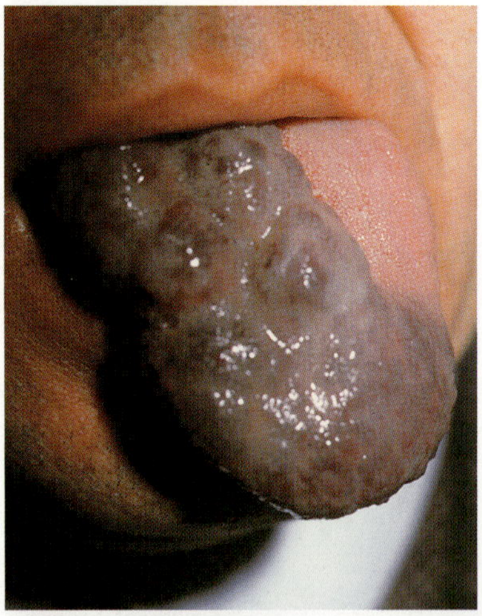

12-29

Fig. 12-29. Large cavernous hemangioma of the tongue in a 64 year old man. The patient had trouble swallowing and complained of difficulty breathing

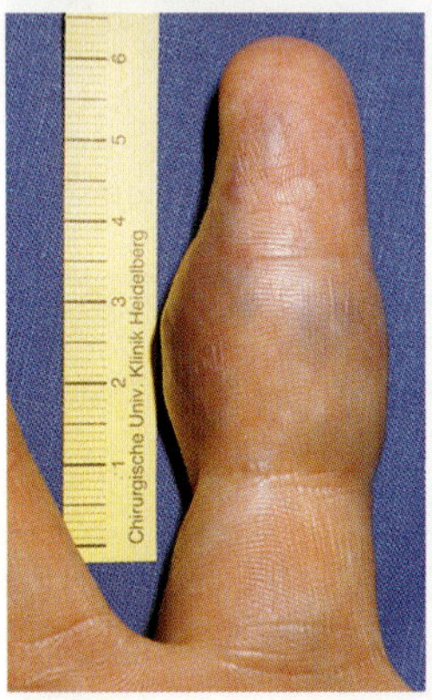

12-30

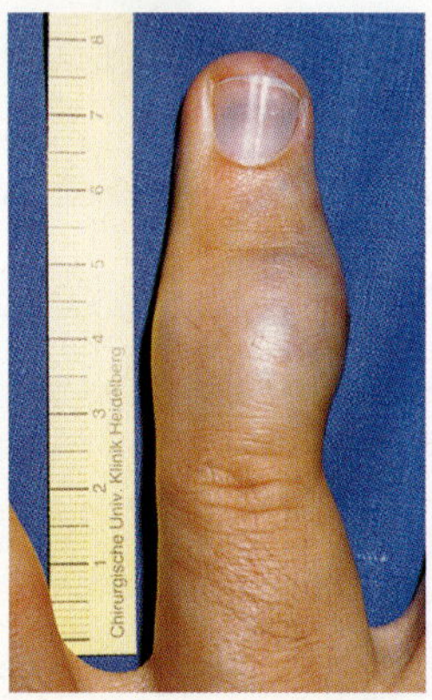

12-31

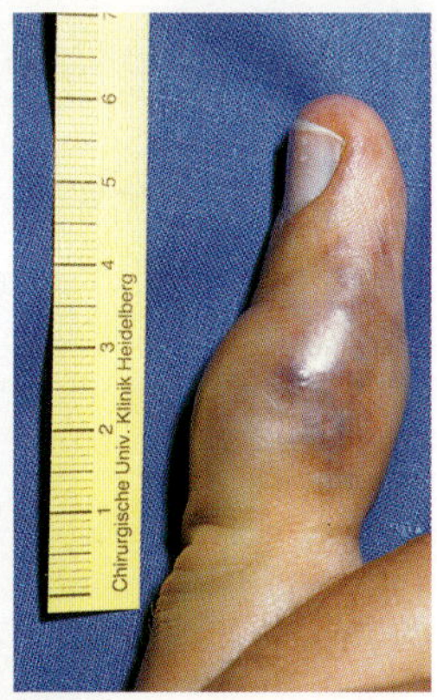

12-32

Figs. 12-30 – 12-32. Cavernous hemangioma of finger

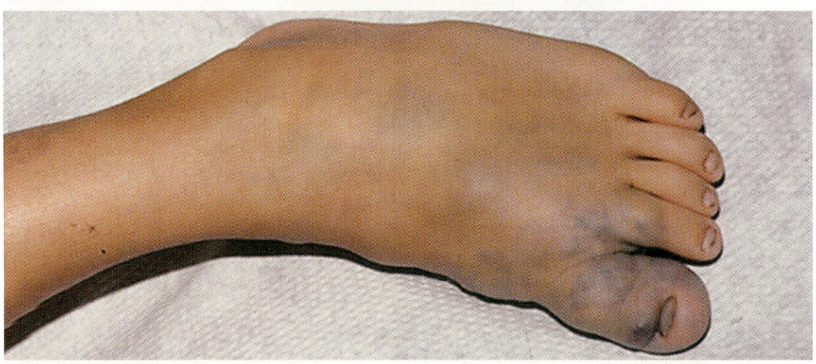

12-33

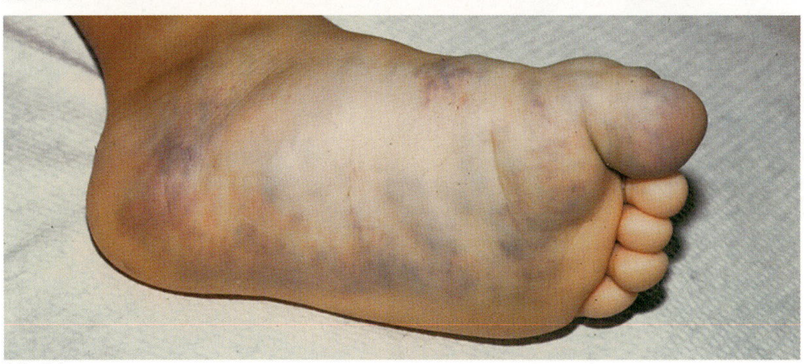

12-34

Figs. 12-23, 12-34. A 3 year old child with a cavernous hemangioma of the left foot, The left great toe is markedly enlarged

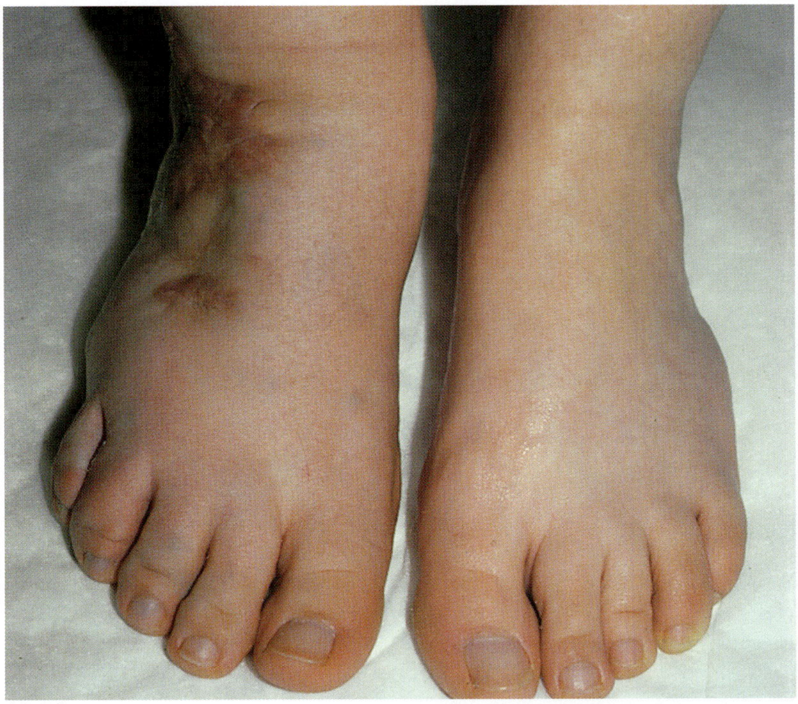

12-35

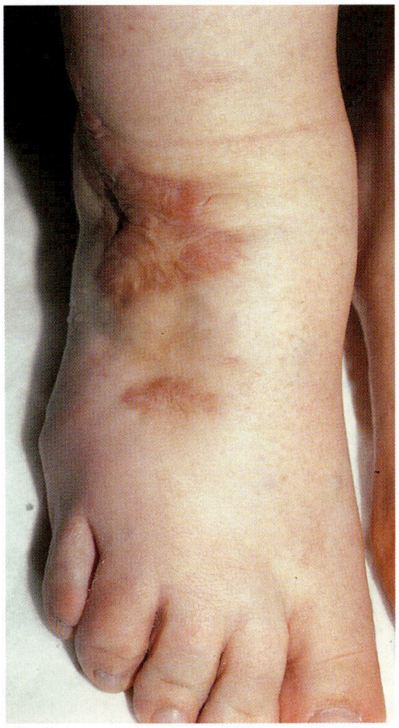

12-36

Figs. 12-35, 12-36. A 24 year old women with cavernous hemangioma of the dorsal aspect of the right foot. A hypertrophic scar developed in this area following surgery

Fig. 12-37. A 4 week old infant with cavernous hemangioma of the left foot

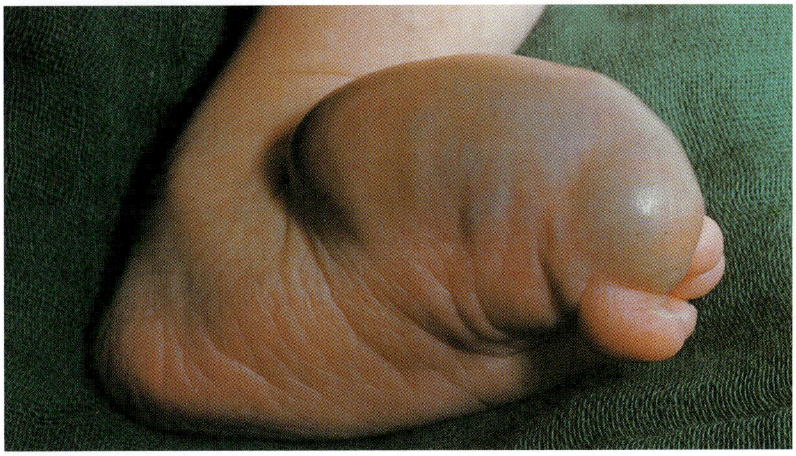

12-37

Fig. 12-38. Cavernous hemangioma of the index and middle fingers of the right hand in a 44 year old woman

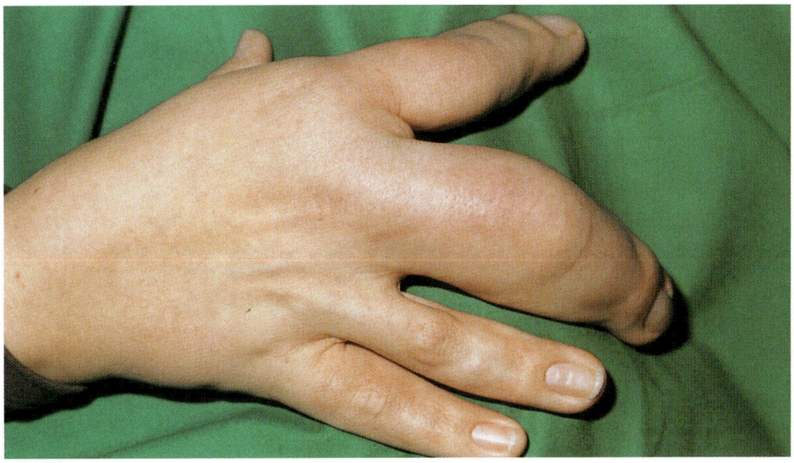

12-38

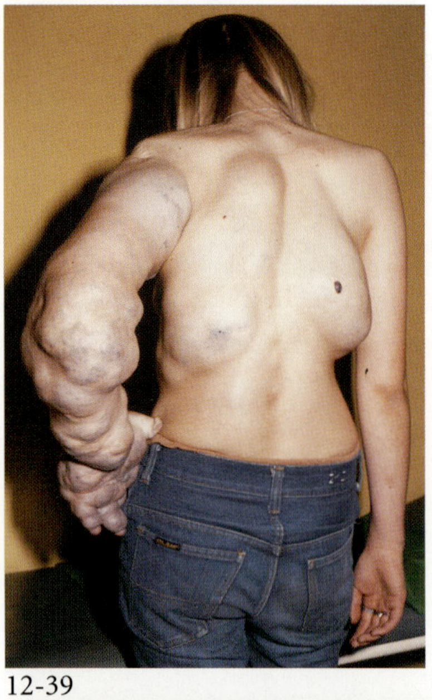

12-39

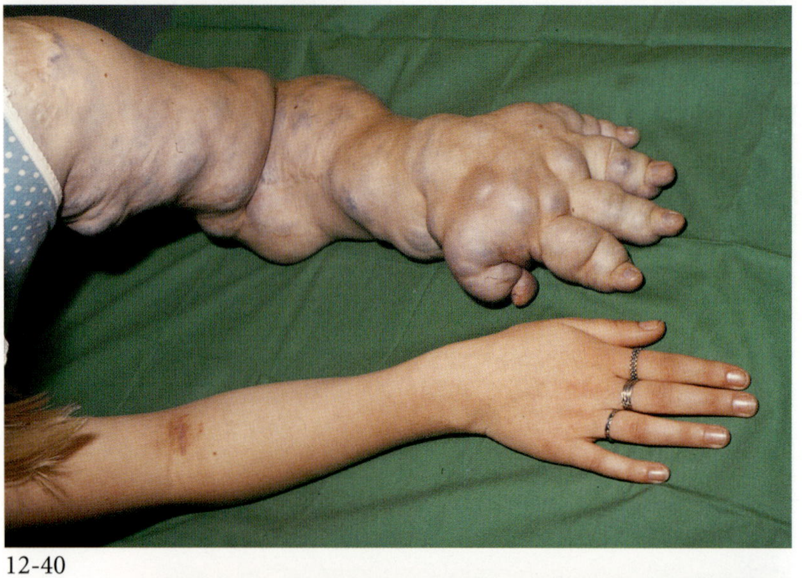

12-40

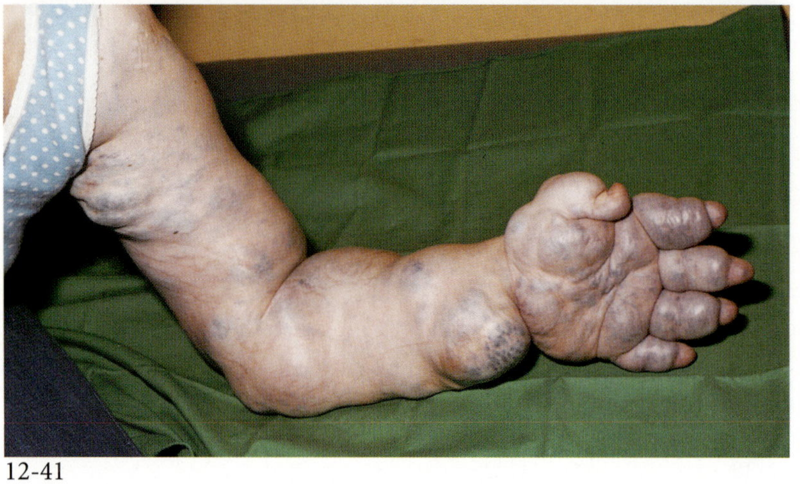

12-41

Figs. 12-39–12-41. A 22 year old patient with multiple large cavernous hemangiomas mainly of the back and left arm. As she changed her body position, the arm either became filled with blood or drained. When she let the arm down into a dependent position, the patient became light-headed as her blood pressure dropped precipitously

Appendix

Anatomic Diagrams

All of the these illustrations have been re-drawn. The following list indicates the original sources upon which the new drawings are based.

Fig. 1	From LANZER	Fig. 3, p. 8
Fig. 2	From SCHIEBLER	Fig. 11.56, p. 465
Fig. 3	From SCHIEBLER	Fig. 10-46, p. 303
Fig. 4	From SCHIEBLER	Fig. 10-47, p. 304
Fig. 5	From SCHIEBLER	Fig. 10-48, p. 304
Fig. 6	From SCHIEBLER	Fig. 13-31, p. 533
Fig. 7	From SCHIEBLER	Fig. 14-60, p. 607
Fig. 8	From SCHIEBLER	Fig. 14-26, p. 575
Fig. 9	From SCHIEBLER	Fig. 10-17, p. 251
Fig. 10	From SCHIEBLER	Fig. 15-7, p. 619
Fig. 11	From SCHIEBLER	Fig. 10-88, p. 366
Fig. 12	From SCHIEBLER	Fig. 10-89, p. 367
Fig. 13	From SCHIEBLER	Fig. 10-90, p. 368
Fig. 14	From SCHIEBLER	Fig. 10-91, p. 369
Fig. 18	From SCHIEBLER	Fig. 10-49, p. 306
Fig. 19	From SCHIEBLER	Fig. 13-32, p. 534
Fig. 20	From SCHIEBLER	Fig. 14-61, p. 608
Fig. 22	From SCHIEBLER	Fig. 10-92, p. 370
Fig. 23	From HACH	Fig. 1, p. 4
Fig. 24	From SCHIEBLER	Fig. 11-58, p. 470

LANZER P, RÖSCH J (eds) (1994) Vascular Diagnostics. Springer, Berlin, Heidelberg, New York, Tokyo

SCHIEBLER TH, SCHMIDT W, ZILLES K (eds) (1997) Anatomie- 7th Edition. Springer, Berlin, Heidelberg, New York, Tokyo

HACH W, HACH-WUNDERLE V (1997) Phlebography and Sonography of the Veins. Springer, Berlin, Heidelberg, New York, Tokyo

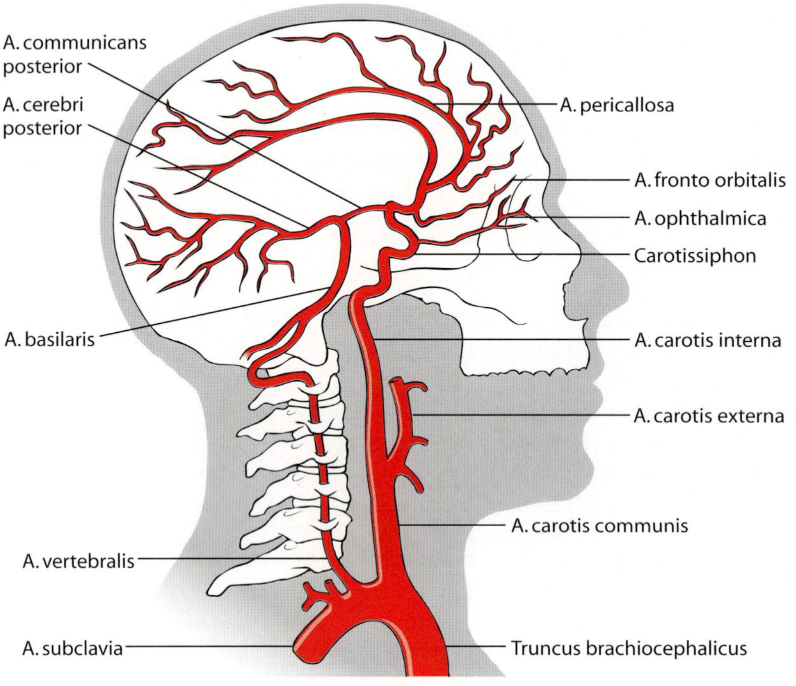

Fig. 1. Common carotid and internal carotid arteries as well as vertebral artery

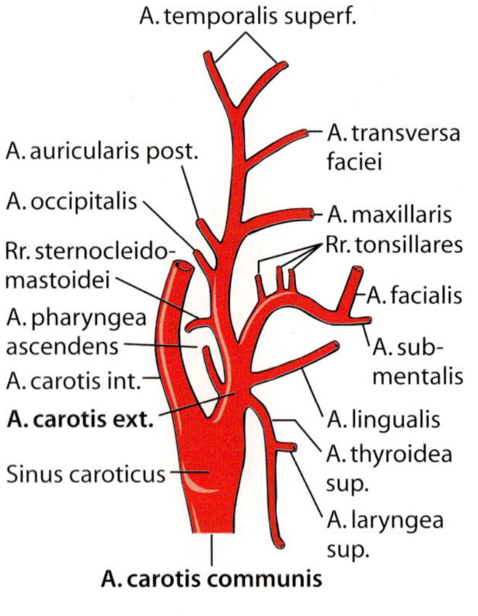

Fig. 2. The branches of the external carotid artery (the carotid branching as seen from anteriorly on the *right*)

Fig. 3. The right subclavian and right axillary arteries and their branches

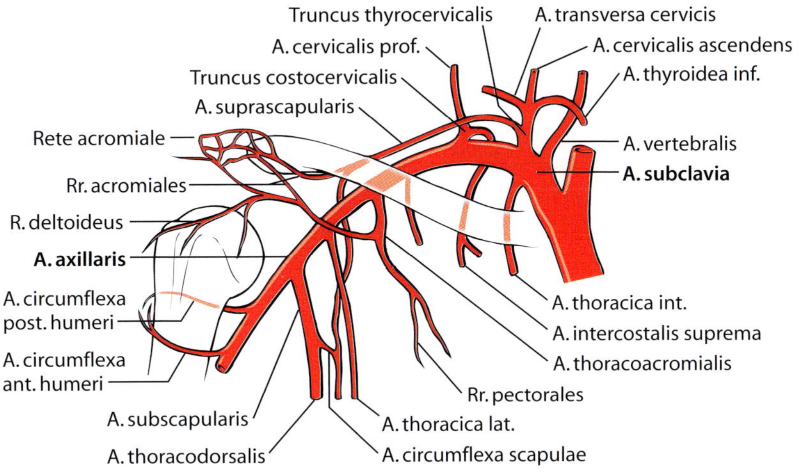

Fig. 4. Arteries of the upper arm and the anastomoses around the elbow

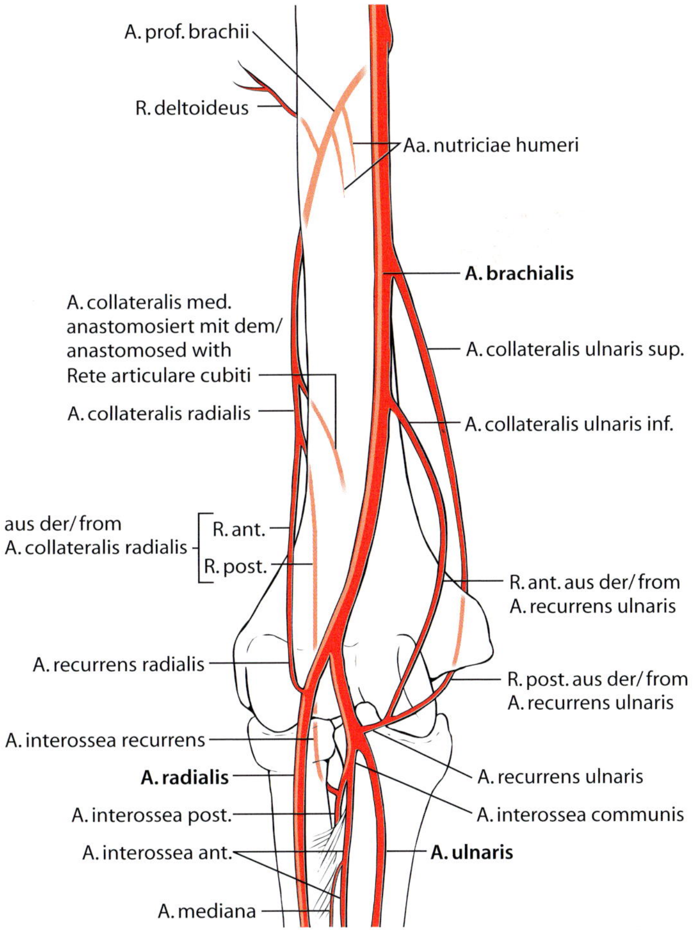

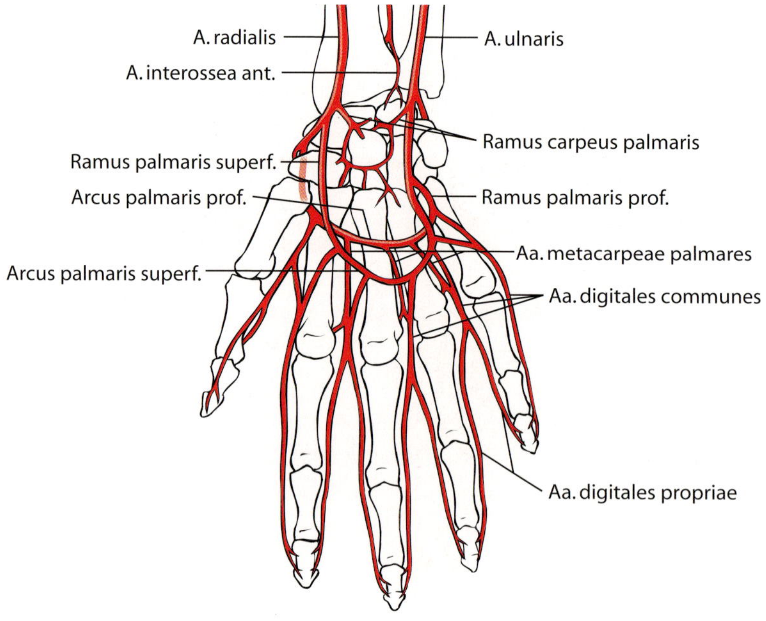

Fig. 5. Arteries of the hand (palmar view)

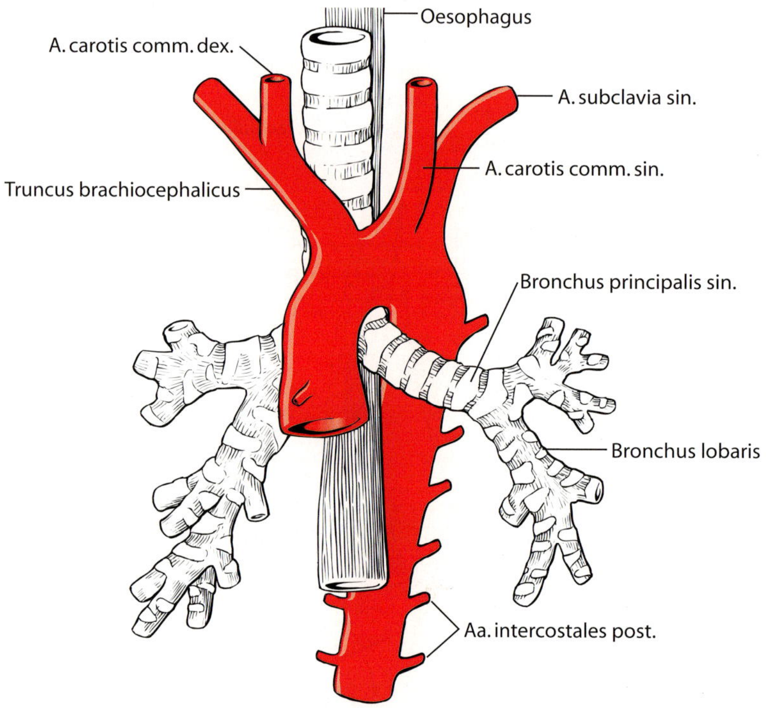

Fig. 6. Ascending and descending thoracic aorta

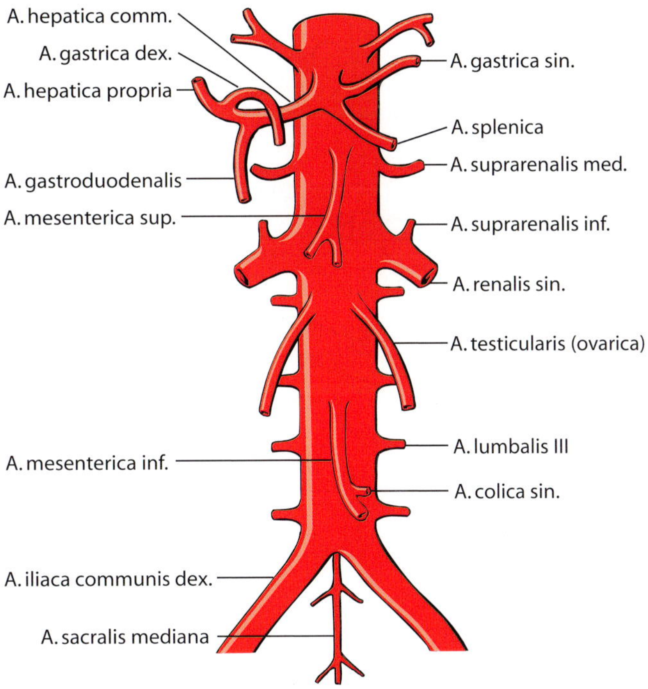

Fig. 7. Abdominal aorta with its branches

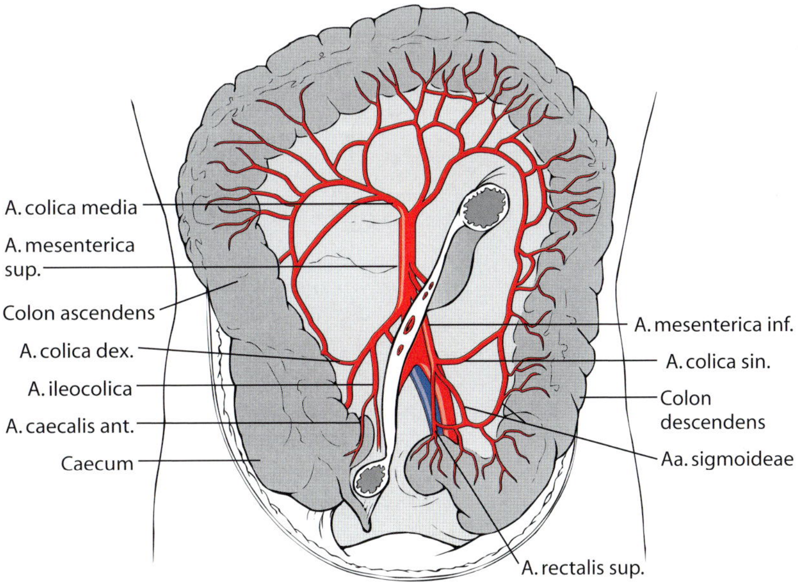

Fig. 8. Vascular supply of the colon

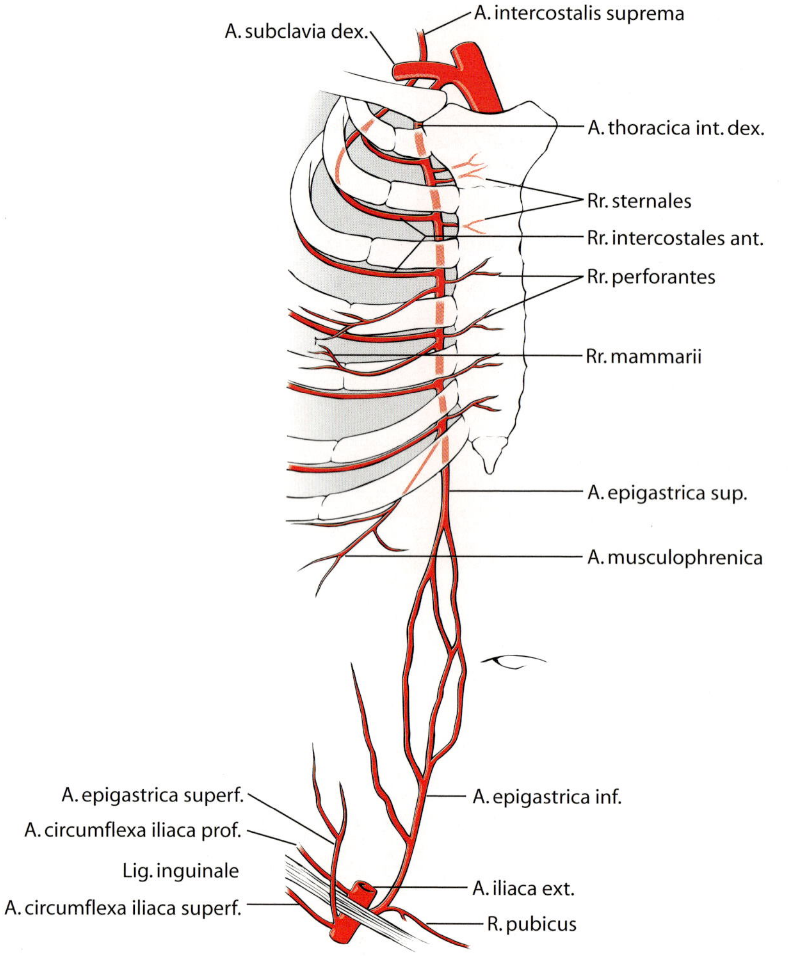

Fig. 9. Arterial supply of the anterior chest and abdominal walls

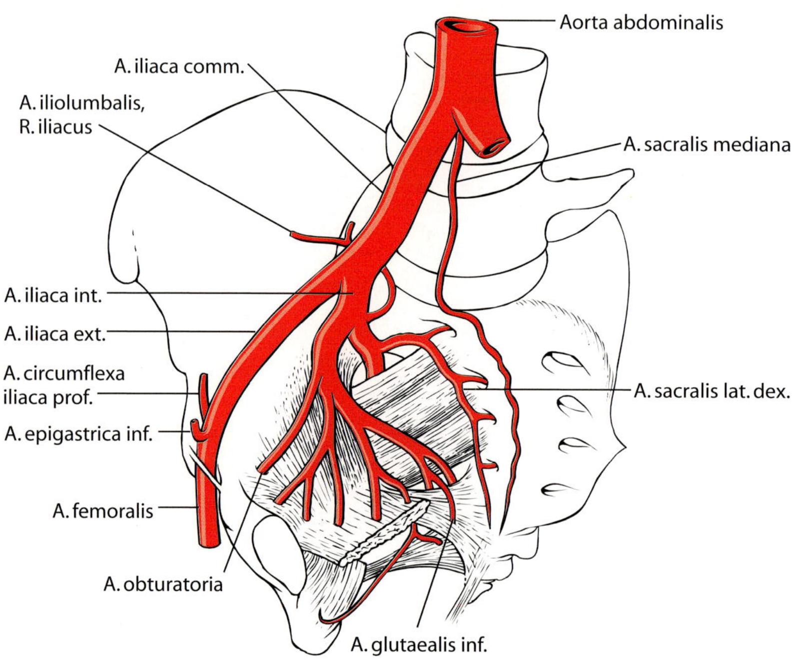

Fig. 10. Pelvic arteries

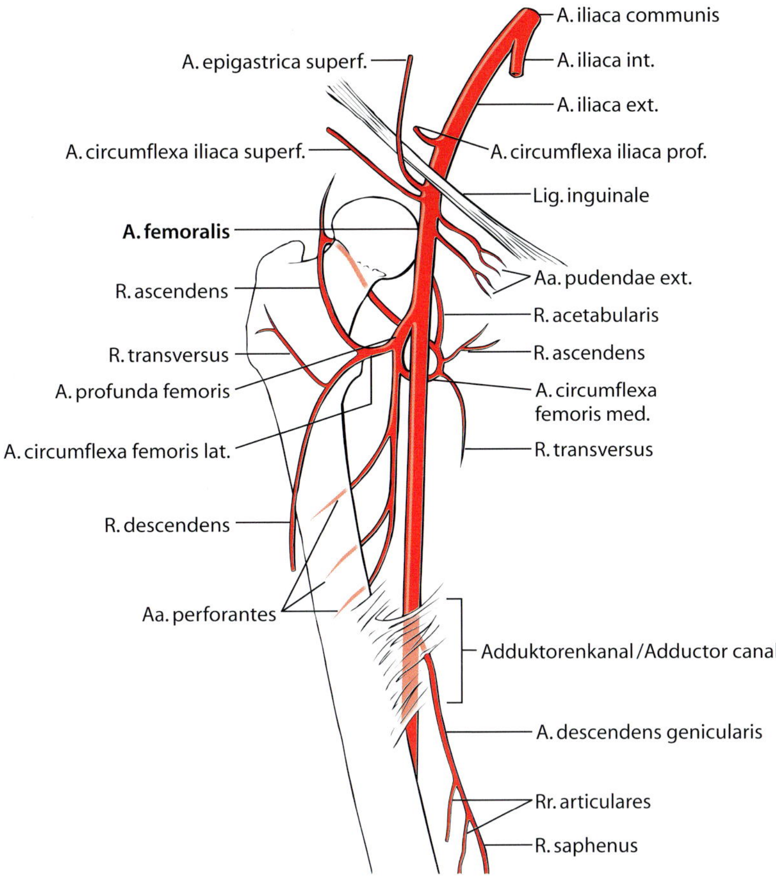

Fig. 11. Femoral artery with its main branches

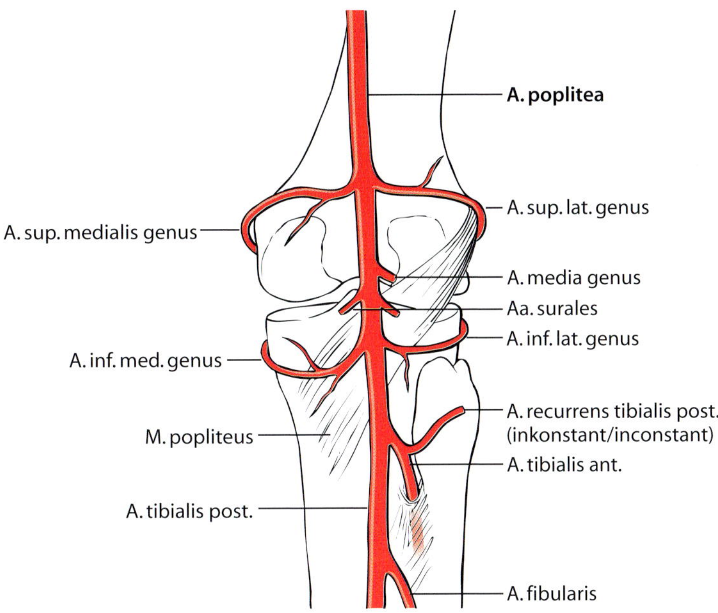

Fig. 12. Popliteal artery with its main branches

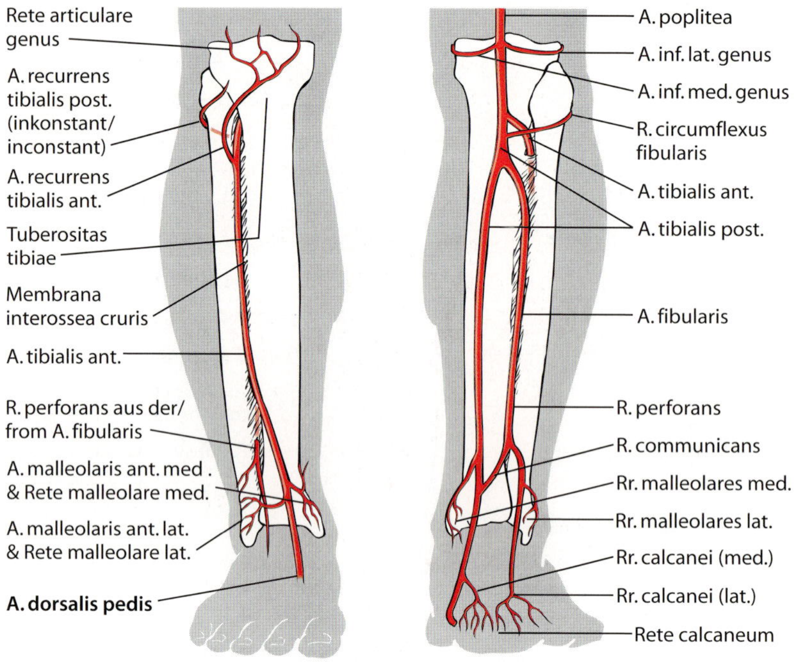

Fig. 13. Arteries of the lower leg

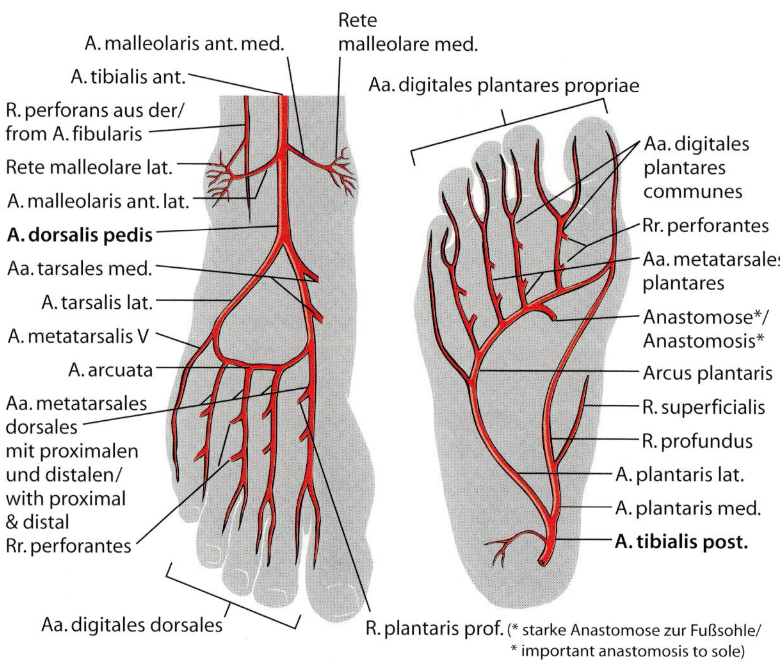

Fig. 14. Arteries of the foot

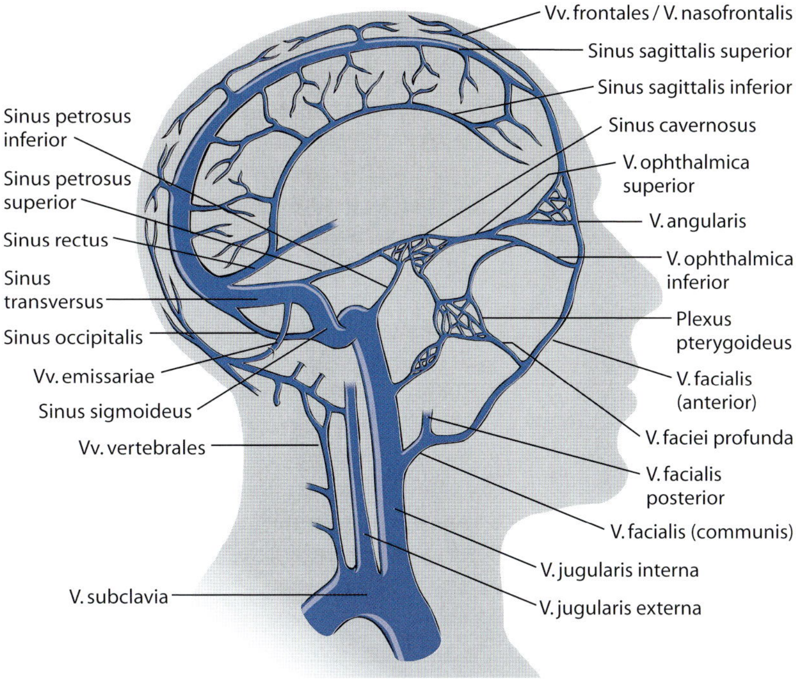

Fig. 15. The extracranial system of the facial vein and the connection with the cavernous sinus

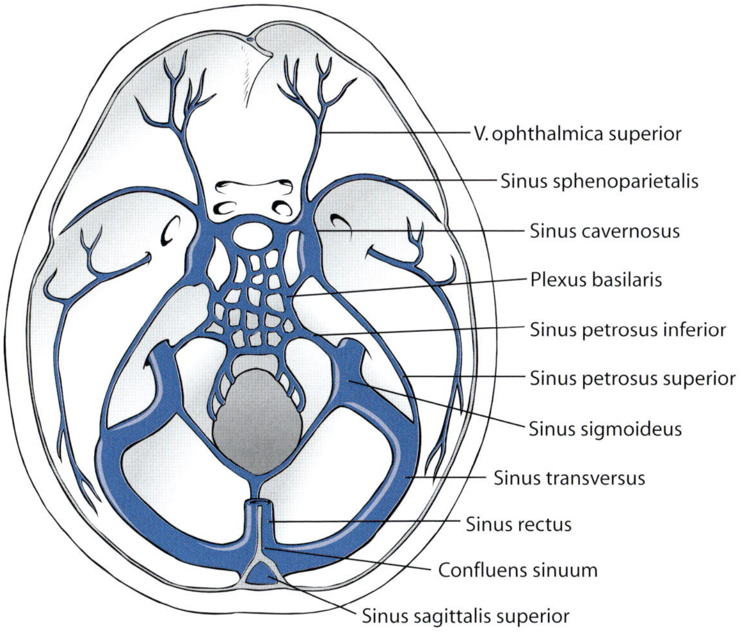

Fig. 16. Intracranial view of the veins of the base of the skull (view from above with the major sinuses and their connections)

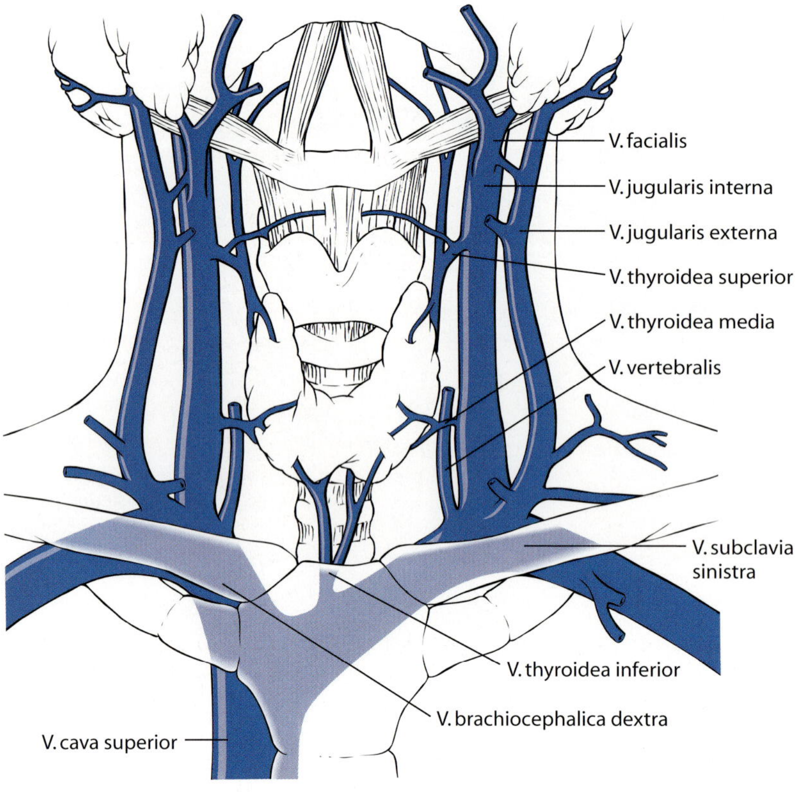

Fig. 17. Veins of the neck

Fig. 18. Veins of the arm

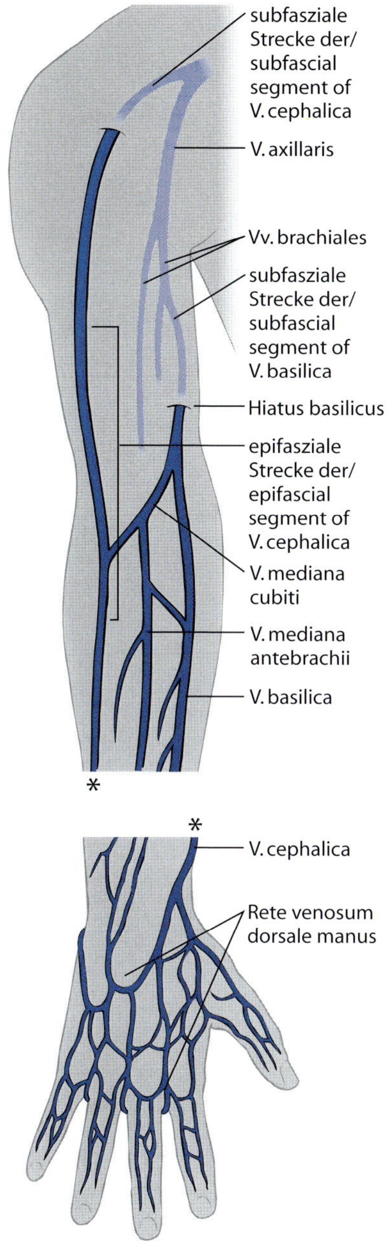

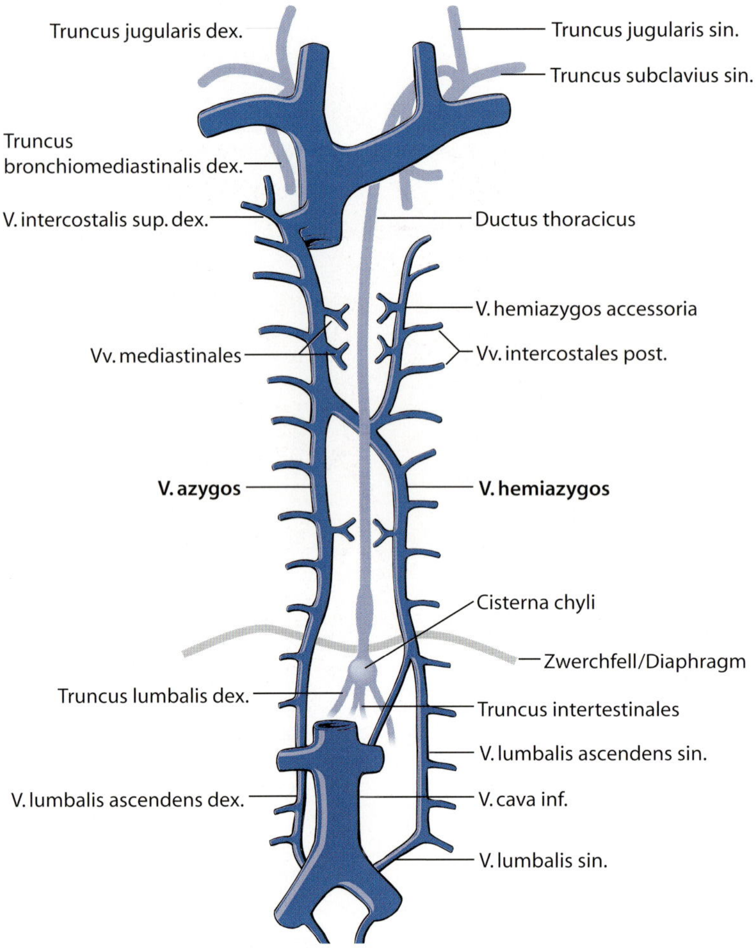

Fig. 19. Azygos and hemiazygos veins with their drainage. Thoracic duct and larger lymphatics are *lighter-colored* and *speckled*

Fig. 20. Portal vein and its supply

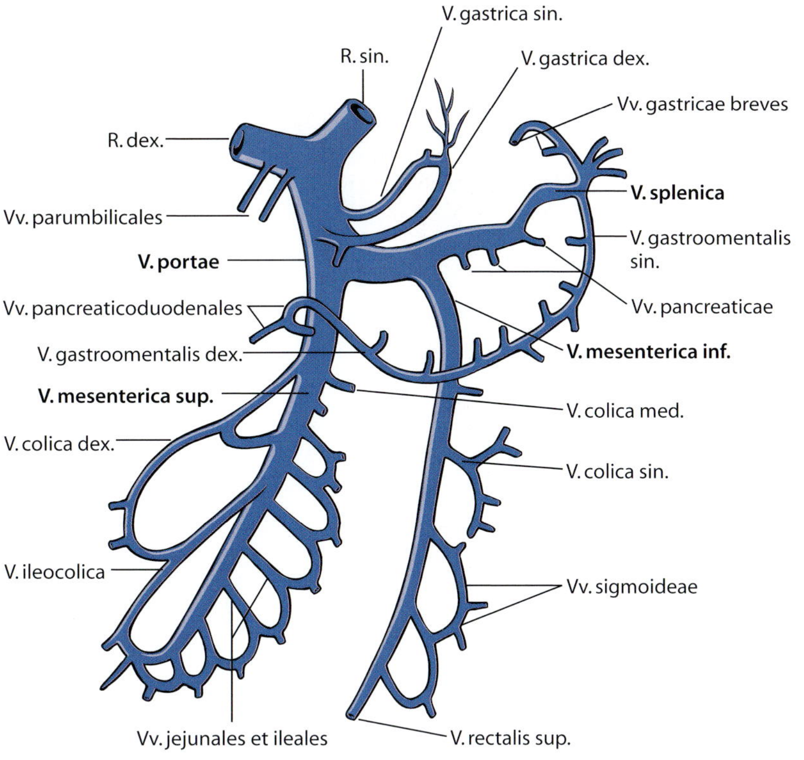

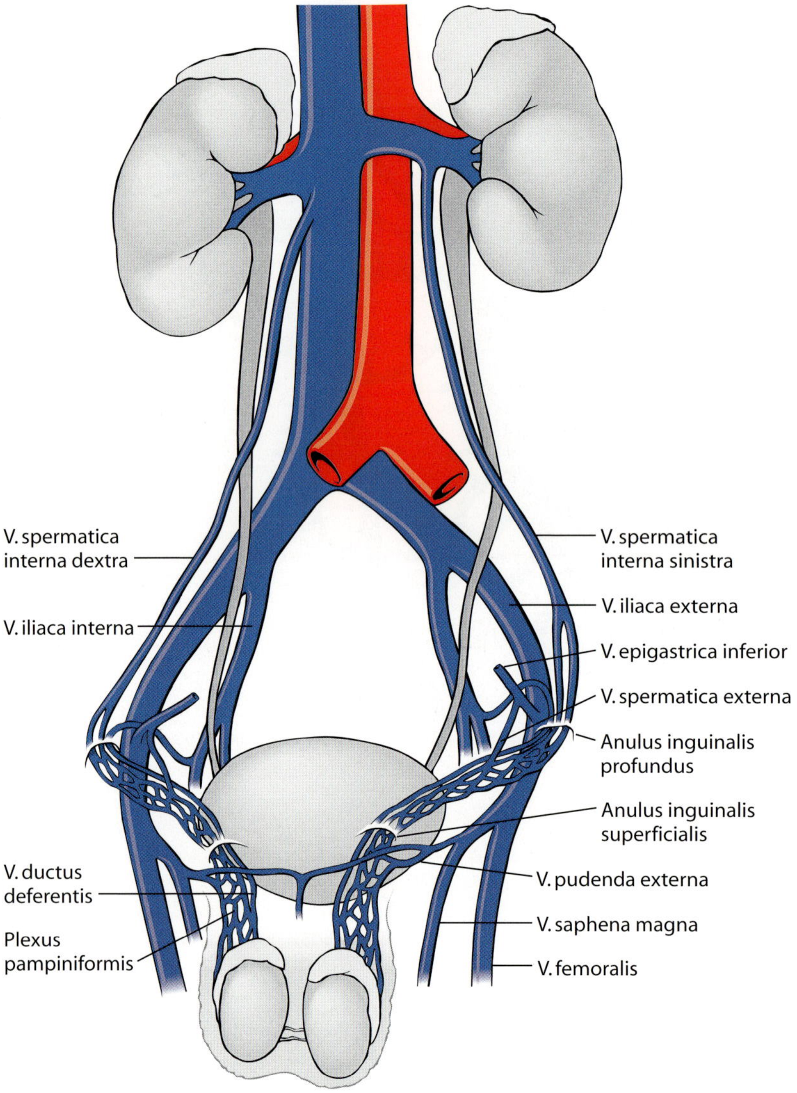

Fig. 21. Veins of the testes and pelvis

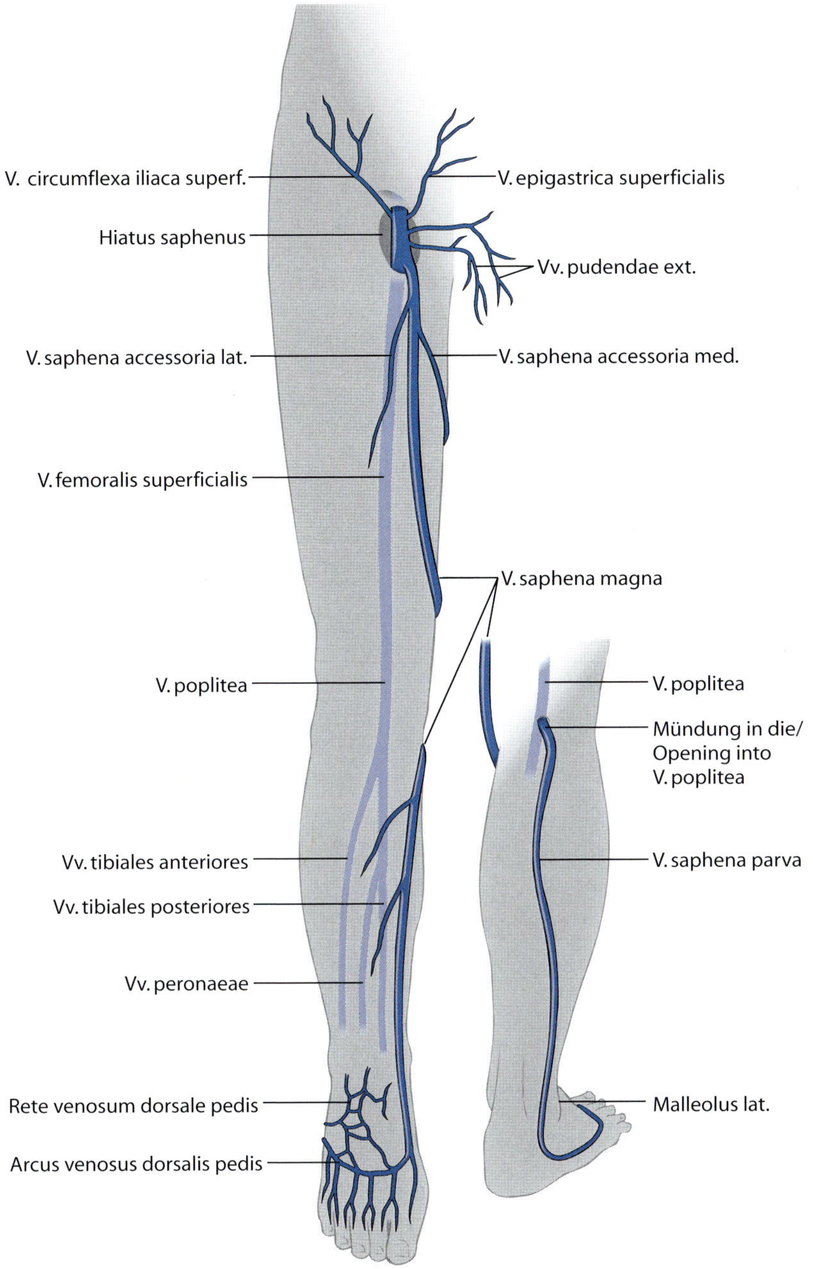

Fig. 22. Deep saphenous vein and its branches, as well as superficial saphenous vein

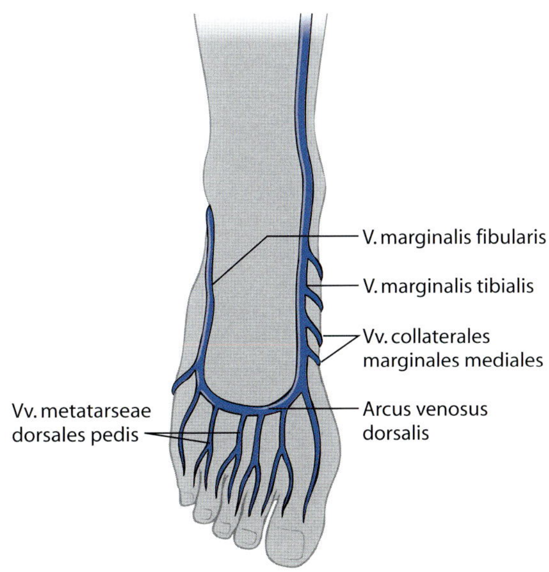

Fig. 23. Superficial veins of foot

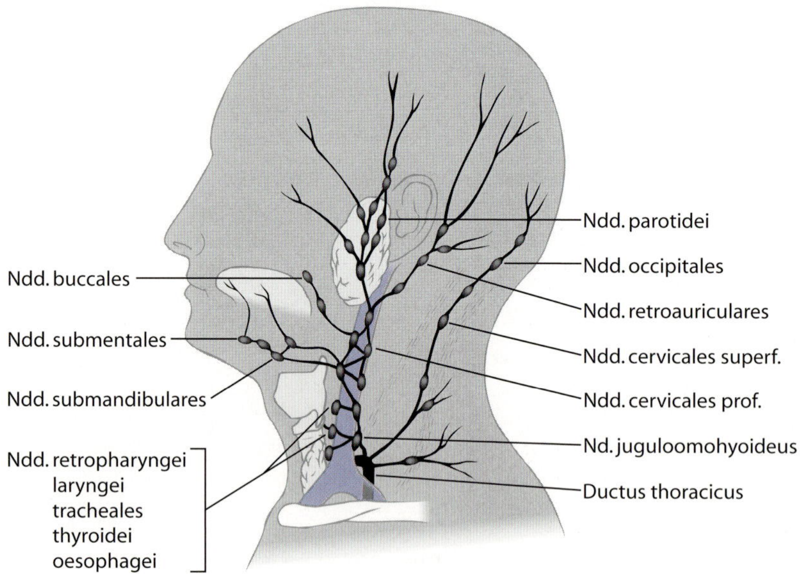

Fig. 24. Lymphatics of the head and neck

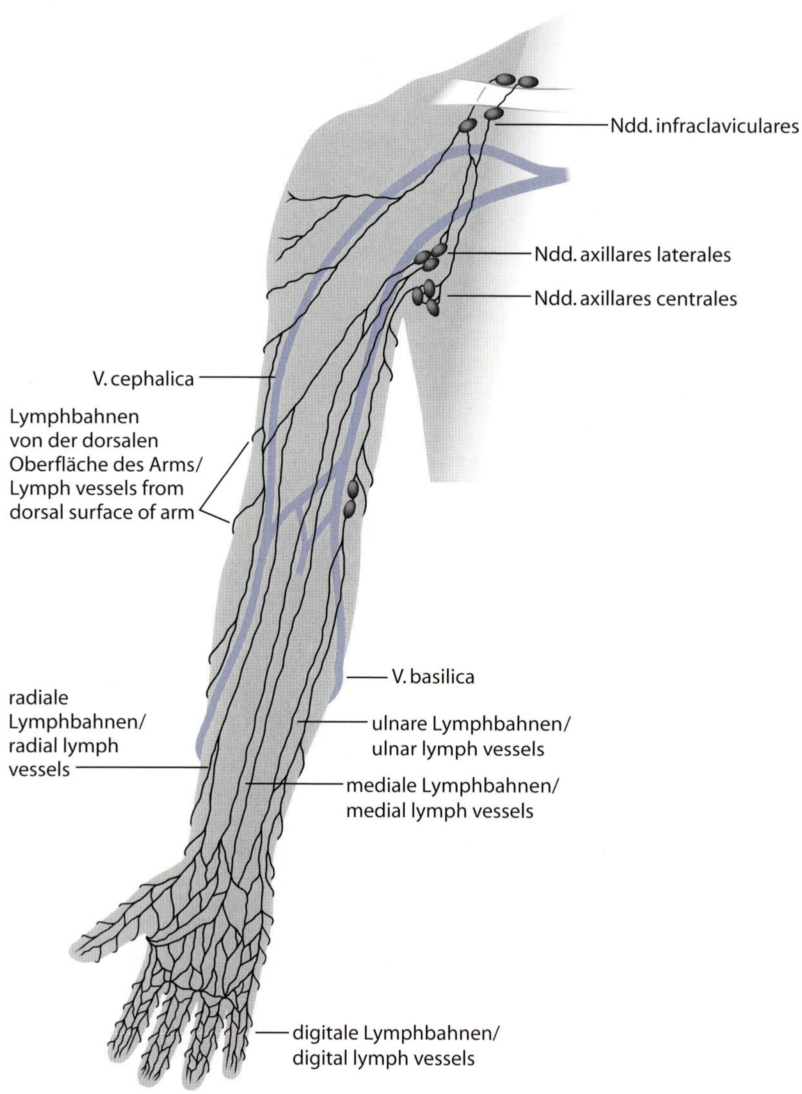

Fig. 25. Lymphatics of the arm and thorax

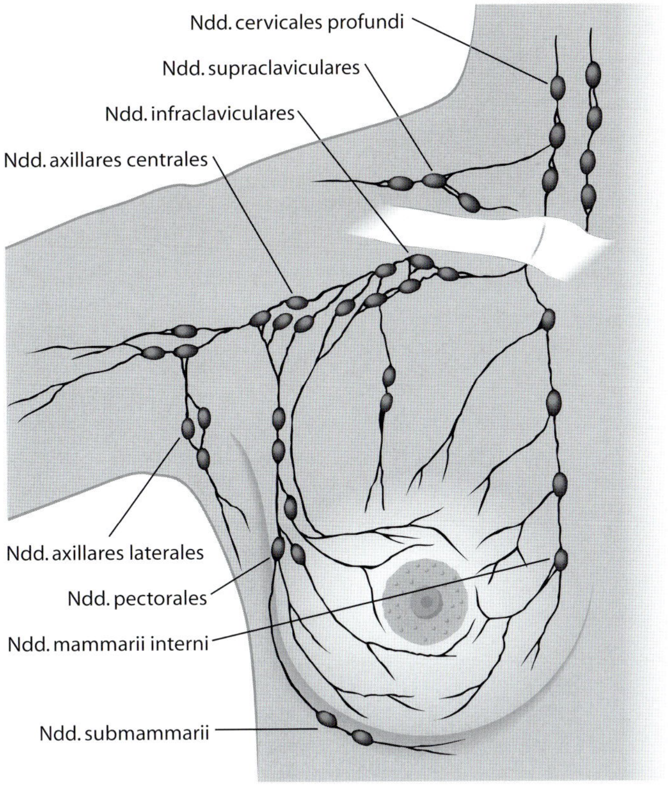

Fig. 26. Lymphatics of the neck and breast

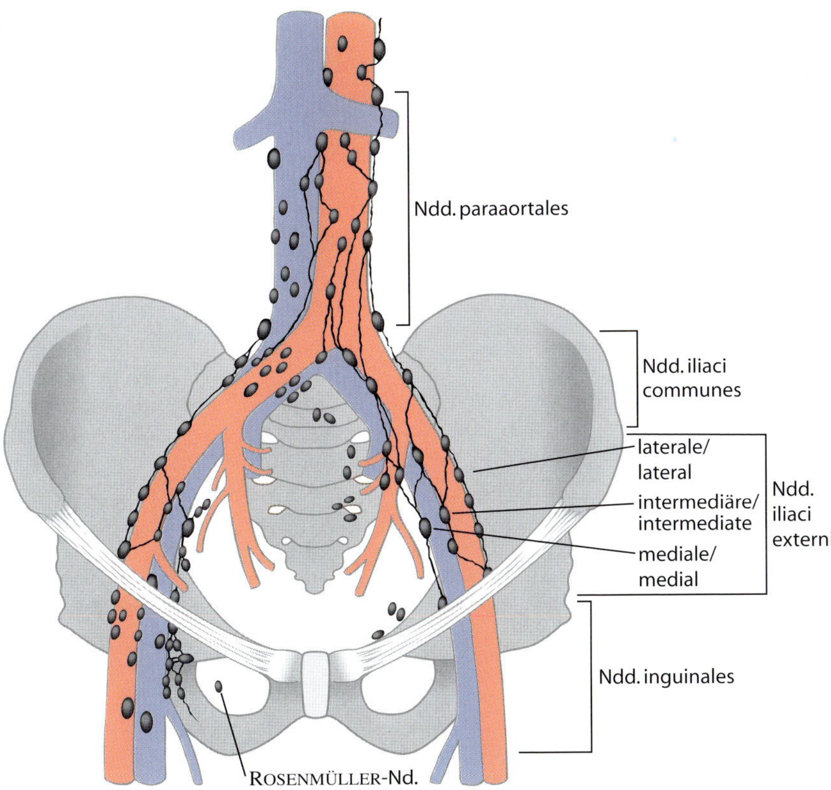

Fig. 27. Lymphatics of the pelvis

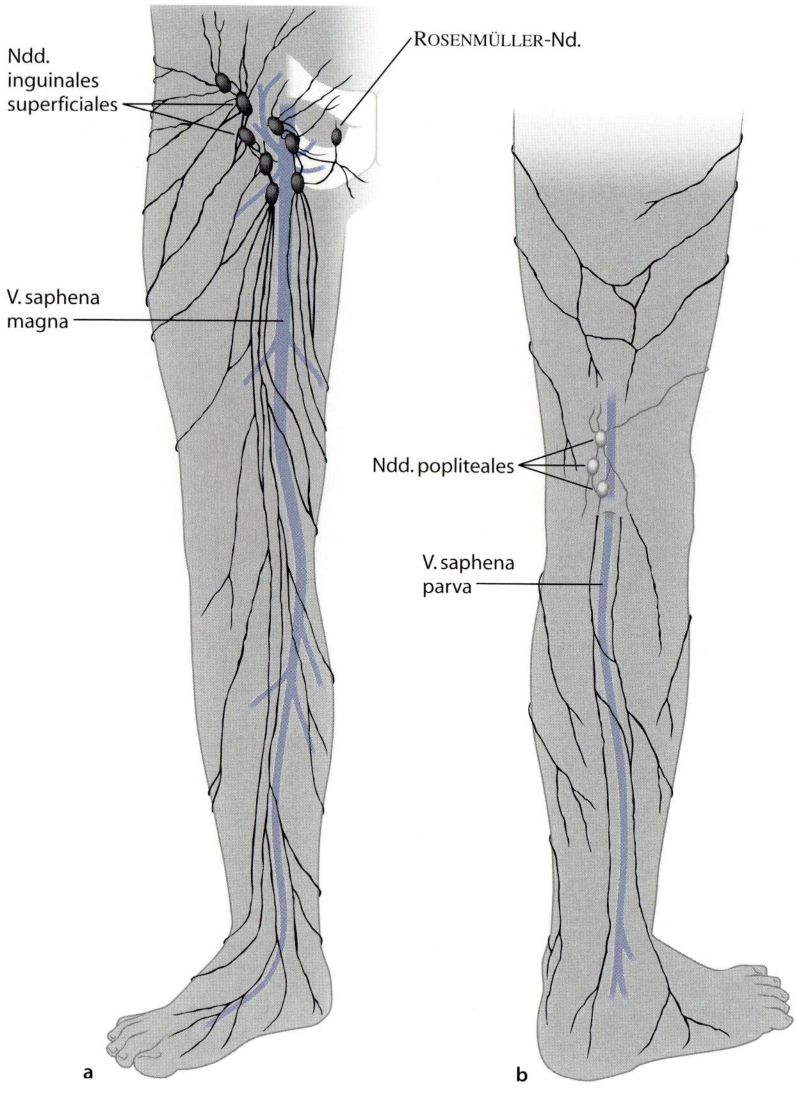

Fig. 28 a, b. Lymphatics of the leg. **a** Medial superficial lymphatics; **b** lateral superficial lymphatics

Subject Index